The Coronavirus Crisis and Challenges to Social Development

Maria do Carmo dos Santos Gonçalves • Rebecca Gutwald
Tanja Kleibl • Ronald Lutz
Ndangwa Noyoo • Janestic Twikirize
Editors

The Coronavirus Crisis and Challenges to Social Development

Global Perspectives

Springer

Editors
Maria do Carmo dos Santos Gonçalves
Centro Scalabriniano de Estudos
Migrató
Brasilia, Brasília, Brazil

Rebecca Gutwald
Munich School of Philosophy
Munich, Germany

Tanja Kleibl
Faculty of Applied Social Sciences
University of Applied Sciences
Würzburg-Schweinfurt
Würzburg, Germany

Ronald Lutz
Faculty of Applied Social Sciences
University of Applied Sciences
Erfurt, Germany

Ndangwa Noyoo
Department of Social Development
University of Cape Town
Rondebosch, South Africa

Janestic Twikirize
Department of Social Work and Social Administration
Makerere University
Kampala, Uganda

ISBN 978-3-030-84677-0 ISBN 978-3-030-84678-7 (eBook)
https://doi.org/10.1007/978-3-030-84678-7

This Springer imprint is published by the registered company Springer Nature Switzerland AG
The registered company address is: Gewerbestrasse 11, 6330 Cham, Switzerland

To all social workers around the world who are struggling to promote social justice and human rights, sometimes having to sacrifice their own freedoms.

Foreword

Gender-based violence, lack of access to basic services, high levels of unemployment, and systemic inequality—these are just some of the iniquities that children of the global South have inherited from colonialism, apartheid, and post-colonial governance failures, for generations. The advent of the coronavirus (COVID-19) pandemic has amplified a number of these societal challenges in many ways. Indeed, out of the shadow of the pandemic have emerged a multitude of other diseases and social ills, which, in truth, have been at crisis level long before this virus swept across the globe in 2020. Furthermore, other than causing untold death and loss across the globe, what the COVID-19 pandemic has effectively managed to do is lay bare the stark inequalities that have existed across the global South since the end of colonialism and apartheid

As the Chief Executive Officer of the Oliver & Adelaide Tambo Foundation, I remember the feeling of doom that overtook me in the first few weeks after the President of South Africa announced the beginning of what turned out to be the harshest lockdown in the world. Here was a disease that was stuck to the root of the failures of our continent to effectively redress the inequalities brought about by hundreds of years of colonial rule and apartheid, and further exacerbated by mismanagement, malfeasance, and corruption thereafter.

I harboured two anchoring fears. The first was based on the spatial politics that exist in South Africa and how challenging it would be in our current state to combat a disease whose most effective treatment was access to clean drinking water and the ability to socially distance. With a great number of South Africans residing in overcrowded areas, such as squatter camps, hostels, and townships that were built on the outskirts of cities to service and perpetuate white privilege, the chance of survival seemed slim. How glaring, then, were the shortcomings of a democratic dispensation that failed to provide adequate access to basic services, that had suddenly become an immediate source of defence from disease and death. How uncomfortable was it to realise that the living conditions for the majority of our population were not just unsuitable but, now, deadly?

My second fear was for the frontline workers across the country, and in frontline I include the community-based workers and advocates who have dedicated their lives to working in the service of others. There are well over 100,000 Community-Based Organisations (CBOs) in South Africa. The current proud and vibrant social work sector in this country was born from a robust network of social workers, activists, and religious and community leaders who provided the delivery of essential services to a population for whom apartheid had made few or no provisions at all. As our democracy grew, these institutions became an essential part of the South African society, firmly embedded in the national consciousness.

Who, I found myself repeatedly wondering, would help the helpers?

This book answers this and so many other important questions that the COVID-19 pandemic has brought to the fore. It looks at the impact of the disease on the poorest of the poor and on the wealthy alike. It examines how the COVID-19 pandemic has compounded some of the greatest global challenges that we were already facing. It assesses the global responses to the pandemic from a political and socioeconomic perspective and seeks to generate critical information on how social workers across the globe are using innovation and courage to save lives and livelihoods.

Oliver & Adelaide Tambo Foundation
B.A., Political Science (University of Cape Town—UCT), Johannesburg, South Africa

Zengeziwe Msimang

Preface

This book discusses the manner in which the social work profession responded to the coronavirus (COVID-19) pandemic and the ways that social development was affected in different parts of the world. In this regard, it highlights the interactions between social work and the COVID-19 pandemic. The chapters cover a multiplicity of these issues pertinent to social work responses to COVID-19 whilst unpacking the pluriversal knowledge and experiences that postcolonial social work can build on to decolonise its past in the era of globalisation.

In late 2019, the global community was alerted to an outbreak of a deadly epidemic in the city of Wuhan in China. This disease was identified as the novel coronavirus COVID-19. At the time, many Chinese citizens had been infected and lost their lives from COVID-19. Subsequently, in early 2020, the virus spread to other parts of the world and claimed many more lives. In January 2020, the World Health Organization (WHO) declared COVID-19 a global pandemic. COVID-19 is now in its second year of wreaking havoc across the world, and in its wake it has afflicted and killed many people. The extent of the damage caused by the pandemic was not limited to the issue of individual health or the extreme wear and tear on health systems around the world, but also had a dramatic impact on the entire functioning of social life. Social detachment and mobility limitations imposed by the health crisis have affected the foundations of the economic systems and beyond in many countries. The change in work regimes with an accelerated integration of remote work technologies, the reduction of jobs resulting from the consumption crisis, and the paralysis of educational services are situations, among others, brought about by the global health crisis that exposed, or rather deepened, economic and social inequalities which were already the subject of attention in the field of social work studies and practices. The chapters in this volume have been written at the end of 2020 and beginning of 2021 in the so-called first and second waves of the pandemic, when many countries had already faced severe measures such as lockdowns of public institutions and the private sector, social distancing orders, rising death rates, and a scarcity of medical resources. As the Preface to this book is being written, that is, as of 13 May 2021, there are already 160,074,267 confirmed cases of COVID-19, including 3,325,260 deaths globally (WHO, 2021).

Given its global magnitude, this pandemic has literally disrupted the lives of people in every country of the world. This crisis is unprecedented in modern times. The last time the world was besieged by a pandemic in this manner was in 1918, when there was an outbreak of a global influenza, pejoratively referred to as the 'Spanish flu' even though it initially emanated from the United States of America (U.S.). This pandemic had claimed the lives of approximately 50,000,000 people. At the time, there was no cure for this pandemic. However, it finally dissipated in 1920 after several waves and many more deaths. In the present scenario, vaccines were developed in 2020 and went on trial later in the same year. Currently, many countries around the world are rolling out some form of vaccination program against COVID-19. Globally, as of 12 May 2021, a total of 1,264,164,553 vaccine doses have been administered (WHO, 2021). Most articles underline the unbroken post-colonial power dynamics in which we are still living. This situation can be clearly observed again in the current unequal distribution of COVID-19 vaccines, which leaves countries of the Global South worse off than Western nations. Hence, we are once more confronted with the deadly impact caused by the crucial interconnections between colonialism and global inequality, which continue to shape the capabilities and opportunities as well as life expectancies of millions of people worldwide.

The pandemic has followed different patterns across the globe, with Europe being severely impacted, whereas COVID-19 was contained in China and several other Asian countries such as Taiwan and South Korea. Thereafter, the U.S. and Brazil registered high infection rates and fatalities. Presently, since spring 2021, it is India that is exhibiting high infection and death rates. It is important to underline the fact that the disruptions engendered by COVID-19 overturned all human activities defining the modern world: from markets, commerce, and industry, and the supply chains that underpin the former, to the entertainment industry and sports, and to the educational and social services sector, everything ground to a resounding halt.

With the aforementioned issues coming to the fore, there was also the loss of livelihoods and sources of income, as companies closed down or wealth-creating opportunities ceased to exist. The highest cost borne by societies is human loss, with countries losing valuable human resources key to running modern industries and other organizations. Thus, countries lost different professionals, the clergy, health workers, teachers, business persons, scientists, and farmers, among others, in large numbers. At the family level, breadwinners and nurturers were lost to the pandemic. The emotional and psychological strain brought on individuals, families, groups, communities, and societies by COVID-19 cannot be easily quantified. Indeed, the psychosocial devastation is incalculable. It is also noteworthy that the initial responses by national governments, across the globe, of instituting lockdowns and quarantines had the unintended consequences of increasing mental health challenges, gender-based violence, child abuse, and other various social ills. The foregoing clearly underscored the fact that COVID-19 was not only a health issue, as important as this was, but it also equally had psychosocial implications. Furthermore, it led to sociopolitical and economic disruptions. In particular, Redondo-Sama, Matulic, Munté-Pascual, and de Vicente (2020, p. 1) point out that social work has fulfilled a crucial role during the COVID-19 crisis, covering the most urgent social needs of vulnerable groups, such as the homeless and elderly people. A great number of articles furthermore point towards the devastating impact of the pandemic on people on the move (e.g., migrants and refugees), as well as women and children who seem to have been neglected as a group by many governments. However, most research has been focused on health professionals, and less is known about social workers on the frontline, including those working in public health institutions.

This skewed appraisal of the professionals confronting or coping with the pandemic leads to the partial rationale for this book, as the editors wanted to present COVID-19 from the prism of the social work profession. To this end, the book is guided by the following objectives:

1. To draw attention to the global impact of COVID-19 and to highlight national responses that affect the global pandemic in southern and northern countries.
2. To assess global and local social work responses to COVID-19 as well as initiatives for social development.
3. To discuss how nations are (not) meeting the needs of the poor and marginalised communities in the Global South and Global North.
4. To examine the coping mechanisms and strategies of poor and vulnerable groups in the Global South and Global North.

These objectives guided the different authors as they wrote their chapters. Therefore, the chapters offer different perspectives and reach into the local context showing how a global pandemic has affected life in almost all corners of the world and how reactions have differed depending on the local conditions. Taking the foregoing issues into critical consideration, this book endeavours to offer a platform for analysing and discussing the perspectives of social work on COVID-19 and related aspects from both the Global South and Global North. It puts a spotlight on the challenges that were brought on by the pandemic in the different countries and regions of the globe, and also examines current developments related to COVID-19 and their impacts thereof.

The book is designed in 38 chapters with different parts covering different themes as they relate to COVID-19 in different regions. In this book, the regions that are covered are Africa, Asia, Europe, Latin America, and North America. Many divergent issues emerge in the respective chapters relative to the local context, but there are also commonalities in the various countries worldwide. The differences mentioned in countries across the globe speak to the uniqueness of culture, political systems, people's resilience, cushioning mechanisms embedded in indigenous knowledge systems, and contextual nuances related to economic activities and resources, political freedoms, and innovations, among others. Despite these differences, the chapters also point to the common heritage of the human race and which the pandemic ironically managed to lay bare. It did not matter which ideologies or political systems we believed in or followed, or how rich, poor, or influential we were. COVID-19 humbled the human race and reminded human beings of how fragile they are on the one hand and how interconnected they are on the other. Even if selfish desires emerged during the manufacture and distribution of vaccines, leading to what has come to be known as 'vaccine nationalism,' human beings of all races, religions, ethnicities, and cultures were all the same and faced the same danger of the pandemic.

For these reasons we have decided to structure the book according to the issues and questions that the chapters raise, not with regard to regions. We have grouped the chapters according to three major themes that arise in research of the pandemic and social work: Analysis: Social Issues and the COVID-19 Pandemic; Strategies and Responses in Social Work: Globally and Locally; and Outlook: Looking Ahead Beyond the Pandemic.

Brasilia, Brazil — Maria do Carmo dos Santos Gonçalves
Munich, Germany — Rebecca Gutwald
Würzburg, Germany — Tanja Kleibl
Erfurt, Germany — Ronald Lutz
Cape Town, South Africa — Ndangwa Noyoo
Kampala, Uganda — Janestic Twikirize

References

Redondo-Sama, G., Matulic, V., Munté-Pascual, A., de Vicente, I. (2020). Social work during the COVID-19 crisis: Responding to urgent social needs. *Sustainability 12*(8595):1–16. https://doi.org/10.3390/su12208595

World Health Organization (WHO). (2021). WHO Coronavirus (COVID-19) Dashboard Overview. https://covid19.who.int/

Contents

Part I Analysis: Social Issues and the COVID-19 Pandemic

1 **COVID and Social Work Voices from India and Australia: Strategic and Meaningful Solidarities for Global Justice** 3
Rimple Mehta and Linda Briskman

2 **Examining Decent Work During COVID-19: With Reference to Female Migrant Workers in South Asia** 17
Sunny Wadhwaniya, Rupa Korde, and Biju Varkkey

3 **The Impact of COVID-19 on the 'Culture of Deportation' for Refugees from African Countries in Germany** 31
Claudia Koehler

4 **Corona Challenging Social Work in Korea and Vietnam** 45
Habin Jung and Quynh Anh Nguyen

5 **COVID-19 Safety Measures and Socioeconomic Status in Urban Zimbabwe** 55
Rose Jaji

6 **Face Mask Wearing in Kampala, Uganda** 67
Paul Bukuluki and Peter Kisaakye

7 **Implications of the COVID-19 Pandemic and Responses on Persons with Disabilities Including Psychosocial Disabilities in the Global South: The Case of Ghana** 77
Magnus Mfoafo-M'Carthy and Augustina Naami

8 **Lockdown in a Dual Society: Exploring the Human Capability Implications of the Coronavirus (COVID-19) in South Africa** .. 87
Minenhle Matela and Alexandre Maaza

9 **The Exposition of the Stark Realities of an Unequal Society Based on the COVID-19 Pandemic** 97
Veronica Nemutandani and Thabisa Matsea

10 **The COVID-19 Crisis: Impact of Social Attitudes and Representations on Social Development in Sub-Saharan Africa** 109
Etienne Serupia Semuhoza and Alexandre Hakizamungu

11 Knowledge, Adherence, and the Lived Experiences of Refugees in COVID-19 119
Gloria Seruwagi, Catherine Nakidde, Eric Awich Ochen, Betty Okot, Stephen Lawoko, Joshua Kayiwa, Dunstan Ddamulira, Andrew Masaba, Brian Luswata, Johnmary Ssekatte, and Denis Muhangi

12 The Impact of COVID-19 Among the Vulnerable Population of Children and Youth in Lesotho: The Circle of Courage Perspective 133
Katiso Samuel Sehlabane and Thandie Keromamang Hlabana

13 Analysing the Situation of Migrants and Social Work Interventions in South Africa During the Coronavirus (COVID-19) Pandemic 143
Nomcebo Dlamini, Thabisa Matsea, and Ndangwa Noyoo

14 Impacts of the COVID-19 Pandemic on International Migration in Brazil: Normative, Economic, and Social Issues 153
Eveline Vieira Brigido, Roberto Rodolfo Georg Uebel, and Vítor Eduardo Alessandri Ribeiro

15 From the Absence of Public Policies to a State of Emergency: The COVID-19 Pandemic and the Migrant Subject Condition 163
Giuliana Redin and Maria do Carmo dos Santos Gonçalves

16 Social Justice in the Time of COVID-19: Transcend Borders—From the Micro to the Macro, from Patagonia Argentina to the World 171
Marina Anahí Curzio

17 Colombian Women Between the Pandemic and Armed Conflict and Poverty 187
Maria Mauersberger

Part II Strategies and Responses in Social Work: Globally and Locally

18 Ecuador's and Iran's Response to Protect Refugees and Migrants in Vulnerable Situations During the COVID-19 Pandemic 201
Cesar Castilla and Samaneh Kachouie

19 "Am I an Essential Worker?" COVID-19 and (Re)shaping of the Social Work Profession in Uganda 211
Laban Kashaija Musinguzi, Janestic Twikirize, Agnes Kyamulabi, and Denis Muhangi

20 Responses of Social Work Students and Teachers to COVID-19: Experiences from Crisis Relief in Urban Slum and Rural Communities of Maharashtra, India 223
Sanaya Singh, Prabha Tirmare, and Apurva Shinde

21 **COVID-19, Hyper Vulnerabilities, Silenced Traumas, and Colonial Scars: Social Work Scholars Engaging in Critical Dialogue with Racialized Communities** 237
Sophie Hamisultane, Edward Ou Jin Lee, and Roxane Caron

22 **The Kerala, India Experience of Facing the COVID-19 Pandemic** 251
Anu George

23 **Responding to COVID-19 and Beyond: Key Recommendations for the Effective Public and Mental Health Response to Support the Well-Being of Aboriginal and Torres Strait Islander Peoples in Australia** 263
Pat Dudgeon, Joanna Alexi, Kate Derry, Emma Carlin, and Rob McPhee

24 **COVID-19 Pandemic in Nigeria: A Story Worth Telling from the Eyes of Social Workers** 281
Uzoma Odera Okoye and Uche Louisa Nwatu

25 **COVID-19 Pandemic and the Urban Poor: The Relevancy of Uganda's Social Protection Measures** 295
Deborah Atwine and John A. Mushomi

26 **Social Work as an Unwitting Enabler of Oppression and Disenfranchisement of the Masses: A Freirean Analysis of Social Workers' Perspectives on the Government of Zimbabwe's COVID-19 Response** 307
Victor Chikadzi and Ajwang' Warria

27 **The Professional Practice of the Brazilian Social Worker: Problems About the Impacts of the COVID-19 Pandemic** 323
Evelyn Secco Faquin, Líria Maria Bettiol Lanza, Eliezer Rodrigues dos Santos, Fabrício da Silva Campanucci, and Carolina Camilo da Silva

28 **Front-Line Social Workers' Practices Under the Political and Sanitary Crisis in Chile** 335
Taly Reininger, Gianinna Muñoz Arce, Cristóbal Villalobos Dintrans, and Ignacio Wyman

Part III Outlook: Looking Ahead Beyond the Pandemic

29 **Time for New Epistemological Inquiries, the Global South, and Resilience in the Time of COVID-19** 347
Lars Bedurke

30 **Decolonising Safeguarding During a Pandemic: Lessons for Research Praxis in International Social Work** 357
Leona Vaughn, Jassi Sandhar, and Geoffrey Omony

31 Participatory Photography, Ethical Storytelling, and Modern Slavery Survivor Voices: Adapting to COVID-19 371
Aisha Ali Haji, Rehema Baya, Emily Brady, Helen McCabe, Yasmin Manji, and Sophie Otiende

32 Social Work in the Time of a Pandemic: COVID-19 and the Need for Resilience-Critical Thinking 381
Anna Pfaffenstaller and Jacques Love Babatoundé Zannou

33 A Social Work and Social Development Perspective on the Need to Decolonise African Economies in Light of the COVID-19 Pandemic: Lessons for Africa 389
Victor Chikadzi

34 Critiquing Western Development Paradigms and Theories in the Age of the Coronavirus (COVID-19): An African Perspective 399
Ndangwa Noyoo

35 How Has Population Health Been Amplified Through Integrated Indigenous Community Networks? Opportunities During the COVID-19 Pandemic 409
Claudia Ortiz-Rico

36 Soup Kitchens and Radical Social Work Against COVID-19 from Liberation Theology in Chile 421
Francisca Valdebenito-Acosta, Paulo Álvarez Bravo, and Julio Hasbún-Mancilla

37 Overcoming the Socioeconomic Impacts of the Coronavirus Pandemic: Social Work Perspectives and Postcolonial Reflections from Ethiopia 431
Robel Afeworki Abay, Demelash Kassaye, and Tanja Kleibl

38 Concluding Remarks and Summation 443
Maria do Carmo dos Santos Gonçalves, Rebecca Gutwald, Tanja Kleibl, Ronald Lutz, Ndangwa Noyoo, and Janestic Twikirize

Epilogue 447

Index 451

Contributors

Robel Afeworki Abay Department of Rehabilitation Sciences, Humboldt University of Berlin, Berlin, Germany

Joanna Alexi School of Indigenous Studies, University of Western Australia, Crawley, WA, Australia

Gianinna Muñoz Arce Department of Social Work, Universidad de Chile, Santiago, Chile

Deborah Atwine Faculty of Arts and Social Science, Kyambogo University, Kampala, Uganda

Rehema Baya Freelance Writer, Nairobi, Kenya

Lars Bedurke Brot für die Welt, Berlin, Germany

Emily Brady Department of History, University of Leeds, Leeds, UK

Paulo Álvarez Bravo Architecture and Urban Studies, Pontificia Universidad Católica de Chile, Santiago, Chile

Eveline Vieira Brigido Escola Superior de Propaganda e Marketing, Porto Alegre, RS, Brazil

Linda Briskman School of Social Sciences, Western Sydney University, Liverpool, NSW, Australia

Paul Bukuluki Department of Social Work and Social Administration, School of Social Sciences, Makerere University, Kampala, Uganda

Fabrício da Silva Campanucci Social Work and Health: training and professional practice, State University of Londrina (UEL), Londrina, Paraná, Brazil

Emma Carlin Rural Clinical School Western Australia, University of Western Australia and Kimberley Aboriginal Medical Services, Broome, WA, Australia

Roxane Caron School of Social Work, Université de Montréal, QC, Canada

Cesar Castilla CLACSO's Research Group in the Middle East and North of Africa, Buenos Aires, Argentina

Victor Chikadzi Department of Social Work, University of Namibia, Windhoek, Namibia

Marina Anahí Curzio Graduate in Social Work, National, Faculty of Humanities and Social Sciencies, University of Patagonia San Juan Bosco (UNPSJB), Chubut, Argentina

Research Group: Action and Territory Research Group (GIGAT-Patagonia Geographical Research Institute-UNPSJB), Cultural Heritage Research Group (LUPAT Civil Association "Activate from Knowledge"—UNPSJB)—Comprehensive Learning and Development Center (CADI-Inclusion Support Program), Chubut, Argentina

Carolina Camilo da Silva Social Work and Health: training and professional practice, State University of Londrina (UEL), Londrina, Paraná, Brazil

Dunstan Ddamulira Agency for Cooperation in Research and Development (ACORD), Kampala, Uganda

Kate Derry School of Indigenous Studies, University of Western Australia, Crawley, WA, Australia

Nomcebo Dlamini Faculty of Humanities, Community Development Unit, University of the Free State, Phuthaditjhaba, South Africa

Pat Dudgeon School of Indigenous Studies, University of Western Australia, Crawley, WA, Australia

Evelyn Secco Faquin Department of Social Work, Graduate Program in Social Work and Social Policy; Research Group: "Social Work and Health: training and professional practice", State University of Londrina (UEL), Londrina, Paraná, Brazil

Anu George Christ (Deemed to be) University, Bangalore, India

Maria do Carmo dos Santos Gonçalves Centro Scalabriniano de Estudos Migrató, Brasilia, Brasília, Brazil

Rebecca Gutwald Munich School of Philosophy, Munich, Germany

Aisha Ali Haji Freelance Photographer, Nairobi, Kenya

Alexandre Hakizamungu Department of Social Sciences, School of Governance, University of Rwanda, Kigali, Rwanda

Sophie Hamisultane School of Social Work, Université de Montréal, Montréal, QC, Canada

Julio Hasbún-Mancilla Department of Industrial Engineering, Universidad de Chile, Santiago, Chile

Symbolon Consulting, Santiago, Chile

Human Development and Capability Association (HDCA), Santiago, Chile

Thandie Keromamang Hlabana Department of Sociology and Social Work, National University of Lesotho, Rome, Lesotho

Rose Jaji Department of Sociology, University of Zimbabwe, Harare, Zimbabwe

Habin Jung University of Appllied Sciences Würzburg-Schweinfurt, Würzburg, Germany

Samaneh Kachouie Kish—International Campus, University of Tehran (UT-KIC), Kish, Iran

Laban Kashaija Musinguzi Department of Social Work and Social Administration, Makerere University, Kampala, Uganda

Demelash Kassaye College of Social Sciences, School of Social Work, Addis Ababa University, Addis Ababa, Ethiopia

Joshua Kayiwa Ministry of Health (MoH), Kampala, Uganda

Peter Kisaakye Department of Population Studies, School of Statistics and Planning, Makerere University, Kampala, Uganda

Tanja Kleibl Faculty of Applied Social Sciences, University of Applied Sciences, Würzburg-Schweinfurt, Würzburg, Germany

Claudia Koehler Farafina Institute, Bamberg, Germany

Rupa Korde Faculty, Economics Area, FLAME University, Pune, Maharashtra, India

Agnes Kyamulabi Department of Social Work and Social Administration, Makerere University, Kampala, Uganda

Líria Maria Bettiol Lanza Department of Social Work, Graduate Program in Social Work and Social Policy; Research Group: 'Social Work and Health: training and professional practice", State University of Londrina (UEL), Londrina, Paraná, Brazil

Stephen Lawoko Department of Public Health, Faculty of Medicine, Gulu University, Gulu, Uganda

Edward Ou Jin Lee School of Social Work, Université de Montréal, Montréal, QC, Canada

Brian Luswata Ministry of Health (MoH), Kampala, Uganda

Ronald Lutz Faculty of Applied Social Sciences, University of Applied Sciences, Erfurt, Germany

Alexandre Maaza Southern African Policy and Development Nexus, Cape Town, South Africa

Yasmin Manji Clinical Psychologist registered under the Kenya Psychological Association (KPA), Nairobi, Kenya

Andrew Masaba The Lutheran World Federation (LWF), Kampala, Uganda

Minenhle Matela Southern African Policy and Development Nexus, Cape Town, South Africa

Thabisa Matsea Faculty of Humanities, Social Sciences and Education, Department of Social Work, University of Venda, Thohoyandou, South Africa

Maria Mauersberger Fundación Mujeres en Paz Colombia (Women Peace Fountation), Barrio Recreo, Cundinamarca, Colombia

Helen McCabe Rights Lab, The University of Nottingham, Nottingham, UK

Rob McPhee Kimberley Aboriginal Medical Services, Broome, WA, Australia

Rimple Mehta School of Social Sciences, Western Sydney University, Parramatta, NSW, Australia

Magnus Mfoafo-M'Carthy Lyle S. Hallman Faculty of Social Work, Wilfrid Laurier University, Waterloo, ON, Canada

Denis Muhangi Department of Social Work and Social Administration, Makerere University, Kampala, Uganda

John A. Mushomi College of Business and Management Sciences, Makerere University, Kampala, Uganda

Augustina Naami Department of Social Work, University of Ghana, Accra, Ghana

Catherine Nakidde Centre for Health and Social Economic Improvement (CHASE-i), Kampala, Uganda

Veronica Nemutandani Department of Social Work, Faculty of Humanities, Social Sciences and Education, University of Venda, Thohoyandou, South Africa

Quynh Anh Nguyen University of Appllied Sciences Würzburg-Schweinfurt, Würzburg, Germany

Ndangwa Noyoo Department of Social Development, University of Cape Town, Cape Town, South Africa

Uche Louisa Nwatu Department of Social Work, University of Nigeria, Nsukka, Enugu State, Nigeria

Eric Awich Ochen Department of Social Work and Social Administration, Makerere University, Kampala, Uganda

Betty Okot Centre for Health and Social Economic Improvement (CHASE-i), Kampala, Uganda

Uzoma Odera Okoye Department of Social Work, Faculty of the Social Sciences, University of Nigeria, Nsukka, Enugu State, Nigeria

Geoffrey Omony YOLRED, Gulu, Uganda

Claudia Ortiz-Rico Salud Comunidudes Group, Facultad de Ciencias de la Salud, Universidad de Santander, Bucaramanga, Colombia

Red GRAAL—Grups de Recerca d'Amèrica i Àfrica Llatines, Barcelona, Spain

Sophie Otiende Azadi Resource Center, Nairobi, Kenya

Anna Pfaffenstaller University of Bamberg and KSH München University of Applied Sciences, Munich, Germany

Giuliana Redin Department of Law, Universidade Federal de Santa Maria—UFSM, Santa Maria, Brazil

MIGRAIDH, International Human Mobility and Human Rights, Santa Maria, Brazil

Taly Reininger Department of Social Work, Universidad de Chile, Santiago, Chile

Vítor Eduardo Alessandri Ribeiro Escola Superior de Propaganda e Marketing, Porto Alegre, RS, Brazil

Eliezer Rodrigues dos Santos Social Work and Health: training and professional practice, State University of Londrina (UEL), Londrina, Paraná, Brazil

Jassi Sandhar The Goldin Institute, Chicago, IL, USA

Katiso Samuel Sehlabane Department of Sociology and Social Work, National University of Lesotho, Rome, Lesotho

Etienne Serupia Semuhoza School of Governance, Department of Social Sciences, University of Rwanda, Kigali, Rwanda

Gloria Seruwagi Centre for Health and Social Economic Improvement (CHASE-i), Department of Social Work and Social Administration, Makerere University, Kampala, Uganda

Makerere University School of Public Health (MakSPH), Kampala, Uganda

Apurva Shinde ICMR Indo-Swedish Ageing Care Project; Non-Profit Organization Consultant on Environment, Health, and Educational Issues, Mumbai, Maharashtra, India

Sanaya Singh Department of Social Work and Psychology, University of Gävle, Gävle, Sweden

Johnmary Ssekatte National Association of Social Workers of Uganda (NASWU), Bunga, Uganda

Prabha Tirmare Nirmala Niketan College of Social Work, Mumbai, India

Janestic Twikirize Department of Social Work and Social Administration, Makerere University, Kampala, Uganda

Roberto Rodolfo Georg Uebel Escola Superior de Propaganda e Marketing, Porto Alegre, RS, Brazil

Francisca Valdebenito-Acosta Symbolon Consulting, Santiago, Chile

Human Development and Capability Association (HDCA), Santiago, Chile

Biju Varkkey Faculty, Human Resource Management Area, Indian Institute of Management Ahmedabad, Ahmedabad, Gujarat, India

Leona Vaughn Faculty of Humanities and Social Sciences, University of Liverpool, Liverpool, UK

Cristóbal Villalobos Dintrans Centro de Estudios de Políticas y Prácticas en Educación (CEPPE-UC), Pontificia Universidad Catolica de Chile, Santiago, Chile

Sunny Wadhwaniya Head of Operations, Institute of Defence Studies and Research, Gujarat University, Ahmedabad, Gujarat, India

Ajwang' Warria Department of Social Work, University of the Witwatersrand, Johannesburg, South Africa

Ignacio Wyman Centro de Estudios de Políticas y Prácticas en Educación (CEPPE-UC), Pontificia Universidad Catolica de Chile, Santiago, Chile

Jacques Love Babatoundé Zannou Universität der Bundeswehr München, Abomey-Calavi, Benin

About the Editors

Maria do Carmo dos Santos Gonçalves is director and researcher at the Scalabrinian Center for Migratory Studies in Brazil. She has a long experience in the field of social work in Brazil, working in the care of migrants and refugees. Her research interests include biographical and ethnographic narrative research, studies on contemporary diasporas, migration and refugees, the Middle East and Islam.

Rebecca Gutwald is a senior researcher at the Munich School of Philosophy, Germany, in a collaborative research project on the ethical use of algorithms in social work and child protection services. Previously, she was academic director of the graduate school on *Ethics, Culture and Education* at the Munich School of Philosophy, as well as associate professor of philosophy at the University of Munich, Germany. Her main areas of research are political philosophy, the capability approach and the normative foundations of social justice. Her current focus lies on the topic of disadvantage, resilience and global social justice.

Tanja Kleibl is currently Professor of Social Work, Migration and Diversity at the University of Applied Sciences Würzburg-Schweinfurt (FHWS), Germany, and Research Associate at the University of Johannesburg, South Africa. She is also Director of the Master's Programme 'International Social Work with Refugees and Migrants'. Previously, she was Professor of Scientific Foundations of Social Work at the University of Applied Sciences Augsburg and Associate Professor of Social Work at the Catholic University of Applied Sciences Munich. Her main research and teaching promotes knowledge and debate about discourses and concepts of development, migration and mobility, civil society as well as governance from postcolonial perspectives. Her emphasis is on social development and social work in the Global South whilst applying a political economy lens to enquiring about differences and contestations in the Global North. She brings together 15 years of extensive practice and research experience in development cooperation and migration.

Ronald Lutz, Dr. phil. Sociologist and Anthropologist, is Lecturer at the University of Applied Sciences of Würzburg-Schweinfurt, Germany; Lecturer at the University of Applied Sciences of Erfurt, Germany; and Research Associate at the School of Social Work, University of Johannesburg, South

Africa. From 1993 to March 2019, he was Professor at the Faculty of Applied Social Sciences at the Erfurt University of Applied Sciences, Germany. His fields of interest include poverty, social politics, social development, and international relations.

Ndangwa Noyoo is a Professor in the Department of Social Development at the University of Cape Town, South Africa, and former Head of the Department of Social Development. He previously worked at the University of Johannesburg in the Department of Social Work as an Associate Professor. He was also employed by the South African Government in the Department of Social Development as a Chief Director/Social Policy Specialist, and the University of the Witwatersrand's Department of Social Work as a Senior Lecturer and Deputy Head of Department. He holds a PhD from the University of the Witwatersrand, Master of Philosophy (MPhil) in Development Studies from Cambridge University and Bachelor of Social Work (BSW) from the University of Zambia. He was a postdoctoral fellow at the Fondation Maison des Sciences de l'Homme (FMSH) Paris, France. He has published widely in the areas of social policy, social development, social work, human rights, corporate social responsibility and indigenous knowledge systems. He has also researched in the foregoing areas. His recent publications include *Social Welfare and Social Work in Southern Africa*. Stellenbosch: Sun Media Press (2021) (Editor); *Promoting Healthy Human Relationships* in *Post-Apartheid South Africa*: *Social Work and Social Development Perspectives*. Cham: Springer (2020) (Editor); and *Social Policy in Post-Apartheid South Africa: Social Re-engineering for Inclusive Development* (1st ed.). Oxon: Routledge.

Janestic Twikirize is Senior Lecturer in the Department of Social Work and Social Administration, Makerere University, Uganda. She holds a PhD in Social Work and Social Development and an MA in Social Sector Planning and Management. She has also served as a visiting Lecturer at Gothenburg University in Sweden, University of Stavanger in Norway and Lincoln University in the UK. She has published over 20 scientific papers including four books and has made over 30 presentations in international conferences in the past 5 years. She was previously Vice President of the Association of Schools of Social Work in Africa and a board member of the International Association of Schools of Social Work (IASSW) until 2018. Between 2012 and 2018, she served as the East Africa regional Coordinator of PROSOWO, a 6-member advanced academic partnership that worked to strengthen professional social work in East Africa.

Part I

Analysis: Social Issues and the COVID-19 Pandemic

1 COVID and Social Work Voices from India and Australia: Strategic and Meaningful Solidarities for Global Justice

Rimple Mehta and Linda Briskman

1.1 Introduction: A World Turned Upside Down

The year of 2020 has been like no other for many of the world's inhabitants. Although humankind differentially experiences ongoing crises such as wars, environmental catastrophes, and extreme poverty, the COVID-19 pandemic was seen by some as the 'great leveller' as barely any country or class or creed within was not affected. Social workers have been among those impacted directly through their work or through contemplating what the pandemic has meant for its social justice leanings, at country-specific levels and globally. Although social work approaches have not had the visibility of health responses, it is timely to re-vision our profession's value base, which is concerned with challenging structural inequalities and promoting social justice. In doing so, we contest the idea of COVID as the 'great leveller' to show how COVID has distinct consequences for those living in the Global South and the Global North. We concur with Soutphommasane (2021, p. 24) that the pandemic has revealed how much inequality exists that is being further accelerated by COVID-19. We have selected two countries to illustrate our points—India and Australia—our own countries of citizenship and where our collegial conversations led to this exploration. The chapter gives primacy to the voices of a small group of social work practitioners and academics from each country as a co-production. For this chapter, co-production is defined as deliberative collaborative research based on professional observations and reflections.[1]

1.2 Turning Around Dominance of Health Responses

In the global quest to minimise and even eradicate the virus, the perspectives and voices of health professionals have been privileged. Media reportage reinforces a health paradigm and scans of news items reveal constant attention to numbers, sites, protective equipment, hospital settings, and the quest for a vaccine. Although we acknowledge that the pandemic is a public health issue, we argue that the lack of focus on its socio-economic impact has deepened marginalisation of already excluded people and communities. Although some attention is given to severe social consequences, such as increased mental health concerns, internal migrations, unemployment,

R. Mehta (✉)
School of Social Sciences, Western Sydney University, Parramatta, NSW, Australia
e-mail: R.Mehta2@westernsydney.edu.au

L. Briskman
School of Social Sciences, Western Sydney University, Liverpool, NSW, Australia

[1] We thank the co-producers of this chapter: Sivan Barak, Parul Chaudhury, Dheeraj, Jerome D'Souza, Susie Latham, Shubhada Maitra, Christine Morley, Carolyn Noble, Kim Robinson, Deborah Rosenberg, Emily Stuart, Prabha Tirmare and Penelope Tong.

M. C. S. Gonçalves et al. (eds.), *The Coronavirus Crisis and Challenges to Social Development*,
https://doi.org/10.1007/978-3-030-84678-7_1

and domestic/family violence, governments around the world have handled these inconsistently, with a lag behind public health responses.

We argue that social work has much to offer: the pandemic can create lessons for handling not only the present crisis but also possible future events. Attention to poverty alleviation, structural disadvantage, community development, social justice, and equity can create a strong edifice for cultivating a society in which equitable distribution of resources is the norm. It is promising to observe that emerging literature in social work on the pandemic is located in theorising on poverty and structural disadvantage, arguing for the need to work at both the micro and macro level (Amadasun, 2020b; Walter-McCabe, 2020; Bright, 2020). Gerontological social work (Berg-Weger & Morley, 2020; Cudjoe & Abdullah, 2020; Seifert, 2020) and family and domestic violence have also received much attention. There has also been a focus on the need for social work to reflect on its practices (O'Leary & Tsui, 2020; Amadasun, 2020a). We add to this emerging body of literature by looking at the Global South and Global North and highlight how inequities are starkly revealed within country and global contexts, and among 'the south that lives in the Global North'—migrants, refugees, and asylum seekers. Through this chapter we, as do several others, debunk the myth of the virus as a 'great leveller' (Zarkov, 2020) by highlighting the interconnectedness of the globalised world where "the fate of the countries and people are irrevocably intertwined" (Carrington et al., 2018) and focus on the most marginalised communities in India and Australia. It is also our intention to invoke the idea of ethics of care, which is often confined to micro work or localised work, as one that can address large-scale social or global problems. Robinson (1997, p. 114) argues: "The idea of an ethics of care can be relevant to the question of relations among moral agents on a global scale, provided that it takes account of the social relations, institutional arrangements, norms, and structures through which perceptions of difference and moral exclusion are created in the global system." Such an understanding of an ethic of care can enable us to call on countries to engage in global duty of care to facilitate the idea of global justice.

1.3 Methodology

To gain a snapshot of inequality within and across borders, we asked a small number of social work academics and practitioners in India and Australia to be co-producers of the study, an ideas fest. We emailed six broad questions to each and requested succinct and focused responses to the questions. The areas of inquiry included: Specific field of practice or research interest; Impact of COVID-19 on this field or interest; Nature of inequalities that have surfaced; What helped social workers in pandemic work; Challenges faced by social workers; and Lessons for social work academics and practitioners for the post-COVID future. We used convenience sampling from those we were aware were overtly working within a social justice framework. The questions were framed in such a way that they were reflective and forward looking. Responses were received from three social work academics/educators from India, four social work academics/educators from Australia, three social work practitioners from India, and three social work practitioners from Australia.

From the narratives of contributors in India and Australia, we singled out four thematic areas of social and public policy that feature in contemporary social work:

- People and the State: Migrants, Refugees, and Citizens
- Women, Mobility, and Violence
- Digital Divide: Access to Communities and Social Work Practice
- Role of Social Workers: Relief and Systemic Interventions

1.4 People and the State: Migrants, Refugees, and Citizens

The pandemic has justified punitive and surveillance actions of the state, which would in 'normal' times be resisted and immediately garner a civil society response. In both India and Australia, the relationship between the citizens and the state became even more fraught and tilted with power towards the state. Refugees, migrants, and asylum seekers, who also inhabit the space of the state along with the citizens, have limited opportunities to lay claim to rights.

Amongst the citizens, a particular group that stood out in the Indian context were the migrant labourers who worked in different parts of urban India. According to Census of India 2011, interstate and intrastate migrants are estimated to number 177.5 million. Nearly 88% of India's employed population works in the informal sector (ILO, 2018) and contributes about half the GDP. A sudden lockdown declared in India left the migrant workers employed in the informal sector scrambling for their survival (Xavier, 2020). Labour migrants in urban areas were forced to go back to their homes in rural areas because of the loss of jobs and daily wages. The urban poor were also left to their own devices to find resources for their everyday survival.

Dr. Prabha Tirmare is an Associate Professor at Nirmala Niketan College of Social Work, Mumbai. She is the co-founder of Jeevan Pravaah: Life Stream, a project initiated during COVID-19 relief work in Mumbai slums for ragpicker women and their children. She observes:

> In urban slums there are slum dwellers, construction workers, vendors, domestic workers, and waste workers. In rural communities there are poor villagers, those who are landless, and marginal farmers and other unskilled labourers. Most are illiterate and engaged in the unorganized sector. They do not live in a conducive environment because they subsist on no or low daily wages, with no health and hygiene facilities, no recreation, and service conditions without any resources (land, water, or forest). All these groups have been suffering quite a lot during the pandemic to manage their daily food, water, health, hygiene, and mobility.

She further adds:

> Community youth became unemployed, directionless. Children discontinued their schooling. Women domestic workers were banned from continuing their job. However, the most vulnerable group, that is, waste workers/ragpickers, continued their engagement in collecting and disposing of garbage. The long lockdown period meant that most of the industrial areas, shops, schools, and offices were closed; hence, women found it hard to collect garbage, which is part of their livelihood. This condition became very challenging and a risk factor to the waste workers during the pandemic.

While Prabha highlights the issues faced by rural–urban migrants and urban slum dwellers, *Dheeraj, Programme Manager in Research and Capacity Building at Praxis—Institute for Participatory Practices, emphasises the vulnerable position of Dalits, Adivasis, Minorities, Denotified Tribes, and sexual minorities. As an over-arching theme of his work, democratising policy spaces through participatory methods has been significant in bringing the voices of the most marginalised to the fore.* He says:

> In labour rights and business responsibility space, the exodus of the large number of migrants, back to villages, exposed the skewed levels of disparity with fragile social security for informal sector workers, which hampered their ability to make ends meet. It was clear that large businesses have flourished by exploiting the informal workforce, and at this stage businesses did not own their workers in their extended supply chains. Further, with return to villages families had to access loans for making ends meet and this also posed a risk as there is a clear danger of children being pushed into the labour market at low wage rates. The situation has been critical for adolescent girls, as instances of child marriage have also increased.
>
> The relationship between state and citizens was not defined on equal footing, and in the name of controlling the spread of the virus various restrictions were put on the liberties of the citizens. Citizens found it difficult to apply for accessing social security programmes or to raise grievances with appropriate authorities. Access to food, health, shelter, and other necessities were disrupted by limited mobility or shrinking resource capacity. Many of the processes were completed online but limited access to online facilities meant workers or migrants found themselves at a loss. This limitation of access has been particularly difficult for Dalits, Adivasis, Minorities, and Denotified Tribes as they are already amongst the most disadvantaged in the Indian social structure.

The pandemic has had a cascading impact on the marginalisation of particular groups of citizens. It has led to emerging realities that will require an interdisciplinary and intersectional lens to understand and then work through them.

In the Australian context, Islamophobia shook the claim to citizenship for a number of groups. Apart from recognised citizens, a population that already has a fraught relationship with the state is that of asylum seekers and refugees, some of whom are Muslim, who await bestowal of rights afforded to others. This issue was flagged as an important one by social workers in Australia. The area of migration has become one of global contention, especially in the field of forced migration. This area has become one of social policy conflict in Australia with the measures applied to asylum seekers, particularly immigration detention, being seen as among the harshest in the world (Global Detention Project, 2017–2018). During the pandemic a number of countries released people from detention settings because of concerns about virus spread; Australia was not among them. Although Australia has been said to be more generous to settlement (invited) refugees, and is also a multicultural country of migration, the pandemic revealed gaps in the extent of this welcome. An area alluded to by contributors is the differential treatment of migrants during the pandemic, particularly the harsh and sudden lockdown that occurred in inner Melbourne when public housing tenants in highrise apartments were, without notice, forbidden to leave their homes. A panicked public health response trumped social well-being and service provision.

Dr. Susie Latham is an adjunct research fellow in the School of Social Sciences at Western Sydney University. She is co-author of Human Rights Overboard: Seeking Asylum in Australia (Briskma, 2008). Currently, Susie conducts research and writes about Islamophobia.

Susie's response centres on both political and media commentary, which targeted Muslim groups both explicitly and implicitly. Susie argues that social workers can amplify the voices of communities affected by the type of injustices outlined next.

As she notes:

> The comments of political leaders and media reporting on COVID-19 has drawn attention to cases involving Muslims and migrant communities in a way it has not done for white Australians.

On politicians:

> Even progressive politicians such as Victorian Premier Daniel Andrews made coded references to Muslims and migrants. On June 30 Andrews drew attention to suburbs with high levels of migrants and Muslims saying, "I do feel obliged to tell you that in Broadmeadows and Keilor Downs alone, some 929 people refused to be tested."

On 14 September, Victoria's Chief Health Officer Brett Sutton referred to cases in the multicultural council of Casey. "I have made an offer to personally speak to that community," he said. "Having been to Afghanistan a couple of times… I want to be able to reflect on my cultural experiences…I know there are universal motivations that every family has to do the right thing to protect their own families and the wider community." Sutton apologised after the Afghan Australian community published a statement condemning their community being singled out.

On media:

> Commentary on a cluster at a Melbourne abattoir, Cedar Meats, included the fact that it was halal certified, and television coverage included shots lingering on the Lebanese flag on its premises. An article in *The Australian* newspaper cited a medical centre receptionist as a source for the claim in late June 2020 that a spike in cases which became the "second wave" emerged from "a large family Eid celebration." The Islamic Council of Victoria issued a press release at the time calling for more balanced reporting, and it later emerged that the cases had entered the community as the result of a failure in government systems in hotel quarantine. Conservative media commentator Andrew Bolt wrote a column titled Diversity and Death, in which he wrote 'many of the sick are probably from immigrant families.'

Deborah Rosenberg is the student program coordinator at Community Information and Support Victoria (CISVic), a peak body for the community information and support sector. CISVic and its member organisations provide financial and material aid to people in crisis, within a supportive service model that includes the provision of tailored information, referrals and advocacy.

Her response provides leads to understanding how asylum seekers have experienced the pandemic. She says:

> …almost all people of colour in short-term casual work have been hit particularly hard by job loss yet are ineligible for government support payments. Already marginalised groups have been further disadvantaged by inequitable government responses.

Furthermore:

> Marginalised people are always hit hardest by any negative social or economic change. Many government responses were in opposition to social work values. Responding to quarantine issues from a custodial-punitive perspective (armed police at housing towers,[2] security guards at hotels, harsh fines) rather than a social health perspective is in stark contrast to social work framing.

An old adage applies:

> When the only tool you have is a hammer, every problem looks like a nail. When you purposefully deplete the health and community sectors, the only 'tool' that remains for responding to social issues is an aggressive one.

Carolyn Noble is a retired Australian social work academic interested in progressive politics and social work's capacity to influence social change in terms of human rights, gender and distributive justice and environmental activism. She holds two Emeritus Professor positions in social work, one at the Australian College of Applied Psychology (ACAP) and the other at Victoria University.

Carolyn's narrative also captures migration:

> Many migrants are experiencing discrimination and accusations of poor health regimes and being scapegoated as people feel the frustration of the restrictions and public health warnings/fear campaigns.

Dr. Kim Robinson is a Senior Lecturer in Social Work at Deakin University in Australia. She has been a social work practitioner and manager in community health and refugee services in Australia, Timor Leste and the UK. The three main areas of interest in her current work are working with asylum seekers and refugees, and settlement issues; family violence; and social work students returning to study in neoliberal university settings.

She maintains:

> Working in the space of refugees we know that many have been impacted due to their current working arrangements in the gig economy. Many people have not had access to financial supports, which has impacted on their ability to pay for basic goods and services. Communities have relied on emergency relief, often provided by other refugee communities, and we know that those services have been oversubscribed

Parul Chaudhury's area of work for the past 10 years has been rights-based community organising with low-income single women—widows, separated, never married, and other single women in Rajasthan, India. She is also actively involved in bringing in gender concerns in rights-based organising work with indigenous communities.

Parul succinctly sums up the scenario based on her work and observations in India. However, this may be applied to understanding the approach of the state towards people within it in different parts of the world. She adds:

> Many of the policy decisions taken by the government in this time have made it clear that a large section of the public – is invisible to the government. This blind-sidedness is not limited to a particular party in power, but is rather much more systemic, as social work practitioners we have to work with those we serve to find ways to make our democracy work for all.

1.5 Women, Mobility, and Violence

In April 2020, UN Women reported that 243 million women and girls in the age group of 14–59 years had been subjected to sexual and/or physical violence by an intimate partner in the previous 12 months. Based on the emerging data, they highlighted that violence against women and girls had intensified the world over because of the pandemic and hence referred to it as 'the shadow pandemic' (Mlamb-Ngcuka, 2020). Increase in instances of domestic violence during the pandemic are not confined to specific countries. It was a feature of contributor responses in both India and Australia, as reflected in their narratives. It is prevalent across both the Global South and Global North. Despite program development and the work of the advocacy sector, the home

[2] Note that a significant number of tower residents are from refugee backgrounds.

remains a dangerous place for women and children. The area of family violence is one of the most fraught areas of social policy in Australia.

Professor Christine Morley is a social work educator at the Queensland University of Technology (QUT) in Australia. Her broad area of research interest is critical social work practice and education. She has a specific focus on violence against women. During 2020, Christine was involved in a collaborative research project on the impact of COVID-19 on domestic and family violence services in Australia.

Christine reports on the impact of COVID-19 in this research and practice area.

> Our national survey involving 362 respondents [service providers] indicated that COVID has significantly increased the prevalence and severity of domestic and family violence (both incidences of physical violence and more extreme behaviours) (Carrington et al., 2020). Travel restrictions and physical/social distancing rules during COVID increased victims/survivors' level of isolation and reduced access to outside supports (formal, personal, and community based). This resulted in victims/survivors being locked down with perpetrators, and in greater stress for families for a range of reasons (including job loss, financial precarity, and housing instability, home-schooling children), which correlated with an increase in new forms of family violence that occurred as perpetrators have 'weaponised' COVID to intensify coercive and controlling behaviours during the pandemic (Carrington et al., 2020). Consequently, the combination of these factors during the pandemic has had terrible consequences for people's mental health and emotional well-being (Carrington et al., 2020).

Professor Shubhada Maitra, School of Social Work, Tata Institute of Social Sciences (TISS), Mumbai, focuses on mental health, recovery and reintegration of women living with long-term mental illness, gender, sexualities, and gender-based violence and child and adolescent mental health. She is the Project Director for two field action projects in TISS: Tarasha, which is a community-based recovery and reintegration project and Muskaan, the Child and Adolescent Guidance Centre of TISS. Tarasha works towards recovery and reintegration within the Regional Mental Hospital. As part of the deinstitutionalisation process, the organisation conducts intensive group and individual therapeutic sessions with women diagnosed with a mental illness and admitted to the mental hospital to prepare them for a life outside the institution.

Shubhada talks about the challenges of working with women in mental health institutions and the increase in domestic violence:

> With COVID-19 and the subsequent lockdown, access to women in the hospital was stopped. It was impossible to continue the therapeutic sessions in the hospital, to track women's mental health status and their journey towards recovery. We are sure that for women residents of the mental hospital, being locked up within the hospital with minimal contact with mental health workers must also have been very difficult. However, some follow-up was done indirectly by connecting with Hospital Social Workers and Occupational Therapists.
>
> While online mental health work with different groups has suddenly become popular in the context of COVID-19, those with long-term mental illness both within and outside the mental hospital have been completely invisibilised. The first 3–4 months of lockdown were extremely difficult in terms of addressing their mental health needs. The burden on caregivers increased manifold. Women living with mental illness/mental health issues, like many other women, have been victims of increased domestic violence.

Parul Chaudhury highlights the complexities that the pandemic presented for single women:

> Organizing work in this context relies heavily on field work – travelling, holding meetings, workshops, etc. In our work with women, mobility through this organizing work has been a very effective strategy for encouraging critical reflection, building confidence, and widening the world view of individual women. The biggest impact COVID-19 has had has been on mobility. Women who had challenged cultural practices restricting their mobility have once again found themselves unable to move out of the house. Many report feeling sad, depressed, stressed, and insecure. Among single women, those who live in the same households as extended family, many contribute through wage labour and other work; the pandemic and the lockdown resulted in loss of work for them, as well as other members in the household. The economic crunch felt by many families in some cases increased the level of unwantedness, alienation, and isolation that some single women feel from their families. Several elder widowed women reported being harassed and pressurized into parting with their meagre monthly pension amount.

> In aiding and supporting single women facing harassment and violence in their homes, help is sought from local public resources and other organizations. In the lockdown period and even up until now, such support is severely limited. Law enforcement, health workers, and those employed in grassroots delivery of public services have been overburdened during this time as they have formed the backbone of the public pandemic response, and issues being faced by women have taken a back seat. Police stations not registering complaints, shelter homes not taking in people in need, and hospitals turning away patients have all been challenges that have been difficult to solve in this period.

The increase in cases of domestic violence and family violence world over is referred to as a 'pandemic within a pandemic' (Evans et al., 2020). The advances made by social workers, activists, and the civil society in curbing domestic and family violence seemed to have taken a blow as a result of the pandemic. The confinement of women back in the domestic sphere often with their perpetrators, this time in a legitimised lockdown, has had serious implications for their well-being. The gendered impact of the pandemic will have implications long after the virus has been managed.

1.6 Digital Divide: Access to Communities and Social Work Practice

Prospects afforded through digital access have been extolled during the pandemic. These range from workplace flexibility, means of maintaining family connection, and the pursuit of recreational activity. Less considered is the divide between those with access to resources and those without, an area that has always been of concern to social workers, but in pre-COVID times there was little reference to the digital divide. In both India and Australia, contributors spoke of interrelated barriers of the digital divide for client groups, social work practitioners, and students.

Social work practitioners were vocal in expressing views on how modified ways of working impacted negatively on practice and, at times, conveyed cautious optimism.

Sivan Barak is a family services social worker at the Dandenong and District Aborigines Co Operative in Australia. As a family support worker her role traverses the breadth of issues experienced by the family: housing, mental health, family violence, financial hardship, and legal. Her field of work is underpinned by culturally safe practice working in the best interests of children through support and advocacy alongside families who identify as Aboriginal.

Sivan states the difficulties in social work practice in her setting where trust and engagement are central and where informal conversations in family homes is foundational to the work. With the advent of COVID restrictions, support was provided remotely through telephone calls, SMS, or emails.

> In the case of clients who already knew me it has been a smoother transition as we have built trust and familiarity with the specific capabilities and needs of the family, such as literacy levels and access to electronic gadgets and data. New referrals have been extremely difficult to initiate particularly with the backdrop of deep distrust and trauma within the community towards service providers.
> Our organisation has no prior experience in remote service provision and so we have all had to be creative and inventive on the go.

On inequalities that surfaced:

> Transitioning to remote or distant services has increased the interaction for my clients with online service, which requires a level of numeracy, literacy, and computer accessibility which they often lack. Children's home-schooling has been stressful for parents who are unable to provide suitable electronic gadgets for their children or to help with their learning. Much of my work requires forms to be sighted and signed by clients: consent, assessments, support letters, legal documents, etc. My clients do not have computers or printers and are often reading documents on their mobile phone and are unable to understand them, causing anxiety and misunderstandings.

Sivan also refers to important Aboriginal cultural practices that are increasingly recognised by social workers (Briskman, 2014):

> Physical isolation from family and broader community has had a deeply negative effect on decision-making capacity and conflict resolution

which is usually overseen by Uncles, Aunties, and Elders. Many of my families expressed feeling lost without their extended family to sort out problems and give advice from the cultural perspective.

Of help to social workers, Sivan stated:

Social workers carry their tools of trade within themselves and have had to adapt creatively to the new reality. Home visits and face-to-face meetings allow for 'reading the room' gauging body language and noticing details in the environment which cannot be observed via p/c or SMS. Flexible communication skills have been vital to navigate the levels of confusion and anxiety of clients. I share a photograph of myself in front of the computer with each new client after my first phone call so they have an idea of what I look like; they have often reciprocated with a family photograph. Strengthening networks with colleagues and resources has been vital for positive outcomes with access to services.

Shubhada Maitra articulates the problems of working in the digital space and proposes solutions:

The need as always was far greater than the availability of resources. But this was particularly seen during this pandemic. Reaching out to the most needy was a challenge. The only means of communication was virtual and remote; this had its own difficulties. Working from congested homes, sudden disappearance of a 'work space' affected productivity, perhaps in the initial months of the pandemic, until everyone got used to the 'new normal.'

Linkages with civil society organisations and professional networks particularly with the police, medical and allied professionals, and the State were important to address issues that were thrown up as a result of COVID-19. Whether it was the migrants' crisis and loss of livelihoods, facilitating return of students and migrants back home, dealing with emergencies and crises, procuring prescriptions and medicines for those living with mental illness, it was these linkages and networks that helped social workers continue their work during the pandemic. Not to mention the strong sense of purpose and motivation to reach out to those in need.

Kim Robinson steps back from the everyday working environment that online approaches have created to raising broader questions about inequalities:

One of the challenges is to think about how we come together as practitioners and as educators, and how we navigate privilege. For many people, working from home has been less stressful, with less travelling and commuting, being able to work in a quiet working space, and more time to exercise and relax. For others, home is not a safe space, nor is it one that is conducive to work and reflection. It may involve caring responsibilities, home-schooling, juggling limited time outdoors, shopping for food, and feeling anxious and unsafe. In some cases, we are confronted with colleagues and friends for whom the latter is their reality. We have all gained insight and understanding of how we are working, in that we have all been confined to home, with a view into our more intimate space.

Emily Stuart is a recent Bachelor of Social Work graduate from Western Sydney University. Unemployed for the most part during COVID-19, she has now obtained employment in the policy/research and disability sector.

On an encouraging note, Emily notes how lockdown during COVID-19 opened up opportunities for people with disability:

As lockdown began and only essential workers were allowed to attend their workplace, the capacity for people with a disability to work from home opened up. This was an exciting development as for years, people with a disability have been requesting the ability to work from home but were always told it was not possible. However, since the need arose for services to continue during lockdown via phone or online, employers are now understanding that this could be a possibility for social workers with a disability.

I believe one of the lessons that social work practitioners and educators need to carry forward in their work is that there is a capacity for social workers with disabilities to work from home: this has occurred with the introduction of telehealth appointments and connecting with clients and other staff via online video conferencing programs like Zoom, Skype, and Microsoft Teams.

Emily further speaks of her personal experience of obtaining work during lockdown that supports the idea of flexibility for people with disability.

During the pandemic I found employment with a government agency writing policy in the disability sector. When applying for this position, all the interviews and tasks were conducted online. I felt this process actually reduced some of the nerves I had before the interview. I was successful and offered the position. I commenced at the end of October, so most of the issues with working remotely had already been resolved. Although we were still able to come into the office, we weren't required to. We used video calling platforms for meetings and we also have an instant messaging service on our laptops called Microsoft Lync. This help was fantastic as I was able to quickly message a colleague to ask for clarification on work matters or even just to check in with someone and ask them how their day was. Using both these platforms assisted me in feeling connected with my colleagues even though I still have not met all of them yet.

In January 2021, we were asked to return to the office; however, we could also put in an application for home-based work. This process was relatively easy, and I was approved to work two days in the office and two days at home. My supervisor has made it clear that if I am feeling tired, sore, or if I am nervous about catching public transport during the pandemic to not feel pressured to come into the office as we can connect quite easily over Cisco or Lync. For someone with a physical disability, it was wonderful to work in such a positive and flexible environment and for our supervisors to understand that sometimes you may have to work from home due to pain or tiredness is really refreshing too. I hope in the future other employers will be understanding and flexible to allow people with disability to work from home since this pandemic has proved it is possible.

From a climate change perspective, Kim Robinson also reflects on re-visioning from the pandemic, an area that is receiving increasing attention in social work:

Climate change and the warming of the planet – reduce travel and movement of people is one way of doing this, give people the option of working at home, if they can/want to. Look more at online education, online healthcare, and other services, meetings and appointments and where this can be moved online/or other modes.

Penelope Tong is a social work practice educator in School of Social Work, TISS, specialising in fields of criminal justice—women prisoners and mental health of prisoners, interpersonal conflict and violence. In her field education role, she identifies the disquiet that emerges for students on the pathway to become professional social workers, despite measures put in place to accommodate pandemic requirements.

In India and many other parts of the world, educational instruction has been transported from a physical sphere to a virtual one. For educational programmes that are theoretically concentrated, the virtual location still provides for a learning conducive environment. However, the challenges to learning within virtual spaces increase when components of the programme require live skill development.

The indispensability of fieldwork to social work education is undeniable. COVID-19 has resulted in the introduction of mandatory social distancing, wearing of masks and other protective gear, and caution with regard to entering densely populated or containment spaces. Fieldwork in social work education by its very nature requires in-person contact with marginalised and economically and socially disadvantaged groups, who often inhabit areas that do not have the luxury of space, sanitation, and sometimes even the privilege of being cautious. Fieldwork has thus had to be converted to a block programme from a concurrent one or has had to take the form of a less potent version that happens virtually; this undoubtedly obstructs the development of people skills which are so imperative to social work. Needless to say, without the field, a social work education programme remains incomplete.

Furthermore, the digital divide exists in student cohorts:

For students coming from backgrounds that enable the study from home option, the education process still carries on largely unabated, albeit without the full experience. However, for students coming from educationally unconducive backgrounds, the very process of accessing the educational programme becomes a struggle. Not possessing devices necessary for a remote education and having to rely on mobile phones, constraints related to the cost of adequate data, a lack of internet connectivity in their locations, etc. are what render them physically as well as virtually disadvantaged, unconnected, and confronted with a challenged access to a virtual education.

Aligned with Penelope's reservations, Carolyn Noble raises the question of what the pandemic means for the next generation of social workers:

Student social workers have been dramatically impacted by courses going online but agencies closing and leaving them without real-life practice experience to explore the link with theory is of great concern.

1.7 Role of Social Workers: Relief and Systemic Interventions

The purpose of social work remains divided in ways identified more than two decades ago by Dominelli (1998), as therapeutic helping approaches, maintenance approaches, and emancipatory approaches. To some extent, as narrated by contributors, these divisions have been challenged during the pandemic, as social workers have had to bridge the conceptual divide and micro and macro elements of practice have merged in social work responses. Structural social work paradigms have re-surfaced more directly, in the way its founder Maurice Moreau (1979) posited that social work practice needed to consider the structural oppression of individuals while still considering the individual, because of the interconnection between personal aspects of a problem and the institutional and political elements (Allan, 2003).

Dheeraj speaks of how:

> The pandemic led to infusion of a lot of energies from the social sector into providing for immediate relief to families and this also predominantly moved attention towards the service delivery rather than on rights-based work, seeking accountability from the state. It needs to be recognised that rights-based work cannot be ignored during the times of such pandemics as accountability of the systems would largely depend on the nature of this engagement. In many instances, the relationship between NGOs and communities was defined in a way where NGOs were more of a donor of relief services, giving power to them vis-à-vis the communities. Social work practice needs to focus on structural inequalities and engage with power structures rather than just focusing on filling the gaps in service delivery.

Moreover:

> The social sector over the period has evolved as a professional field and in that pursuit created systems for ensuring credibility. However, the sector has also been a victim of bureaucratisation. It was found that during the relief, at many places, focus remained on clicking pictures for either maintaining records or gaining public appreciation to generate more resources. Communities challenged this attitude, and this surely needs to be recognised in future engagement.

Much of the response during the crisis was based on short-term crisis intervention approaches. A number of contributors expressed concern about the place of social work values in policy responses to COVID-19, which are antithetical to social work tenets, particularly social justice. As Deborah Rosenberg comments in relation to emergency relief:

> It responds only to immediate need, rather than systemic change. Being part of a peak body that is simultaneously involved with social justice campaigns, is a partial salve to the ethical dilemmas of emergency relief.

For Deborah, there were other dilemmas for social workers and their constituents:

> As agencies moved to remote service provision it was challenging to find processes that did not add further oppressive loads to people already struggling with job loss and the emotional impact of lockdown. How do you create systems that make it easy for people seeking help, while ensuring you maintain program integrity and meet your funding obligations?
>
> There are aspects of service delivery in this sector that clearly align with social work values, and others, which by necessity relate to funding accountability.
>
> Marginalised people are always hit hardest by any negative social or economic change. Many government responses were in opposition to social work values. Social workers must highlight the different outcomes that could have been achieved if another perspective had been taken and alternate resources had been available. Social workers and the sectors that employ them, need to loudly call out structural racism in government policy, take their lead from activists of colour, and work alongside them for social justice.

The time of the pandemic has opened up for Kim Robinson opportunities to reflect on what matters:

> I think for me it is reinforcing that communities matter however they are defined and drawing on the strengths and communication that exists in communities is essential.

The direct impact on social workers is raised by Sivan Barak, which brings to the forefront questions of industrial justice, a concern of social workers that ought to be a centrepiece of social work's critique of neoliberalism.

> Stress and work levels for social workers has been overwhelming with little to no support. Supervision is most often focused on case work rather than on the well-being of the worker, there must be counselling and supports in place for the workers which are easily accessible to avoid burn out.
>
> Over the last 7 months, work has been intense and relentless, with increases in client need and little planning regarding the impact on social workers. The intersection of working from home with ever-increasing workload has made the separation between the professional and personal difficult to manage. It is unsustainable for long periods of time without harm caused to the well-being of social workers and their families.

This is reinforced by Kim Robinson:

> Services and supports have also had to respond to the needs of their own staff and teams, and to ensure that workers do not burn out or get too over-loaded when working from home.

From India, Shubhada also speaks of social worker stress:

> The core job of social workers is to connect with people, to work closely with systems and structures to bring about change that is grounded in social justice, equality, dignity and empowerment. With the enforced lockdown and mandatory 'stay-at-home,' and 'work from home,' social workers needed to shift gears to ensure continued contact with their communities, and this was extremely difficult in the initial months of the lockdown. The nature of their work also changed. Some became active in organising relief and repatriation for those who had lost their livelihoods and were stuck in Mumbai. There were concerns about their communities, loss of contact with the 'field.' Social workers' own mental health needs altered daily routines, the double burden of work and domestic responsibilities, an added demand for a 'workplace' within a household with other members, uncertainty about job, and the future and fear of infection led to high stress, exhaustion, and fatigue among some workers.

Parul Chaudhury says:

> Activists and social workers have done what they can, setting up pan-national networks, collecting charity, relief support, undertaking large-scale distribution, setting up mobile clinics, etc. all with no public support, rather faced with many hindrances.

Additionally:

> Economic fallouts of the pandemic and changes in government regulations have seen funding dry up for many nongovernment organizations (NGOs), putting social workers out of work. Many have continued their work under enormous stress. There was very little to no psychosocial support available for social workers, counsellors, and activists.
> During the lockdown, permissions had to be sought at the district level to provide essential services, as many of the services provided by social workers and NGOs were not included in the list of essential services exempt from lockdown restrictions. We have had sometimes to cope with law enforcement, fines, etc. while engaging in important work to provide essential relief to the most vulnerable, or to aid women facing violence.

Jerome D'Souza is a social work practitioner working as a consultant for a community organisation in rural Bengal, Wild Chhotonagpur PlateauTrust (WCPT), which focuses on innovative approaches for access to education. He adopts a community participation approach, for example, in the selection of teachers and pedagogy.[3]

He discusses the consequences of moving from the mission of his organisation to one of handling crisis:

> The major concern for the NGO was scarcity of food material in the adjoining villages and lack of accessibility to rations. Very soon the NGO started receiving calls regarding starvation and the funds remaining in its account were inadequate. WCPT was successful in coordinating with local administration in reaching out to the communities in need. The funds that the NGO had accumulated for education and research were diverted towards food, health, and essential items for the community. COVID-19 had also rendered many households without income and had to be supported by WCPT. A result of COVID-19 is that the education system is losing steam, which could be a major cause for rising inequalities in the long term. The lockdown during the pandemic has swallowed opportunities for work and, with falling income, increasing frustration is leading to many accounts of domestic violence. It is also seen that girls in the family get married off very soon because of this lack of income and such cases may increase in the near future.
>
> This problem provides opportunities for WCPT to reinvent its design but also causes the challenge of lack of funds and rearranged community dynamics.

[3] Jerome D'Souza passed away in July 2021, a few months after he read the final version of this chapter. He was much loved by fellow social workers and alumni of Tata Institute of Social Sciences where he did a Master of Arts in Social Work.

For Jerome, consistent with some of the Australian contributors, this necessitates the importance of rethinking social work's value system and approach and not just in a material sense.

> It is critical for a development practitioner to think from the perspective of a value system in the broader sense and not in a materialistic aspect. Doing the best for the community requires empathetic and human centric thinking. The pandemic has reinforced the need for planning, coordination, and implementation in a dynamic setting. Responding after having studied and understood the significance of the situation is very important for social workers working with grassroots organizations.

Carolyn Noble throws down the gauntlet to social workers:

> The most pressing challenge social workers face, and it seems it is more obvious now, is their relevancy! I am not sure social work practitioners have the wherewithal to stand up against the politics of fear and the short- and long-term consequences on people's welfare and health because of these imposed lockdowns and restrictive health measures and to publicly advocate for the most vulnerable impacted by these events. If the time ever came for social work to step up for its constituencies, it is now!!!!
>
> The major lesson is for social work to strengthen its advocacy base and its critique of right-wing politics that have contributed to the economic and environmental destruction linked to this and other potential pandemics.
>
> I am concerned that the authoritarianism that has emerged to keep people well and confined to their houses has empowered this discourse and any recovery will only give more legitimacy to right-wing conservative politics. It seems conservative governments cannot abide public policies that help people cope with these social and economic changes but return to old mantra of jobs and neoliberal economics!

As Penelope Tong says, 'it is the socially and economically marginalised that are most adversely affected by crises.' She has, however, some optimism in how 'the pandemic has reinforced the need and importance of flexibility, adaptability, collaboration, community, and resilience as values in social work' and how it is possible to 'work against the odds with conviction and optimism.' Deliberating globally, she adds that the future needs to confront the race for resources and exploitation of the environment. Pointing out that the pandemic altered the very nature of how social work was transacted, she observed:

> Reaching people, connecting with them, and experiencing the connect was something that had to be reimagined and conducted within a physically restricted or 'virtual space.' It involved uncertainty, difficulty in reaching people, and generating resources so as to keep everyone on board.

In the context of India where the population is large and public support systems skeletal, the pandemic has underlined for Parul Chaudhury the need for these concerns:

> Large-scale community organising efforts, especially amongst the most poor and vulnerable, so that they are better able to collectively face and deal with challenges. Community organising coupled with capacity building and leadership development are the interventions most required.

1.8 Conclusion

Throughout this chapter we have engaged with the views and experiences of a small number of experienced social workers in India and Australia to foreground social issues that have been magnified by COVID-19. We argue that it is important to engage social workers during the pandemic and after, given their depth of understanding of issues and their ability to see the interconnection between different issues and different levels of practice. Also, it is crucial to acknowledge connections between particularities of injustice in different parts of the world. The reason for putting the social workers from India and Australia together in the different themes is not to suggest that the issues confronting them in the two countries are the same. The deep divide between the realities of the two countries is evident from the narratives, but what is also evident are the continuities between the experiences of the most marginalised in both these countries. This caveat calls for a meaningful and strategic dialogue amongst social workers to acknowledge the principles of social work which tie them together and the strategies that helped them carry out their work during the pandemic. Collaboration and effective communication amongst social workers in different parts of the world can enable the struggles for more just and equitable societies through a globalised ethic of care. By focusing on practice and interests, we are able to delve into intimate spaces of striving for contextual, national, and global justice.

References

Allan, J. (2003). Practising critical social work. In J. Allan, B. Pease, & L. Briskman (Eds.), *Critical social work: An introduction to theories and practices* (pp. 52–71). Allen & Unwin.

Amadasun, S. (2020a). COVID-19 pandemic in Africa: What lessons for social work education and practice? *International Social Work, 64*(2). https://doi.org/10.1177/0020872820949620

Amadasun, S. (2020b). Social work and COVID-19 pandemic: An action call. *International Social Work, 63*, 753–756. https://doi.org/10.1177/0020872820959357

Berg-Weger, M., & Morley, J. E. (2020). Loneliness and social isolation in older adults during the Covid-19 pandemic: Implications for gerontological social work. *The Journal of Nutrition Health and Aging, 24*(3), 456–458. https://doi.org/10.1007/s12603-020-1366-8

Bright, C. L. (2020). *Social work in the age of a global pandemic*. Oxford University Press.

Briskman, L., Latham, S., Goddard, C. (2008). Human Rights Overboard: seeking asylum in Australia. Melbourne: Scribe Publishing.

Briskman, L. (2014). *Social work with indigenous communities: A human rights approach* (2nd ed.). The Federation Press.

Carrington, K., Hogg, R., Scott, J., & Sozzo, M. (2018). *The Palgrave handbook of criminology and the global south*. Springer International.

Carrington, K., Morley, C., Warren, S., Harris, B., Vitis, L., Ball, M., Clarke, J., & Ryan, V. (2020). *The impact of COVID-19 pandemic on domestic and family violence services*. QUT Centre for Justice.

Cudjoe, E., & Abdullah, A. (2020). Drawing on kinship care support for older people during a pandemic (COVID-19): Practice considerations for social workers in Ghana. *Journal of Gerontological Social Work, 63*, 254–256.

Dominelli, L. (1998). Anti-oppressive practice in context. In R. Adams, L. Dominelli, & M. Payne (Eds.), *Social work: Themes, issues and critical debates* (pp. 3–22). Macmillan.

Evans, M. L., Lindauer, M. & Farrell, M. E. (2020). A pandemic within a pandemic—Intimate partner violence during Covid-19. *New England Journal of Medicine, 383*, 2302–2304.

Global Detention Project. (2017–2018). Australia immigration detention. *Country profiles*. https://www.globaldetentionproject.org/countries/asia-pacific/australia

International Labour Organisation. (2018). *Statistics on the informal economy*. https://ilostat.ilo.org/topics/informality/

Mlamb-Ngcuka, P. (2020). *Violence against women and girls: The shadow pandemic*. https://www.unwomen.org/en/news/stories/2020/4/statement-ed-phumzile-violence-against-women-during-pandemic

Moreau, M. (1979). A structural approach to social work practice. *Canadian Journal of Social Work Practice, 5*(1), 78–94.

O'Leary, P., & Tsui, M. S. (2020). *Ten gentle reminders to social workers in the pandemic*. SAGE.

Robinson, F. (1997). Globalizing care: Ethics, feminist theory and international relations. *Alternatives: Global, Local, Political, 22*(1), 113–133.

Seifert, A. (2020). The digital exclusion of older adults during the COVID-19 pandemic. *Journal of Gerontological Social Work, 63*, 674–676.

Soutphommasane, T. (2021, January 18). *Virus wipes out of myth of equality* (p. 24). The Age.

Walter-McCabe, H. A. (2020). Coronavirus pandemic calls for an immediate social work response. *Social Work in Public Health, 35*(3), 69–72. https://doi.org/10.1080/19371918.2020.1751533

Xavier, J. (2020). *Walking with the migrants: Beyond the COVID-19 pandemic*. IIST Bengaluru, Caritas India, Indo Global Social Service Society. https://www.caritasindia.org/wp-content/uploads/2020/08/Walking-with-the-migrants-beyond-COVID-19-pandemic.pdf

Zarkov, D. (2020). On economy, health and politics of the Covid 19 pandemic. *European Journal of Women's Studies, 27*, 213–217.

Examining Decent Work During COVID-19: With Reference to Female Migrant Workers in South Asia

2

Sunny Wadhwaniya, Rupa Korde, and Biju Varkkey

2.1 Introduction

History's deadliest pandemics such as SARS (February 2003), Swine flu (January 2009), HIV/AIDS (June 1981), Ebola (November 1976), and MERS (September 2012) had an acute and lasting impact globally, often with devastating consequences. However, the ongoing COVID-19 outbreak is one of the most crucial global health calamities, triggering longer, more profound, and more pervasive social and economic crises worldwide (Suresh et al., 2020). The pandemic spread globally with alarming speed, infecting about 90,054,813 people, and taking 1,945,610 lives so far (as of 13 January 2021) (WHO COVID-19, Dashboard). In terms of public response, enforcement of containment measures such as strict public lockdowns and social distancing by countries worldwide crippled the global supply chain, the economy, and the livelihoods of millions of migrant workers (Azeez et al., 2020).

Migrant workers have a significant role in the socioeconomic development of a country. At the same time, they also face challenges in accessing social protection, including healthcare and income security, making them more vulnerable to pandemic adverse impacts (such as COVID-19) (Testaverde, 2020). According to International Labour Organization (ILO) and the International Social Security Association (ISSA) estimates, migrant workers are 4.7% of the global workforce (164 million workers worldwide) (ILO and ISSA, 2020). Almost half of them were affected by full or partial lockdown measures imposed by governments to contain the pandemic (ILO, 2020a). Governments worldwide are making efforts to protect workers' lives and livelihood; however, in very few cases are measures are taken to address the unique challenges of migrant workers and their families (Testaverde, 2020).

Although all migrant workers faced the adverse impacts of the COVID-19 pandemic, mostly women migrant workers (WMWs) worldwide are more adversely affected. Furthermore, because of pandemic containment measures in many countries, WMWs have fewer options to access support services in domestic violence or harassment situations in their accommodations, in workplaces during retrenchment, or while returning home (ILO, 2020a). The adverse impact

S. Wadhwaniya (✉)
Head of Operations, Institute of Defence Studies and Research, Gujarat University, Ahmedabad, Gujarat, India
e-mail: sunny.cug@gmail.com

R. Korde
Faculty, Economics Area, FLAME University, Pune, Maharashtra, India

B. Varkkey
Faculty, Human Resource Management Area, Indian Institute of Management, Ahmedabad, Gujarat, India

M. C. S. Gonçalves et al. (eds.), *The Coronavirus Crisis and Challenges to Social Development*,
https://doi.org/10.1007/978-3-030-84678-7_2

of the COVID-19 crises was significantly higher for WMWs in the South Asian countries (Bangladesh, India, Nepal, and Pakistan). The majority of women in these countries are engaged in the informal sector with precarious working conditions without any formal employment contracts, and with limited coverage by labour laws (UN Women, 2020; Rajan et al., 2020). These women are also deprived of access to social protection, as well as decent work standards, minimum rights, and safety (Rao et al., 2020).

Many reported incidences portraying the marginalization and exploitation of WMWs resulted from containment measures imposed in response to the pandemic from the South Asian countries. For instance, several WMWs in countries such as Nepal, India, and Bangladesh were subject to various forms of exploitation, including trafficking and sexual abuse, while being stranded for months by the imposed lockdown and other restrictions forced by sub-agents and illegal recruiters, thus resulting in psychological distress among WMWs (South Asia Monitor, 2020).

Furthermore, containment measures such as the lockdown in India have pushed Dalit[1] WMWs even further to the margins. WMWs were denied access to the government relief packages by the lack of documents or exclusion because of their affiliation with lower social strata. Such discrimination based on caste and religion has also exacerbated the existing vulnerabilities of returning WMWs in their home settlements, being perceived as the carrier of the virus even if they have not tested positive for COVID-19 (Srivastava, 2020).

Another issue has been living conditions of WMWs attempting to return to their homes from uncertainty and possibilities of future lockdowns. For example, the abrupt announcement of lockdown by the Indian government left WMWs with no choice than to walk home, because they could not survive without daily wages. However, these women were intercepted and sent to shelters/facilities with inadequate food, water, and sanitation (Bhattacharjee, 2020). Similarly, countries such as Nepal, Bangladesh, and Pakistan could not handle the issues faced by the WMWs entering the country upon reopening of the international borders. Quarantine facilities set up to accommodate the influx migrant workers were often primary schools with a lack of sufficient safe water, toilets, or hygiene facilities, increasing COVID-19 transmission risk rather than preventing it (Bhattacharjee, 2020). Further, incidents of rape and harassment of WMWs have raised serious questions about the security arrangements of these quarantine facilities. For example, three volunteers at the quarantine facility in Nepal raped a WMW after she was left alone in the centre (The Rising Nepal, 2020). A similar incident was reported in Rajasthan, India, where a WMW was allegedly gang-raped by three men staying at a quarantine centre (Arora, 2020).

The COVID-19 pandemic has adverse impacts on people across the globe. The WMWs, however, have disproportionately borne the burden of the pandemic, especially in South Asian countries. Preliminary evidence indicates an overall dearth of social welfare-oriented policy-making initiatives and lack of preparedness. However, to our knowledge, no research has been conducted in this area. Using the social work and decent work perspective, this chapter seeks to comparatively examine government policies, both proactive and reactive, specifically impacting WMWs in the South Asian countries, particularly internal migrants. In the broader context, it aims to understand the country-level strategies and provide policy recommendations concerning WMWs in the region.

2.2 Review of Related Literature

2.2.1 Impact of Pandemic on Migrant Workers

Migration is an intrinsic phenomenon of population dynamics and as old as humankind (Castelli, 2018; Castelli & Sulis, 2017). Migrant workers are often involved in casual wage work with very

[1]The term Dalit refers to socially, economically and historically marginalized communities in India.

Table 2.1 Economic and noneconomic factors for migration

Category	Factors
Macro factors	• Environmental • Political • Socioeconomic • Demographic
Meso factors	• Living and working conditions in destination country • Diasporic links
Micro factors	• Personal characteristics – Education – Religion – Marital status

Source: Castelli (2018)

little savings, coupled with limited social protection (Rao et al., 2020). The literature on the impact of pandemics on migrant workers starts with understanding the critical factors behind migration (Rao et al., 2020). Castelli (2018) notes an array of economic and noneconomic factors that act together to inform the final decision to migrate. These factors are further subdivided into macro, meso, and micro factors by Castelli (2018) (Table 2.1).

The impact of macro factors on people's movements, such as extreme environmental events, including natural hazards, is now a critical concern and extensively debated (McMichael, 2015). Natural hazards such as pandemics occur with little or no warning and exacerbate current vulnerability, making it difficult for people to survive (IOM, 2009). Therefore, results in 'forced' displacement are often linked to the socioeconomic conditions of migrant workers, lack of rights to health coverage, lack of social protection, and, in most cases, partly attributed to economic crises primarily caused by standard control measures adopted by the government to control the disease (Testaverde, 2020; Castelli, 2018). There has been evidence in the past about how pandemics have significantly impacted the lives and living conditions of migrant workers and forced them to leave their habitual homes, either temporarily or permanently within their country or abroad.

A cross-sectional study of 797 migrant workers carried out by Hickey et al. (2016) revealed some facts about how the 2009 H1N1 pandemic impacted the migrant workers in Thailand. According to the authors one in four respondents reported barriers such as cost of treatment, fear of arrest, and language barriers in accessing healthcare services in their country.

Another study indicated that Latino migrant workers in the United States (Spana et al., 2009) during the 2009 H1N1 influenza pandemic often faced social threats to their health and well-being, including disgrace, limited access to healthcare facilities, and economic conditions interfering with disease containment guidelines. Further, lack of health insurance or social protection prevents them from seeking medical care for disease prevention because they cannot afford the cost of treatment even at reduced rates. Moreover, meagre living conditions inhibit these workers to comply with official guidelines on disease containment issued by the government.

Similarly, a study by Steege et al. (2009) highlights migrant farm workers in the United States are at a higher risk of morbidity and mortality owing to several socioeconomic factors such as low language proficiency, low literacy level, lower income levels, limited resources, inadequate access to healthcare services, cultural barriers, mistreatment in government shelter homes, discrimination, and exclusion from the federal assistance programme. A survey from the American University in Cairo, Egypt, on the impact of the influenza pandemic on 293 Sudanese migrant workers in Greater Cairo found that 61.1% of Sudanese migrant workers do not have access to public hospitals and that treatment in these hospitals is discriminatory and below the standards. Another 67.6% of the Sudanese migrant workers have no ability to stock food and other essential commodities in pandemic times because their low income barely covers basic needs (Ahmed & Dibb, 2008).

Koser (2014) also highlighted the discrimination faced by migrant workers when they were perceived as vectors of disease during the 2014 Ebola pandemic in West Africa, which resulted in travel restrictions that made it difficult for migrant workers to survive on trivial savings and to support their family.

2.2.2 Impact of Pandemics on Women Migrant Workers

Research on the impact of past pandemics on internal migrant workers in Asian countries is relatively sparse, and research on WMW vulnerability in pandemics is further limited. Thus, in the present section, we provide scoping review of the studies that do not have an explicit Asian focus but do have clear relevance to the challenges faced by WMWs in past pandemics. However, the impact of pandemics on WMWs is because they are less valued and have lower social status, resulting from rigid gender norms and prevalent gender inequalities (Wenham et al., 2020; Azeez et al., 2020).

Further, studies have also shown that even though women constitute a significant part of the migrant worker population, the issues and challenges faced by WMWs remain primarily ignored in policy and programme interventions. An interesting example of a clear and visible ignorance of issues/challenges faced by WMWs in both the long-term strategies on health system strengthening and in emergency response during the 2014 Ebola outbreak in West Africa is given by Harman (2016), who observed that in the short term and long-term strategies of crises management during Ebola, issues/challenges faced by WMWs were often forgotten and as best viewed as a side issue, rendering them invisible in health governance in the epidemic.

Such ignorance by government predisposes WMWs to discrimination and exploitation, making them vulnerable to human rights abuse. Thus, the protection of WMWs in pandemics must be considered a priority in intervention programmes adopted by the governments to stop the disease spread. In this context, Amparita (2005) examine the reasons for intervention programmes failure to protect WMWs from vulnerability to the HIV AIDS epidemic. According to the authors, two primary reasons are responsible for the failure of interventions programmes adequate to implementing mechanisms:

1. Policy infirmity coupled with lack of gender-sensitive approach in designing the programmes for WMWs.
2. Noncompliance of human rights obligations (under the constitutional mandate, especially regarding the right to access health facilities and services, and the right to seek health issues).

The authors further observed that poor implementation and noncompliances prevented WMWs from receiving adequate health information and services, which rendered them more vulnerable to the disease.

2.3 Impact Assessment of COVID-19 on Women Migrant Workers in India, Nepal, Pakistan, and Bangladesh

2.3.1 India

As of 17 January 2021, India recorded 10,542,841 active cases, with 1,52,093 deaths so far as the infection multiplies unabated (WHO COVID-19 Dashboard, 2020). To combat the spread of the pandemic, the Indian government resorted to mandatory precautionary measures relatively early at the onset of the infection such as stringent public lockdown from 24 March 2020 to 31 May 2020, which includes closure of economic activities, restrictions on inter- and intrastate movements, and other measures (Ghosh, 2020; Acharya & Porwal, 2020). The announcement of lockdown in India resulted in a dramatic economic collapse and humanitarian catastrophe, which ravaged millions of people in the informal sector, especially migrant workers (Suresh et al., 2020).

Migration is a livelihood strategy for millions of people in India and is considered the backbone of India's economy (Bhagat et al., 2020). According to one estimate, there are more than 450 million internal migrants in India, thus accounting for 37.7% of the total population, with nearly half being WMWs (Rajan et al.,

2020). Rao et al. (2020) argue that migration's primary reason is the lag in development of a particular region development. Often, migration is from a backward region to a relatively developed region in searching for better employment and livelihood options. The majority of the WMWs are from remote and poor rural locations in the Indian states of Bihar, Jharkhand, Odisha, and West Bengal to better-off key destination areas in Gujarat, Maharashtra, Delhi, Haryana, Punjab, and Karnataka, seeking better employment and livelihood options.

2.3.2 Nepal

Similarly to many other South Asia countries, Nepal faces unprecedented health and economic impact in the unfolding COVID-19 pandemic (IIDS, 2020; Raut, 2020). As of 17 January 2021, more than 266,816 cases had been recorded, with 1948 deaths so far (WHO COVID-19 Dashboard, 2020). The Government of Nepal enforced a nationwide lockdown from 24 March to 21 July 2020 (120 days) (Bhattarai & Baniya, 2020). The government suspended all domestic and international travels to close borders. The closure of nonessential services severely disrupted economic activity, especially in the construction, manufacturing, and trade sectors (ILO, 2020b). This closure brought the economy to a virtual standstill, resulting in job loss, reduced wages, and fewer working hours for workers engaged in these sectors (ILO, 2020b; IIDS, 2020). Estimates show that approximately 5.7 million or 80.8% of workers in these sectors are in informal employment, lacking the basic benefits of formal jobs including social protection coverage (Sharma, 2020a; ILO, 2020b). As estimated by ILO and Amnesty International (2011), close to 2.6 million are internal migrants, with more than 30% WMWs.

2.3.3 Bangladesh

Bangladesh is among the top 30 countries in confirmed cases of COVID-19 with a total of 525,485 confirmed cases and 7862 deaths as of 17 January 2021 (WHO COVID-19 Dashboard). It is the most densely populated country globally with a total population of 161.3 million (Islam et al., 2020), of whom about 106.1 million belong to the working-age population. Estimates reveal that approximately only 13.8% among the working-age population work in formal employment, whereas the rest (86.2%) work in informal jobs, mostly in Bangladesh's rural areas (BBS, 2017). Of these, 53.1% are internal migrant workers (urban–urban or rural–urban) (Hasan, 2019). Further, according to an estimate, WMWs constitute 13.85% of the total percentage of internal migrant workers in Bangladesh (Siddique et al., 2019).

Bangladesh has followed the same trend as almost every country in adopting aggressive measures to prevent and control COVID-19 virus transmission. However, initial steps such as shutting down of borders and enforcement of 65 days of lockdown (26 March to 30 May 2020), were sharply criticized because of corruption and the lack of a proper mechanism to deliver aid to vulnerable populations, especially workers engaged in informal work in the ready-made garment (RMG) industry and other export-oriented industries (Anwar et al., 2020. These industries contribute roughly 65% of the country's GDP and employ about five million workers, of whom 90% are women, including WMWs (Anam, 2020).

2.3.4 Pakistan

The first case of COVID-19 was reported on 26 February 2020 from Karachi. Successively, the virus has spread nationwide in various regions, and currently the total tally has reached 514,338 confirmed cases with 10,863 deaths (as of 17 January 2021) (WHO COVID-19 dashboard, 2020). In response to the surging infection rates, the federal and provisional governments in Pakistan imposed a full lockdown from 1 April to 9 May 2020. However, as cases rose, the lockdown was re-imposed in some parts of the country (Markhof & Arif, 2020). The announcement and enforcement of abrupt lockdown in response to the COVID-19 pandemic posed an unprecedented challenge to Pakistan's large informal economy, which contributes almost one third of their GDP and more than 80% of total employment (Sareen, 2020).

Experts estimate that the labour-intensive manufacturing sector and wholesale and retail trade have been affected adversely by both supply and demand shocks from restrictions imposed on the cross-border movement of goods and people (Ahmed, 2020a, b; Pakistan Worker's Federation, 2020). This restriction has exacerbated the strain of the crises, leading to adverse impacts on the livelihood of approximately 22 million workers engaged in the informal sector. Of these, 8.5 million are internal seasonal labour migrants, many not covered by mainstream social protection, especially WMWs in Sindh and Punjab provinces working in garment and textile industries (UNDP, 2020; Markhof & Arif, 2020; Khan, 2020). The impact on WMWs is compounded by the lack of adequate system or support services, particularly addressing human and labour rights abuse such as domestic or intimate partner violence (ILO, 2020a; Khan, 2020).

2.3.5 Summary of Impact of COVID-19 Pandemic on Women Migrant Workers

The pandemic and subsequent containment measures adopted by various governments added considerable burden with multiple hardships of WMWs and their families (Panwar & Mishra, 2020). A summary of the impact of COVID-19 Pandemic on WMWs, before and after the lockdown, is presented in Table 2.2.

Such a situation of WMWs signals the absences of decent working conditions and social welfare policies necessary to address the challenges faced by WMWs.

2.4 Decent Work, COVID-19 Pandemic, and Women Migrant Workers

2.4.1 Decent Work: The Concept

ILO introduced the multidimensional concept of Decent Work (DW) in June 1999 with the following four key components (ILO, 1999):

Table 2.2 Country-wise summary of the impact of the COVID-19 pandemic on women migrant workers

Impact		India	Nepal	Bangladesh	Pakistan
Economic	Loss of jobs	X		X	X
	Pay cuts in existing jobs		X	X	X
	Exhausted savings	X		X	
	Increased debt	X		X	
	Difficulty in access to basic facilities/essential services	X	X	X	
	Increased unpaid work			X	
	Increased hours of work		X		
	Adverse effect on health		X	X	
	Discrimination in access to healthcare		X	X	
Social	Gender-based violence	X	X	X	X
	Social stigma		X		
	Human rights violation		X	X	
	Lack of family support		X		
	Social wellbeing		X		
	Nonavailability of insurance coverage		X	X	
	Nonavailability of decent working conditions		X	X	X
	Noncompliance of pandemic-related safety		X		
Psychological	Emotional bearing	X	X	X	X
	Mental well-being affected	X	X	X	X

Source: Author's data

(a) Employment conditions
(b) Workplace rights
(c) Social protection
(d) Social dialogue[2]

2.4.2 COVID-19 Pandemic and Decent Work

Migrant workers, in particular, WMWs, face elevated challenges within each of the aforementioned DW components, as analysed in this section.

2.4.2.1 Employment Conditions and Workplace Rights

Studies have shown that the pandemic and measures to prevent its spread have worsened WMW employment overall. WMWs, mostly employed as domestic help, at construction sites, the handicraft sector, and retail units, have lost their jobs or been forced to accept unpaid leaves and reduced wages, which has pushed their families even further into poverty (Bhandare, 2020; Thomas & Jayaram, 2020).

A study by Aajeevika Bureau, a labour rights organization, on WMWs in the textile and garment industry of Ahmedabad (one of the textile hubs in India) mentions that WMWs from the rural areas of Rajasthan, Uttar Pradesh, and Bihar belong to the oppressed caste groups and are engaged as daily wage workers. The study found that more than 95% of the surveyed WMWs worked for as little as INR[3] 10–15 for more than 8 hours a day during the pandemic. On many occasions, they also spent time in organizing raw materials from the companies over and above their regular working hours. Many WMWs reported irregular payment of their wages and thus struggled to survive the financial crises to pay the rent or buy essential goods. The study also found that many of the surveyed WMWs, even during the time of the pandemic, were expected to manage the responsibilities of their families, which they do by either using their little savings or mortgaging small amounts of gold jewellery, for which they have to pay high rates of interest (Thomas and Jayaram 2020).

2.4.2.2 Social Protection (Social Security and Occupational Safety and Health)

Limited access to social protection coverage by millions of informal workers in the pandemic highlights the huge decent work deficits that still prevail in 2020 (UN Global Impact, 2020). Adequate and accessible social protection mechanisms are crucial to protect the poor vulnerable population from the pandemic adverse impacts. However, such mechanisms have limited coverage in many countries and need significant policy interventions to protect vulnerable populations, mainly migrant workers, from the pandemic's adverse impact (World Bank, 2020).

Access to healthcare, including tests and treatment, is an essential aspect of social protection, particularly during the pandemic (ILO, 2020a). Recent studies have found that migrant workers, particularly WMWs in the informal sector, face barriers in accessing healthcare in countries of destination, making them more vulnerable to the exposure of COVID-19 (WHO, 2020).

Further, available evidence also indicates that many WMWs are exposed to undue risks in their workplace by compromise in Occupational Safety and Health standards (OSH) by employers in COVID-19 pandemic (UN Women, 2020). WMWs employed in hospitals and other frontline sectors often are exposed to biological hazard by the unavailability of personal protective equipment (PPE) (Franklin, 2020). This lack has increased COVID-19 cases among WMWs in such countries as Singapore and Malaysia (ILO, 2020a).

Another major problem for WMWs during the pandemic is lack of access to adequate information, coupled with language barriers, which prevent them from claiming their social protection benefits or obtaining access to various grievances mechanisms, which is the case with WMWs in most of the EU 15 and border transit countries (as observed by Kluge et al , 2020).

---

[2]Copyright © International Labour Organization 1999.

[3]1 Indian Rupee (INR) = 0.011 Euro.

2.4.2.3 Social Dialogue

The ILO defines social dialogue as *"all types of negotiation, consultation and information sharing among representatives of governments, social partners or between social partners on issues of common interest relating to economic and social policy"* (ILO, 2013).[4] Although the importance of social dialogue is repeated by ILO, we found that literature on social dialogue with respect to WMWs in a pandemic is absent and that not much evidence has been reported so far.

2.4.3 Policy Response by Countries

The governments of India, Nepal, Bangladesh, and Pakistan announced various schemes and packages to address the challenges faced by migrant workers, including WMWs, amid COVID-19 crises (Table 2.3). However, these policy responses were limited in nature given the scale of the problem and severe impact faced by WMWs from the pandemic. Administrative lags result in a delay in policy measure implementation desired by the governments. Therefore, social work interventions are critical in combating public health emergency effects by responding to the most urgent social problems such as loss of jobs and income, gender violence, depression, and anxiety, or the homelessness of vulnerable populations such as the migrant workers (Sama et al., 2020).

2.5 Social Work, COVID-19 Pandemic, and Women Migrant Workers

Since the beginning of the pandemic, to improve the well-being and living conditions of migrant workers, particularly WMWs, social work response has been primarily at a local level, through CBOs (community-based organizations), NGOs (nongovernmental organizations), and other international social work organizations (Sama et al., 2020; IFSW, 2020; BASW, 2020). Volunteers, along with CBOs and NGOs, have responded to the urgent social problems/challenges faced by WMWs, through diverse social work interventions such as the use of digital technologies to guide, support, and counsel WMWs who have mental health concerns, facing domestic violence (Sama et al., 2020). For instance, in India, Jan Sahas Foundation—an NGO collaborated with 40 organizations—in its COVID relief initiatives to reach more than 10 lakhs migrant workers, including WMWs in 120 districts across India during the lockdown, supported them with dry rations, cooked food, mobile recharges, cash transfers, water, and transportation (Sharma, 2020b).

Resonating with this approach, at the regional level in Bangladesh, there are examples of collaboration between the government and NGOs; for example, the Bangladesh Rural Advancement Committee (BARC), the world's largest NGO operating in 11 countries in Asia and Africa with its headquarters in Bangladesh, along with the Government of Bangladesh coordinated relief work for migrant workers with humanitarian interventions, socioeconomic rehabilitation, and development programmes (Dhaka Tribune, 2020; BARC, 2020).

Similarly in Nepal, CARE Nepal in partnership with State agencies and research institutes has worked to address social issues such as gender-based violence for WMWs. Also, the distribution of free soap and sanitizers, installing hand-washing stations to protect the migrant workers from COVID-19, has been provided. One of the central social work interventions of NGOs focused on spreading awareness on the spread of the diseases considering the prevalent myths and misinformation related to the symptoms, treatment, and transmission of the diseases that can have severe outcomes for migrant workers (Sama et al., 2020; Ali, 2020). In this background, it is essential to highlight the Al-Khidmat foundation's efforts, a Pakistan-based NGO, which has carried out a massive awareness campaign for migrant workers and the general population about the disease, its hazards, and preventive measures since the beginning of the pandemic. Also, 7200 trained volunteers of the

[4]Copyright © International Labour Organization 2013.

Table 2.3 Summary of policy response by country

Policy response (long term and short term)	Decent work interventions			General policy measures
	Employment conditions and fundamental rights at the workplace	Social protection (social security and occupational safety and health)	Social dialogue	
India	Garib Kalyan Rojgar Abhiyaan (GKRA) scheme of INR 50,000 crore in 116 districts of 6 states (Bihar, Uttar Pradesh, Madhya Pradesh, Rajasthan, Odhisa, Jharkhand) to address the employment and livelihood crises of returnee migrant workers	Free ration support and distribution to migrants for 2 months. Migrant workers not registered under the National Food Security Act or without ration card are also covered under this scheme. Government of India allocated INR 3500 crore for this scheme	–	• One Nation One Ration Card' (ONORC) scheme implemented to provide migrant workers and family members access to PDS (Public Distribution System) from any Fair Price Shop in the country, even during their transit • To provide decent housing at an affordable rate for returnee migrant workers, Ministry of Housing and Urban Affairs launched Affordable Rental Housing Complexes (ARHCs), a sub-scheme under Pradhan Mantri AWAS Yojna (Prime Minister Urban Housing Scheme)
Nepal	Migrant workers who lost their jobs or who had a work permit for employment in foreign countries but could not travel due to pandemic were included in the Prime Minister Employment Project (a wage employment programme which ensures minimum 100 days of employment to unemployed citizens). Government of Nepal has allocated a total of NRP five million for this project	–	–	• Counselling services for migrant workers and their families were provided by a dedicated grievance call centre set up Ministry of Labour, Employment and Social Security (MoLESS) daily • The National Human Rights Commission (NHRC) of Nepal set up a mechanism to monitor the violation of rights of migrant workers in various countries of destination
Bangladesh	–	–	–	• As a relief package for migrant workers, the Government of Bangladesh came up with a policy package of BDT 700 crore funds for rehabilitation and reemployment returnee migrant workers from overseas who lost jobs owing to COVID-19 pandemic

(continued)

Table 2.3 (continued)

Policy response (long term and short term)	Decent work interventions			General policy measures
	Employment conditions and fundamental rights at the workplace	Social protection (social security and occupational safety and health)	Social dialogue	
Pakistan	–	–	–	• Ehsaas Emergency Cash (EEC) programme to provide urgent cash payments to 12 million most impoverished and hardest hit families to weather the initial shock of the crises. The federal government announced the fiscal stimulus of PKR 50 billion to provide food items at subsidized rates to the poorest people, including migrant workers. Besides, the Provisional government announced small financial packages and cash transfers of PKR 150 billion for low-income families and migrant workers

Source: Authors' data

foundation helped the government better manage resources in the pandemic (Latif, 2020).

Therefore, social work interventions help handle long-term effects of the pandemic and are essential in approaching the problems/challenges faced by WMWs with an eye on long-term stabilization, in contrast to short-term economic interventions by the governments.

2.6 Conclusion

Whether it is economic crises or massive health crises such as the COVID-19 pandemic, a country needs to protect its population effectively, particularly the vulnerable groups, minimise human loss, recover economic hardship and suffering, reduce the economic impact of the crisis, and work towards improving the capacity to handle such events. COVID-19 has created extraordinary intense uncertainty for governments worldwide, resulting in a struggle to find the most effective response to protect their people and the economy.

In this chapter, we attempted to understand the impact of the COVID-19 pandemic on WMWs in the South Asian countries of Bangladesh, India, Nepal, and Pakistan using Decent Work and Social Work perspectives. Our research shows that the voice for WMWs has been relatively silent in government policy responses. COVID-19 increased the risk of violence and harassment of WMWs, which had severe consequences not only on their physical, mental, sexual, and reproductive health but also for their personal and social well-being. In general, policy measures announced by each South Asian country's governments were limited to mostly short-term measures such as providing free shelter and relief camps with food, healthcare, and other necessities. However, although this effort is laudable, we argue that these measures are neither sufficient nor targeted, considering the intensity of the pandemic's adverse impacts on WMWs. Further, the policy responses also lacked a transformative agenda strengthening worker rights, trade union participation, and ensuring decent work conditions.

Based on our findings, we conclude that the active participation of social workers working with disasters such as the COVID-19 pandemic was missing in practice and is also limited in the literature. Recent studies and reports focusing on the pandemic's impact on WMWs mainly highlight the role of healthcare workers, government officials, and law enforcement agencies, whereas contribution of social worker professionals is missing. The negative impact of the pandemic on individuals and families naturally calls for social work professionals also to be included in the mitigation efforts.

In similar situations earlier, social workers and Civil Society Organisations have been actively involved in the work of reaching out to vulnerable groups and communities, assessing their critical needs, and delivering the required materials and services. These are areas in which social workers could have contributed significantly during this crisis. Given the nature and scope of such crisis, and the probability of its occurrence in future, the governments should recognise the social worker's role in targeted interventions for dealing with WMWs.

Acknowledgments We acknowledge the contribution of Ms. Ashni Patel in initial data collection and literature compilation.

References

Acharya, R., & Porwal, A. (2020). A vulnerability index for the management of and response to the COVID-19 epidemic in India: An ecological study. *The Lancet Global Health, 8*(9), 1142–1151.

Ahmed, A. (2020a). COVID-19: Millions of migrant workers in Pakistan face threat of layoffs due to lockdown. *World Asia*. https://gulfnews.com/world/asia/pakistan/covid-19-millions-of-migrant-workers-in-pakistan-face-threat-of-layoffs-due-to-lockdown-1.70870067

Ahmed, S. (2020b). Covid-19 and women workers. *The News International*. https://www.thenews.com.pk/print/697005-covid-19-and-women-workers

Ahmed, Y., & Dibb, R. (2008). *Pandemic preparedness among Sudanese migrant workers in great Cairo*. Centre for Migration and Refugee studies. The American University in Cairo. https://www.google.co.in/books/edition/Pandemic_Preparedness_Among_Sudanese_Mig/_NK2DcaD9CUC?hl=en&gbpv=1

Ali, S. (2020). Combating against Covid-19 & misinformation: A systematic review. *Human Arenas*, 3–6.

Amnesty International. (2011). *Nepal: False promises. Exploitation and forced labour of Nepalese migrant workers*. Amnesty International. https://www.amnesty.org/en/documents/ASA31/007/2011/en/

Amparita, M. (2005). *An analysis of the Philippine legal and policy frameworks for the protection of women migrant workers, particularly the domestic workers and entertainers, from vulnerability to HIV/AIDS*. Thesis. University of Toronto. http://rizal.library.ateneo.edu/node/9607

Anam, S. (2020, March). What about workers in the informal sector? *The Daily Star*. https://www.thedailystar.net/opinion/perspective/news/what-about-workers-the-informal-sector-1887409

Anwar, S., Nasrullah, M., & Hosen, M. (2020). COVID-19 and Bangladesh: Challenges and how to address them *Frontiers of Public Health, 8*, 1–8.

Arora, N. (2020, April). Indian women gang raped after being quarantined alone in school, say police *Independent*. https://www.independent.co.uk/news/world/asia/gang-rape-india-woman-quarantine-school-rajasthan-a9485726.html

Azeez, A., Negi, D., Rani, A., & Kumar, S. (2020). The impact of migrant women workers in India. *Eurasian Geography and Economics*, 1–21.

BARC. (2020). *Our response strategy*. https://covid19.bracinternational.nl/our-response-strategy/

BASW (2020). *The role of social workers in a pandemic and its aftermath: Learning from Covid-19*. https://www.basw.co.uk/role-social-workers-pandemic-and-its-aftermath-learning-covid-19

BBS (Bangladesh Bureau of Statistics). (2017). *Quarterly Labour Force Survey 2015–16*. BBS https://www.ilo.org/surveyLib/index.php/catalog/2214/study-description

Bhagat, B. R., Reshmi, R., Sahoo, H., Roy, A., & Govil, D. (2020). *The COVID-19, migration and livelihood in India. A background paper for policy makers*. International Institute for Population Sciences. https://iipsindia.ac.in/sites/default/files/iips_covid19_mll.pdf

Bhandare, N. (2020, December). Although men too lost jobs, the pandemic affected Indian women in the workforce harder. *Scroll*. https://scroll.in/article/981291/although-men-too-lost-jobs-the-pandemic-affected-indian-women-in-the-workforce-harder

Bhattacharjee, S. (2020, March). Migrants want to return despite getting amenities at shelters. *The Hindu*. https://www.thehindu.com/news/cities/Visakhapatnam/migrants-want-to-return-despite-getting-amenities-at-shelters/article31211664.ece

Bhattarai, G., & Baniya, J. (2020). Nepali migrant workers amid covid-19 in major destination countries: A human security approach. *Tribhuvan University Journal, 34*, 123–146.

Castelli, F. (2018). Drivers of migration: Why do people move? *Journal of Travel Medicine, 25*(1), 1–7.

Castelli, F., & Sulis, S. (2017). Migration and infectious diseases. *Clinical Microbiology and Infection, 23*, 283–288.

Dhaka Tribune. (2020, July). *ALAP webinar discusses role of NGOs during Covid-19 in Bangladesh.* https://www.dhakatribune.com/bangladesh/2020/07/10/live-discussion-on-the-role-of-ngos-during-covid-19-regulatory-practical-challenges

Franklin, P. (2020). Hazardous! Occupational safety and health in the care economy during the pandemic. *Social Europe*. https://www.socialeurope.eu/hazardous-occupational-safety-and-health-in-the-care-economy-during-the-pandemic

Ghosh, J. (2020). A critique of the Indian government's response to the COVID-19 pandemic. *Journal of Industrial and Business Economics, 47*, 519–530.

Harman, S. (2016). Ebola, gender and conspicuously invisible women in global health governance. *Third World Quarterly, 37*(3), 524–541.

Hasan, A. (2019). Internal migration and employment in Bangladesh: An economic evaluation of rickshaw pulling in Dhaka City. In K. Jayanthakumran, R. Verma, G. Wan, & E. Wilson (Eds.), *Internal migration, urbanization, and poverty in Asia: Dynamics and interrelationships* (pp. 339–359). Springer.

Hickey, J., Gagnon, A., & Jitthai, N. (2016). Knowledge about pandemic influenza preparedness among vulnerable migrants in Thailand. *Health Promotion International, 31*(1), 124–132.

IFSW. (2020). International Federation of Social Workers. *Update information on IFSW and COVID 19.* https://www.ifsw.org/covid-19/

IIDS (Institute of Integrated Developmental Studies). (2020). *Rapid assessment of socioeconomic impact on COVID 19 in Nepal: United Nation Development Programme.* https://www.np.undp.org/content/nepal/en/home/library/rapid-assessment-of-socio-economic-impact.html#:~:text=The%20uncertain%20impact%20of%20the,or%20when%20the%20spread%20of

ILO. (1999). *Decent work. Report of the Director General (87th Meeting).* International Labour Conference. https://www.ilo.org/public/english/standards/relm/ilc/ilc87/rep-i.htm

ILO. (2013). *National Tripartite Social Dialogue—An ILO guide for improved governance* (pp. 1–306). International Labour Organisation.

ILO. (2020a). *Impact of lockdown measures on the informal economy: A summary.* International Labour Organisation. https://www.ilo.org/wcmsp5/groups/public/%2D%2D-ed_protect/%2D%2D-protrav/%2D%2D-travail/documents/briefingnote/wcms_743534.pdf

ILO. (2020b). *COVID 19 labour market impact in Nepal.* https://www.ilo.org/wcmsp5/groups/public/%2D%2D-asia/%2D%2D-ro-bangkok/%2D%2D-ilo-kathmandu/documents/briefingnote/wcms_745439.pdf

ILO and ISSA (International Society for Security Association). (2020). *Migrant workers and COVID 19.* https://ww1.issa.int/news/migrant-workers-and-covid-19

IOM (International Organisation for Migration). (2009). *Migration, environment and climate change: Assessing the evidence.* https://publications.iom.int/system/files/pdf/migration_and_environment.pdf

Islam, S., Islam, R., Mannan, F., Rahman, S., & Islam, T. (2020). COVID-19 pandemic: An analysis of the healthcare, social and economic challenges in Bangladesh. *Progress in Disaster Science, 8*, 100–135.

Khan, T. (2020). *Labour migration governance in Pakistan: Protecting Pakistan's overseas labour migrants.* LSE South Asia Centre. https://blogs.lse.ac.uk/southasia/2020/06/03/labour-migration-governance-in-pakistan-protecting-pakistans-overseas-labour-migrants/

Kluge, P., Zsuzsanna, J., Jozef, B., Veronika, D., & Santino, S. (2020). Refugee and migrant health in the COVID-19 response. *The Lancet, 395*(10232), 1237–1239.

Koser, K. (2014). Why travel bans will not stop the spread of Ebola. *World economic forum.* https://www.weforum.org/agenda/2014/11/why-travel-bans-will-not-stop-the-spread-of-ebola/

Latif, A. (2020). *Pakistan's charities assist in fight against coronavirus.* Anadolu Agency. https://www.aa.com.tr/en/asia-pacific/pakistans-charities-assist-in-fight-against-coronavirus/1780046#

Markhof, Y., & Arif, K. (2020). *COVID-19 and social protection in South Asia: Pakistan.* International Policy Centre for Inclusive Growth. https://ipcig.org/pub/eng/OP453_COVID_19_and_social_protection_in_South_Asia,_Pakistan.pdf

McMichael, C. (2015). Climate change-related migration and infectious disease. *Virulence, 6*(6), 548–553.

Pakistani Workers Federation. (2020). *COVID-19 and world of work: A position paper.* https://www.ituc-csi.org/pakistan-covid-19-and-the-world-of-3

Panwar, N., & Mishra, A. (2020). COVID-19 crisis and urbanization, migration and inclusive city policies in India: A new theoretical framework. *Journal of Public Affairs: An International Journal, 20*(4), 1–13.

Rajan, I., Sivakumar, P., & Srinivasan, A. (2020). The COVID 19 pandemic and internal labour migration in India. *The Indian Journal of Labour Economics*, 1–20.

Raut, K. (2020). A Review of the Economic Impacts of the COVID-19 Pandemic and Economic Policies in Nepal. MPRA Paper No. 102778. 1–18

Rao, N., Narain, N., Chakraborty, S., Bhanjdo, A., & Pattnaik, A. (2020). Destinations matter: Social policy and migrant workers in the times of Covid. *The European Journal of Development Research, 54*, 1–23.

Sama, G., Matulic, V., Pascual, A., & Vicente, I. (2020). Social work during the COVID 19 crises: Responding to urgent social needs. *Sustainability, 12*, 1–16.

Sareen, S. (2020). COVID-19 and Pakistan: The Economic Fallout, ORF Occasional Paper No. 251, June 2020, Observer Research Foundation.

Sharma, G. (2020a, June). Nepal arrests 3 men for quarantine rape, amid protests over unsafe conditions. *South Asia News*. https://in.reuters.com/article/health-coronavirus-nepal-rape/nepal-arrests-3-men-for-quarantine-rape-amid-protests-over-unsafe-conditions-idINKBN23M2C9

Sharma, I. (2020b, November). Uneven pandemic impact on Nepali women. *The Nepali times*. https://www.nepalitimes.com/opinion/uneven-pandemic-impact-on-nepali-women/

Siddiqui, T., Sultana, M., Sultana, R., and Akhter (2019). Labour Migration from Bangladesh 2018: Achievements and Challanges. RMMRU. https://www.forum-asia.org/uploads/wp/2019/05/Migration-Trend-Analysis-2018-RMMRU.pdf.

South Asia Monitor. (2020). *Exploitation risk for women migrant workers has increased during pandemic*. https://southasiamonitor.org/nepal/exploitation-risk-women-migrant-workers-has-increased-during-pandemic

Spana, M., Bouri, N., Norwood, A., & Rambhia K. (2009). Preliminary findings: Study of the impact of the 2009 H1N1 influenza pandemic on Latino migrant farm workers in the *U.S. Clinicians Biosecurity News*. https://www.centerforhealthsecurity.org/cbn/2009/2009-SW-H1N1-Issue-Briefs/2009-11-23-RschBrf_msfw_stigma.html

Srivastava, S. (2020, August). For millions of migrant workers, Covid-19 brought caste discrimination back. *Business Standard*. https://www.business-standard.com/article/current-affairs/for-millions-of-migrant-workers-covid-19-brought-caste-discrimination-back-120082100542_1.html

Steege, A., Baron, S., Davis, S., Kilgore, J., & Sweeney, M. (2009). Pandemic influenza and farm workers: The effects of employment, social, and economic factors. *American Journal of Public Health, 99*, S308–S315.

Suresh, R., James, J., & Balaraju, S. (2020). Migrant workers at cross roads. The COVID 19 pandemic and migrant experience in India. *Social Work in Public Health, 35*(7), 633–643.

Testaverde, M. (2020). Social protection for migrants during the COVID-19 crisis: The right and smart choice. *World Bank blogs*. https://blogs.worldbank.org/voices/social-protection-migrants-during-covid-19-crisis-right-and-smart-choice

The Rising Nepal. (2020, June). *NA members demand stern action against alleged rapists in quarantine*. https://risingnepaldaily.com/main-news/na-members-demand-stern-action-against-alleged-rapists-in-quarantine

Thomas, C., & Jayaram, N. (2020). Pandemic crisis: Migrant home-based women workers work 8 hours/day for Rs 10–15. *India Spend*. https://www.indiaspend.com/pandemic-crisis-migrant-home-based-women-workers-work-8-hours-day-for-rs-10-15/

UN Global Impact. (2020). *COVID 19 impact brief. Decent work* https://unglobalcompact.org/take-action/20th-anniversary-campaign/uniting-business-to-tackle-covid-19/decentwork

UN Women. (2020). *Guidance note on addressing the impact of COVID 19 pandemic on migrant women workers*. https://www.unwomen.org/en/digital-library/publications/2020/04/guidance-note-addressing-the-impacts-of-the-covid-19-pandemic-on-women-migrant-workers

UNDP. (2020). *COVID 19. Pakistan socioeconomic impact: Assessment and response plan*. https://www.undp.org/content/dam/undp/library/covid19/Pakistan%20-%20COVID-19%20Socio-economic%20Impact%20Assessment%20and%20Response%20Plan%201%20May%202020.pdf

Wenham, C., Smith, J., Davies, S., Feng, H., Grepin, K., Harman, S., Crabb, A., & Morgan, R. (2020). Women are most affected by pandemics—Lessons from past outbreaks. *Nature (London), 583*(7815), 194–198.

WHO (World Health Organization). (2020). *Interim guidance for refugee and migrant health in relation to COVID 19 in the WHO European Region*. https://www.euro.who.int/__data/assets/pdf_file/0008/434978/Interim-guidance-refugee-and-migrant-health-COVID-19.pdf

WHO COVID-19 Dashboard. (2020). https://covid19.who.int/

World Bank. (2020). *Social protection and COVID-19 (coronavirus)*. https://www.worldbank.org/en/topic/socialprotection/brief/social-protection-and-covid-19

3 The Impact of COVID-19 on the 'Culture of Deportation' for Refugees from African Countries in Germany

Claudia Koehler

3.1 Introduction

At the end of 2019, 79.5 million people worldwide were forcibly displaced. The top hosting countries worldwide were Turkey, Colombia, Pakistan, Uganda, and Germany (UNHCR, 2020a). The procedures for accepting displaced people in a host country usually include the assessment whether the person is in need for international protection, such as a recognised refugee.

There are two options for people who are not officially recognised as a refugee: "return [voluntary or involuntary] to the country of origin or access to alternative legal migration options (e.g., regularization in the host country or legal onward movement to another country)" (UNHCR, 2020b). The way in which host countries prioritise, provide opportunities for, and implement these two options differ and impact the lives of refugees profoundly. Although some countries provide options for regularisation and only in rare cases implement forced returns, other countries prioritise return; for example, they provide incentives for voluntary return, and threaten with and implement forced returns, also called deportations. As a coercive state act, deportation is a highly sensitive political and human rights issue (Ellermann, 2009). It is related to normative ideas of state sovereignty, political positions on border control, migration policies, and the inclusion and exclusion of certain categories of people (Nyers, 2003), as well as to the concept of the nation state versus concepts of globalization.

This chapter takes the spotlight on the fifth major host country of refugees—Germany—and its principles and practices of deportations of people from African countries.

The public discourse on asylum and deportation in Germany became rather polarised following the arrival of larger numbers of asylum seekers since 2015. On the one hand, right-wing groups have been gaining ground. On the other hand, a fraction of the population has been in favor of liberal asylum and migration policies. The pro-migrant and antiracist movements that started in the 1980s brought out influential actors: Refugee Councils and the lobbying group, Pro Asyl, consisting of refugee councils, church representatives, unions, and human rights organizations. These groups have been positioning themselves as voices countering the anti-immigrant discourse, as advocates against restrictive migration policies, and as a direct support network for refugees, mainly those with precarious legal status (Kirchhoff & Lorenz, 2018). Movements of resistance—solidarity protests and refugee activism—have been gaining in qualitative and quantitative importance (Rosenberger, 2018). In line with the self-perception of those actors as advocates for refugees, this

C. Koehler (✉)
Farafina Institute, Bamberg, Germany
e-mail: claudia.koehler@farafina-institute.org

M. C. S. Gonçalves et al. (eds.), *The Coronavirus Crisis and Challenges to Social Development*,
https://doi.org/10.1007/978-3-030-84678-7_3

Table 3.1 List of interviews and observations

Interviewee /observation	Interviewee/observation number	Date of interview/ observation
Migrant (Nigerian, male, 38, living in refugee first reception center [ANKER-Zentrum] in Germany)	Interviewee 5	21 July 2018
Migrant (Ghanaian, male, 28, living in refugee first reception center [ANKER-Zentrum] in Germany)	Interviewee 6	21 July 2018
Migrant (Nigerian, male, 32, living in refugee first reception center [ANKER-Zentrum] in Germany)	Interviewee 7	21 July 2018
Migrant (Ghanaian, male, 42, living in refugee first reception center [ANKER-Zentrum] in Germany)	Interviewee 9	21 July 2018
Migrant (Nigerian, male, 27, living in refugee first reception center [ANKER-Zentrum] in Germany)	Interviewee 10	16 October 2019
Migrant (Nigerian, male, 36, living in refugee first reception center [ANKER-Zentrum] in Germany)	Interviewee 11	24 June 2019
Migrant (Nigerian, female, 25, living in refugee first reception center [ANKER-Zentrum] in Germany)	Interviewee 12	15 May 2020
Migrant (Nigerian, male, 34, living in shared accommodation center for refugees in Germany)	Interviewee 13	30 April 2021
Expert (Volunteer counselor, female, 46, Bamberg)	Interviewee 14	28 February 2020
Demonstration 'Mahnwache Asyl' in Bamberg, Germany	Observation 1	14 June 2020

chapter discusses the issue of deportations from the perspective of people with a precarious legal status in Germany, as opposed to debates that argue from the perspective of the mainstream society without adequate consideration of the perspective of noncitizens.

The chapter is based on the analysis of documents (academic analyses, reports, and analyses by refugee and civil society activists), interviews, observations (Table 3.1), remote consultations with volunteers working with refugees, and the personal experiences of the author from her work with African refugee activists and asylum seekers in Germany before and during the COVID-19 pandemic.

3.2 Culture of Deportation

"When a deportation is executed, it is the last ring of the Slavery and Colonial chain." (The Voice Refugee Forum, 2017).

The term 'culture of deportation' was first used by activists from the VOICE Refugee Forum[1] and Karawane Network in Germany. The cultural element of the term is based on the understanding of a reproduction of an old tradition, a maintenance of the status quo that continues by the support by a larger majority of the society. This support is enabled by a shared understanding that a certain type of mobility is illegal per se whereas other types are legal. This understanding, or culture, can be traced back to the colonial mentality that Europeans are entitled to go and settle down wherever they wish (Happelmann & Zólyom, 2019), but people from other regions in the world are refused the same rights when wanting to come to Europe. According to The Voice Refugee Forum (2017), deportation "has been an instrument of power by the oppressor against the subalterns. … [It] is the added manifestation of […] slavery and colonial powers."

The societal support of this understanding legitimates the policies and their administrative enforcement to the point where even many of those who claim to be in solidarity with refugees consider deportations as legitimate (Happelmann & Zólyom, 2019). They believe that a form of selection has to take place dividing foreigners by those who have a right to enter or to stay and those who have no right to do so. In other words, deportations are framed as a removal of undesired

[1]The Voice Refugee Forum was founded by five African asylum seekers in 1994.

migrants to make room for the desired ones (Oulios, 2013, p. 220).

According to Happelmann and Zólyom (Happelmann & Zólyom, 2019, pp. 136–137), the 'culture of deportation' is the counterpart of Germany's much celebrated 'welcome culture' that promotes Germany as a migrant- and refugee-welcoming country. In reality, the 'welcome' applies only to a selected few, those who are considered as 'beneficial' to the country, such as highly educated people, business people, or people who have qualifications that Germany needs, and the small number of people whose asylum is approved. Those who are in asylum procedures and whose claims for asylum are rejected are illegalised and made subject to deportation.

The hierarchy of rights that come along with a certain passport can be traced back to its colonial roots. The German passport is one of the most powerful passports in the world, allowing its holders to travel to most countries, whereas Germany, through its culture of deportation, systematically prevents the entry and mobility for people with other passports. This attitude is part of what Happelmann and Zólyom (2019, p. 135) call the 'double logic' of the European Union's (EU) Schengen area: for EU citizens it is a zone of free movement and trade, whereas for non-EU citizens, Schengen is a zone of external and internal borders. For people in asylum procedures and undocumented people internal borders entail mobility restrictions through residence obligation and refugee camps, and controls that often come along with racial profiling by the police. Üstün (2019, p. 23) establishes, therefore, that some of the EU's internal policies on migrants have a negative impact on its image as 'normative actorness and self-constructed force-for-good' as these policies demonstrate the "EU's preference for interest-based policies rather than rights-based ones."

The EU's external borders often block people's entry through restrictive visa policies and the physical protection of the EU land and sea borders. In 2016, the overall rejection rate of visa applications was only 6.71%, but for countries with high numbers of asylum applicants, including many African countries, the visa rejection rate was almost 50%. For example, the German embassy and consulates in Nigeria rejected 45.71% of all Schengen visa applications in 2017 (Deutscher Bundestag, 2018). The lack of legal opportunities to enter Europe leads some people to embark on the irregular route (Koehler, 2018), forcing most non-EU migration into the asylum system while denying asylum status to most applicants (Happelmann & Zólyom, 2019).

Increasingly, border policing is being moved away from the actual border of the EU and into the territory of the African continent to prevent Africans from migrating to Europe and to facilitate deportations back to Africa (Korvensyrjä, 2019). Several instruments are used for this strategy.

Efforts have been undertaken to interrupt the zone of free mobility within the Economic Union of West Africa (ECOWAS) to make it more difficult for people to reach the northern shores of the African continent as a starting point for crossing the Mediterranean, mainly through agreements with individual ECOWAS countries on national border policing (Happelmann & Zólyom, 2019, p. 140). Such measures are in contradiction with regional integration; they bring harm to intra-African trade with affected traders who lose their businesses becoming potential migrants, as well as increased dangers on migration routes because people no longer can travel on the regular roads and have to use the services of smugglers.

To keep those who have reached the northern shores of Africa from entering Europe, the EU has been shutting down and criminalising rescue operations of nongovernmental organisations (NGOs) and refusing their embarkation (Cusumano & Gombeer, 2018). At the same time, they have been providing financial support to border police of the northern African countries, including military groups of the contested Libyan Government of National Accord (GNA). As a result, people who try to cross the Mediterranean are captured by militias and are taken to Libyan prisons where they suffer multiple forms of abuse while the same action is labeled as humanitarian "search and rescue" (Lemberg-Pedersen, 2019). The reverse logic used by the EU is evident: While it is justifying its measures with 'fighting human trafficking and the root causes of illegal migration,' it is effectively contributing to the said dangers.

The lack of passports identifying people as citizens of their country of origin means people in Germany cannot be deported (Kirchhoff & Lorenz, 2018), because when moving along the irregular migration routes, most people carry no passport or hide it. Biometric databases in the countries of origin would make it possible to retrieve identification data for the purpose of deportation. For this reason, the EU has been pressuring African countries into readmission agreements and biometric passport conditions (Happelmann & Zólyom, 2019, p. 140). Assisted, or voluntary returns with financial incentives, have been presented as a humane alternative to deportations (Kirchhoff & Lorenz, 2018).

These practices of externalization and deportation delocalise off-shore and outsource sovereign power in the pursuit of particular interests (Bialasiewicz, 2012) and parallel colonial practices during the transatlantic slave trade (Lemberg-Pedersen, 2019).

3.3 Impact of the 'Culture of Deportation' on African Refugees in Germany

The majority of refugees from African countries (except for people from Eritrea and Somalia) have only very low prospects for attaining a stable residence status on the basis of asylum[2] (Bundesamt für Migration und Flüchtlinge, 2019). Among asylum seekers from Africa, Nigerians are the largest group, with 3303 new asylum requests in 2020. The numbers of newly arriving Nigerian refugees have steadily been rising over the past few years, making them the fifth major country of origin of asylum seekers in Germany (Statista, 2021).

[2]Nationals of Ghana and Senegal are per se nearly excluded from the access to asylum as these two countries are classified as 'safe countries of origin', hence it is assumed that a person from there would not suffer any form of persecution that would provide grounds for asylum.

In EU Member States (MS), the assessment on the need for international protection is preceded by the so-called Dublin-III assessment, where the MS responsible for the examination of the asylum application is established, mostly the first country of entering the EU (European Commission, 2020). If a different MS than the host country is identified as responsible for the asylum procedures, the person is usually transferred back to that country. The majority of refugees from Africa who reach Germany have passed through Italy or another EU country, which is then responsible for their asylum application. If a 'Dublin-decision' is taken, the person can be deported to the responsible EU MS during the period of 6 months. If the person cannot be found at the time of deportation, the period for the Dublin-transfer is extended, usually for another 12 months.

If a person remains in Germany throughout this time without being deported, Germany takes over the asylum case. If no 'Dublin-decision' is taken, the asylum case is directly taken over following the asylum interview upon arrival. In many cases, the asylum interview takes place only a few days after arrival, leaving the person no time to be counselled on the asylum procedures or to recover from traumatic experiences.

The majority of asylum applications are rejected (~57%), against which most people file an appeal. A period of roughly 1 year passes until the court decides about the appeal. If the court's decision confirms the rejection of asylum and no grounds for a ban of deportation are established, the person is formally obliged to leave the country (Bundesamt für Justiz, 1992). At this point German authorities start preparations for the person to leave the country. This is, the person is urged to 'clarify their identity,' which means submitting their passport or birth certificate so that the country of origin will accept him/her back. Legally the person is now obliged to cooperate with the German authorities in identifying themselves through documents, such as a passport, which means facilitating their own deportation. If the person fails to 'cooperate' according to the authorities' expectations, they implement measures of force, such as taking the person for forced embassy hearings, gradually reducing the payments to the person up to their complete termination, and sentencing the person for illegal stay in the country (Happelmann & Zólyom, 2019). Some people are arrested and held in deportation detention. Courts have ruled in several cases on the unlawfulness of this measure. In some cases, even people who agree to voluntarily return to their countries are deported before the voluntary return.

In 2019, 22,097 people were deported from Germany, among them were 8423 people who were transferred to other EU countries through the Dublin-Regulation (Bundestagsdrucksachen 19/8021 and 19/18021). In the same year, Germany requested Italy to accept 14,175 people back for Dublin-transfers; 2575 were actually transferred to Italy (Pro Asyl, 2020b). Deportations have increasingly been enforced with more severity. During the past few years there have repeatedly been reports about police violence, captivation, and forced medication in the course of deportations (Bundestagsdrucksachen 19/4960, 19/7401 and 19/21149). In 1764 cases of deportees in 2019, handcuffs, foot cuffs, steel cuffs, or body cuffs were used to enforce the deportation against their will: this is a considerable increase, compared to 135 of such cases in 2015 (Bundestagsdrucksache 19/18201). The Anti-Torture Committee of the Council of Europe recently requested Germany to cease the inappropriate use of violence in the course of deportations (Der Spiegel, 2019).

In the terminology used by refugees in Germany, anybody who can be deported, to another EU MS or to their country of origin, is 'under deportation.' In June 2020, this applied to 271,767 people in Germany who were legally obliged to leave the country; among them about 35,000 people with the nationality of an African country (Bundestagsdrucksache 19/21149).

This section identifies the impact of the 'culture of deportation' on African refugees in Germany on three levels: (1) threat of deportation as a legal barrier to participation in society; (2) physical insecurity; and (3) status insecurity and threat of deportation as a cause for mental disorders.

3.3.1 Threat of Deportation as a Legal Barrier to Participation in Society

While people are 'under deportation,' they usually receive a so-called 'toleration' ('Duldung'), which is not a residence permit but a temporary suspension of deportation. With this status, access to the core institutions of society (e.g., education and training system, labour market, comprehensive healthcare) is basically impossible (Kirchhoff & Lorenz, 2018). The persons cannot legally leave the city limits and are deprived of elements of personal autonomy and privacy (Happelmann & Zólyom, 2019). The same applies almost with the same severity to people who are waiting for a decision on their asylum requests, unless they are from a country categorised as 'high prospects to stay in Germany.' Understandably enough, this regulation is not comprehensible by refugees, who majorly do not wish to receive social benefits but want to work or acquire education (Sindani, 2018), as one interviewee from Nigeria explains: "We want to work and pay taxes. Why does the German government not allow us to do that? We don't want to receive money from them." [Interviewee 5].

En route, most refugees could provide for the needs of the family, despite the difficulties of the travel and hard working conditions. They do not understand why, once arrived at their destination, they have no permission to work. By forcing them to stay idle, especially without work and education, they have the impression that in Germany the reasons why they risked their lives to be there are being ignored (Koehler, 2018). This situation affects people's morale. It is paradoxical to note that it is in reception camps that many people start to lose their spirits. Because for them, idleness is more deadly than anything they have endured so far. They feel as prisoners in golden cages. Doubts settle in their minds that overcome courage, strength, and resilience.

A man from Cameroon describes: "The life in the camps is an additional suffering because I see every day people getting crazy, crazy into madness. Indeed, how is it possible to abandon people who risked their lives to find work to take care of their families, one or two years, without doing anything? For many of us, the families got into debt, especially to get them out of the hands of the Libyan militias. You have to pay back that money." During a demonstration against camps in Bamberg in August 2018, a speaker from Ghana said: "All the hardship and pain that we had to go through during our journeys and on the sea were not as painful as what we are now going through in the camps in Germany" (interviews in Koehler, 2018).

Hence, even though Germany has declared the integration of refugees as one of their top priorities, it is out ruling any form of integration for many of them, as the refugee activist Rex Osa explains: "An integration policy that undermines our active participation is racist and colonial" (Happelmann & Zólyom, 2019).

3.3.2 Physical Insecurity

The physical insecurity from the danger of deportation is ever present among those who are 'under deportation.' The danger of deportation can be unpredictable and may even appear as 'by chance' as the legal processes that might culminate in a deportation are highly complex and not transparent for those concerned. Hence, many people are not in the position to estimate their risk of being deported. Rumors that spread among refugee communities contribute to this insecurity.

In first reception camps, deportations are a sad reality in people's everyday lives (Koehler, 2018), as expressed by a refugee from Ghana: "Life in camp is a hellfire, at any moment you can be deported." [Interviewee 9].

Deportations are done mostly at night and in the early morning hours, so that people are on constant alert and suffer from sleeplessness (Bayerischer Flüchtlingsrat, 2021a), as described by two refugees from Nigeria: "Every night we sleep with our eyes open. When we see lights shining through our windows we hide." [Interviewee 7]; "I can't remember the last time I slept at night. I always sleep after 6 a.m. During the night I stay close to my window so I can jump in case they come." [Interviewee 13].

Deportations also happen in regular situations during the day. Several interviewed refugees have observed others being picked up by the police for deportation as they were collecting their monthly payments, eating in the camp canteen, or praying [Interviewee 5, 7].

In many instances, physical force is applied in the different stages of a deportation. Violent police actions also happen in a seemingly arbitrary manner in camps, often upon accusing refugees for inciting violence or preventing a deportation, and also in response to organized activism among refugees. It appears as if African refugees are purposely, and more than others, targeted. Such form of 'legal violence is supposedly justified violence effected by and through the law' (Happelmann & Zólyom, 2019). The systemic elements of discrimination and intimidation become apparent when refugees are not given a chance to explain the situation from their perspective or their statements are not considered as credible by authorities, including courts, after such incidents.

To protect each other, residents of reception camps find different forms of collective support, such as watching out for the police at night, as explained by a refugee from Nigeria: "One of us always stays up at night and warns the others when a police car approaches our building." [Interviewee 11].

Some refugees even report of threats by individual police officers, as one Nigerian refugee narrates: "The last time they [the local foreigners office] called me for an appointment, one police officer told me 'If the authorities do not deport you, I will make sure that I deport you personally.'" [Interviewee 13].

Any person who is involved with public authorities is perceived by refugees as a potential accomplice for a deportation. This perception is confirmed by experiences they make, such as the case of a Nigerian refugee: "One day I was in the car with the caretaker [of the reception camp] because I had to move into another room. While we drove, he made a phone call. When we parked in front of the building, he told me to wait for a moment. Then I saw police driving up. I jumped out of the car and ran towards the exit gate of the camp. I thought my life in Germany had come to an end." [Interviewee 10].

Some people, however, who are not directly linked to authorities, may offer some support in limiting chances for a deportation, as the experience of a Ghanaian refugee demonstrates: "The teacher [of my German class] told me it might be safer for me if I didn't come back to class because police might come and pick me from there. She said they are looking for me. I was a good student; it pains me that I had to stop German class." [Interviewee 6].

Solidarity groups are further engaged for the rights of refugees, with local variations in the level of activity. Refugee activism takes place but is hampered by the threat of deportation as many people are afraid to speak out for their rights in fear of deportation as a punitive action (Happelmann & Zólyom, 2019).

The constant threat of deportation leads many people to leave the reception camps (Hess et al., 2018). Some of them move on to other EU countries; others move to larger cities in Germany where they try to find unregistered work. Sources indicate that most people whose asylum requests were rejected remain in the country without a regular status (Sindani, 2018; Koehler, 2018). Those people are disconnected from any social and legal support systems; this makes them highly vulnerable for exploitation and even trafficking (Koehler, 2018). Legally they have basic rights, and some NGOs offer services for them, but often they are not informed about them (Vogel, 2015) and are afraid to make use of them for fear of deportation.

Since 2015, laws on the stay of people living in Germany irregularly have been tightened, especially related to deportations. The 'Asylverfahrensbeschleunigungsgesetz' (Law for accelerated asylum procedures) specifies that deportations must take place without first informing the person who will be deported about the exact date and time (Section 59, Residence Act). Thus, people living in irregularity now have to fear deportation at any time, which applies to the estimated 200,000–500,000 people in Germany (Link, 2019).

3.3.3 Status Insecurity and Threat of Deportation as a Cause for Mental Disorders

Many refugees from African countries who live in Germany with an insecure status and are threatened by deportation suffer from depression; they complain of nightmares, are not able to sleep, and are unable to concentrate on studying. Many people develop mental disorders; some even attempt suicide. Hess et al. (2018) establish that the living situation in camps, which includes the threat of deportation, leads to psychological disorders. Insecurity of residence status can lead to depression and anxiety (Demiralay & Haasen, 2011; Schenk, 2007) and fear of having to return to the country of origin fear of deportation, and insecurity about the future lead to extreme psychological stress (Schouler-Ocak & Kurmeyer, 2017). Because of such conditions, some refugees even attempt suicide.

A common saying among African refugees living in first reception camps is 'When I get transfer, I will start learning German.' They connect being transferred from a first reception to a more permanent camp with status security. In reality, however, such a transfer does not automatically come with the assurance of a safe status. It is the perceived feeling of being save from deportation that enables people to study and concentrate. While the feeling of insecurity continues, most people are unable to make plans for their future.

In some cases, a medical condition, including psychological disorders, can give rise to a ban of deportation. However, in 2016, a new asylum law change, Asylum Package II, was adopted. It exacerbated the exception regulations concerning the protection against deportations. It is now generally assumed that medical reasons are no longer obstacles for deportations, only in the case of a life-threatening or severe illness. Thus, post-traumatic stress disorders are no longer obstacles for deportations (see §60(7), Residence Act). This decision worsens the situation of traumatised refugees dramatically.

3.4 Impact of the 'Culture of Deportation' on Involuntary Returnees in African Countries

This section discusses how a forced return impacts deportees upon the actual deportation and after their return to the country of origin.

3.4.1 Forceful Discontinuation of a Stage of Life

For most refugees from African countries in Germany, returning to their country of origin is not an option (Koehler, 2018). In their 2020 reflections on deportations from Germany, Pro Asyl (2020a) writes "with every deportation, the life of a human being is thrown out of joint – often not for the first time." This statement can best be illustrated by two exemplary cases: Mira[3] from Ethiopia was deported in prison clothes from deportation detention and in a wheelchair, which she needed because of her poor health, to Addis Ababa on 28 December 2020 (Bayerischer Flüchtlingsrat, 2020). Gloria, a single mother of two, passed through 2 painful years of asylum rejection, forced embassy hearings, and fearful living in a first reception camp, before she was transferred to a second-stage camp where her daughter was finally allowed to attend school and the family felt a sense of security. Shortly after, she and her kids were deported to Ghana; as she had resisted the deportation, she was held in hand- and foot cuffs throughout the whole flight (Interviewee 14). Gloria and her children as well as Mira were left at the airport without any support. Only through the help of volunteers (Mira) and a group of former deportees who got together to meet new deportees at the airport to help them to at least make phone calls to family members and friends (Gloria) were they able to find a first shelter.

The practice of 'dropping' deportees at the airport of their country of origin without any first support or guidance is quite common. Even though international and governmental organisations are on the ground to provide such first support, in practical terms and upon first arrival, support is often not available.

Obviously, the harder and the more dangerous the journey to Europe was, the more tragic it is to be forcefully be returned. Refugees from Sub-Saharan African countries have no choice but to embark on the deadly journey through the Sahara Desert and across the Mediterranean Sea, unless they find one of the extremely rare opportunities to enter Europe regularly. Chances are high that we will never know which of the two dreadful stages of the journey has claimed more lives of mainly young Africans. A man from Senegal explains: "Many will prefer to spend their whole lives here [in Germany] trying to find something, but hardly will they agree to return. Indeed, many think that looking back at the suffering endured to get here to Europe, they deserve to be here, to stay." (Interview in Koehler, 2018).

People from Africa who enter Europe along the irregular routes do not only put their lives in extreme danger but are also carriers of hopes and expectations of their families; some are sent by them. Often during their journeys, but at the latest after they arrive in Europe, family members expect the migrant to send money home to help out with the family's needs (Sindani, 2018). Throughout their stay in Germany, the hope to 1 day make it through the difficult time of work prohibition, have an income, and be able to support the family back home, is what gives many refugees a sense of strength (Koehler, 2018). Hence, being deported means that risking one's life was meaningless and the hopes and expectations of the family and local community were disappointed.

Many people who are returned from Germany to Italy end up on the street and are forced into irregular and exploitive labour, mostly in agriculture (Happelmann & Zólyom, 2019). Large numbers of people have been living under these conditions for many years; some of them want to return home but do not have the means and papers to do so, but many prefer to stay.

[3]All names and other personal identifiers in the chapter have been changed to protect privacy and confidentiality.

3.4.2 Disconnection from Local Communities and Barriers to Reintegration

Many forcefully returned people have been away from their countries of origin for many years. Societal changes have happened in the meantime, and social connections with friends and family members have suffered from the distance and from circumstances related to the reasons they leave the country.

People who return from Europe without 'having made it in life' (e.g., having built a house, bought a car, or have accumulated) are often considered as 'losers' and are blamed for coming home 'empty-handed' and disappointing the expectations of the family; some are blamed of bringing shame over the family (Koehler, 2018). A man from Senegal explains: "What is worse, when you return without having reached your goal, it is a failure that many do not accept. … In addition, there is the pressure of the family. Every day many are returning empty handed. Because of their failures and their difficult journey, unlucky migrants are weakened psychologically, rejected by their families and relatives, considered as crazy, they are ostracised and often see family ties broken… Those who fail are low profile" (Interview in Koehler, 2018).

In some cases, groups of returnees try to bridge the gap of social and economic connections by forming returnee self-help groups to reintegrate socially and economically. A group discussion with forcefully returned people in Accra, Ghana in January 2020 revealed that all returnees in the group did not return to their local communities after having been deported but instead remained in Accra and formed an activist group because they felt disconnected from and rejected by their local communities, while the people they could relate to and associate with the most are those who spent some years in Europe and had similar experiences to theirs.

Support mechanism, such as training and business start-up support, by international and German-governmental organisations in countries of origin until recently limited most of their reintegration support to voluntary returnees but have started to open up for deportees. However, there are a number of obstacles that those in need of support encounter: complicated processes of application, conditions and approval of support often lack transparency and take a long time, contact offices of the respective organisations are only based in large cities.

If efforts to reintegrate fail, numerous returnees start considering to reembark on the irregular journey to Europe, and many of them actually do so.

3.5 Impact of COVID-19 on the 'Culture of Deportation'

This section discusses the ways the COVID-19 pandemic impacted the 'culture of deportation' for refugees from African countries in Germany in regard to (1) the suspension and continuation of deportations, (2) health risks, and (3) lack of information and counselling.

3.5.1 Suspension and Continuation of Deportations

As international airports in Europe and Africa closed, many people with an insecure status started hoping that deportations would be suspended. Finally, on 25 February 2020, a ban of Dublin-transfers to Italy and later to other EU countries until at least April was declared. Several Federal States of Germany decided in March 2020 to suspend deportations of 'people at risk' to countries that were categorized as corona-risk areas. Others decided on a case-by-case level on a temporary suspension of deportation, often in response to the closure of international airports. 'Duldung' papers were issued to some people (Pro Asyl, 2021). Those who were subject of an official suspension of deportation were informed in writing by the Ministry of Migration and Refugees.

The reactions among those 'under deportation' were characterized by overwhelming joy and relief. The statement by a Nigerian refugee at a demonstration in June 2020 expresses this feeling: “God has blessed us. We can finally sleep in peace.” [Observation 1].

People no longer needed to fear that police may come at night to deport them. Some of those who were temporarily hiding to avoid deportation reentered the official system and were able to continue their asylum cases, access housing, social benefits, and health coverage, or do simple things like travelling on the train without fear. People who were subject to Dublin transfers and who had been staying in the reception center, but not collecting their monthly payments and not sleeping in their rooms to avoid being deported, were able to move back into their rooms and collect their payments. A calm, almost peaceful atmosphere emerged in the camps that often appear hostile, as one refugee from Nigeria narrated during the suspension of deportations: “The camp is so calm now; we hardly see police around and when we see them, we are not afraid. It’s good now.” [Interviewee 12].

Hence, a deadly pandemic turned out as a carrier of hope for many thousands in danger of deportation. The relief from being out of danger of deportation outweighed the fear of the COVID-19 disease for many.

However, there has been no moment during the COVID-19 pandemic when Germany completely suspended its ‘culture of deportation.’ A general suspension of deportations, strongly demanded for by human rights organisations such as Pro Asyl, was never declared despite the disastrous impact of the pandemic on some of the countries of origin, as established by an EASO special report on “Asylum trends and COVID-19” (EASO, 2020). People were still in deportation detention during the spread of the pandemic in Germany and were only released after repeated calls by human rights organisations or following court decisions. Thus, many people remained in insecurity (Pro Asyl, 2020b). While Portugal granted temporary residency with full access to social and health services to asylum seekers during the pandemic, multiple lawyers in Germany tried to achieve the issuing of ‘Duldung’ papers for their clients for the time of the suspension of Dublin-transfers ito enable them to exercise at least the very limited rights of people who are being ‘tolerated,’ but mostly without success.

Even though a considerable drop in deportations was notable during the pandemic, there was not a single month during the first half of 2020 when no deportations happened. After in January as well as in February 2020 about 1600 people were deported, numbers dropped to 923 in March and 30 in April, before they rose to 92 in May and 406 in June 2020. Even though Italy was the European country that was hit the hardest by the first wave of COVID-19, 384 people were deported to Italy. 509 people were deported to African countries, most of them to Morocco (138), Algeria (106), Nigeria (71), and Ghana (52). Among the 4616 people deported to other EU countries and to countries of origin between January and June 2020, 1129 had a citizenship of an African country; the majority of them were Nigerians (231), including 42 women and 20 children. Nigerians are also the largest nationality group (163) among those who were transferred to other EU countries according to the Dublin-regulation during the first six months of 2020 (Bundestagsdrucksache 19/21149, own calculations). During the same time 4616 police officers were involved in deportations and approximately 1500 people were deported in the scope of mass deportations by chartered flights, sometimes in collaboration with other EU countries. These deportations cost about five million Euro, of which about two million was spent for deportations to African countries. Most of these costs are borne by the European Border and Coast Guard Agency FRONTEX, a small part by Germany alone (Bundestagsdrucksache 19/21149, own calculations). Some of the deportation flights took place even while international airports of the countries of destination were still closed.

The second wave of the pandemic, starting around October 2020, hit Europe and many other parts of the world even harder than the first one. Numbers of COVID-19 cases were up to ten times higher than during the first wave. Nevertheless, an official suspension of deportations to any country never took place in Germany. Deportations have been taking place regardless of the COVID-19 situation in the countries of destination and despite repeated demands of civil society organisations for the suspension of deportations. Pro Asyl (2020a) states the case of the 19-year-old Abdul from Guinea who was picked up by police on 15 September 2020 from the vocational school that he was attending. He was placed in deportation detention, where he was refused any contact, even with his lawyer. Only after his deportation to Spain, which was at the time officially a COVID-19 risk area, was he able to use his phone and communicate. Others who were deported to a neighbouring EU country were simply dropped at the border by German police officers and were left to make their own way.

For people living in reception camps, being requested to take a COVID-19 test now triggers fears as it could be a sign of authorities preparing to deport the person.

3.5.2 Health Risks

People living in reception camps as well as undocumented people have been exposed to particular health risks during the pandemic. Living conditions in camps, where people 'on deportation' have to stay, imply that many people live together in a narrow space. Sanitary, eating, and sleeping areas have to be shared with multiple people. Hence, the risk to a rapid spread of the virus has been large (Pro Asyl, 2020b). As larger outbreaks of COVID-19 occurred in camps during the first and second wave of COVID-19, such as in the Ellwangen camp where at one point every second person was infected, human rights groups demanded the ending of the camp system as such (Pro Asyl, 2020b). The limited space in camps leads to more crowded living conditions when certain areas have to be transferred into quarantine zones for infected people. The high occupancy means many people have to be assigned to contact quarantine spaces following positive cases (Bayerischer Flüchtlingsrat, 2021b).

The situation of people who live in the country with an irregular status has been even worse: they have often remained without health assistance during the COVID-19 crisis. Even when they have symptoms of a possible COVID-19 infection, they often do not seek the attendance of a doctor or hospitals from fear of deportation. Hence, in the event of an infection, they may infect others not knowing that they are sick (Grunau, 2020).

3.5.3 Lack of Information and Counselling

Lockdowns and consequent closures of counselling services and the interruption of voluntary support systems mean refugees and asylum seekers have been facing an immense information void that has led to high levels of fears and insecurity, especially among those who have been 'on deportation.' Regardless of the nonavailability of translation and counselling services, public authorities have been sending out decisions and appointments, often with short deadlines for responses or legal action. This practice led to situations where concerned people were not aware of the date of the appeal hearing for their asylum case, could not seek legal advice in time, or could not submit the requested documents to authorities in time, which in turn impacted their asylum procedures negatively and thereby increased their risk of deportation.

The official information that was being circulated about the various and frequently changing contact restrictions, lockdowns, and curfews has primarily been in German. People who do not speak German have had to rely on the information passed on by others and have often felt insecure and in fear of unknowingly breaking a regulation.

3.6 The Role of International Social Work

As Popescu and Libal (2018) state "Social work […] has an important (if largely unfulfilled) role to play in advancing the human rights of migrants and refugees. […] It is time for a renewal of solidarity work in alliance with targeted groups of refugees and migrants."

The harshness with which deportations are enforced, mostly without consideration of the personal circumstances of the concerned people, including efforts to integrate into the German society, causes not only fears and trauma for those in danger of and affected by deportations but also despair for social workers and activists who are engaged for the rights and integration of refugees in Germany. Often, the 'Culture of Deportation' as a counterpart of the 'Welcome Culture' of Germany becomes more strongly evident for them: While they invest multiple efforts into welcoming refugees and assisting their integration 'against the odds,' the threat of deportation is a constant obstacle to their efforts before the actual deportation undoes most of the integration achievements those whom they assist have made. Hence, to a certain extent they share a part of the frustrating experience of deportations with refugees.

It is this understanding of what the 'Culture of Deportation' means for the lives of people that social work has to capitalise on to protect and advocate against inhumane policies and practices and for the rights of migrants and refugees: in particular:

- There is a need for better collaboration on the national level between NGOs, welfare organisations, volunteers, and (refugee) activist groups to raise awareness of the inhumane effects of the 'Culture of Deportation' on the lives of refugees and advocate advance refugees' human rights. These collaborations should become more engaged in governmental levels of response and policy-making or within local or international humanitarian NGOs; they should also intensify their solidarity work with refugees and their self-organisations.
- On an international level, social work should form alliances to ensure collaboration between social workers and NGOs in countries of origin, transit, and destination. These alliances should advocate for human rights for refugees and provide guidance and support across borders. This provision includes setting up support networks for returnees in countries of origin; these can ease the hardship of a forced return where such cannot be prevented. The project Deportees Emergency Reception and Support (DERS) in Lagos, Nigeria, founded by the Network for Critical Migration Consciousness in Nigeria and the Network Refugees4Refugees in Germany, is an example of such a support mechanism. DERS provides first shelter and transport for the most vulnerable deportees from Germany who arrive in Nigeria (Network for Critical Migration Consciousness, 2021).
- To enable appropriate responses by social workers, there is the need for an increased focus in preparing a qualified workforce to effectively work with asylum seekers. Also needed is the fostering of the understanding of the complex political and social context, such as the 'Culture of Deportation,' that shape social work with migrants and refugees.
- The COVID-19 pandemic has demonstrated clearly that some traditional forms of social work require transformation. Core services closed down, leaving refugees without support networks. Guidance and advocacy work have to be ensured even under conditions that do not allow personal interaction. Social work has to become flexible enough to adapt to swiftly changing contexts. In times of crisis, the stability of the connection between social workers and refugees and the guarding of their human rights is even more important than usual.

3.7 Discussion

This chapter demonstrated the impact that the 'Culture of Deportation' has on refugees from African countries in Germany as well as on those who were deported to their countries of origin or to other EU countries. The fear and risk of deportation impacts their everyday life; it inhibits their participation and inclusion in society and their exercise of basic rights, triggers psychological issues, and exposes them to intimidation, force, and isolation, not only for a few months but for many years.

The role of international social work in this context should reach beyond service delivery for refugees. Social work should form national and international alliances in close collaboration with refugees and clearly advocate against policies and practices that jeopardise refugees' human rights.

As Pro Asyl (2020a) rightly assess, the lives of deportees are "thrown out of joint"; they suffer trauma that comes with a forced deportation, including the frequent use of forceful methods in the process. Upon return, many deportees are disconnected and excluded from their societies; reintegration is difficult for many of them to the point where some consider a repeated irregular migration to Europe.

For a short time, relieve came with the temporary suspension of Dublin-deportations during the COVID-19 pandemic. However, contrary to hopes of refugees who were 'on deportation' and contrary to the demands by human rights and activist groups, deportations from Germany to countries of origins of refugees, among them several African countries, continued, yet in smaller numbers. The continuation of deportations, irrespective of the pandemic and its impact on countries of origin, confirms the cultural element of the practice of deportations in Germany as a reproduction of an old tradition and a maintenance of the status quo that is being retained at any time and at any cost.

The chapter also demonstrated that the 'Culture of Deportation' is not limited to its interior dimension but is equally enshrined in its exterior dimension. The post-coloniality of the 'Culture of Deportation' is to be understood in the concurrence of visa policies, border controls, naval interceptions, externalization of borders, readmission and biometric passport agreements, isolation, intimidation and criminalization of refugees in Europe and their selection into 'desired' and 'undesired' ones, the actual deportation, including the use of forceful methods in the process, and the framing of these in the context of 'fighting the root causes of migration,' 'fighting human smuggling,' and others that lead to the social acceptance of the practices and even the legalisation of violence.

This is why, in the words of the Voice Refugee Forum (2017), "The fights to stop deportation … should be a fight that should go beyond the justification against persecution in [countries of origin] or for integrationist […] reasons. It should be seen as a fight against imperialism, capitalism, racism, slavery and colonialism. It is a fight against impunity and for a different world order."

References

Bayerischer Flüchtlingsrat. (2020). Rollstuhl und Gefängniskleidung nach Äthiopien. In T. Der Fall von Mimi (Ed.), *Abschiebewahnsinn gegen jede Vernunft*. https://www.fluechtlingsrat-bayern.de/in-rollstuhl-und-gefaengniskleidung-nach-aethiopien/

Bayerischer Flüchtlingsrat. (2021a). *Abschiebungen—Themeninfo*. https://www.fluechtlingsrat-bayern.de/themen/abschiebungen/#themeninfo

Bayerischer Flüchtlingsrat. (2021b). *Corona-Pandemie wütet in bayerischen Unterkünften für Geflüchtete*. https://www.fluechtlingsrat-bayern.de/corona-pandemie-wuetet-in-bayerischen-unterkuenften/

Bialasiewicz, L. (2012). Off shoring and out-sourcing the borders of Europe: Libya and EU border work in the Mediterranean. *Geopolitics, 17*(4), 843–866.

Bundesamt für Justiz. (1992). *Asylverfahrensgesetz*. https://www.gesetze-im-internet.de/asylvfg_1992/

Bundesamt für Migration und Flüchtlinge. (2019). Sichere Herkunftsstaaten. *Asyl und Flüchtlingsschutz*. https://www.bamf.de/DE/Themen/AsylFluechtlingsschutz/Sonderverfahren/SichereHerkunftsstaaten/sichereherkunftsstaaten-node.html

Cusumano, E., & Gombeer, K. (2018). In deep waters: The legal, humanitarian and political implications of closing Italian ports to migrant rescuers. *Mediterranean Politics, 25*, 245–253.

Demiralay, C., & Haasen, C. (2011). Acculturation. In W. Machleidt & A. Heinz (Eds.), *Praxis der interkulturellen Psychiatrie und Psychotherapie. Migration und Psychische Gesundheit* (pp. 63–66). Elsevier, Urban & Fischer.

Der Spiegel. (2019). Europarat kritisiert deutsche Abschiebepraxis. *Bericht des Anti-Folter-Komitees*. https://www.spiegel.de/politik/deutschland/abschiebungen-europarat-kritisiert-deutschland-bericht-des-anti-folter-komitees-cpt-a-1266507.html

Deutscher Bundestag. (2018). Visaerteilungen im Jahr 2017. *Antwort der Bundesregierung auf eine Kleine Anfrage, Bundestags-Drucksache 19/2035*. http://dip21.bundestag.de/dip21/btd/19/020/1902035.pdf

EASO. (2020). EASO special report: Asylum trends and COVID-19. *PUBLIC*. https://www.easo.europa.eu/sites/default/files/easo-special-report-asylum-covid-june-2020.pdf

Ellermann, A. (2009). *States against migrants: Deportation in Germany and the United States*. Cambridge University Press.

European Commission—Migration and Home Affairs. (2020). *Country responsible for asylum application (Dublin)*. https://ec.europa.eu/home-affairs/what-we-do/policies/asylum/examination-of-applicants_en

Grunau, A. (2020). Corona-Crise gefährdet Menschen ohne Papiere. *Deutsche Welle*. https://www.dw.com/de/corona-krise-gef%C3%A4hrdet-menschen-ohne-papiere/a-53366474

Happelmann, N. S., & Zólyom, F. (2019). *Ankersentrum—Surviving the ruinous Buin*. Archive Books.

Hess, S., Pott, A., Schammann, H., Scherr, A., & Schiffauer, W. (2018). *Welche Auswirkungen haben "Anker-Zentren"?—Eine Kurzstudie für den Mediendienst Integration*. Mediendienst Integration.

Kirchhoff, M., & Lorenz, D. (2018). Between illegalization, toleration, and recognition: Contested asylum and deportation policies in Germany. In S. Rosenberger, V. Stern, & N. Merhaut (Eds.), *Protest movements in asylum and deportation. IMISCOE Research Series*. Springer Open.

Koehler, C. (2018). Study on trafficking resilience and vulnerability en route to Europe—STRIVE: National Report Germany. ICMPD. (unpublished).

Korvensyrjä, A. (2019). Activist perspectives on the "made in Germany" culture of deportation.

Lemberg-Pedersen, M. (2019). Manufacturing displacement. Externalization and postcoloniality in European migration control. *Global Affairs, 5*(3), 247–271.

Link, R. (2019). Leben in der Schattenwelt—Papierlose in Deutschland. *Deutschlandfunk*. https://www.deutschlandfunk.de/papierlose-in-deutschland-leben-in-der-schattenwelt.724.de.html?dram:article_id=459359

Network for Critical Migration Consciousness. (2021). *Deportees emergency reception and support*. https://www.nfcmc.org/de/ders/

Nyers, P. (2003). Abject cosmopolitanism: The politics of protection in the anti-deportation movement. *Third World Quarterly, 24*(6), 1069–1093.

Oulios, M. (2013). *Blackbox Abschiebung. Geschichten und Bilder von Leuten, die gerne geblieben wären*. Suhrkamp.

Popescu, M., & Libal, K. (2018). Social work with migrants and refugees: Challenges, best practices, and future directions. Editorial. *Advances in Social Work, 18*(3).

Pro Asyl. (2020a). *Schicksal Abschiebung: Zehn Schlaglichter aus 2020*. https://www.proasyl.de/news/schicksal-abschiebung-zehn-schlaglichter-aus-2020/.

Pro Asyl. (2020b). Flüchtlingspolitische Anliegen in Zeiten von Covid-19 zur Tagung zur Tagung der Innenministerkonferenz vom.

Pro Asyl. (2021). *Newsticker Coronavirus: Informationen für Geflüchtete und Unterstützer*innen—Hintergrund*. https://www.proasyl.de/hintergrund/newsticker-coronavirus-informationen-fuer-gefluechtete-unterstuetzerinnen./

Rosenberger, S. (2018). Political protest in asylum and deportation. An introduction. In S. Rosenberger, V. Stern, & N. Merhaut (Eds.), *Protest movements in asylum and deportation. IMISCOE Research Series*. Springer Open.

Schenk, L. (2007). Migration and health–developing an explanatory and analytical model for epidemiological studies. [migration und gesundheit–Entwicklung eines Erklärungs- und Analysemodells für epidemiologische Studien]. *International Journal of Public Health, 52*, 87–96. https://doi.org/10.1007/s00038-007-6002-4

Schouler-Ocak, M., & Kurmeyer, C. (2017). *Study on female refugees: Repräsentative Untersuchung von geflüchteten frauen in unterschiedlichen Bundesländern in Deutschland*. Charité.

Sindani, J.-M. (2018). *Gestrandet im "Paradies." Erfahrungen aus der Caritas-Asylberatung*. Lambertus-Verlag.

Statista. (2021). *Hauptherkunftsländer von Asylbewerbern in Deutschland im Jahr 2020*. https://de.statista.com/statistik/daten/studie/154287/umfrage/hauptherkunftslaender-von-asylbewerbern/#professional

The Voice Refugee Forum. (2017). *The slave and colonial culture of deportation (Updated)*. http://thevoiceforum.org/node/4400

UNHCR. (2020a). *Figures at a glance*. https://www.unhcr.org/figures-at-a-glance.html

UNHCR. (2020b). *Return of people not in need of international protection*. https://www.unhcr.org/return-of-people-not-in-need-of-international-protection.html

Üstün, C. (2019). *The impact of migration policies on the EU's image as a value-driven normative actor. EuroMeSCo series, 46 papers*. IEMed., European Institute of the Mediterranean.

Vogel, D. (2015). *Update report Germany: Estimated number of irregular foreign residents in Germany (2014)*. Database on irregular migration. Update report. http://irregular-migration.net/

4 Corona Challenging Social Work in Korea and Vietnam

Habin Jung and Quynh Anh Nguyen

4.1 Introduction

Towards the end of 2019 there was an outbreak of a deadly epidemic in the city of Wuhan in China known as the coronavirus (COVID-19). At that time, many Chinese citizens already were either infected by the virus or suffering in the hospital. Some had already died. Then in early 2020, the virus spread to other parts of the world and killed many more people. In January 2020, the World Health Organization (WHO) declared COVID-19 a global pandemic. This chapter discusses the way COVID-19 broke out in Korea and Vietnam, which are two countries in Asia. These countries are also in close proximity to China, where the pandemic originated. This chapter is divided into two parts: Korea and Vietnam.

4.2 Korea

South Korea's economy has grown rapidly; it is currently the 12th largest economy in the world. Based on this economic growth, the health sector also improved considerably. South Korea put in place social and health insurance in the 1970s, universal healthcare coverage in 1989, and a single-payer system in 2004 (June-ho, 2020, p. 3). South Korea's health system is based on hospital-based care. The number of hospital beds per capita, 12.3 beds per 1000 of the population, is two times higher than the average in the Organisation of Economic Co-operation and Development (OECD) countries. The country excels not only in hospital capacity but also in interactions with doctors, with an OECD-leading score of 16.6 consultations annually per capita. Although some critics suggest that South Korea's health system is overly dependent on secondary or tertiary facilities instead of primary facilities, this extra capacity enabled hospitals to respond quickly to COVID-19 without sacrificing care for non-COVID-19 patients (June-ho, 2020, p. 3).

Despite Korea's sufficient health system, South Korea had battled to handle previous outbreaks of other pandemics such as the Middle East respiratory syndrome (MERS) in 2015. MERS had 17,000 suspected cases and 38 deaths. With this experience, Korea started to prepare for future pandemics such as COVID-19. The government of Korea established the country's Disease Control and Prevention Agency (KDCA) to handle the pandemic. Under this new system, the Korean state managed the pandemic quickly, with approximately 600 screening and testing centers and 150 diagnostic laboratories. With this infrastructure, at the height of the pandemic the total number of patients was 132,000: 122,000 people recovered, and 1903 people died.

H. Jung (✉) · Q. A. Nguyen
University of Applied Sciences, Würzburg-Schweinfurt, Würzburg, Germany
e-mail: habin.jung@student.fhws.de

M. C. S. Gonçalves et al. (eds.), *The Coronavirus Crisis and Challenges to Social Development*,
https://doi.org/10.1007/978-3-030-84678-7_4

4.2.1 COVID-19 Outbreak in Korea

Korea was one of the first countries to experience the COVID-19 outbreak. Korea is located close to China, so many people worried about the hazard of the pandemic, especially after the MERS experience. Thus, many people cared more about preventing the disease. The first case was reported on January 20, 2020. Media reported the COVID-19 symptoms several times, and people were sensitive about the border closure policy. The majority of the people wanted the government to close the border but at the same time, many people were concerned about the economic issues related to trade. After the first case was discovered, it seemed quite peaceful for a while; however, there was a huge outbreak in the city of Daegu. On February 19, there were 15 cases from one church called Shincheonji Church of Jesus. From this one church, there was a huge outbreak that reached a peak of 909 cases on February 29. At that time, people were in a panic and there was chaos, especially in Daegu. People who were involved in the Shincheonji Church lost their jobs and could not get enough protection from society. They were accused of spreading the disease. To handle this outbreak, the government tried to expand the capacity of testing. Korea's Disease Control and Prevention Agency directed private companies to produce a diagnostic reagent (June-ho, 2020, p. 5). With this expanded testing capacity, the Korean state focused on screening. To prevent the spread of disease, COVID-19 screening clinics were set up outside entrances with drive-through centers. During the surge of cases in Daegu in February 2020, health officials opened 600 screening centers using innovative approaches to increase capacity June-ho, 2020, p. 5).

4.2.2 Main Impacts of the Pandemic

COVID-19 affected Korea as follows:

4.2.2.1 Travel Restrictions

In late January 2020, South Korea enforced entry procedures for travelers coming from Wuhan. In the summer and fall of 2020, South Korea tightened travel restrictions. In October 2020, Korea required visas for nearly all foreign nationals. It suspended visa-waiver countries and visa-free countries, with some exceptions (June-ho, 2020, p. 7). Visa applicants were required to submit forms about their health status and show symptom-free certification from a medical professional.

4.2.2.2 Isolation and Quarantine

To cope with the outbreak in Daegu, the South Korean government transformed public facilities and private corporation places of residence into temporary isolation spaces. There were two reasons for this transformation: first, to treat the patient without spreading the disease; second, to manage the hospital system. Since the outbreak, there were more than 5000 patients at the same time. To handle this huge number in a short period, treating all of them in the hospitals was impossible. Patients who were staying at these spaces reported their symptoms and got a regular checkup. As a result, 15 community treatment centers, including several in dormitories for training institutes of private companies such as Samsung and LG, admitted 3033 people between March 3 and March 26, 2020. Health professionals monitored the centers, and patients reported their symptoms regularly by a smartphone application or by phone. The facilities were equipped with pulse oximeters, X-ray machines, and RT-PCR tests for SARS-CoV-2. Only 81 of 3033 (2.67%) cases were transferred to a hospital for higher-level care (June-ho, 2020, p. 7). Quarantine policies are strict but supportive to prevent the disease. People needed to self-quarantine if they had been in contact with a confirmed case, traveled internationally, or had symptoms and risk factors for getting the disease. Using the Self-Quarantine Safety Protection app was mandatory for the people who had to quarantine. Case officers monitor the app and they can check the location tracking. If people break quarantine, they are required to wear "safety bands." The electronic wristbands are connected to the app and case officers can get the location information. There is also a fine for violating self-quarantine of US$8217. But the quarantine policy actually helped people to cope with the quarantine. Officers delivered a full box of food, medical aid devices such as masks, sanitizers, thermometer, psychological counseling, and video-streaming services for entertainment. Furthermore, South Korea focused on mental health throughout the pandemic, creating hotlines and maintaining a national psychological support team.

4.2.2.3 Contact Tracing

South Korea did aggressive tracing to prevent the virus. South Korea expanded its usual workforce of Epidemic Intelligence Service (EIS) officers by quickly training staff at approximately 250 local public health centers, hiring 300 private epidemiologists, and leveraging staff at 11 nongovernmental organizations that train and support EIS officers. This multilevel approach was effective, and it led to earlier case detection, kept the rate of new infections low, and potentially reduced estimated mortality rates by preventing hospital overcrowding and infections among high-risk populations (June-ho, 2020, p. 8).

The work of the EIS officers was further facilitated by legal changes following the 2015 MERS outbreak. When necessary, the officers were permitted to draw on four major types of information in addition to patient and doctor interviews:

- Facility visit records, including pharmacies and medical facilities
- Cellular GPS data from cell phones
- Credit card transaction logs
- Closed-circuit television

This information was combined with interviews and cross-checked with other data to trace contacts and take appropriate containment measures.

4.2.2.4 Social Distancing

Korea implemented the social distancing policy during the pandemic even though it did not institute an entire lockdown. Thus, it allowed limited periods for businesses to operate. For example, restaurants could not be open after 9 p.m. In particular areas that had an outbreak, no more than five people could gather at one time in a restaurant. All citizens had to wear a mask all the time. During the second outbreak in Seoul, public places were temporarily closed. Furthermore, all schools closed for a long time, and the KDCA and Education department tried to cope and respond to the pandemic. An online education system was created for students to have online classes in their homes.

4.2.2.5 Treatment

Regardless of Korea's sufficient medical system, it was difficult to respond to all patients in the month of March 2020. In Daegu, there were more than 5000 people who needed to be checked and treated. KDCA and health officials developed a special system and classified the patients into four levels: mild, moderate, severe, and critical. Many ill people or those with adverse symptoms were sent to the community treatment centers where medical teams could check and monitor them frequently. Severe patients were taken into intensive care, and all patients from the outbreak were provided with almost-free treatment. Korea's health officials used portable negative pressure devices so that the government could easily expand the supply of temporary airborne infection isolation rooms. In Daegu, officials created about 400 additional negative pressure beds during the crisis (June-ho, 2020, p. 9).

Daegu officials also recruited about 2400 additional healthcare workers who were spread out among screening clinics, infectious disease hospitals, and community treatment centers. In addition, 327 physicians volunteered without pay to participate in the public health response, with 30 volunteering for the centralized COVID-19 response team and 250 volunteering for phone triage centers (June-ho, 2020, p. 9).

At the time of the first outbreak, all citizens tried to buy as many masks as they could, which resulted in a shortage of masks. The government tried to control the supply of masks to prevent a panic among citizens. The government further banned the export of masks and made a rule to buy masks for the needs of each citizen. This policy was enforced by the development of a shared database that logged purchases across markets, post offices, and pharmacies.

After the Daegu surge, South Korea took a series of steps to manage the capacity in the health system. The Central Disaster and Safety Countermeasure Committee restructured the healthcare system to form 6 regional clusters (instead of 17 state and city jurisdictions) to make it easier to transfer patients between facilities and manage capacity (June-ho, 2020, p. 10). Currently, a variation of the severity scoring system first used in Daegu is in use nationwide, with four different categories: asymptomatic, mild, moderate, or severe. Asymptomatic and mild cases are placed in one of five residential treatment centers instead of hospitals (June-ho, 2020, p. 11).

4.2.2.6 State Planning and Public and Private Cooperation

Korea employed large-scale testing and tracing in a short period efficiently. These measures were possible because testing and tracing were done locally and the state had the ability to cooperate with the productive sector for national objectives.In the early stage of the COVID-19 outbreak, citizens rushed to buy stocks of masks, as mentioned earlier, and this risked a shortage in masks. The government intervened in late February 2020 and announced that it would buy 50% of the masks produced by national companies. With the Korean pharmacists' associations, the government could control the stock and the sale prices of masks ahead of their commercialization. The government also outlawed the export of masks and requested that national companies increase their production (Schwak & Nardon, 2020, p. 13).

At the same time, there was a campaign by the Seoul metropolitan government on mask use to handle the distribution of masks.

4.2.2.7 Economy

Economically, South Korea is expected to be one of the better-performing countries in 2020. In August, the OECD projected that it would face the least economic impact, as measured by the percentage decrease in GDP for all 37 OECD member countries. In October 2020, South Korea reported a growth of 1.9% from the previous quarter. Much of this growth has been driven by exports of memory chips for electronics and of automobiles to Europe and the United States.

Part of the explanation for this success is that South Korea was able to avoid some of the severe long-term restrictions, such as lockdowns and business closures, that have led to troubled economies in many high-income countries. For example, after the government tightened restrictions in August because of the church outbreak and in late September because of a national holiday, it relaxed them again in October. In fact, the country never activated its highest level of restriction, which would have barred gatherings with more than 10 people and closed gyms and other high-traffic businesses. South Korea faced significant economic disruption, however, including large job losses. The government responded by providing subsidies to businesses for payroll and to unemployment insurance and low-interest loans to low-income job seekers. The Government also lowered insurance premiums for social safety net programmes for individuals and businesses. All households, regardless of income, received a disaster relief payment of KRW 400,000 (US$344) for single-person households, KRW 600,000 (US$516) for two-person households, KRW 800,000 (US$688) for three-person households, and KRW one million (US$859) for households with four or more members (Kim, n.d. p. 2).

4.2.3 Role of Social Work in Korea During the Pandemic

After the pandemic, social problems emerged. In particular, the elderly faced many difficulties. The majority of social workers visited the elderly and took care of them before the pandemic. After the pandemic and social distancing, the fear of getting the disease made this impossible. The vulnerable people who were unable to move easily and needed to be given care faced considerable difficulties. Korea tried to make an 'un-tact' society even before the pandemic. 'Un-tact' is the combination of words of prefix 'un' and the word 'contact.' After the pandemic, an 'un-tact' society seemed to come about more quickly. An 'un-tact' society lets people do many things in their own place without contacting people in person. It also allows people to get information quickly and easily with only one touch or one click. During the pandemic many people easily got tracing information of disease and could get information on where to buy a mask or find out how many stocks were available and when they could buy them. But this 'un-tact' society and the pandemic excluded elders from society and social protection. One 79-year-old person who lives alone in Seoul complained that he had been stuck at home alone for months. Pre-coronavirus, he was a regular at his local senior center but since early February he had stayed home. He is fearful of getting the virus and only ventures out when he absolutely must to get groceries or go to a hospital appointment (Lee, n.d. p. 2).

To solve this kind of isolation and exclusiveness, Korea needed to approach social work in a new way that could adjust under an 'un-tact' society. After the Daegu outbreak, most of the cities closed schools temporarily and students stayed at home. The online education system posed big problems for children. Many children whose parents could not stay home because of work literally stayed home by themselves, and they had a hard time getting online access by themselves. But it was not only that kind of education gap: more dangerous situations occurred. Children were exposed to many dangers. They did not have food if they could not eat at their school. Also, they were exposed to domestic violence more often than before. School systems could not check properly the students' circumstances and this weakness caused severe child abuse. Thus far, the Government has proposed online health promotion programmes for children, emergency care services and allowances, and school meal delivery services. Based on these findings, we recommend the establishment of mental health, sexual abuse, and child abuse online messaging services; allocation of additional financial and educational support to low-income families; and prioritisation of childcare services. Taken together, these recommendations highlight the need for multidimensional services to ensure children's safety and well-being. Because children become more vulnerable during emergency situations and disasters, we must continue to explore ways to protect children during the COVID-19 pandemic while simultaneously preparing them for potential future pandemics (Chun & Kim, 2020).

The Central Government's Supplementary Budget, approved by the National Assembly, will provide livelihood support to all nations (about 21.7 million households). This single project is about 12.2 trillion won in central budget and 2.1 trillion won in local government budget, totaling 14.3 trillion won. It is expected to pay 400,000 won for single-person households, 600,000 won for two-person households, 800,000 won for three-person households, and up to 1000,000 won for four-person households. The payment method is expected to be paid in local currency, and local gift certificates to activate the local economy, in addition to the existing credit and check cards. The expiration date is the end of August 2020, when the unused amount automatically loses all value. In addition, donations can be made through non-receipt of disaster basic income, not only to Korean citizens; the Korean state has not pursued xenophobic policies. Indeed, the state exhorted the 380,000 illegal immigrants living in Korea to seek medical help, tests, and masks, guaranteeing that they would not face legal consequences.

4.3 Vietnam

Vietnam is a Southeast Asia country bordering China, Laos, and Cambodia. It has the longest border line with China, 1200 km. The population of Vietnam (April 2019) is 96.21 million and 65% of its population lives in rural areas. The quality of life has improved significantly over the two decades between 2002 and 2018. Gross domestic product (GDP) per capita has more than doubled, to more than $2500 in 2018, when the country saw real GDP growth of 7.1% (World Economic Forum, 2020). The healthcare system also witnessed improvement, however, there is still room for the national healthcare performance to grow. Vietnam has only about 8 doctors to every 10,000 people, whereas the ratios are 41 doctors per 10,000 people in both Italy and Spain, 26 doctors per 10,000 people in the U.S., and 18 doctors per 10,000 people in China. This background has shaped the Vietnam strategies in managing the coronavirus, which urged the country to act quickly and proactively to avoid a national crisis.

In the early days of 2020, the Government of Vietnam had been highly concerned about a strange virus in Wuhan, China. Having a shared border with China resulted in Vietnam announcing the first COVID-19 case on 23 January 2020, and this was a 60-year-old Chinese man coming from Wuhan. By the second quarter of 2021, Vietnam had reported 9292 cases with 55 deaths (Ministry of Health, 2021). At the time of the third wave of the outbreak, the number of COVID-19 cases in Vietnam stood at 1300, then experienced a significant growth during the fourth wave of the pandemic to reach 9292 cases by the beginning of June 2021. This figure had increased tremendously over a 2-month period from April to June 2021 because of the appearance of the new variant from India. The common view in health management has always been that the ranking of the healthcare system's performance, size of the population, and the financial competence of a nation is correlated with the effectiveness in controlling a pandemic. However, evidence has shown that Vietnam can have a successful coronavirus prevention with no such advantages.

The success of Vietnam in controlling the pandemic and bringing safety to the country is dependent on the involvement and effort of all stakeholders to minimize the spread of the virus and treat the infected people or prevent deaths. In general, the Vietnamese stakeholders made concerted efforts to contain and control the scale of the pandemic. In particular in Vietnam, the role of the government is considered to be the motive force in containing the pandemic by showing a high sense of responsibility from the government to restrict the introduction and spread of the virus (Nguyen, 2020). By the first week, after the Lunar New Year, when the World Health Organization (WHO) reported that there was an outbreak in Wuhan, China that was killing thousands of people, the Vietnamese government decided to close the border with China, including mainland and air travel. All flights from and to Wuhan, China were canceled. In addition, the government began to track the visitors coming from Wuhan within 14 days, and the first 16 cases infected with the virus were identified by the government, police, and local authorities. The first wave of the pandemic was stopped quickly by fast action from the government to restrict contacts with China and isolate these infected patients from the community. It can be argued that the Vietnamese government is considered as an effective leader in delivering appropriate responses to contain the pandemic. The government quickly took action to find and isolate the infected cases and to localize specific areas to end the outbreak faster (Nguyen, 2020). Further, the government decided to sacrifice the economic profits of the country by closing all tourism, hospitality, and events activities and borders to foreign countries such as China and the United Kingdom, to restrict the entrance of the virus from external sources. The fast actions of the government allowed for more time to prepare the health infrastructure such as field hospitals; oxygen therapy devices, ventilators, and other devices; medicines and medical equipment; personal protective equipment (PPE) such as face masks and medical gloves; and transportation vehicles (Nguyen, 2020).

Specifically, when several confirmed patients were discovered in Da Nang on 25 July 2020 and in Hanoi on 7 March 2020, the government decided to enforce these cities under immediate lockdown. All unnecessary activities and services were closed to limit the spread of the virus, and food and other essential commodities were controlled tightly to support the 'new normal.' The national health system implemented third-degree contact tracing to find and isolate people who had close contact with the confirmed patients known to be F0. These people who had come into close contact with this person were known to be F1, F2, and F3. In reality, F1 and F2 were identified and isolated in the specific isolation areas with regular health checks whereas F3s were forced to self-quarantine at home with regular health checks by social workers (Boudreau & Nguyen, 2020). It must be emphasised that the Vietnamese Government organized the quarantine by focusing on exposure instead of finding individuals with clear systems (Boudreau & Nguyen, 2020). The government consulted with the top professionals and experts in virology to decide on concentrating on exposure and providing mandatory testing for the close contacts of confirmed cases.

In addition, the government regularly updated information of the pandemic and announced formally on television, newspapers, and the Internet to warn people about the appearance and expansion of the virus by providing formal information relevant to the coronavirus to the citizens (Pham et al., 2020). The hard efforts of the government helped to avoid panic and affect the stability of Vietnamese society. Furthermore, the government also issued urgent acts, regulations, and policies such as social distancing, quarantine, and lockdown in a short period to ensure that the pandemic was contained by identifying and isolating the infected cases living in the community for treatment and cure (Pham et al., 2020). The Vietnamese government showed consistency in containing the pandemic to reach effectiveness in controlling the virus. Moreover, the government also commended the involvement of the national healthcare system, soldiers, police, and community to lend a hand to contain the pandemic. The Vietnamese Government has boosted the dedicated traditions of fighting against foreign invaders, showing the high spirit of national unity and patriotism of the Vietnamese people to contain the pandemic quickly and efficiently. The Prime Minister of Vietnam has raised the slogan that to stay at home is to fulfill the patriotic duty. The Government informed and offered the community and people to switch from a normal lifestyle to a 'new normal' of wearing a face mask in public places, social distancing 3 meters apart, avoiding direct contact and communication such as handshaking, and washing the hands frequently (Nguyen et al., 2020). Similarly, the government quickly built field hospitals and took advantage of university dormitories for COVID-19 treatment and isolation. These actions show that Vietnam seriously concentrates on restricting the spread of the virus in the community by taking strong, quick, and consistent actions at the same time.

Furthermore, along with the government, people, health workers, enterprises, and organizations in Vietnam also joined to stop the spread of the pandemic and protect the health of the community. Particularly, Vietnamese people were following all guidelines and instructions from the health minister, avoiding crowds and trying to stay at home as much as possible (Pham et al., 2020). The participation of the Vietnamese, from generation to generation worked effectively with the efforts of the government to control the pandemic.

Moreover, Vietnamese people were self-aware and self-disciplined to fulfill the health declaration on the tokhaiyte.com website, created by the government, by reporting on their 14-day routine and supporting social workers and the government to track the infected cases for quarantine, isolation, and treatment (Pham et al., 2020). Practically, the Vietnamese people also showed their positive attitudes to fight against the pandemic by sharing the formal information of the COVID-19 pandemic on social media and the Internet (Diep, 2020). It turns out that wrong information on the pandemic might create a severe panic in society. For example, the panic that happened in the United Kingdom (UK) when a small group of people misunderstood the cause of the pandemic and began to destroy the 5G cable towers in remote areas of the UK. In the case of Vietnam, the involvement of the people to read and share formal information about the pandemic has brought a benefit to the fight against it, helping the government to stabilize society and achieve success in complying with the policies of containing the pandemic. Additionally, the Vietnamese committed deeply in preventing the pandemic by complying with all rules, orders, and regulations from the Government (Nong et al., 2021). Also, the celebrities and billionaires in Vietnam were willing to donate billions of dollars to COVID-19 prevention, building infrastructure, laboratory rooms, and breathing machines or ventilators, lending a hand to prevent and control the pandemic effectively. It can be noted that the consistent socially strong approaches, while encouraging the involvement of multidisciplinary stakeholders, facilitated the development of appropriate solutions and strategies in each phase of the pandemic.

4.3.1 Role of Social Work

Although the government has become a motive force to lead and run the country in the COVID-19 battle, social workers hold a major role in ensuring that the operations of hospitals run smoothly alongside health workers. In general, social work is considered the soul of the process in enhancing patients' experiences at medical facilities. Specifically, throughout the pandemic social workers do the tasks of screening people entering hospitals and teaching preventive measures to patients (Viet Nam News, 2020).

Moreover, during the second and third waves of the pandemic in Hanoi and Danang, social workers were ready to participate in the battle to contain the pandemic. The front-line social workers working in the hospitals sacrificed themselves and pushed themselves into high-risk situations to make sure the communication between COVID-19 patients and doctors was as effective as possible. The high concentration and collaboration between social workers and healthcare staff to stop the growth of the outbreak also showed the serious attitudes of social workers to handle the pandemic in Vietnam.

The social workers also engaged with the Ministry of Labour – Invalids and Social Affairs to assist vulnerable citizens who suffered from the economic impact of the pandemic. Social workers were in charge of providing people living in poverty, the elderly, the unemployed, etc., with correct information about government assistance to Vietnamese. It is an effort to fulfil the motto of 'Leave no one behind' in Vietnam by emphasizing the role of the social work profession to enable effective and equitable distribution of public and private financial aid to vulnerable people. The Ministry of Labour – Invalids and Social Affairs regularly updated the information on government assistance to the citizens on social media, television, and formal newspapers to encourage the Vietnamese during hard times.

4.4 Conclusion

This chapter discussed the COVID-19 outbreak in Korea and Vietnam and how it affected the social work profession to adapt to the situation. The success of Korea and Vietnam in controlling the pandemic refers to the role of the government as the motive force. Another factor that has contributed to the success is the compliance of Vietnamese to all the rules and regulations to prevent the severe spread of the virus. Social workers are considered to have a major role in maintaining the well-being of patients and vulnerable people during the hard times of COVID crises. Also, Korea could handle the pandemic without a nationwide lockdown. Economic activities were diminished but there was little damage compared to other countries. "The K-model," a term referring to Korea's successful COVID-19 response, has made Koreans proud. Still, challenges remain. Social welfare policies need to be double-checked. Social welfare policies for the elderly and children need to be revised and complemented. Lessons from MERS have helped Korea to cope with the pandemic properly. The Korean state handled the pandemic with cooperation with various other departments and Korean citizens also complied well. Economic losses were inevitable, and there were many social problems as well. However, this pandemic also showed which parts needed to be updated and double-checked to make Korean society better. The Korean state learned how to handle the disease and the economic situation at the same time. So, this is the time when the Korean state focuses on social problems and makes better policies for vulnerable people.

References

Boudreau, J., & Nguyen, X. Q. (2020). Hanoi's largest hospital locked down on virus outbreak fears. https://www.bloomberg.com/news/articles/2020-03-28/hanoi-s-largest-hospital-locked-down-on-virus-outbreak-fears. https://www.bloomberg.com/news/articles/2020-03-28/hanoi-s-largest-hospital-locked-down-on-virus-outbreak-fears.

Chun, J. S., & Kim, J. (2020). Child welfare policies and services during the COVID-19 pandemic in South Korea. *Asia Pacific Journal of Social Work and Development, 31*(1–2), 38–44. https://doi.org/10.1080/02185385.2020.1859407

Diep, U. (2020). COVID-19: For Vietnam, information is a public-health weapon. https://www.reportingasean.net/covid-19-vietnam-iinformation-public-health-weapon/. https://www.reportingasean.net/covid-19-vietnam-iinformation-public-health-weapon/

Kim, J. (n.d.). Emerging covid-19 success story: South Korea learned the lessons of mers. Our World in Data. Retrieved November 10, 2021, from https://ourworldindata.org/covid-exemplar-south-korea

Lee, Y. L. (n.d.). The South Koreans left behind in a contact-free society. BBC Worklife. Retrieved November 10, 2021, from https://www.bbc.com/worklife/article/20200803-south-korea-contact-free-untact-society-after-coronavirus

June-ho, K. (2020). Emerging COVID-19 success story: South Korea learned the lessons of MERS. Our World in Data. https://ourworldindata.org/covid-exemplar-south-korea#note-62

Ministry of Health. (2021). Bo Y te: Trang tin ve dich benh viem duong ho hap cap Covid-19. https://ncov.moh.gov.vn/

Nguyen, S. (2020). Vietnam's pandemic success is a lesson for the world. Global Asia, 15(3) https://www.globalasia.org/v15no3/cover/vietnams-pandemic-success-is-a-lesson-for-the-world_sen-nguyen

Nguyen, T., Nguyen, D. C., Nguyen, A., Nguyen, L. H., Vu, G. T., Nguyen, C. T., Nguyen, T. H., & Le, H. T. (2020). Fake news affecting the adherence of national response measures during the COVID-19 lockdown period: The experience of Vietnam. *Frontiers in Public Health, 8*, 589872. https://doi.org/10.3389/fpubh.2020.589872

Nong, V. M., Le Thi Nguyen, Q., Doan, T. T, Van Do, T., Nguyen, T. Q., Dao, C. X., Thi Nguyen, T. H., & Do, C. D. (2021). The second wave of COVID-19 in a tourist hotspot in Vietnam. *Journal of Travel Medicine, 28*(2), taaa174. https://doi.org/10.1093/jtm/taaa174

Park, J. (2020). Changes in subway ridership in response to COVID-19 in Seoul, South Korea: Implications for social distancing. Cureus. https://doi.org/10.7759/cureus.7668

Pham, T. Q., Rabaa, M., Duong, L. H., et al. (2020). The first 100 days of SARS- CoV-2 control in Vietnam. Clinical infectious diseases. https://doi.org/10.1093/cid/ciaa1130

Schwak, J., & Nardon, L. (2020). A democratic tour de force: How the Korean State successfully limited the spread of COVID-19. https://www.ifri.org/en/publications/notes-de-lifri/asie-visions/democratic-tour-de-how-korean-state-successfully-limited

Social Work Action. (2020). International Federation of Social Workers. https://www.ifsw.org/south-korea-sharing-social-workactivities-to-intervent-during-covid-19/

Viet Nam News. (2020, December). Hospitals benefit from great development in social work system. https://vietnamnews.vn/society/831498/hospitals-benefit-from-great-development-in-social-work-system.html

World Economic Forum. (2020). Viet Nam shows how you can contain COVID-19 with limited resources. https://www.weforum.org/agenda/2020/03/vietnam-contain-covid-19.

COVID-19 Safety Measures and Socioeconomic Status in Urban Zimbabwe

5

Rose Jaji

5.1 Introduction

As a novel medical condition, the coronavirus disease (COVID-19) has generated much debate and controversy. However, one area where there is consensus is that when people are exposed to the coronavirus, which causes COVID-19, the virus is somatically oblivious to class or socioeconomic status, among other categories. The virus has infected people from all backgrounds and identity categories under which people can be classified whether one considers infection from a racial, ethnic, gender, age, nationality, and rank or class perspective. Yet, beyond this generalized organic vulnerability, observation of safety measures recommended by the World Health Organization and Centers for Disease Control and Prevention around the world to prevent infection follows the contours of socioeconomic inequalities entrenched by lack of capacity, neglect, or policy indifference to a wide range of issues pertinent to the well-being of the poor. People's socioeconomic circumstances are apposite to practicability of the recommended safety measures to curb the spread of the coronavirus. This chapter specifically focuses on limited mobility, the practice of social distancing, self-isolation, handwashing/sanitizing, and wearing of masks as the main recommended safety measures, paying particular attention to how these practices are mediated by differential socioeconomic circumstances in urban Zimbabwe. The recommended safety measures are to a great degree naturally occurring aspects of everyday life in the homes and residential areas inhabited by the rich, which were designed to guarantee secession from the public and crowded areas, although mainly for reasons other than anticipation of highly infectious diseases such as COVID-19. In contrast, social distancing, self-isolation, handwashing/sanitizing, and wearing of masks require an almost impracticable and radical change in the routines and way of life in the homes and neighborhoods inhabited by the poor as well as in the informal sector where they eke out a living.

5.2 Mobility, A Global Pandemic, and Zimbabwe's Reaction

For many decades, antiimmigration discourses have associated mobility, especially from the poor to more affluent parts of the world, with the spread of diseases. Indeed, this has fueled xenophobia, racism, and other antiimmigration sentiments observable in contemporary times (Feinstein & Bonikowski, 2019; Gorodzeisky et al., 2015; Vaughan, 2020). This association of mobility with the spread of transmissible diseases

R. Jaji (✉)
Department of Sociology, University of Zimbabwe, Harare, Zimbabwe
e-mail: rjaji@sociol.uz.ac.zw

M. C. S. Gonçalves et al. (eds.), *The Coronavirus Crisis and Challenges to Social Development*,
https://doi.org/10.1007/978-3-030-84678-7_5

became particularly salient with the outbreak of COVID-19 in Wuhan, China. In the United States, COVID-19 saw a spike in racism, xenophobia, and anti-Asian hate crimes (Gover et al., 2020). As cases of the highly infectious virus started to be recorded outside China, travelers and governments found themselves in a quandary with the latter having to do a delicate balancing act as they tried to address the mobility aspect of the disease and simultaneously ensure that their economies would not experience the negative effects of a total shutdown of both international and domestic mobility, considering the debilitating impact of global travel restrictions on economic activities such as tourism (see Gössling et al., 2021). This concern is salient for African countries where lockdowns have crippling effects on export-oriented economies, people's livelihoods, and food security (Yaya et al., 2020).

Governments also found themselves treading a fine line between keeping the virus outside their borders and the need to deflect accusations of racism and xenophobia in the process of doing so. This dilemma happened at a time of heightened "anti-" sentiments directed to mobile people, especially those who are conspicuously different in spaces where they presumably do not belong in a nativist scheme of things (see Comaroff & Comaroff, 2005). Interestingly, COVID-19 is being used by right-wing parties in the European Union to champion the narrative that migrants pose a public health danger (Reynolds, 2020), notwithstanding that the EU has had more cases than, for example, the whole continent of Africa. China found itself in a diplomatic row with Nigeria following accusations that Chinese authorities had racialized COVID-19, which ironically started in China, by linking it to African migrants who were forced out of their apartments by Chinese authorities, leading to protest by an official from the Nigerian embassy in China and the summoning by the Nigerian federal government of the Chinese ambassador in Nigeria.[1] Many Africans with online platforms chimed in, reminding China that there were more Chinese citizens in Africa than there were Africans in China.[2]

In an increasingly interconnected world, curbing international mobility as a precautionary measure taken by many governments around the world could not completely deter global mobility, which explains the spread of COVID-19 across the globe, prompting the World Health Organization to declare it a global pandemic. In this respect, COVID-19 provides a reality check on the sobering fact that the advantages that interconnectedness as a hallmark of globalization entails are accompanied by challenges such as those which are observable in the event of infectious diseases (Saker et al., 2004; Wilson, 1995). Reverse logic suggested that a virus that spreads through human mobility would be contained by stopping, reducing, and monitoring mobility.

As much as Zimbabwe reduced international travel by closing its international borders and partially closing its airports, international mobility, although reduced in volume, still occurred. Through globalized mobility, COVID-19 eventually found its way into Zimbabwe as it did to the rest of Africa. There were Zimbabweans who were coming back home, and the country recorded its first case of infection in Victoria Falls and its first death in Harare, both in March 2020. The first death in Harare induced panic and jolted the country into action. Some Zimbabweans who had initially dismissed the coronavirus under the erroneous impression that it would only infect people who traveled outside the country or those who interacted with them, suddenly realized that the disease had become a real threat to everyone in the country. With nonadherence to quarantine

[1]MSN, (2020, April 10). FG summons Chinese ambassador over maltreatment of Nigerians in China. https://www.msn.com/en-xl/africa/nigeria/fg-summons-chinese-ambassador-over-maltreatment-of-nigerians-in-china/ar-BB12qX87. Accessed 02 Dec 2020.

[2]Among the people who spoke out on the discrimination against African migrants in China was former African Union ambassador to the United States, Dr. Arikana Chihombori-Quao, who exhorted President Xi Jinping of China to take the right decisions and extend the same hospitality to Africans that Africa had extended to Chinese living on the continent. See *Oak TV*. President Xi stop the abuse of Africans in China – Amb. Arikana Chihombori-Quao. https://dai.ly/x7tbihq. Accessed 21 Jun 2021.

and self-isolation by people coming into the country, the virus started spreading, and the country inevitably started recording cases of local transmissions. At this point, COVID-19 ceased to be a disease of the mobile as assumed by some sections of the population in the country. The dividing line between the mobile and the immobile became blurred as family members traveling back to the country infected those who had not traveled. As of 3 June 2021, there was a total of 39,031 infections of which there were 36,661 recoveries and 1599 deaths.[3]

Reduction in the number of international travelers was complemented by measures requiring people to change their everyday routines and reorganize their lives under conditions akin to house arrest. As the specter of local infections became reality, restrictions on international mobility were extended to local mobility involving people leaving their homes to go to work, to the supermarket, or to attend to other basic necessities. Many countries around the world accordingly went into lockdown whose logic was to curb infections by limiting mobility and interaction with the world outside the home. Against the backdrop of intermittent strikes by medical staff and an underfunded and ill-equipped public health system incapable of handling the pandemic if infections kept rising, Zimbabwe went into lockdown on 30 March 2020, which was extended twice, on 20 April and again on 3 May 2020. Law enforcement and security personnel were deployed to enforce the lockdown. High-traffic workplaces and supermarkets also recorded cases of infections, which compelled them to temporarily close as they took measures to contain the spread of the virus. Media reports on Zimbabwe between April and July 2020 indicated that many people, including those who had tested positive for the virus, were escaping quarantine centers because of the poor living and sanitary conditions (Mutsaka, 2020). The Zimbabwe Republic Police reported that 270 people returning from outside the country had fled quarantine centers before the lapse of the 21 days that they were mandated to remain at these centers. Some of these people had tested positive, and 30 of them were arrested for fleeing the quarantine centers.[4]

As the government of Zimbabwe placed the country under lockdown, it took into cognizance the fact that the first cases were recorded in urban Zimbabwe and it accordingly banned urban–rural travel to ensure that the virus would not find its way to rural areas where access to health facilities is even more limited and where care is nowhere near the standards required for COVID-19 patients. The government also banned intercity travel to curb the spread of the virus to cities and towns that had not yet been affected. Within the cities, services provided by minibuses used for public transport were suspended as part of the lockdown. Public buses in which people could observe some social distancing remained on the roads to ferry predominantly workers in the essential service category to work. This measure reduced intracity mobility mostly by the poor who rely on public transport. People were required to have official letters from their employers or the police authorizing them to move, and this posed challenges for many people considering that the majority of urban dwellers are self-employed in the informal sector (FinScope, 2012) and their economic activities had been deemed nonessential by the government and therefore prohibited.

5.3 Socioeconomic Status and Access to Information

As the virus started spreading, many urban Zimbabweans with access to the Internet spent a lot of time online for regular updates on ongoing research on the virus, conditions under which infections occur, symptoms, and what to do when the disease became manifest. They also sought information on which masks are effective and how long the virus can survive under various

[3] Worldometer, 22 December 2020. https://www.worldometers.info/coronavirus/country/zimbabwe/. Accessed 03 June 2021.

[4] *Africa News* (2020, July 20). https://www.youtube.com/watch?v=Ala5fEZQLJc. Accessed 24 Nov 2020

conditions, among other concerns associated with the virus. People with access to the Internet can easily search online for information provided by experts and answers to questions they may have, all of which enables them to better protect themselves. While the Internet has proved to be a double-edged sword providing both information and misinformation, it is the people with reliable access to the Internet who could better inform themselves and separate reality from falsehoods in an environment where various conspiracy theories were being thrown around. A couple of these included the idea that COVID-19 vaccines were intended to depopulate Africa and that they were microchip implants connected to the "mark of the beast" in the Bible. Sections of urban Zimbabweans who do not have access to the Internet were left to rely on people such as religious leaders, some of whom were pushing these theories, prompting the state-run newspaper, *The Herald*, to rebuke and ask them to confine themselves to preaching religious messages and leave communication on the disease and the country's vaccination program to scientists.[5]

In countries where it takes time to mobilize resources for outreach and awareness campaigns, most of the poor rely on what filters to them through relevant government offices, local health experts, and the media where they have access to the latter. The poor tend to be the last to get comprehensive and accurate information on how to protect themselves. Limited access to both print and electronic media means that in most cases, the poor rely on rumor and information provided by other citizens, which can result in distortion or misunderstanding. Street interviews by local media showed that some ordinary citizens were not sure about the veracity of the information they had on the virus because it was based on hearsay, as indicated by most of them starting with "We are hearing that…" when they talked about the virus.

Lack of accurate information especially on how the virus is transmitted is illustrated by behavior in public spaces. Safety measures such as social distancing and wearing masks are either not observed or wrongly followed. For example, it is not unusual to find people in public spaces not observing social distancing and at the same time either without masks or wearing them over their chins or around necks. Some cover the mouth and leave the nose outside and greet each other with handshakes and hugs. In some instances, people wear masks in crowded places but after some time they simply take them off or push them down to their chins or necks. People also rely on rumor, distortion, and misinterpretation of information on issues relating to who gets infected and suffers severe symptoms in terms of demographic characteristics such as age and even race. The reckless and unconcerned behavior in public places suggests limited understanding of the virus, which requires constant adherence to the safety measures instead of inconsistent observation.

It does not help that police officers deployed to enforce the lockdown sometimes do not observe the recommended precautions. For example, when Zimbabwe went into lockdown at the end of March 2020, ordinary citizens raised concern with some of them wondering whether the virus spared police officers as they moved around in crowded police trucks without masks. Enforcing the safety measures would be easier if those tasked to do so adhered to them. Nonadherence by law enforcement officers creates, for people without adequate information about the virus, the impression that the virus is not serious or deadly. Indeed, in a country where the poor disproportionately bear the brunt of police brutality, especially when political tensions rise, the severity with which the unmasked police dealt with people who defied the lockdown was interpreted by the public not as strict enforcement of the lockdown but as a case of the "trigger-happy" police using the virus as a pretext to brutalize citizens. There is thus the need to avoid situations in which people observe safety measures because of fear of the police rather than because they have adequate information on the

[5]Fungai Kwaramba, (2021, March 10). Covid-19 vaccinations: experts red-flag sceptical church leaders. *The Herald*. https://www.herald.co.zw/covid-19-vaccination-experts-red-flag-sceptical-church-leaders/. Accessed on 03 June 2021.

danger posed by the coronavirus. Many Zimbabweans tend to wear car seatbelts because of fear of traffic police rather than out of appreciation of their utility as a safety measure, and there is need to avoid replication of the "seat belt" attitude under the coronavirus and COVID-19. It should be fear of COVID-19 rather than fear of the police that motivates observation of the recommended safety measures to curb the spread of the coronavirus but this is unlikely to happen if the police themselves do not practice the same measures that they compel citizens to observe.

5.4 Mobility-Based Livelihoods, Precarity, and the Lockdown

The economic problems that Zimbabwe has experienced in the past two decades and the concomitant high unemployment rate have pushed the majority of urban Zimbabweans into the informal sector (FinScope, 2012). The nature of their economic activities requires them to work outside their homes, mostly in public spaces where they can easily find customers. People who sell fresh farm produce in their neighborhoods or in the Central Business District (CBD) need to travel to the main supply markets where they buy the produce in bulk for resale. As they sell perishables, they have to go to the main market regularly so that they can purchase and sell fresh produce and avoid incurring losses from buying more produce than can be sold before it perishes. Small to medium entrepreneurs need to be in their workshops to earn an income as their economic activities are not readily transferable to their homes. Considering that informal sector activities were deemed "nonessential" under the lockdown, movement became difficult, which resulted in people who survive on the informal sector losing incomes. The requirement that people moving around and traveling have letters authorizing their movement also complicated the situation for people in the informal sector as they could no longer sell their wares at their usual selling points frequented by customers.

Mostly formally employed people with authorization letters and those with cars could still travel without facing hurdles such as being turned back home by police officers and soldiers deployed to enforce the lockdown or not finding transport in the first instance. People who traded in locally available goods thus found themselves in the same situation as cross-border traders who could not leave Zimbabwe to purchase goods for resale back in the country. Although borders were re-opened in December 2020, cross-border traders, just like other cross-border travelers, were required to have COVID-19 test certificates, pegged at between US$50 and US$60. These amounts are beyond the reach of many cross-border traders, most of whom do not have alternative sources of income. The result was some unscrupulous individuals selling forged certificates to travelers at a lower price some of them were found out and arrested.[6]

In the first week of April 2020, which was the first week of the lockdown, the police reported that close to 2000 people had been arrested around the country for defying the lockdown (Marima, 2020). In some cases, beatings by police officers of people who defied the lockdown were recorded.[7] A combination of lack of transport and the sometimes violent enforcement of the lockdown meant that people who relied on the informal sector for incomes and could not work from home were the most affected. Under

[6] Anadolu Agency, (2020, December 08). Zimbabwe: 2 arrested for selling fake COVID-19 test results. https://www.aa.com.tr/en/africa/zimbabwe-2-arrested-for-selling-fake-covid-19-results/2068910 (Accessed on 03 June 2021.

[7] On 16 April 2020, two sisters were arrested at a supermarket in Bulawayo and brutally assaulted by the police for "defying the lockdown". Images of the battered women circulate on social media causing outrage by human rights activists. Opposition Members of Parliament called for an investigation into the incident. The national police spokesperson, Assistant Commissioner Paul Nyathi, stated that six police officers had been arrested for the heavy-handed manner in which the women had been treated. This is according to an article penned by Tshili, N. (2020, May 09). Police "brutality" –women "battered" for lockdown defiance. *The Chronicle*. https://www.chronicle.co.zw/police-brutality-women-battered-for--lockdown-defiance/. Accessed on 26 November 2020.

the lockdown and the ban on "unnecessary" travel or movement, there was no transport for them to go to the main markets to replenish supplies of the goods they traded in or to the city centers where they sold their merchandise. The government deemed informal sectors activities "nonessential" and banned them because they occur in environments where it is difficult to enforce social distancing and handwashing/sanitizing. As the number of cases of infections kept growing, the country remained under lockdown until September 2020 when the lockdown measures were eased to allow for economic activities to take place and schools to reopen. The ban on intercity travel, which started when the lockdown was announced on 30 March 2020, was only lifted on 15 September 2020 when the government relaxed the restrictions and re-opened the economy by, among others, extending business hours from 4:30 p.m. to 6:30 p.m. The easing of the lockdown saw a spike in cases of infections in November 2020, with a number of infections being recorded at boarding schools. The government stated that law enforcement would be deployed again to enforce compliance with the safety measures based on its assessment that many Zimbabweans had stopped practicing them.

Notwithstanding the sometimes brutal enforcement of the lockdown, there were differences in adherence to the lockdown that can be linked to socioeconomic circumstances. The lockdown and the accompanying precautionary measures were introduced at a time when Zimbabwe was experiencing shortages of cash and basic commodities such as fuel, and, in the early days of the lockdown, the staple corn meal. As a result of these shortages, many Zimbabweans spent much of their time in queues where social distancing proved difficult to enforce as jostling for the scarce commodities was the order of the day. The long queues meant that people spent more time in crowded spaces where they were exposed to the virus than in their homes. Considering the low incomes in both the formal and informal sectors, many people cannot afford to buy supplies in bulk and their precarious existence compels them to visit grocery stores or the open-air food markets on a regular basis when they have scraped together enough cash to buy food. This factor counteracts the requirement for people to reduce visits to supermarkets and open-air markets. Although people in the formal sector with access to the Internet can work from home, many Zimbabweans in the informal sector lead a hand-to-mouth existence and need to go out onto the streets every day to sell their wares.

When people defied the lockdown and went to the markets to buy farm produce for resale, these markets, which are usually crowded spaces, made it difficult for social distancing to be enforced. Images of many deserted cities around the world juxtaposed with pictures of crowded streets in Harare circulated on online media platforms as Zimbabweans expressed concern that people in the country seemed oblivious to the pandemic as they were moving around instead of staying at home. Most of the people either did not have face masks or wore them around their necks as they moved around in crowded spaces. In interviews conducted with ordinary citizens by the media, many explained that their choice was between starving to death or dying of COVID-19 and that staying indoors was "luxury" for them.[8] Some of these people rationalized their mobility in spite of the lockdown by stating that there was a higher chance of recovering from COVID-19 than of surviving hunger. The problems that many urban Zimbabweans, especially the poor, face in adhering to the requirement to stay at home were illustrated by the number of arrests for violation of the lockdown. Between March and July 2020, more than 100,000 people were arrested for "unnecessary movement" and not wearing masks.[9] The more economically stable sections of urban dwellers easily bought masks and even face shields for some, but the poorer sections of the population struggled to buy masks for every

[8]Muronzi C. (2020, March 30). "We'll die of hunger first." Despair as Zimbabwe lockdown begins. *Al Jazeera*. https://www.aljazeera.com/economy/2020/3/30/well-die-of-hunger-first-despair-as-zimbabwe-lockdown-begins. Accessed 18 Dec 2020.

[9]*Africa News*, (2020, July 20). Zimbabwe arrests 100,000 for flouting lockdown rules –Police. https://www.youtube.com/watch?v=Ala5fEZQLJc. Accessed 24.11.20.

family member and the majority could only buy surgical masks. Although these masks are effective in protecting people from the coronavirus (see Fischer et al., 2020), they are disposable and require replenishment, which is expensive for many people. The difference in the circumstances of the economically stable and unstable in relation to COVID-19 is aptly captured by Ioannidis (2020, p. 26):

> "The poor, the homeless, people in prisons, and low-wage workers in meat-processing plants and other essential jobs are among the hardest hit, while privileged people like me are videoconferencing in safety. That is a tragic disparity.

The poor's income-generating activities require their physical presence in the places where they run their small businesses, and they most often work in overcrowded spaces that make it difficult for them to protect themselves from infectious diseases such as COVID-19. In contrast, the rich can work from home and avoid gatherings and crowded spaces.

5.5 Physical Space, Personal Hygiene, and COVID-19

Physical space is not neutral because socioeconomic text can be deciphered on it. Like many cities around the world, physical space in urban Zimbabwe is structured around socioeconomic status, which can be traced back to colonial era demarcation of space based on racial ideologies in which the presumed hierarchy among the races was reflected by a corresponding hierarchization of physical space. In terms of residential space under the "colonial ordering of space" (Porter & Yiftachel, 2019, p. 179), the sparsely populated neighborhoods locally referred to as low-density suburbs were historically reserved for white people. Indians had their own suburb in this cluster of urban residential space. Middle-density suburbs were the halfway space inhabited mostly by biracial people and a few "rich" black people while high-density suburbs accommodated black people in Rhodesia as Zimbabwe was known before independence (see Jaji, 2020 for detailed information on these suburbs). The demarcation of residential space in post-independence Zimbabwe continues although the racial dimension has been superseded by socioeconomic status, which means that people of different races can now live in the same suburbs in the low-density cluster based on high income. Notwithstanding official deracialization of space, the crowded high-density suburbs remain poor and black.

The structuring of space in urban Zimbabwe along socioeconomic status creates disparities in capacity to observe the recommended safety measures because of reasons relating to infrastructure and income. Social distancing is easier to observe in the low-density suburbs where fewer people have more space to themselves. In the spacious homes with many rooms found in residential areas inhabited by the financially stable, maintenance of social distance is largely a naturally occurring way of life. In these airy homes, individuals who need to self-isolate have rooms and other facilities all to themselves. The houses are also built on large tracts of land that sometimes have private swimming pools, sport courts, and other amenities. In these suburbs, residents can spend time outdoors because they have the space to exercise and walk in the spacious gardens, which renders the lockdown less stressful. For some rich people, the lockdown has provided the opportunity to enjoy their homes, discover new hobbies, and nurture those that lay dormant when their schedules were busy. For the rich who own large houses with numerous rooms on spacious grounds usually enclosed by high walls, failure to practice social distancing is not a matter of impracticability but of carelessness and choice not to observe the recommended safety precautions. The gated community creates physical and social barriers between the residents within and the people outside (Blandy & Lister, 2005). In the context of COVID-19, this secessionist characteristic of the gated community functions as a naturally occurring form of self-isolation, which provides a level of safety from infectious diseases beyond the reach of the poor living in the crowded high-density suburbs and informal settlements.

In contrast, high-density residential areas, as the name suggests, are overcrowded with many people sharing cramped and claustrophobic living space. The high level of poverty and overcrowding in the high-density suburbs have implications on measures to curb the spread of the coronavirus in urban Zimbabwe. Pathogens naturally thrive in unsanitary and squalid conditions in which many poor people in urban Zimbabwe and, indeed, in many other urban spaces around the world, live. Overcrowding in indoor spaces translates into high concentration of exhaled or emitted microscopic droplets/aerosols and high risk of infection for co-residents of the infected person(s). The high-density areas in Zimbabwe tend to have large families whose members have low levels of education and are not formally employed (Manjengwa et al., 2016). There can be as many as four or more households in a 100-m^2 house sharing confined living space and ablution facilities. In recent years, more accommodation quarters have been built, usually without city council approval, on the small spaces available around the formal houses. Since 2005 when the government launched Operation *Murambatsvina* (Drive Out Filth), under which it demolished these unauthorized structures (see Bratton & Masunungure, 2006; Potts, 2006; Tibaijuka, 2005), they are increasingly being built with the very basic minimum, which means that these are not the most hospitable residences, especially where ablution facilities, which have to be shared by more people, are concerned. Although the government stated that it would build houses for victims of the demolitions under Operation *Garikai/Hlalani Kuhle*, almost none of the victims benefited from this housing scheme.[10] The building of additional unauthorized structures leaves high-density homes with very small spaces outside, which are often used for growing vegetables. There is therefore not much space both inside and outside the houses, and this forces residents to go into the streets, where they encounter sometimes brutal reactions from law enforcement for violating the lockdown.

Social distancing requires a complete overhaul of life, which is almost impracticable in the homes and neighborhoods inhabited by the poor who often share bedrooms as well. In cases where there is need for self-isolation, there simply is no space for people to self-isolate, thus exposing more people to possible infection than would be the case in the low-density suburbs where fewer people live in more spacious houses in which they can have their own living space during self-isolation. The conditions in which the poor live in urban Zimbabwe and around the world diminish their capacity to protect themselves from infectious diseases such as COVID-19 by a combination of factors (Mahabir et al., 2016; Mberu et al., 2016). Lipsitch (2020) clearly explains the circumstances of the poor thus:

> [..] exposure to high doses of virus tends to cause severe disease, and disadvantaged people are often exposed to higher doses due to confined living and working conditions, [and] comorbidities such as heart disease and obesity are higher among disadvantaged people, and lead to more severe outcomes.

Hand sanitizers are a necessity for people who spend much of their time in shared spaces with high human traffic. Yet, it is the people who share much of the spaces they live in or occupy who can least afford hand sanitizers. Exacerbating the situation of the urban poor in Zimbabwe is the fact that the supply of clean water is erratic, thus making regular handwashing difficult to practice. Handwashing is a key aspect of protecting oneself from coronavirus infection, yet people who live in spaces where facilities are shared do not have much water to practice it. Clean water is a basic necessity, but many urban areas in Zimbabwe have gone for many years without a consistent supply of water. When the urban councils provide the water, there is concern among residents especially in the capital city, Harare, that the water is contaminated and not suitable for human consumption (Nhiwatiwa et al., 2011; Teta et al., 2017). The poor have resorted to fetching water from sometimes unsafe sources such as

[10] Reliefweb, 2006, September 08, Zimbabwe: housing policy built on foundation of failures and lies. https://reliefweb.int/report/zimbabwe/zimbabwe-housing-policy-built-foundation-failures-and-lies. Accessed 03 June 2021.

wells they dig on their own. In contrast, the economically stable who can afford hand sanitizers are the same people who also have the means to buy large tanks of water or drill boreholes and have a consistent supply of water, provided that these sources do not dry up in the long dry seasons. Personal hygiene through consistent handwashing or sanitizing is impracticable for people who have limited access to clean water and no money to buy hand sanitizers.

One of the issues raised in relation to COVID-19 is lifestyle, which creates comorbidities that set hurdles for people with unhealthy lifestyles and compromised immune systems to fight the virus. Although much has been written about obesity as a comorbidity, in Zimbabwe, unhealthy diets and a sedentary lifestyle, which are the main culprits for obesity, are not major issues among the poor, to most of whom a sedentary lifestyle and fast food are an indulgence. In urban Zimbabwe, obesity is a threat to the rich who can afford to buy fast food and neglect exercise because they can drive themselves around. A study by Mukora-Mutseyekwa et al., (2019) showed that in Zimbabwe, obesity was related to high wealth status, urban residence, and having a job. In contrast, obesity is not as much of a comorbidity among the poor as is the absence of adequate and nutritious food, which compromises their immune systems. Limited incomes and lack of their own means of transportation also compel the poor to walk long distances. This, in addition to some of the activities they engage in in the informal sector, requires physical exertion, which provides exercise, although much more strenuous physical exertion becomes detrimental to their physical health. As such, obesity in Zimbabwe is a major problem for the economically stable whereas inadequate food lacking in protein and other vital nutrients combined with lack of access to the best healthcare facilities is the main threat to the poor's capacity to fight the virus once infected. People living in economic precarity are also least able to know whether they have underlying conditions or comorbidities because they can hardly afford regular health check-ups as well as tests for COVID-19 itself. Although much has been said about "diseases of affluence" and how they play out with COVID-19, the circumstances of the poor in Zimbabwe and in other parts of the world require that questions be directed to undernourishment and "diseases of poverty" and their interplay with COVID-19.

5.6 Conclusion

The coronavirus, which biologically infects everyone, is a much more potent threat to people living in economic precarity in urban Zimbabwe because the conditions under which they live and work are detrimental to their capacity to practice the recommended safety measures. Various factors interconnect to place people from low socioeconomic statuses in a particularly vulnerable situation. While the rich have access to the Internet, which enables them to access updates on the coronavirus and COVID-19 as well as work from home, the poor whose access to information is limited in addition to the fact that they earn a living in the informal sector seek people as customers instead of shunning them as potential vectors of the highly infectious pathogen. As the economically stable residents of urban Zimbabwe retreat into their airy residences where numerous and spacious rooms enable them to practice social distancing and self-isolation, the urban poor who live in cramped conditions in the crowded neighborhoods of Zimbabwe's cities and towns are forced by their physical environment to unintentionally defy social distancing and self-isolation measures. They live in neighborhoods where personal hygiene is difficult to maintain because overcrowding is combined with an erratic or no supply of clean water. Their economic circumstances limit their capacity to remedy the erratic water supply situation in Zimbabwe's urban areas or buy hand sanitizers as an alternative to handwashing. Buying for the family the most efficacious masks, which may seem basic, is, for the poor, an expense requiring sacrifice of other basic needs. Although fewer people than predicted have been infected or died of COVID-19 in Zimbabwe, the circumstances under which many urban poor live are highly risky. The fact that many of them have not been infected by the virus in spite of their living and working conditions merits research. Indeed, the lower-than-projected numbers of infections and deaths so far across Africa at large merit in-depth study beyond the current, predominantly confounded, and speculative explanations.

References

Blandy, S., & Lister, D. (2005). Gated communities: (ne) gating community development? *Housing Studies, 20*(2), 287–301. https://doi.org/10.1080/0267303030 42000331781

Bratton, M., & Masunungure, E. (2006). Popular reactions to state repression: Operation Murambatsvina in Zimbabwe. *African Affairs, 106*(422), 21–45.

Comaroff, J., & Comaroff, J. L. (2005). Naturing the nation: Aliens, apocalypse, and the postcolonial state. In T. B. Hansen & F. Steppulat (Eds.), *Sovereign bodies: Citizens, migrants, and states in the postcolonial world* (pp. 120–147). Princeton University Press.

Feinstein, Y., & Bonikowski, B. (2019). Nationalist narratives and anti-immigrant attitudes: Exceptionalism and collective victimhood in contemporary Israel. *Journal of Ethnic and Migration Studies, 47*(3), 1–21. https://doi.org/10.1080/1369183X.2019.1620596

FinScope. (2012). *MSME survey Zimbabwe 2012*. Fin MarkTrust. http://documents1.worldbank.org/curated/en/780081468137402417/pdf/945050WP0Box38544 2B0P12644800PUBLIC00ACS.pdf

Fischer, E. P., Fischer, M. C., Grass, D., Henrion, I., Warren, W. S., & Westman, E. (2020). Low-cost measurement of face mask efficacy for filtering expelled droplets during speech. *Science Advances, 6*(36), 1–5.

Gorodzeisky, A., Glikman, A., & Maskileyson, D. (2015). The nature of anti-immigrant sentiment in post-socialist Russia. *Soviet Affairs, 31*(2), 115–135.

Gössling, S., Scott, D., & Hall, C. M. (2021). Pandemics, tourism and global change: A rapid assessment of COVID-19. *Journal of Sustainable Tourism, 29*(1), 1–20. https://doi.org/10.1080/09669582.2020.17587 08

Gover, A. R., Harper, S. B., & Langton, L. (2020). Anti-Asian hate crime during the COVID-19 pandemic: Exploring the reproduction of inequality. *American Journal of Criminal Justice*, 1–21. https://doi.org/10.1007/s12103-020-09545-1

Ioannidis, J. P. A. (2020). *The totality of the evidence. The great disruption: COVID-19 and the global health crisis*. https://papers.ssrn.com/sol3/papers.cfm?abstract_id=3670455&download=yes

Jaji, R. (2020). *Deviant destinations: Zimbabwe and north to south migration*. Lexington Books.

Lipsitch, M. (2020). Good science is good science. In *The great disruption: COVID-19 and the global health crisis*. https://papers.ssrn.com/sol3/papers.cfm?abstract_id=3670455&download=yes

Mahabir, R., Crooks, A., Croitoru, A., & Agouris, P. (2016). The study of slums as social and physical constructs: Challenges and emerging research opportunities. *Regional Studies, Regional Science, 3*(1), 399–419. https://doi.org/10.1080/21681376.2016.12 29130

Manjengwa, J., Matema, C., & Tirivanhu, D. (2016). Understanding urban poverty in two high-density suburbs of Harare, Zimbabwe. *Development Southern Africa, 33*(1), 23–38.

Marima, T. (2020, April). Anxiety over rights violations as Zimbabwe enforces lockdown. *Al Jaazera*. https://www.aljazeera.com/news/2020/4/6/anxiety-over-rights-violations-as-zimbabwe-enforces-lockdown

Mberu, B. U., Haregu, T. N., Kyobutungi, C., & Ezeh, A. C. (2016). Health and health-related indicators in slum, rural, and urban communities: A comparative analysis. *Global Health Action, 9*(1), 33163. https://doi.org/10.3402/gha.v9.33163

Mukora-Mutseyekwa, F., Zeeb, H., Nengomasha, L., & Adjei, N. K. (2019). Trends in prevalence and related risk factors of overweight and obesity among women of reproductive age in Zimbabwe, 2005–2015. *International Journal of Environmental Research and Public Health, 16*(15), 1–13. https://doi.org/10.3390/ijerph16152758

Mutsaka, F. (2020, July). Zimbabwe names people who escaped filthy quarantine centres. *CTV News*. https://www.ctvnews.ca/world/zimbabwe-names-people-who-escaped-filthy-quarantine-centres-1.4977665

Nhiwatiwa, T., Barson, M., Harrison, A. P., Utete, B., & Cooper, R. G. (2011). Metal concentrations in water, sediment and sharptooth catfish *Clarias gariepinus* from three peri-urban rivers in the upper Manyame catchment, Zimbabwe. *African Journal of Aquatic Science, 36*(3), 243–252. https://doi.org/10.2989/160 85914.2011.636906

Porter, L., & Yiftachel, O. (2019). Urbanizing settler-colonial studies: Introduction to the special issue. *Settler Colonial Studies, 9*(2), 177–186. https://doi.org/10.1080/2201473X.2017.1409394

Potts, D. (2006). "Restoring order"? Operation Murambatsvina and the urban crisis in Zimbabwe. *Journal of Southern African Studies, 32*(2), 273–291. https://doi.org/10.1080/03057070600656200

Reynolds, J. (2020). Fortress Europe, global migration and the global pandemic. *Symposium on COVID-19. Global Mobility and International Law*. https://doi.org/10.1017/aju.2020.64

Saker, L., Lee, K., Cannito, B., Gilmore, A., & Campbell-Lendrum, D. (2004). Globalization and infectious diseases: A review of the linkages. UNICEF/UNDP/World Bank/WHO special Programme for Research & Training in tropical diseases (TDR), social, economic and Behavioural (SEB) research, special topics no. 3. https://www.who.int/tdr/publications/documents/seb_topic3.pdf

Teta, C., Ncube, M., & Naik, Y. S. (2017). Heavy metal contamination of water and fish in peri-urban dams around Bulawayo, Zimbabwe. *African Journal of Aquatic Science, 42*(4), 351–358. https://doi.org/10.2989/16085914.2017.1392925

Tibaijuka, A. K. (2005). *Report of the fact-finding mission to Zimbabwe to assess the scope and impact of operation Murambatsvina*. United Nations.

Vaughan, K. R. (2020). Anti-immigrant sentiment and opposition to democracy in Europe. *Journal of Immigrant & Refugee Studies*. https://doi.org/10.1080/15562948.2020.1843749

Wilson, M. E. (1995). Travel and the emergence of infectious diseases. *Emerging Infectious Diseases, 1*(2), 39–46. https://doi.org/10.3201/eid0102.950201

Yaya, S., Otu, A., & Labonte, R. (2020). Globalisation in the time of COVID-19: Repositioning Africa to meet the immediate and remote challenges. *Globalization and Health, 16*(1). https://doi.org/10.1186/s12992-020-00581-4

Face Mask Wearing in Kampala, Uganda

6

Paul Bukuluki and Peter Kisaakye

Abbreviations

CDC	Centre for Disease Control
KCCA	Kampala Capital City Authority
LICs	Low-Income Countries
NASW	National Association of Social Workers
SSA	sub-Saharan Africa
WHO	World Health Organization

6.1 Introduction

The emergence of COVID-19 as a result of acute respiratory infection (Kumar et al., 2020) in December 2019 (Yee et al., 2020) called for behavioral protective measures to prevent its spread (Balachandar et al., 2020). Some of the behavioral protective practices that prevent the spread of COVID-19 include social distancing (Lewnard & Lo, 2020), restricted movement (Atalan, 2020), handwashing (Desai & Aronoff, 2020; Kisaakye et al., 2020), and the use of face masks (Abdullahi et al., 2020; Brainard et al., 2020; Kumar et al., 2020; Landi et al., 2021; Mitze et al., 2020).

A face mask is a low-cost, nonpharmaceutical behavioral protective practice (Li et al., 2020). Face mask wearing protects against cross-contamination among medical practitioners, patients, and health workers (Kumar et al., 2020). The use of face masks also prevents infection among people in crowded places from inhaling infected viral particles (Carbon, 2020; Kähler & Hain, 2020; Leung et al., 2020; O'Dowd et al., 2020). Other benefits of face mask wearing include protection against inhaling poisonous fumes or touching the mouth or nose with dirty or infected hands (Chua et al., 2020; Khadka et al., 2020).

Despite the benefits of face mask wearing, previous studies (Aloui-Zarrouk et al., 2020; Cheng et al., 2020; Machida et al., 2020; Missoni et al., 2020; Sookaromdee & Wiwanitkit, 2020) point to uncertainty surrounding the quality of face masks, poor use, and their shortage and efficiency in low-income countries. Moreover, a sizeable number of people have not embraced the idea of face mask wearing in public spaces (Howard, 2020; Tucho & Kumsa, 2021) despite having knowledge about the spread of COVID-19 and the effectiveness of face mask wearing (Dzisi & Dei, 2020). For example, previous research

P. Bukuluki (✉)
Department of Social Work and Social Administration, School of Social Sciences, Makerere University, Kampala, Uganda
e-mail: pbukuluki@chuss.mak.ac.ug; pbukuluki@gmail.com

P. Kisaakye
Department of Population Studies, School of Statistics and Planning, Makerere University, Kampala, Uganda

M. C. S. Gonçalves et al. (eds.), *The Coronavirus Crisis and Challenges to Social Development*,
https://doi.org/10.1007/978-3-030-84678-7_6

(Adesegun et al., 2020) reported low frequency of face mask wearing among Nigerians despite knowing about the spread of COVID-19. In Sudan, only a third of residents was reported to be practicing face mask wearing (Hezima et al., 2020). In Ethiopia, about 50% of respondents did not wear a face mask while leaving home although they were going to a crowded place (Haftom et al., 2020). Results from a survey in Uganda reported that only 68% of respondents had correct information about face mask wearing (Mboowa et al., 2021).

Reasons for non-use of face masks include cost (Dzisi & Dei, 2020), lack of correct education (Khadka et al., 2020; Olum et al., 2020; Tso & Cowling, 2020), poor understanding about face mask wearing (Yıldırım & Güler, 2020), myths related to COVID-19 infection (Naeem & Bhatti, 2020; Sahoo et al., 2020), and stigma related to face mask wearing (Song et al., 2020).

This study examined the factors that influence face mask wearing inside public spaces among urban dwellers in the greater Kampala metropolitan area [areas under Kampala Capital City Authority (KCCA) and its surrounding suburbs of Mpigi, Mukono, and Wakiso] in Uganda. The greater Kampala metropolitan geographic area was considered for the study because it is a high-risk area for COVID-19 infection (Government of Uganda, 2020) and represents different environmental settings such as slums, congestion, and traffic jams, which facilitate the easy spread of COVID-19 (Janusz et al., 2019; Ssemugabo et al., 2021). Further, the greater Kampala area is one of the most densely populated areas in Uganda, which facilitates congestion or overcrowding (Uganda Bureau of Statistics, 2016).

Therefore, this study aimed to present the design of effective strategies aimed at promoting face mask wearing among urban dwellers in low-income countries such as Kampala, Uganda. The results from this study can also provide better insights in understanding the myths related to face mask wearing (Greenhalgh et al., 2020; Howard, 2020).

6.2 Data and Methods

This study formed part of the project whose aim was to investigate the impact of COVID-19 on social support systems. We analyzed data collected for a period of 3 months (August–November 2020) during which lockdown and mobility restrictions were lifted (Development Initiatives, 2020; Government of Uganda, 2020). We collected information from 1054 urban respondents from Greater Kampala Metropolitan, which includes areas under Kampala Capital City Authority (KCCA) and its surrounding suburbs of Mpigi, Mukono, and Wakiso.

We used accidental sampling to recruit respondents for interview. The accidental sampling method is mostly used by researchers when the researcher wants to take advantage of easy access, geographic proximity, and the availability and willingness of people to participate in the study (Etikan et al., 2016). We adopted such a sampling approach given the prevailing circumstances of COVID-19 (for example, minimal movements to people's households, shorter hours of daily work because of curfew). Interviewers positioned themselves in busy spots to interview people passing by who were willing and consented to participate in the study.

All standard operating procedures (SOPs) for collecting data during the COVID-19 pandemic as guided by the World Health Organization were followed (WHO, 2020). For emphasis, all respondents wore a face mask during the consenting process and during the interview. The response rate for this study was 81%, given that we had estimated a total sample of 1300 respondents.

We collected information on the age (18 years and older) and sex of the respondents (female or male), if wearing a face mask evokes emotional feelings (yes or no), seeing someone wear a face mask evokes emotional feelings (yes or no), and wearing a face mask has meaning related to culture (yes or no). Respondents were asked whether they wear a face mask inside public spaces (yes or no) to prevent COVID-19 infection. This question was used to measure knowledge, perception of risk to COVID-19 infection, and efficacy of face masks (as the outcome variable).

Stata software version 15.0 (StataCorp, 2017) was used for data analysis to present frequency distributions, bivariate relationships, and multivariate results. We fitted a binary logistic regression model to examine the determinants of knowledge, perception of risk to COVID-19 infection, and the efficacy of face masks.

Permission to conduct this study was granted by the School of Social Sciences Research Ethics Committee at Makerere University. We sought consent from all respondents who participated in the study. The interview duration ranged from 30 to 45 min.

6.3 Results

6.3.1 Distribution of Respondents

Table 6.1 shows the distribution of respondents in the study. Slightly more than half (53%) of respondents were female and nearly half of respondents (49%) were in the age group 25–34 years. About 90% of respondents said that wearing a face mask or seeing someone wear a face mask does not evoke any emotional feelings. The majority of respondents (95%) said that wearing a face mask has no meaning related to culture.

Table 6.1 Distribution of respondents

Variable(s)	Number	Percent
Sex of respondent		
Female	559	53.3
Male	489	46.7
Age of respondent (years)		
18–24	209	20.0
25–34	509	48.6
35–44	243	23.2
45+	86	8.2
Wearing a face mask evokes emotional feelings		
No	934	89.6
Yes	109	10.4
Seeing someone wear a face mask evokes emotional feelings		
No	944	90.2
Yes	103	9.8
Wearing a face mask has meaning related to culture		
No	996	95.1
Yes	51	4.9
Total	1054	100

Note: Missing cases are not shown. Figures may not add up to 100% due to rounding errors

6.3.2 Proportion of Respondents Wearing a Face Mask in Public Spaces to Prevent COVID-19 Infection

Respondents were asked whether wearing a face mask inside or outside public spaces can prevent COVID-19 infection. These questions were used to measure knowledge, perception of risk to COVID-19 infection, and efficacy of face masks. Figure 6.1 shows that the majority of female (92%) and male (91%) respondents wore a face mask inside public spaces to prevent COVID-19 infection.

6.3.3 Relationship Between Selected Variables and Knowledge, Perception of Risk to COVID-19 Infection, and the Efficacy of Face Masks

Table 6.2 shows results of bivariate relationships between selected variables and whether wearing a face mask inside public spaces can prevent COVID-19 infection. The results indicate a significant relationship between 'seeing someone wear a face mask evokes emotional feelings' and wearing a face mask inside public spaces to prevent COVID-19 infection. Overall, the majority of respondents (91%) wore a face mask inside public spaces to prevent COVID-19 infection.

6.3.4 Determinants of Knowledge, Perception of Risk to COVID-19 Infection, and Efficacy of Face Masks

The results presented in Table 6.3 are from a binary logistic regression model. Results indicate that 'seeing someone wear a face mask evokes

Fig. 6.1 Wearing a face mask in public spaces

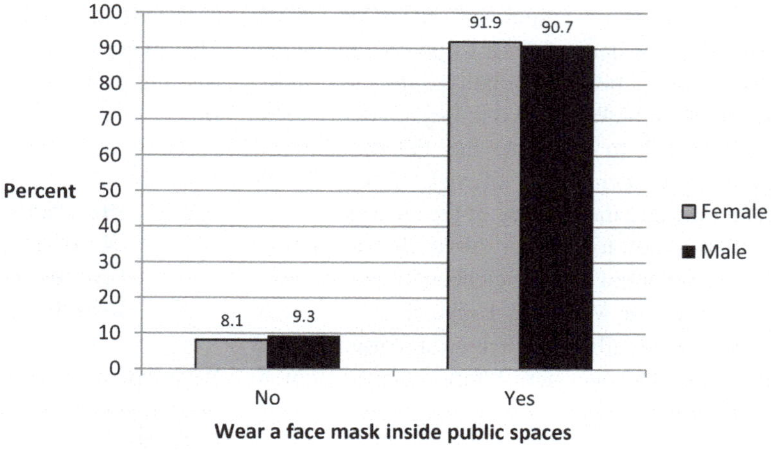

Table 6.2 Relationship between selected variables and wearing a face mask in public spaces

Variable(s)	Wear a face mask inside public spaces: No	Yes	Chi-square (*P*-value)
Sex of respondent			0.43 (0.510)
Female	8.1	91.9	
Male	9.3	90.7	
Age of respondent			3.51 (0.319)
18–24	6.7	93.3	
25–34	9.7	90.3	
35–44	9.1	90.9	
45+	4.7	95.3	
Wearing a face mask evokes emotional feelings			0.03 (0.854)
No	8.7	91.3	
Yes	9.3	90.7	
Seeing someone wear a face mask evokes emotional feelings			6.41** (0.011)
No	9.4	90.6	
Yes	2.0	98.0	
Wearing a face mask has meaning related to culture			0.09 (0.765)
No	8.6	91.4	
Yes	9.8	90.2	
Total (%)	8.7	91.3	
Total (*N*)	91	954	

Note: ***P* < 0.05. Missing cases are not shown. Figures may not add up to 100% due to rounding errors

emotional feelings' emerged as the only significant determinant of wearing a face mask inside public spaces. Respondents who agreed (yes) that wearing a face mask evokes emotional feelings were more likely (OR = 1.73; 95% CI = 1.16–2.59) to wear a face mask inside public spaces than their counterparts who disagreed that wearing a face mask evokes emotional feelings.

6.4 Discussion

Our study demonstrates that the majority of the respondents wore a face mask inside public spaces. Overall, the majority of respondents (91%) wore a face mask inside public spaces to prevent COVID-19 infection. Therefore, our findings have shown that that most of the respon-

Table 6.3 Relationship between selected variables and wearing a face mask in public spaces

Variable	Odds ratio (95% CI)
Sex of respondent (RC = female)	
Male	0.93 (0.79–1.10)
Age of respondent (RC = 45+)	
18–24	0.88 (0.60–1.29)
25–34	0.77 (0.54–1.09)
35–44	0.77 (0.53–1.12)
Wearing a face mask evokes emotional feelings (RC = No)	
Yes	0.83 (0.60–1.13)
Seeing someone wear a face mask evokes emotional feelings (RC = No)	
Yes	1.73*** (1.16–2.59)
Wearing a face mask meaning related to culture (RC = No)	
Yes	0.95 (0.65–1.40)
Constant	3.11**** (2.19–4.40)
Number of observations	1026
Likelihood ratio chi-squared (Probability)	12.88 (0.075)

Note: RC Reference category; confidence intervals (CI) in parentheses: ***$P < 0.01$; **** $P < 0.001$

dents appreciate the need to wear face masks to prevent COVID-19. However, our results also demonstrate that wearing face masks in public places is not universal (Adesegun et al., 2020; Dzisi & Dei, 2020). Other studies in Sub-Saharan Africa also show similar findings (Adesegun et al., 2020; Haftom et al., 2020; Hezima et al., 2020; Mboowa et al., 2021).

Our study shows a higher percentage of respondents who were knowledgeable about face mask wearing. These results are quite different from the findings of Mboowa et al. (2021) in a study in Uganda. It shows a relatively lower proportion (68%) of respondents in their study had received information about the use of face masks (Mboowa et al., 2021). The difference in findings may be attributed to methodological differences, especially in sampling. For example, the study by Mboowa and colleagues targeted only high-risk populations whereas this current study targeted all categories of people. Our study may also differ from those carried out in remote rural areas that could have challenges related to meeting the cost of face masks (Dzisi & Dei, 2020), access to information (Khadka et al., 2020; Olum et al., 2020; Tso & Cowling, 2020), and where the perception of risk for COVID-19 is lower than in urban settings where prevalence of COVID-19 is relatively high (Government of Uganda, 2020).

Our results show that psychosocial/emotional feelings related to mask wearing were a key determinant of the likelihood to always wear a face mask inside public spaces. This finding suggests that wearing face masks evokes emotions that should not be taken for granted and that require further exploration. These results further suggest that information education and communication strategies or social behavioral change communication initiatives need to give consideration to psychosocial issues associated with wearing face masks in various contexts, which could be a reflection of empathy as a motivation to wear a face mask to protect self and others from COVID-19. It could also be feelings linked to stress those who wear masks endure in terms of expressing themselves (without facial expressions) or continuing to maintain their identity with only part of their face seen. Other studies have also pointed to emotional and psychosocial related issues that are associated with wearing face masks in the context of COVID-19 (Carbon, 2020; Song et al., 2020). However, this is an area that requires further investigation, particularly using qualitative research methods to understand the human stories and life experiences linked to wearing face masks in the context of COVID-19.

As in other studies conducted in Sub-Saharan Africa (SSA) contexts (Adesegun et al., 2020; Haftom et al., 2020; Hezima et al., 2020; Mboowa et al., 2021), our results also demonstrate that wearing face masks in public places is not universal. It is likely that particularly groups of people who are vulnerable and at risk, especially in the urban slums of greater Kampala city, are less likely to consistently wear face masks. In fact, studies that have targeted the most at-risk population categories have reported lower face mask wearing (Mboowa et al., 2021). Given the special interest of social work in promoting social justice and equity, there is need for social workers to engage in advocacy campaigns to promote access and use of masks for all, particularly those who are vulnerable and at risk. Social workers should also consider paying attention to structural factors such as social/gender norms and their influence in access and utilization of face masks, particularly in low-income communities. This consideration would also fit within the discourse for universal health coverage and "leaving no one behind" that is promoted under the Sustainable Development Goals and in line with the social work ethics and values.

Given that our results show that psychosocial dimensions related to face mask wearing were a key determinant of the likelihood to always wear a face mask inside public spaces, social workers need to explore in depth the mental health and psychosocial issues related to face mask wearing to prevent COVID-19 transmission. In some communities, it has been documented that face mask wearing can attract stigma and discrimination that can affect psychosocial well-being. Beyond face mask wearing, being a survivor of COVID-19 also has potential for attracting stigma in the family, workplace, and the community (Carbon, 2020; Song et al., 2020). Given the competencies of the social work profession in psychosocial support and offering counselling, there is need for strategic engagement by social workers at different levels including policy engagement, developing guidelines for psychosocial support in the context of COVID-19 and its effects including those related to wearing face masks and in direct service delivery at the health facilities and in the community. This need is especially important given that the other control measures of COVID-19 in countries such as Uganda did not, until recently, recognise and facilitate participation of social workers in response to the COVID-19 pandemic. For example, the probation officers and the community development officers were not among the essential staff during the early months of the lockdown in Uganda, yet they are a critical cadre in providing information, counselling, and psychosocial support particularly to the most vulnerable populations. Social workers should therefore use their role as social activists to ensure that they are granted space at national and sub-national levels to offer professional support and to promote policies that foster equity, social justice, human dignity, and human rights. As rightly emphasised by the National Association of Social Workers (NASW), "social workers are in a unique position to promote disease prevention efforts (including disseminating accurate information from trusted sources), and to help address anxiety and other concerns that are arising as a result of this public health crisis" (NASW, 2021).

6.5 Conclusions

The findings reported in this study indicate that although face mask wearing is not universal, knowledge about face mask wearing as a preventive measure against COVID-19 infection among urban dwellers in Greater Kampala Metropolitan area is relatively high. We argue that universal face mask wearing can be achieved through a combination of approaches such as mass education, peer communication, and community-based approaches. Advocacy campaigns by social workers at different levels (political, social, and individual) are also likely to lead to change in behavior, and promote continuous face mask wearing as a preventive measure against COVID-19 infection. Finally, actors involved in social-behavioral change communication for prevention of transmission of COVID-19 should take into account psychosocial and emotional related factors associated with face mask wearing.

6.6 Limitations

This study highlights two main limitations. First, the results may not be representative because accidental sampling was used to select respondents. Second, results may not be generalisable to the entire population because the sample includes only respondents from Greater Kampala Metropolitan area.

6.7 Recommendations

The results presented in this study suggest an information gap. We therefore recommend raising awareness about the dangers of COVID-19, infection pathways, and prevention to increase use of face masks or even lead to embracing the idea of face mask wearing inside public spaces. Raising awareness can be in the form of mass education through information sharing, and distribution of sanitation materials such as soap and sanitizers as well as face masks (Khadka et al., 2020).

Acknowledgments We thank Dr. Hadijah Mwenyango and Dr. Diane Gardsbane for their contribution to development of tools for the study on which this manuscript is based.

Availability of Data and Materials The datasets used in this study are available from the corresponding author on request.

Competing Interest The authors declare that they have no competing interests.

Funding We received no funding for this study.

References

Abdullahi, L., Onyango, J. J., Mukiira, C., Wamicwe, J., Githiomi, R., Kariuki, D., & Mayieka, L. (2020). Community interventions in low-and middle-income countries to inform COVID-19 control implementation decisions in Kenya: A rapid systematic review. *PLoS One, 15*(12), e0242403. https://doi.org/10.1371/journal.pone.0242403

Adesegun, O. A., Binuyo, T., Adeyemi, O., Ehioghae, O., Rabor, D. F., Amusan, O., & Abiodun, O. (2020). The COVID-19 crisis in sub-Saharan Africa: Knowledge, attitudes, and practices of the Nigerian public. *The American Journal of Tropical Medicine and Hygiene, 103*(5), 1997–2004. https://doi.org/10.4269/ajtmh.20-0461

Aloui-Zarrouk, Z., El Youssfi, L., Badu, K., Francis Fagbamigbe, A., Matoke-Muhia, D., Ngugi, C., & Mwaura, G. (2020). The wearing of face masks in African countries under the COVID-19 crisis: Luxury or necessity? [version 1; peer review: 1 approved, 1 approved with reservations]. *AAS Open Research, 3*(36). https://doi.org/10.12688/aasopenres.13079.1

Atalan, A. (2020). Is the lockdown important to prevent the COVID-19 pandemic? Effects on psychology, environment and economy-perspective. *Annals of Medicine and Surgery, 56*, 38–42. https://doi.org/10.1016/j.amsu.2020.06.010

Balachandar, V., Mahalaxmi, I., Kaavya, J., Vivekanandhan, G., Ajithkumar, S., Arul, N., & Mohana Dev, S. (2020) COVID-19: Emerging protective measures. *European Review for Medical and Pharmacological Sciences, 24*(6), 3422–3425. https://doi.org/10.26355/eurrev_202003_20713

Brainard, J., Jones, N., Lake, I., Hooper, L., & Hunter, P. R. (2020). Facemasks and similar barriers to prevent respiratory illness such as COVID-19: A rapid systematic review. In *medRxiv*. https://doi.org/10.1101/2020.04.01 20049528

Carbon, C.-C. (2020). Wearing face masks strongly confuses counterparts in reading emotions *Frontiers in Psychology, 11*(2526), 566886. https://doi.org/10.3389/fpsyg.2020.566886

Cheng, K. K., Lam, T. H., & Leung, C. C. (2020). Wearing face masks in the community during the COVID-19 pandemic: Altruism and solidarity. *The Lancet*. https://doi.org/10.1016/S0140-6736(20)30918-1

Chua, M. H., Cheng, W., Goh, S. S., Kong, J., Li, B., Lim, J. Y. C., & Loh, X. J. (2020). Face masks in the new COVID-19 normal: Materials, testing, and perspectives. *Research 2020*, 7286735. https://doi.org/10.34133/2020/7286735

Desai, A. N., & Aronoff, D. M. (2020). Masks and coronavirus disease 2019 (COVID-19). *JAMA, 323*(20), 2103–2103. https://doi.org/10.1001/jama.2020.6437

Development Initiatives. (2020). Socioeconomic impact of Covid-19 in Uganda. How has the government allocated public expenditure for FY2020/21?

Dzisi, E. K. J., & Dei, O. A. (2020). Adherence to social distancing and wearing of masks within public transportation during the COVID 19 pandemic. *Transportation Research Interdisciplinary Perspectives, 7*, 100191. https://doi.org/10.1016/j.trip.2020.100191

Etikan, I., Musa, S. A. & Alkassim, R. S. (2016). Comparison of convenience sampling and purposive sampling. *American Journal of Theoretical and Applied Statistics, 5*(1), 1–4. https://doi.org/10.11648/j.ajtas.20160501.11

Government of Uganda. (2020). Update on COVID-19 response in Uganda Available: https://www.health.go.ug/cause/update-on-covid-19-response-in-uganda-22-december-2020/ Accessed 14 February 2021

Greenhalgh, T., Schmid, M. B., Czypionka, T., Bassler, D., & Gruer, L. (2020). Face masks for the public during the covid-19 crisis. *BMJ, 369*, m1435. https://doi.org/10.1136/bmj.m1435

Haftom, M., Petrucka, P., Gemechu, K., Mamo, H., Tsegay, T., Amare, E., & Gebremariam, A. (2020). Knowledge, attitudes, and practices towards COVID-19 pandemic among quarantined adults in Tigrai region, Ethiopia. *Infection and Drug Resistance, 13*, 3727–3737. https://doi.org/10.2147/IDR.S275744

Hezima, A., Aljafari, A., Aljafari, A., Mohammad, A., & Adel, I. (2020). Knowledge, attitudes, and practices of Sudanese residents towards COVID-19. *Eastern Mediterranean Health Journal, 26*(6), 646–651. https://doi.org/10.26719/emhj.20.076

Howard, M. C. (2020). Understanding face mask use to prevent coronavirus and other illnesses: Development of a multidimensional face mask perceptions scale. *British Journal of Health Psychology, 25*(4), 912–924. https://doi.org/10.1111/bjhp.12453

Janusz, K., Kesteloot, C., Vermeiren, K., & Van Rompaey, A. (2019). Daily mobility, livelihoods and transport policies in Kampala, Uganda: A Hägerstrandian analysis. *Tijdschrift voor Economische en Sociale Geografie, 110*(4), 412–427. https://doi.org/10.1111/tesg.12349

Kähler, C. J., & Hain, R. (2020). Fundamental protective mechanisms of face masks against droplet infections. *Journal of Aerosol Science, 148*, 105617. https://doi.org/10.1016/j.jaerosci.2020.105617

Khadka, S., Hashmi, F. K., & Usman, M. (2020). Preventing COVID-19 in low- and middle-income countries. *Drugs & Therapy Perspectives, 36*(6), 250–252. https://doi.org/10.1007/s40267-020-00728-8

Kisaakye, P., Ndagurwa, P., & Mushomi, J. (2020). An assessment of availability of handwashing facilities in households from four east African countries. *Journal of Water, Sanitation and Hygiene for Development, 11*(1), 75–90. https://doi.org/10.2166/washdev.2020.129

Kumar, J., Katto, M. S., Siddiqui, A. A., Sahito, B., Jamil, M., Rasheed, N., & Ali, M. (2020). Knowledge, attitude, and practices of healthcare workers regarding the use of face mask to limit the spread of the new coronavirus disease (COVID-19). *Cureus, 12*(4), e7737. https://doi.org/10.7759/cureus.7737

Landi, F., Marzetti, E., Sanguinetti, M., Ciciarello, F., Tritto, M., Benvenuto, F., & Bernabei, O. B. (2021). Should face masks be worn to contain the spread of COVID-19 in the postlockdown phase? *Transactions of the Royal Society of Tropical Medicine and Hygiene, 115*(1), 74–77. https://doi.org/10.1093/trstmh/traa085

Leung, N. H. L., Chu, D. K. W., Shiu, E. Y. C., Chan, K.-H., McDevitt, J. J., Hau, B. J. P., & Cowling, B. J. (2020). Respiratory virus shedding in exhaled breath and efficacy of face masks. *Nature Medicine, 26*(5), 676–680. https://doi.org/10.1038/s41591-020-0843-2

Lewnard, J. A., & Lo, N. C. (2020). Scientific and ethical basis for social-distancing interventions against COVID-19. *The Lancet Infectious Diseases, 20*(6), 631–633. https://doi.org/10.1016/S1473-3099(20)30190-0

Li, T., Liu, Y., Li, M., Qian, X., & Dai, S. Y. (2020). Mask or no mask for COVID-19: A public health and market study. *PLoS One, 15*(8), e0237691. https://doi.org/10.1371/journal.pone.0237691

Machida, M., Nakamura, I., Saito, R., Nakaya, T., Hanibuchi, T., Takamiya, T., & Inoue, S. (2020). Incorrect use of face masks during the current COVID-19 pandemic among the general public in Japan. *International Journal of Environmental Research and Public Health, 17*(18), 6484. https://doi.org/10.3390/ijerph17186484

Mboowa, G., Musoke, D., Bulafu, D., & Aruhomukama, D. (2021). Face-masking, an acceptable protective measure against COVID-19 in Ugandan high-risk groups. *The American Journal of Tropical Medicine and Hygiene, 104*(2), 502–513. https://doi.org/10.4269/ajtmh.20-1174

Missoni, E., Armocida, B., & Formenti, B. (2020). Face masks for all and all for face masks in the COVID-19 pandemic: Community level production to face the global shortage and shorten the epidemic. *Disaster Medicine and Public Health Preparedness*, 1–5. https://doi.org/10.1017/dmp.2020.207

Mitze, T., Kosfeld, R., Rode, J., & Wälde, K. (2020). Face masks considerably reduce COVID-19 cases in Germany. *Proceedings of the National Academy of Sciences, 117*(51), 32293. https://doi.org/10.1073/pnas.2015954117

Naeem, S. B., & Bhatti, R. (2020). The Covid-19 'infodemic': A new front for information professionals. *Health Information and Libraries Journal, 37*(3), 233–239. https://doi.org/10.1111/hir.12311

NASW. (2021). *Coronavirus (COVID-19)*. https://www.socialworkers.org/Practice/Infectious-Diseases/Coronavirus

O'Dowd, K., Nair, K. M., Forouzandeh, P., Mathew, S., Grant, J., & Moran, R. (2020). Face masks and respirators in the fight against the COVID-19 pandemic: A review of current materials, advances and future perspectives. *Materials, 13*(15), 3363. https://doi.org/10.3390/ma13153363

Olum, R., Chekwech, G., Wekha, G., Nassozi, D. R., & Bongomin, F. (2020). Coronavirus Disease-2019: Knowledge, attitude, and practices of health care workers at Makerere University teaching hospitals, Uganda. *Frontiers in Public Health, 8*, 181. https://doi.org/10.3389/fpubh.2020.00181

Sahoo, S., Padhy, S. K., Ipsita, J., Mehra, A., & Grover, S. (2020). Demystifying the myths about COVID-19 infection and its societal importance. *Asian Journal of Psychiatry, 54*, 102244–102244. https://doi.org/10.1016/j.ajp.2020.102244

Song, L. J., Xu, S., Xu, S. L., Sun, Z., & Liu, W. (2020). Psychology of wearing face masks to prevent transition of COVID-19. *General Psychiatry, 33*(6), e100297. https://doi.org/10.1136/gpsych-2020-100297

Sookaromdee, P., & Wiwanitkit, V. (2020). Limited supply of face masks for use in healthcare settings. *Influenza and Other Respiratory Viruses, 15*, 419. https://doi.org/10.1111/irv.12817

Ssemugabo, C., Nalinya, S., Lubega, G. B., Ndejjo, R., & Musoke, D. (2021). Health risks in our environment: Urban slum youth' perspectives using photovoice in Kampala, Uganda. *Sustainability, 13*(1), 248.

StataCorp. (2017). *Stata statistical software: Release 15*. StataCorp LLC.

Tso, R. V., & Cowling, B. J. (2020). Importance of face masks for COVID-19: A call for effective public education. *Clinical Infectious Diseases, 71*(16), 2195–2198. https://doi.org/10.1093/cid/ciaa593

Tucho, G. T., & Kumsa, D. M. (2021). Universal use of face masks and related challenges during COVID-19 in developing countries. *Risk Management and Healthcare Policy, 14*, 511.

Uganda Bureau of Statistics. (2016). The National Population and Housing Census 2014.

WHO. (2020). *Ethical standards for research during public health emergencies: Distilling existing guidance to support COVID-19 R&D*.

Yee, J., Unger, L., Zadravecz, F., Cariello, P., Seibert, A., Johnson, M. A., & Fuller, M. J. (2020). Novel coronavirus 2019 (COVID-19): Emergence and implications for emergency care. *Journal of the American College of Emergency Physicians Open, 1*(2), 63–69. https://doi.org/10.1002/emp2.12034

Yıldırım, M., & Güler, A. (2020). Factor analysis of the COVID-19 perceived risk scale: A preliminary study. *Death Studies*, 1–8. https://doi.org/10.1080/07481187.2020.1784311

7 Implications of the COVID-19 Pandemic and Responses on Persons with Disabilities Including Psychosocial Disabilities in the Global South: The Case of Ghana

Magnus Mfoafo-M'Carthy and Augustina Naami

7.1 Introduction

According to the World Health Organization (WHO), there are more than 1 billion persons with disabilities (PWDs) worldwide (2011). Researchers believe that almost 80% of PWDs live in low-income/middle-income countries—the Global South. PWDs are often marginalized by their condition of disability and the lack of support from families, communities, and government institutions. The WHO approximates that disability affects 15–20% of every population. The Human Rights Watch report estimates that more than five million Ghanaians live with disabilities; of these, 2.8 million are people with mental or psychosocial disability (individuals living with mental illness) (2012). Although the exact number of individuals with disability in Ghana is unknown (Kassah, 2008; Mfoafo-M'Carthy et al., 2020). For Ghana, with a population of approximately 30 million (The World Bank, 2019), having more than five million PWDs is a substantially high number that should be factored in any country's development agenda. It should be borne in mind that individuals with disabilities, including those with psychosocial disabilities, continue to encounter barriers to participation and inclusion in socioeconomic activities because of the stigma and discrimination associated with these conditions (Mfoafo-M'Carthy & Grischow, 2020). Challenges faced by PWDs tend to increase their susceptibility to the COVID-19 infection and worsen its impact on their lives based on the lack of support systems created specifically for PWDs. In Ghana, for instance, government measures to address the impact of the pandemic do not adequately address the needs of persons with disabilities.

Before the pandemic, PWDs in Ghana reported feeling a lack of support for their well-being (den Besten et al., 2016); this problem is likely to be exacerbated during the pandemic as there would not be additional support. Moreover, the weight of caregiving and pressure from family members negatively affect PWDs in times of crisis like the pandemic. Meanwhile, PWDs reported feeling stigmatized from their own family members as they were often left at home instead of being assisted to navigate support, including economic and educational opportunities, and were viewed as liabilities (Opoku et al., 2018; Tijm et al., 2011). These feelings of stigma contribute to the challenges faced by PWDs in

M. Mfoafo-M'Carthy (✉)
Lyle S. Hallman Faculty of Social Work, Wilfrid Laurier University, Waterloo, ON, Canada
e-mail: mmfoafomcarthy@wlu.ca

A. Naami
Department of Social Work, University of Ghana, Accra, Ghana

M. C. S. Gonçalves et al. (eds.), *The Coronavirus Crisis and Challenges to Social Development*,
https://doi.org/10.1007/978-3-030-84678-7_7

times of crisis. As well, being perceived as a financial burden on families and society (den Besten et al., 2016; Opoku et al., 2020) could, in times of a pandemic or any crisis, have a negative impact on these individuals. Thus, ensuring that society's perception of PWDs is transformed requires intense psychoeducation and government intervention. This shift is of great importance in a period when the COVID-19 pandemic is causing so much global havoc.

The pandemic, although it is believed to have originated in China in the latter part of 2019, began having a global effect economically, socially, and in other ways both in the Global North and in the Global South around the beginning of March 2020, which required the shutting down of global economies including the truncation of most air travel. These measures seriously impacted lives in many ways at a global level. Amid the pandemic was the implementation of social/physical distancing and health measures including the wearing of masks and the washing of hands on a consistent basis. PWDs tend to have been disproportionately affected by most of these measures with many individuals with disability, and specifically those with physical disability, facing the brunt of it (Human Rights, 2020; Naami & Mfoafo-M'Carthy, 2020). In Ghana, because of the lack of disability-friendly infrastructures/environment, PWDs have difficulty adhering to these measures based on their physical dependence on structures such as wheelchair-accessible buildings and public transportation to assist with mobility and access to resources or means of support. Based on these conditions, PWDs are seriously affected because of the precarious economic, health, and social locus in which they find themselves.

7.1.1 Impact of the Global Pandemic on PWDs

The impact of the pandemic is on a global proportion and has affected every aspect of society as we know it. As scientists and researchers continue to explore vaccines and other forms of treatment for the virus, the world continues to be inundated with COVID infection at astronomical levels. Although the rate of death in the Global South is minimal compared to that in the Global North, the infection rates continue to increase, and the majority of PWDs are the ones caught in the crossfire of the pandemic (Human Rights, 2020).

In this chapter, we attempt to discuss the impact of COVID-19 on PWDs in Ghana and the challenges they face amid the pandemic. We then propose recommendations to ensure that government measures are more inclusive and discerning in mitigating the challenges faced by this population during the pandemic and beyond.

7.1.2 Economic Challenges

The long-term impact of colonialism which caused financial instability for many countries in the Global South can be analyzed when studying how these regions treat their citizens with disabilities. Sparke and Anguelov (2020) explain that "previous pandemics, such as Ebola and H1N1, have made clear many countries and regions impacted by decades of neoliberalism are especially vulnerable" (p. 500). Many countries in the Global South including Ghana are indebted to foreign banks with strict regulations by large governing bodies such as the International Monetary Fund (IMF) regarding cutbacks to government expenditure and social programs (Sparke & Anguelov, 2020). This restriction could be likened to the structural adjustment programs in Ghana, Nigeria, and other African countries. These cutbacks can be related to the notion of the McKinnely et al. (2020) of a triage system, whereby individuals with preexisting conditions fall to the end of the priority list. Especially during a global health crisis, PWDs are inclined to be seriously impacted as they fall within this category. With privatization and a profits-over-all-else mentality, PWDs are typically considered to be "sub-citizens" according to health policies (Sparke & Anguelov, 2020, p. 500). The authors explain that this mistreatment can be analyzed as an unintentional outcome as neoliberalism pushes toward a free-market economy and less government influence, thereby leaving those who are vulnerable with little to no consideration. They explain this changing economic model as a kind of "disaster capitalism" where mortality is accepted in the name of economic freedom (Sparke & Anguelov, 2020).

Banks et al. (2020) argue that it is difficult to analyze the coping strategies used by persons with physical and psychosocial disabilities during the COVID-19 pandemic because of the lack of available mechanisms. From a financial perspective, the authors contend that those living with disabilities and their families have few avenues to cope with the current economic climate as they were already living in poverty before COVID-19 (Banks et al., 2020). This idea begs the question: if alternative coping strategies were not accessible to PWDs before COVID-19, how might their financial stability and health improve under increased restrictions during and after the pandemic?

Community has a significant role in explaining the resilience of someone who is living with a disability. PWDs tend to have weaker social networks, thus limiting the number of people who are not only able to assist with meeting their daily needs but also advocate for their rights (Banks et al., 2020). Banks et al. (2020) looked at the percentages of enrolment in government subsidy programs for those with disabilities in different countries in the Global South and found the numbers to be extremely low, for example, 25% in the Maldives and 13% in Tanahun, Nepal. Assuming an individual diagnosed with a psychosocial disability is unable to understand the financial subsidies for which they are eligible and has few social networks to ensure they are receiving the assistance needed, this individual (and the population they represent) could easily fall through the cracks of the system. Barriers to accessing support, whether health related or financial, become increasingly difficult for those PWDs in these regions including Ghana.

The pandemic may be a contributing factor preventing PWDs from working in retail or customer service because of their restricted mobility and greater risk of being infected with the virus (Naami & Mfoafo-M'Carthy, 2020). Before the pandemic, the number of PWDs employed by government agencies or established institutions seemed to be limited. The majority of PWDs in Ghana work at menial jobs as toll booth attendants or dressmakers, tailors, handweavers, hairdressers, and petty traders who sell their goods at home, in front of their houses, in kiosks, or on the streets (Naami, 2015). This opportunity has changed since the pandemic and many PWDs are unable to engage in these forms of business activities. Also, the impact of the pandemic in Ghana is enormous, as PWDs are less likely to work in environments that recommend the migration of work to the virtual workspace, which is seemingly becoming the new normal (Naami & Mfoafo-M'Carthy, 2020). The majority of PWDs do not have access to resources that will enable them to participate in this new normal. They are not only unlikely to be employed, but also more likely to lose their jobs because of the measures put in place (Lengnick-Hall et al., 2001), which may in part be caused by attitudinal barriers that remain the major challenge to the employment of PWDs and for those on the job (Naami, 2015; WHO, 2011). Also, the pandemic has created an environment where businesses are compelled to scale down. Such restructuring may require scaling back on the number of employees, which is likely to have a negative impact on PWDs, who may be laid off.

In disability discourses in Ghana and the Global South, gender and disability create multiple levels of oppression or susceptibilities for women and girls. Poverty from unemployment could be worse for women with disabilities because they are less likely to be educated and thus employed compared to their male counterparts; moreover, women with disabilities are more likely to work in the informal sector. In addition to disability-related expenses, women must also incur gender-related expenses such as menstrual hygiene management materials and childcare expenses for single mothers (Naami, 2015).

7.1.3 Educational Challenges

Toquero (2020) highlights the mistreatment of PWDs in the Global South through the suppression of their voices, a reality that is heightened during the COVID-19 pandemic. The author focuses on the policies the Filipino government has created for social engagement for individuals with disabilities, concentrating on the need for equal access to education and lifelong learning (Toquero, 2020). These discrepancies begin with the lack of education provided for children with disabilities which leads to minimal employment opportunities for them in the future. The author explains the necessity for equity, especially during the pandemic, when creating programs for inclusion of PWDs. This can be analyzed through the training teachers receive for students with disabilities and the lack of knowledge of how to structure teaching according to an individual's abilities. Assistive technologies, as an example of structuring teaching according to ability, are proven to be very helpful for students with intellectual disabilities. Despite the evidence that these technologies are beneficial, many teachers and parents are not given proper training in how to use them (Toquero, 2020). If individuals with disabilities are not given the attention and tools needed to succeed from an early age, how would they be educated to advocate for better policies for their community? There must be more representation of individuals with disabilities on the larger stage.

From the perspective of Ghana, PWDs are less likely to be educated, and this may result from several factors including stigma (Mfoafo-M'Carthy et al., 2020). The 'new normal' created by the pandemic requires learning to take place virtually and creates a serious burden for PWDs in the school system. For instance, students with visual and hearing impairments are required to "have access to equipment and services (e.g., screen readers, magnifiers, closed captioning, and subtitle services to make learning materials accessible)" (Naami & Mfoafo-M'Carthy, 2020, p. 11). These services/resources needed by PWDs in the educational system may not be available during the pandemic, and this is worsened for those in rural areas whose families may not have the wherewithal to provide access to the Internet and computers (Naami & Mfoafo-M'Carthy, 2020).

7.1.4 Healthcare Challenges

The pandemic has reinforced many systems of injustice and inequity globally. This is, however, worse in developing countries such as Ghana. With the rate of infection escalating and resources running low, this could create a "survival of the fittest" mentality where those deemed "less fit" (according to society's standards) are marginalized. McKinney et al. (2020) explore the issue of limited resources in public hospitals in South Africa. They argue that in the event of inadequate ventilators for patients, it is likely that patients who have disabilities could be excluded from receiving intensive care and/or gaining access to a ventilator. They explain the persistent fear of this reality amongst disabled people in South Africa, highlighting the injustice of their "second-class medical status" (McKinney et al., 2020, p. 2). This method of prioritizing medical care, known as triage, is not only a reality in the Global South but in the Global North as well where this model is practiced in disaster settings when there are too many patients for a limited number of resources. A difference, however, between the approaches in the developed and developing countries is the support of disabled populations before their possible need for medical attention. The WHO outlined the actions needed to ensure persons with disabilities have access to proper healthcare during the pandemic; however, many of these suggestions are not feasible for citizens of countries in the Global South like South Africa and Ghana (WHO, 2020). For example, one suggestion is to purchase health essentials online, a tip that is not useful for many disabled South Africans who do not have access to credit cards or Internet (McKinney et al., 2020), which may be similar to Ghana where one is required to pay for health services. The lack of financial wherewithal to pay for healthcare in the hospitals makes it difficult for PWDs to access health facilities when they are unwell or affected by the COVID-19 virus.

The WHO recommends less touching of surfaces, social distancing, and certain health practices such as the washing of hands among the measures implemented to minimize the spread of the virus during the pandemic (2020). Despite these measures, PWDs are likely to be more vulnerable to being infected by the COVID-19 virus, based on several factors:

(a) PWDs, particularly those with physical disabilities in Ghana, are more susceptible to the spread of COVID-19 as they are more inclined to hold on to structures or seek the support of caregivers and others.
(b) For follow-up healthcare appointments in the cities, they are required to travel long distances using public transportation, which poses risks of contracting the virus (Naami & Mfoafo-M'Carthy, 2020). The physical condition of many PWDs inhibits their ability to observe social and physical distancing because many are likely to need assistance accessing the built-environment infrastructure, which tends to be disability unfriendly.
(c) The lack of accessibility to transportation and other support makes it challenging for PWDs to utilize the healthcare system (Naami & Mfoafo-M'Carthy, 2020).

In addition, poor infrastructural networks such as non-motorable roads, may make it difficult for most PWDs to commute from one ru,ral community to another. Inaccessible public transport, physical environment, and the distance involved could be more challenging. They may have difficulty observing basic hygiene measures because of their inaccessibility to hand-washing facilities. Social and physical distancing may be difficult for persons with disabilities who need help because of physical, transportation, and information inaccessibility.

The impact may not only be on physical health but on psychosocial support as well. Attitudinal barriers coupled with all the stressors associated with the pandemic can have a devasting impact on the psyche of PWDs. PWDs have less social support and fewer networks and are unlikely to be accorded the social support and sympathy as the virus continues to have a devasting effect on the community.

7.2 Provisions to Protect PWDs

The COVID-19 pandemic has impacted everyone globally, but for persons with disabilities, the effect could be worse because of the many barriers they face. Research shows they are less likely to have jobs (WHO, 2011; Mizunoya & Mitra, 2012; Naami, 2015); more likely to work in precarious employment, which yields less income and is irregular (Mizunoya & Mitra, 2012; WHO, 2011); and more likely to incur high disability-related expenses (WHO, 2020). In a similar vein, children with disabilities are seriously impacted as their families are not able to provide adequate care and resources for their well-being. COVID-19 could add layers of vulnerabilities to persons with disabilities. Those in the formal and informal sectors are more likely to lose their jobs, which could further affect their economic security and resilience. COVID-19 brings additional expenses to everyone, but persons with disabilities must spend more resources on COVID-19-related expenses (hygiene and other safety protocols) because they must touch many objects and structures for support to navigate their inaccessible environment and to compensate those who help them complete their daily chores.

The COVID-19 pandemic has impacted economies globally, resulting in calls for governments across the globe to find better ways of addressing the welfare needs of persons with disabilities. In Ghana, there are very few social protections benefitting persons with disabilities. The only cash transfer in Ghana, Livelihood for Empowerment Against Poverty (LEAP), does not clearly list persons with disabilities in the eligibility criteria. A person with a disability qualifies for LEAP if they are deemed to have severe disability with no productive capacity. This criterion leaves out many persons with disabilities, especially those who are unemployed and have no source of income. The government has not adjusted the cash benefits during the pandemic.

The District Assembly Common Fund (DCAF) for persons with disabilities is the only social protection program earmarked for persons with disabilities. The parliament currently allocates 7.5% of Ghana's total revenue to metropolitan, municipal, and district assemblies (MMDAs) through the Common Fund as mandated under Section 2 of the DCAF Act (Act 455). The MMDAs are required to keep 3% of their allocations of the DCAF to achieve the following objectives related to the well-being of persons with disabilities:

(a) To support the income-generating activities of individual persons with disabilities as a means of economic empowerment.
(b) To provide educational support for children, students, and trainees with disabilities.
(c) To build the capacity of PWDs in the districts to enable them to advocate and assert their rights and undertake awareness-raising and sensitization in relation to disability issues.
(d) To support access for persons with disabilities access to technical aids and other assistive devices and equipment.

It is obvious from the objectives of the DCAF listed here that the support from this source is not aimed directly at meeting the immediate needs of persons with disabilities. However, the meeting of immediate needs is crucial for everyone during any emergency humanitarian situation such as the COVID-19 pandemic. The allocation to the MMDAs is done quarterly. There is evidence that the transfer from the central government is delayed as well as the disbursement by the MMDAs (Agyire-Tettey et al., 2019; Akorlie, 2015). Also, not every person with a disability who needs this kind of support gets it (Agyire-Tettey et al., 2019; Edusei et al., 2017). All of this could worsen the impact of COVID-19 on the overall well-being of persons with disabilities, their caregivers, and their families.

7.3 Addressing Discrepancies in Emergency Responses

Regardless of the clear vulnerabilities of persons with disabilities—which could worsen during the COVID-19 pandemic—and the inadequate social protection to address their needs, the government has yet to put in place measures to address the unique needs of persons with disabilities. During the lockdown, the government provided food and other relief items to vulnerable populations. Anecdotal evidence shows that persons with disabilities queued like everyone else for these necessities. Provisions were not made for persons with disabilities despite being described by the WHO as the major vulnerable population, while the business relief funding under the COVID-19 Alleviation Programme was disbursed by the COVID-19 fund management to support Small and Medium-Scale Enterprises (SMEs). It is thus uncertain how many persons with disabilities benefited from this fund. A question yet to be answered is how persons with disabilities provide for themselves and their households during and after this pandemic, given that they are more likely to be out of a job, not have regular income and savings, and grapple with disability-related expenses. As well, they are less likely to have health insurance.

For effective targeting and development of any population, data are necessary. There is a need for quality quantitative and qualitative data about persons with disabilities and their unique needs. Disaggregated data by type of disability, gender, age, geographic location, and ethnicity is imperative. This information could help develop tailored interventions to address the needs of persons with disabilities. The national response strategies must be inclusive of persons with disabilities as recommended by international bodies such as the International Disability Alliance (IDA), the World Health Organization, and the International Labour Organization (ILO). The International Labour Organization further recommends the need to provide adequate social protection to help minimize disability-related costs.

7.4 Recommendations and Conclusion

The impact of the pandemic on countries like Ghana in the Global South continues to be devastating by the lack of preparedness and making provisions for PWDs including those with psychosocial disabilities. These individuals are thus compelled to bear the brunt of the challenges associated with the virus as they lack a systemic structure to provide for their needs. The impact could be that PWDs are left to their own devices to fend for themselves, which could in many circumstances be disastrous.

The following recommendations are made to mitigate the effects of pandemics or crises on PWDs.

It is necessary for the government and non-governmental organizations (NGOs) to set up a system of support by initially gathering information on PWDs to identify their needs. The data on PWDs would ensure their easy identification and knowledge of the specific needs that must be met. Appropriate and detailed data would enable the government to plan for disasters such as the pandemic and would help in the development of policies to address major issues affecting PWDs. Data are important for targeting the development for policies and programs to better address social problems. The question that one may pose is whether the exact number of PWDs in Ghana is known (this is based on challenges associated with gathering data of PWDs in Ghana). How are the data on these individuals collated and how are they utilized? The pandemic and its resultant lockdown of the economy have revealed the systemic weakness in measures adopted to address challenges faced by individuals from marginalized communities (Naami & Mfoafo-M'Carthy, 2020).

As argued by Naami and Mfoafo-M'Carthy (2020), the creation of a disability emergency response unit is recommended. The creation of a disaster response team would be helpful in galvanizing response for handling challenges faced by PWDs during crises like the COVID-19 pandemic and future crises. It is important for such a unit to be equipped with skilled personnel such as trained social workers to mobilize and coordinate all services and resources to meet the needs of PWDs. They could also partner with faith-based and NGOs and other civic organizations deemed necessary in discharging its mandate. The unit should be set up at the regional, district, and community levels of the country to be optimally helpful for PWDs. It should be ensured that the government can adopt strategies to provide services and resources accessible to all persons with disabilities. This special unit must be equipped with access to special hotlines or video calls designated specifically to meet the needs of all PWDs. In rural areas where there is less access to the Internet and technology, trained professionals could be stationed in these communities to provide the needed assistance.

The inclusion of PWDs in crisis response planning and implementation is suggested. It is worth noting that there is a need for the government to develop emergency response strategies to address future crises similar to COVID-19. The plans must explicitly outline measures to address females, children, and the elderly with different types of disabilities considering their unique needs. It is imperative that persons with different types of disabilities, including psychosocial disabilities, are part of the crisis response team; this should include women who would have a role in identifying needs that are unique to the female gender and to facilitate interventions that could effectively address those needs. The establishment of the crisis team should include PWDs in emergency response planning and implementation throughout every part of the country (Naami & Mfoafo-M'Carthy, 2020).

Amid the pandemic, it is crucial for PWDs to have easy access to hospitals and access to medications in a timely fashion. It is recommended that clinics be established in local communities and municipalities to make healthcare easily accessible. The national healthcare system should be structured in a way that PWDs would not be required to pay for the healthcare services they receive. Hence, medical practitioners or clinicians who discriminate against PWDs by refusing services should be prosecuted. Putting in place such measures will minimize the discriminatory practices against the disability community. Also, NGOs and government should explore the possibility of ensuring that persons with physical disabilities will be provided with wheelchairs to assist with their mobility.

In addition, programs already in existence that assist the poor, such as Livelihood Empowerment Against Poverty (LEAP) (a major social protection program in Ghana), should be revamped to ensure that the needs of PWDs are addressed. The recommendation is that the government makes the effort to expand the program for more disability and disability-gender-specific social protection measures to benefit women with disabilities who tend to be more vulnerable. At present, the LEAP program is not designed to provide support to all PWDs but only those whose condition is described as severe (Naami & Mfoafo-M'Carthy, 2020). The question one may ask is, who makes the determination regarding PWDs meeting the criteria for support amid a pandemic? The fact remains that PWDs are not only less likely to be employed but are more likely to lose their jobs during a global crisis such as a pandemic. They are also more likely to work in jobs that lack security and job-related benefits.

Also, the WHO must put forth support and suggestions that are more suited for countries in the Global South. These suggestions cannot be generalized on a global scale as the resources and norms vary in different parts of the world.

Despite challenges associated with the pandemic, it is important for the government of Ghana as well as community-based organizations including civic organizations to take steps to ease the challenges faced by PWDs. As we know, the impact of the pandemic on one community is likely to affect the entire population. As a community, we are somewhat directly or indirectly interconnected. Thus, the impact of the pandemic on one community is likely to affect the other because of the high rate of infection and the tendency for the virus to spread from one community to the other. Therefore, the government's policies regarding the pandemic should be inclusive of PWDs, engaging them in the decision-making process. It is imperative for the government to put in place measures to promote equal rights to resources and the wellbeing of all to ensure that no one is left behind—the hallmark of the Sustainable Development Goals.

References

Agyire-Tettey, E. E., Naami, A., Wissenbach, L., & Schädler, J. (2019). *Challenges of inclusion: local support systems and social service arrangements for persons with disabilities in Suhum, Ghana: Baseline study report*. University of Siegen. https://dspace.ub.unisiegen.de/bitstream/ubsi/1486/2/ChallengesofInclusionZPE52.pdf. https://doi.org/10.25819/ubsi/33.

Akorlie, C. (2015). *Delays in the disbursement of district assemblies' common fund a bane*. https://www.ghananewsagency.org/features/delay-indisbursement-of-district assemblies-common-fund-a-bane-88669.

Banks, L. M., Davey, C., Shakespeare, T., & Kuper, H. (2020). Disability-inclusive responses to COVID-19: Lessons learnt from research on social protection in low and middle-income countries. *World Development, 137*, 1–4. https://doi.org/10.1016/j.worlddev.2020.105178

den Besten, J., Cornielje, M., Cornielje, H., & Botwey, D. (2016). Supporting parents caring for children with disability in Ghana. *Disability, CBR & Inclusive Development, 27*(3), 87101. https://doi.org/10.5463/dcid.v27i3.530

Edusei, A., Adjei-Domfeh, P., Mprah, W. K., Opoku, M., Badu, E., & Appiah, S. C. (2017). Assessing the impact and uses of the Disability Common Fund among persons with disabilities in Kumasi Metropolis in Ghana. *Review of Disability Studies, 12*(4).

Human Rights Report. (2020). *Impact of COVID-19 on persons with disabilities: European leaders must act now. Extract from the Human Rights Report 2020*. https://www.edffeph.org/content/uploads/2021/01/Final-final-Human-Rights.Published.pdf

Human Rights Watch. (2012). *Ghana: Disability Rights Convention ratified. People with mental disabilities need protection, community-based programs*. https://www.hrw.org/news/2012/08/22/ghana-disability-rights-conventionratified#:~:text=More%20than%205%20million%20people,million%20people%2with%20mental%20disabilities.&text=Human%20Rights%20Watch%20found%2that,and%20subject%20to%20severe%20abuse.

Kassah, A. K. (2008). Begging as work: A study of people with mobility difficulties in Accra, Ghana. *Disability & Society, 23*(2), 163–170. https://doi.org/10.1080/09687590701841208

Lengnick-Hall, M. L., Gaunt, P. M., & Brooks, A. A. (2001). *Why employers don't hire people with disabilities: A survey of the literature*. College of Business, University of Texas at San Antonio. https://www.

cprf.org/studies/why-employersdon't-hirepeoplewith-disabilities–asurvey-oftheliterature

McKinney, E. L., McKinney, V., & Swartz, L. (2020). COVID-19, disability, and the context of healthcare triage in South Africa: Notes in times of pandemic. *African Journal of Disability, 9*, 1–9. https://doi.org/10.4102/ajod.v9i0.766

Mfoafo-M'Carthy, M., & Grischow, J. (2020). "Being Heard": The socio-economic impact of psychiatric care on patients and caregivers in Ghana. *International Social Work*. https://doi.org/10.1177/2F0020872820962177

Mfoafo-M'Carthy, M., Grischow, J., & Stocco, N. (2020). *Cloak of invisibility: A literature review of physical disability in Ghana*. Sage Open. https://doi.org/10.1177/2158244019900567

Mizunoya, S., & Mitra, S. (2012). Is there a disability gap in employment rates in developing countries? *World Development, 42*, 28–43.

Naami, A. (2015). Disability, gender, and employment relationships in Africa: The case of Ghana. *African Journal of Disability Studies, 4*(1), 1–11.

Naami, A., & Mfoafo-M'Carthy, M. (2020). COVID-19: The vulnerabilities of persons with disabilities in Ghana. *African Journal of Social Work, 10*(3), 9–16.

Opoku, M., Alupo, B., Gyamfi, N., Odame, L., Mprah, W., Torgbenu, E., & Eric, B. (2018). The family and disability in Ghana: highlighting gaps in achieving social inclusion. *Disability, CBR & Inclusive Development, 28*(4), 41–59. https://doi.org/10.5463/dcid.v28i4.666

Opoku, M. P., Nketsia, W., Banye, M. A., Mprah, W. K., Dogbe, J. A., & Badu, E. (2020). Caregiving experiences and expectations of parents with in-school children with intellectual disability in Ghana. *Research in Developmental Disabilities, 96*(complete). https://doi.org/10.1016/j.ridd.2019.103524.

Sparke, M., & Anguelov, D. (2020). Contextualising coronavirus geographically. *Transactions of the Institute of British Geographers, 45*, 498–508. https://doi.org/10.1111/tran.12389

The World Bank. (2019) *Population: Ghana data*. https://data.worldbank.org/indicator/SP.POP.TOTL?locations=GH

Tijm, M., Cornielje, H., & Edusei, A. (2011). 'Welcome to my life!' Photovoice to Voice: Needs assessment of, and by, persons with physical disabilities in the Kumasi Metropolis, Ghana. *Disability, CBR & Inclusive Development, 22*(1), 55–72. https://doi.org/10.5463/dcid.v22i1.12

Toquero, C. M. D. (2020). Inclusion of people with disabilities amid COVID-19: Laws, interventions, recommendations. *Multidisciplinary Journal of Educational Research, 10*(2), 158–177. https://doi.org/10.4471/remie.2020.5877

World Health Organization. (2011). *World report on disability*. http://www.who.int/disabilities/world_report/2011/report.pdf

World Health Organization. (2020). *Disability considerations during the COVID-19 outbreak* (No. WHO/2019 nCoV/Disability/2020.1).

8 Lockdown in a Dual Society: Exploring the Human Capability Implications of the Coronavirus (COVID-19) in South Africa

Minenhle Matela and Alexandre Maaza

8.1 Introduction

The COVID-19 pandemic virus literally brought the world to an abrupt halt at the beginning of the year 2020. Based on current reporting, the virus is affecting 215 countries and territories, as well as two International conveyances. COVID was first identified in Wuhan City, Hubei Province, China, and it was first reported on December 31, 2019 (Worldometer, 2021). As a result, the World Health Organization (WHO) declared COVID-19 a Global Public Health Emergency. As of 28 January 2021, globally recorded COVID-19 cases stand at approximately 101 million, 2.1 million deaths, and 73 million recoveries with almost 450,000 new cases recorded daily. Nevertheless, we argued that national governments and global governance institutions have approached this health crisis in a rushed and disjointed manner, somewhat of a failure of multilateral health co-operation. As cases and deaths rapidly increased in the Northern Hemisphere by March 2020, most countries took on harsh measures of nation-wide lockdowns, usually coupled with an almost total closure of national borders. This resultant global decrease in economic activity is expected to shrink by 5.2% in 2020, triggering the biggest global recession since the Great Depression (World Bank 2020). This dire situation is unfolding against a backdrop of high levels of inequalities in income and wealth between states. Inequality between states has enabled developed nations to better secure the necessary emergency medical equipment and provide economic stimulus to buoy their economies much better than developing countries. Surprisingly, the worst health crises related to the pandemic have been punctuated with an overwhelming of public healthcare systems by patients with serious COVID-19 symptoms in developed and developing countries alike. However, the ability to return to postpandemic normalcy, and subsequent economic recovery will hinge on widely accessible vaccines that are presently being rolled out in the developed North. Despite the global co-operation rhetoric around the just acquisition of vaccines, developed states stand in line to receive the most vaccine doses when they become available.

In South Africa, income and wealth inequality levels may be compounded by the pandemic, as early analyses of the distributional impact of the pandemic show (World Inequality Database, 2020). There is already a drop in aggregate spending that coincides with a disproportionate increase in the savings of high-income households. Conversely, we see that the largest drop in earnings with low-income households using their savings or borrowing has caused an increased reliance on government support for their spending. Thus,

M. Matela (✉) · A. Maaza
Southern African Policy and Development Nexus, Cape Town, South Africa
e-mail: minenhle@sapdnafrica.com

M. C. S. Gonçalves et al. (eds.), *The Coronavirus Crisis and Challenges to Social Development*,
https://doi.org/10.1007/978-3-030-84678-7_8

states are required to provide expansive emergency safety nets to their citizens as well as their productive sectors. This need will likely prove challenging for African economies that already held high levels of external debt to their Gross Domestic Products (GDPs) before the pandemic and, like most economies in 2020, will have to run a fiscal deficit. The African Development Bank (AfDB) (2020) predicts that GDP growth in Africa will be between −1.7% and −3.4%, and employment will fall by approximately a third in both the formal and informal sectors. This drop is likely to increase extreme poverty ($1.90) within the 2% range, which would result in a further 28 to 38 million people in Africa falling into this socioeconomic situation. The higher estimates are more likely if "the welfare of the poorest households grows at lower rates" (AfDB, 2020), which could happen given the restricted fiscal space of African states. Furthermore, the pandemic's socioeconomic shock on extreme poverty is most likely to be felt in the services and industrial sectors, whilst the agricultural sector will likely be the most resilient in this aspect (AfDB, 2020). Given these circumstances, it is sensible to expect African households to reduce their consumption until their national economies rebound. This chapter argues that despite a faltering economy, inadequate healthcare, and socioeconomic inequalities, the South African government's response to the pandemic aligns with the capabilities approach.

8.2 Conceptual Framework

The overwhelming negative impact of COVID-19 on the global economy cascading down to the household level should also be understood conversely: from the perspective of individuals and households, local communities, and all the way to the global level. Similarly, we should also seek to view this pandemic's health and socioeconomic implications and perceive the crisis as something that threatens the world's overall well-being as well as human development. In his seminal book *Development as Freedom*, Amartya Sen argues that "development can be seen as a process of expanding the real freedoms that people enjoy" (Sen, 1999, p. 3). Amartya Sen's concept of freedom is based on individual freedoms or capabilities—which are influenced by a wide range of economic and social determinants—to achieve well-being and human development (Robeyns, 2005). Sen asserts that freedom can be used both to assess the improvement or degradation of individual capabilities and to improve the effectiveness of development by advocating for freedom that allows individual agency. Sen (1999) outlines five expansive, nonexhaustive, and interconnected capabilities: political freedoms, economic facilities, social opportunities, transparency guarantees, and protective security. The capability approach is not an explanatory paradigm, but rather a normative framework and tool which seeks to inform policy and social change design that focuses on issues involving poverty and inequality (Robeyns, 2005). It can be seen that globally the responses to curtail the pandemic were quite ad hoc and an iterative process of reducing the real freedoms of individuals. As such, the capability approach offers a valuable paradigm to analyse the bottom-up responses and impacts related to COVID-19.

The capability approach involves a dynamic process, underpinned by personal agency, which seeks to convert capability inputs into achieved capabilities. Thus, each individual will possess a set of capability inputs (nonmarket or market production, net income, transfers) that permit them to purchase certain goods or services. These goods and services are used in a manner that is informed by personal, social, and environmental conversion factors that depend on one's social context to yield a capability set (Sen, 1999). The functionings achieved from an individual's opportunity set depend purely on their choice. This is a choice that is informed by preferences, social context, and innate factors such as personal history and psychology. This process reflects the contextual focus of the capability approach on both material and nonmaterial issues (deprivations) faced by individuals by assessing the economic and social context of their capability sets (Sen, 1999). Before delving into the South African case study, it is important to note that emerging literature links the capability approach to the COVID-19 pandemic. In May 2020, the United Nations Development Programme (UNDP) made use of the capability approach to assess the effect of an accelerating COVID-19 crisis on human development, through its Human Development Index (HDI), an index consisting of education, health, and economic measurements, by recommending a human-centric approach to recovering from the crisis. In envisaging a post-COVID-19 world, the UNDP (2020, p. 3) put forward a three-pillared approach to (1) look at the crisis through an equity lens, (2) focus on people's enhanced capabilities, and (3) follow a coherent multidimensional approach. Anand et al. (2020) list 22 human capabilities that have been impacted by the pandemic while noting the relevance of the capability approach in analysing the depth and breadth of the COVID-19 intensifying impact on preexisting deprivations. Furthermore, Bhorat, and Köhler (2020) argue that the pandemic has elicited responses from governments and individuals which typically take an expanded view of well-being to be successful, thereby potentially entrenching a widespread adoption of policy making based on the capability approach.

In addition, Osmani (2021) operationalises the UNDP approach through policy making that focuses on human capabilities to manage the pandemic in a developing country context. The trade-off in developed countries is a dichotomy: human life versus the economy, whereas developing countries are tied in an inextricable link between economic and human security resulting from the scarcity of social safety nets and large informal sectors relative to developed countries (Osmani, 2021). To best manage this tradeoff in the developing country case of Bangladesh, Osmani (2021) advocates for an adaptive two-phase approach (severe and relaxed lockdowns) and two-sector (essential and nonessential) based on three pillars: (1) physical distancing induced by an economic lockdown; (2) economic support measures, with a focus on financial aid for poor households; and (3) public health system support to ensure its ability to cope with a relaxed lockdown. It is important to note that Bangladesh has a relatively low budget deficit and public debt burden (Osmani, 2021), which is not the case with many countries in Sub-Saharan Africa, including South Africa (Osmani, 2021).

8.3 South Africa: A Dual Economy in Transition

In popular discourse, South Africa is gradually less mentioned as the 'Rainbow Nation' these days and more as the most unequal country in the world, amidst concerning levels of political corruption. According to Statistics South Africa (StatsSA) (2014), South Africa's Gini coefficient was calculated at 0.69 in 2011, based on income data (per capita including salaries, wages, and social grants). The Gini, which measures inequality levels, was the highest in the world at the time and continues to be so even today. This inequality has been increasing since the advent of the country's democracy alongside poverty, which is persistently chronic for its population, particularly the segments that were oppressed by the Apartheid regime. Thabo Mbeki, the country's second democratically elected president, famously described the country's duality in 1998 and constantly referred to it throughout his presidency: he effectively proclaimed South Africa as a country of two nations (Mbeki, 1998).

We can explain a large portion of South Africa's developmental duality as a result of the post-1994 government's historic compromise to ensure economic stability, by recognising the property rights that existed during Apartheid. This deal locked the nation into a path of unequal economic and social structural perpetuity by entrenching structures of capital ownership, sectoral composition, and the distribution of gains between capital and labour (UNDP, 2020). Capital ownership is still concentrated in the hands of white South Africans and foreign investors, with only an estimated 21% black ownership of the top 100 listed companies on the Johannesburg Stock Exchange (JSE). Attempts to increase black ownership through the privatisation of state-owned enterprises and broad-based black economic empowerment (BBBEE), have created a black economic elite without delivering economic freedoms to the historically marginalised population (UNDP, 2014) and increased the concentration of capital in the economy from its 1994 levels (Orthofer, 2016). The sectoral composition of the economy is historically linked to mining and energy and their related sectors. The post-apartheid period has seen a decline in both the mining sector—the main absorber of unskilled labour—and the manufacturing sector, which is typically the sector with the highest economic and labour multipliers (UNDP, 2014). The substantial growth of the tertiary sector has had a modernising effect on the economy, yet its inability to absorb much of the labour force stems from a structural skills gap (UNDP, 2014).

Unequal opportunities, and unequal access to education, and health can offer another lens through which to understand inequality in South Africa and the capabilities of its citizens. The Apartheid regime's education design of racially segregated schools and curricula has a lasting dualistic legacy on the economy, where former black (now public) schools remain dysfunctional, while former white (now private or Model-C) schools stay functional. These divergences result in lower matric pass rates and university success for a large part of the population, translating into negative labour market outcomes with a mismatch of skills in the economy (UNDP, 2014). A similar scenario emerges when looking at the healthcare system, where substantial differences exist between the private and public health facilities. Furthermore, the funding model for the health sector does not account fully for the relative disease burden between different areas. The issue of health is further compounded by the lack of access to basic services by a large portion of the population, which has negative externalities on education and employment (UNDP, 2014).

When discussing the capabilities of South Africans, the main guiding policy document for the country's development is the National Development Plan (NDP). It provides the country's guiding objectives to eliminate poverty and reduce inequality by 2030 as prescribed by the National Planning Commission (NPC) (2011). The NDP is firmly rooted in the capability and human rights approaches to development that subsequently inform policy, planning, and implementation of developmental programmes at all levels of government. The NDP sets out a strategy based on enhancing capabilities through an active citizenry among others. It recognises employment creation, social protection, access to education, and health as critical aspects of reducing poverty and inequality (NPC, 2011). In exploring the human capability implications of the coronavirus (COVID-19) in South Africa, this chapter focuses on the following areas of human development, namely, healthcare and socioeconomic variables.

8.4 South Africa's Dual Healthcare System

According to the Health Systems Trust (1996a, b), the health system inherited by the new government in 1994 was one that was undemocratic and centralised, containing a highly fragmented structure, and disproportionately subjective towards historically 'white' areas and systematically underfunding historically 'non-white' areas such as homelands, rural areas, and townships as a result of Apartheid policies. The spatial segregation of Apartheid continued to affect access to quality healthcare amongst non-white South Africans. Subsequently, the wealthy minority, who were estimated to comprise 23% of the population, was projected to use up to 61% of the total government healthcare expenditure in 1992–1993, thus leaving the remaining 39% of the expenditure to accommodate the 77% disadvantaged majority of the South African population. According to McIntyre et al. (1995), South Africa's healthcare expenditure accounted for approximately 8.5% of the GDP in 1992–1993. A 2015 report by the Department of Health shows that the GDP expenditure remained the same over the years, with 4.1% spent on the public sector and 4.4% on the private sector, as echoed by Perper (2018). In comparison to other middle-income countries, which spend much less of their GDP on healthcare, it is shocking to see that South Africa's healthcare status falls short of its fellow middle-income countries. This difference is largely attributed to an inequitable distribution in healthcare between the public and private sector regarding, amongst other elements, levels of care and geographic location (Perper, 2018).

Before COVID-19, South Africa's public healthcare system was already struggling with rectifying past ills. Its recent history is mired in a chronic deficit of resources, including outdated infrastructure, and several shortages in terms of medicines, general hospital beds, and healthcare workers. The history of healthcare in South Africa can be traced back to the colonial and Apartheid eras, when discrimination and inequality were rampant. A number of the negative forces created by apartheid continued to reproduce inequality, and increase poverty, even after Apartheid policies were formally abolished. These socioeconomic imbalances further contributed to inequalities in healthcare access. South Africa's dual healthcare system comprises the public and private sectors. The public sector is state owned and is separated into primary, secondary, and tertiary healthcare that is managed by nine provincial departments of health, as located in the nine provinces in South Africa, under a centralised National Department of Health (NDoH). The majority of South Africa's hospitals are state/public healthcare facilities, and thus they provide free healthcare services to all South Africans who generally cannot afford private healthcare, in line with the Constitution of South Africa, which guarantees every citizen access to healthcare services (Section 27 of the Bill of Rights) (Republic of South Africa (RSA), 1996). Unfortunately, state hospitals tend to be overcrowded, understaffed, and extremely under-resourced. Furthermore, there are long waiting periods in a state hospital with dysfunctional order and large amounts of paperwork. The reality for South Africans is that in public healthcare the standards of service can go from tolerable to very low, further exacerbated by outdated medical equipment, shortages of staff, and shortage of medicine, according to Van Rensburg, 2014).

On the other hand, private sector users are covered by health insurance in the form of 'medical aid schemes.' These are mutual societies governed by the Medical Schemes Act of 1969, with a smaller number of users paying out of pocket for private services. These medical aid schemes are for the most part employer-based joint contributions by the employer and employee and comprehensively cover the employee and their dependants for the use of private-sector healthcare facilities. Service providers are reimbursed on a fee-for-service basis and employers receive a full tax subsidy for their contributions, according to Wadee et al. (2003). Compared to public healthcare, private healthcare comprises a higher caliber of service delivery for South Africans who can afford the service, which includes excellent hospitals with an increased amount of order, operating on an appointment basis so there are no long lines to receive assistance, no waiting periods, including up-to-date equipment, and a well-trained staff cohort. In 1997, the White Paper for Transformation of the Health System in South Africa adopted Primary Healthcare (PHC) as the foundation of South African Health Policy (National Department of Health, 2011). Through the adoption and restructuring of PHC to the district level, the intended outcome was increased access to healthcare for marginalised populations (National Department of Health, 2015).

Interestingly enough, Statistics South Africa (StatsSA) conducted its October Household Survey between 1993 and 1999 in an effort to establish which healthcare services were used by different populations used and possible reasons why the particular services were used. The survey data included information on morbidity, environmental characteristics, socioeconomic status, and use of health services, and the demographics of the respondents in relationship to the healthcare services they used. The data sets comprised a sample size of 130,787 in 1995 and 106,650 participants in 1999, all of whom had suffered a type of illness or injury in the month before the survey was conducted. Wadee et al. (2003) captivatingly describes the results in this manner: 60.1% of the sample population that used public sector services was mainly African and Coloured (mixed race) respondents; 36.3% who used private sector services mainly included

White and Indian respondents; and 3.6% of Africans consulted a traditional healer. This shows us is that the wealthier, predominantly White and Indian populations had an ease of access to private-sector healthcare services based on their ability to afford these services. African and Coloured people had to rely on public sector healthcare facilities because they could not afford private health care, and Africans further consulted with traditional healers or preferred not to seek medical care because they could not afford it, the state of public healthcare facilities, dissatisfactory service they received at their last visit, and/or the inaccessibility of a public sector healthcare facility near them. In this trend, seen between 1995 and 1999, the presented scenario mirrors Mbeki's two-nations analysis and has not changed much.

In the early 2000s, it was interesting to note that the majority of highly trained health personnel worked under the private sector, serving the minority of the population (Perper, 2018). Private healthcare providers mostly serve the white higher-income groups; this left the public sector serving the largely African lower-income population (Wadee et al., 2003). This picture highlights the highly uneven distribution of human and financial resources in healthcare in the country. To challenge the inequitable distribution of healthcare resources, the Department of Health initiated a number of policies such as the National Human Resources for Planning Framework vision 2015, and the Human Resources Strategy for the Healthcare Sector 2012/2013–2016/2017 (National Department of Health, 2015). Furthermore, in 2011 the National Development Plan was developed to respond to the country's inequities and weak capabilities. Subsequently, the Department of Health initiated the National Health Insurance Plan. These policies encourage public and private sector partnerships and universal healthcare for all citizens of the Republic. According to the Council for Medical Schemes 2015/2016 Annual Report, only 16% of the South African population has medical aid; approximately 72.2% of Whites and 10.5% of Africans reported being on medical aid. Thus, most South Africans must rely on the public healthcare system for their healthcare needs. It is also important to note that the state of public healthcare in the country has not seen major improvements throughout these years.

8.5 South Africa's Socioeconomic Response to COVID-19

South Africa's strict lockdown response was characterised by a systematically underperforming public health system in an already struggling prepandemic economy. The government's initial economic response accompanied its announcement of a national state of disaster in March 2020 with an initial fiscal stimulus package of ZAR59 billion (1.1% of GDP), which served as an emergency bandage. By 21 April 2020, this snowballed into an announcement of the largest fiscal stimulus package for any developing country through a stabilising treatment totaling ZAR500 billion (approximately 10% of GDP). This package is primarily focused at the bottom of the pyramid with approximately ZAR40 billion spent on supporting national health capacities and strengthening basic service delivery of municipalities, and ZAR190 billion was spent on social assistance grants, wage protection through the Unemployment Insurance Fund (UIF), and job protection and creation as stated by Bhorat et al. (2020). The remaining stimulus was focused towards supporting small and informal enterprises, as well as larger employers, largely through a ZAR200 billion Credit Guarantee Scheme (Bhorat et al., 2020). The third stage of the South African government's economic response is anticipatory of a postpandemic national and global economy through the Economic Reconstruction and Recovery Plan (ERRP). This plan hinges on a progression through three phases—Engage and Preserve, Recovery and Reform, Reconstruct and Transform—which successively seek to guide the economy towards President Cyril Ramaphosa's vision to "*not merely to return our economy to where it was before the coronavirus, but to forge a new economy in a new global real-*

ity" (Government Communications & Information Systems, 2020, p. 3). The ERRP seeks to do this through an ambitious variety of measures that include infrastructure investment, localisation of industry, energy security and green economy interventions, economic inclusion of women and youth, mass public employment interventions, agriculture and food security, and macroeconomic policy interventions. The ERRP is aligned to the National Development Plan (NDP) vision to reduce the triple burden of poverty, unemployment, and inequality by seeking to build back better through a refreshed social compact that protects the poor and vulnerable whilst growing the economy in the short run, and in the long run, transforming the patterns of ownership in the economy while making it more competitive through quality services and infrastructure (GCIS, 2020).

It is key to note that despite South Africa's challenging economic circumstances, its government chose to focus on its people rather than industry. This focus was possible by the size of its direct social support package through cash transfers and social grants, which neared 10% of the economic stimulus package announced in April 2020. The government increased the amount of all existing social grants and added a special COVID-19 grant aimed at any adult citizen, permanent resident, or refugee who is unemployed and without any income, social grant, or unemployment payouts (Bhorat et al., 2020). Its poverty-reducing effects and pro-poor distribution led to this special grant being renewed in October 2020 after having reached six million people, the majority of them without any form of support from the government previously. Thus, by the end of 2020, the South African government had extended a social safety net to 61% of its population (Bhorat et al., 2020). This extraordinary social assistance has the potential to morph into a world-first basic income grant. following President Ramaphosa's address at the ruling political party's yearly conference in January 2021. However, the sustainable financing of such an initiative is challenging (Buthelezi, 2021) given South Africa's high debt-to-GDP ratio and minimised fiscal space because of lower tax collection, among other factors.

8.6 Human Capability During COVID-19: A Critical Analysis

In exploring the human capability implications of the coronavirus (COVID-19) in a dual society, such as South Africa, it is important to note that despite the inherited inequities in the health sector, as highlighted earlier, high socioeconomic inequalities. and a faltering economy, the government did not put a premium on the economy but on its people. It can therefore be argued that the government did implement a capability-based and people-centered approach to protect South Africans, especially the poor, marginalised, and most vulnerable from the negative effects of COVID-19. This is in line with the ideological stance of the governing party, the African National Congress (ANC), and the NDP. According to the NDP, to realise its goals of eliminating poverty by reducing inequality and unemployment, it is important to grow an inclusive economy, build human capabilities, and enhance the capability of the state, while promoting partnerships and leadership in society (NPC, 2011). The pandemic required an immediate response and decisive leadership and this is what we saw from the South African government at the onset of COVID-19. Also, the National Department of Health spending approximately 40 billion on supporting national health capacities, allocated to acquiring more medical equipment while also building makeshift hospitals to accommodate an increasing number of patients, and hiring more health care staff is evidence of the government's effort to increase state capabilities in the healthcare sector (Bhorat et al., 2020). These response measures were driven by policies such as the PHC, and Human Resources Strategy for the healthcare sector as part of the pilot phase of the National Health Insurance (NHI) (HST, 2019) in an attempt to increase healthcare access for marginalised communities and create a partnership between the public and private healthcare responses to the pandemic (National department of Health, 2020).

The socioeconomic response towards eliminating poverty and reducing inequality, as stipulated in the NDP, started even before the COVID-19 pandemic. South Africa's government implemented BBBEE, aimed at increasing black business ownership, to create employment opportunities for the previously disadvantaged groups. Although this did not benefit the larger majority, it increased human capabilities for black people to make a contribution to the South African economy. Moreover, with human capabilities in mind, the government continued to make efforts to cushion the consequences of the pandemic through social security relief. The government further provided financial support and social assistance grants, as has been discussed previously. It can be argued that all these measures were aimed at increasing human capabilities for people to survive the COVID-19 pandemic. Furthermore, the NDP promotes self-reliant sustainable development through support that uses people's capabilities and relies on active citizenship. This approach is authenticated by the people's response to the pandemic. Despite challenges that the nation experienced including increased rates of unemployment, corruption, and the looting of COVID-19 relief funds (Bhorat & Köhler, 2020), South Africans made a recognisable effort and displayed active citizenship and solidarity. Evidently, nongovernmental organisations and nonprofit organisations experienced an increase in volunteering as they took an active lead in social assistance initiatives such as the donation of food parcels, the donation of sanitisers, moving people from the streets to shelters, and working together with the government in erecting prefabricated structures for informal settlement dwellers and water infrastructure in communities that had not had water for years. This element of active citizenry further displays the lived experience of the age-old philosophical spirit of *Ubuntu*. Consequently, the pandemic culminated in president Cyril Ramaphosa's announcement of the Economic Reconstruction and Recovery Plan (ERRP), which is designed to help South Africa effectively recover from COVID-19 and forge a new, inclusive, and globally competitive economy (SA Gov, 2020c).

8.7 Conclusion

Despite South Africa's dysfunctional and unequal healthcare sector, a feeble economy, and high socioeconomic inequalities, the country's response to the pandemic was immediate, efficient, and definitive. The response was directed at increasing human capabilities through rapid healthcare initiatives, myriad social assistance packages, increased and ongoing health education, and widespread coronavirus awareness to help curb the virus spread. According to Den Braber (2013), Sen's human development model ties in well with the trajectory of social work, which appeals to putting human well-being at the centre of human developmental thinking. Social work as a practice-based profession understands human development and promotes social change, advancement, cohesion, and community empowerment. Accordingly, the capability approach provides social workers with an execution model that legitimises their actions and evaluates social policy and its implementation (Den Braber, 2013).

This chapter shows that South Africa's responses reflect the capability approach as espoused in the NDP. Therefore, it seems that the capability approach is beginning to take root in South Africa, as this chapter outlines. The government's socioeconomic interventions express a capability and human development-based approach. It is equally important to note the people's responses from a bottom-up perspective, with nonprofit organisations operating from indigenous value systems such as *Ubuntu*; these humanity and solidarity networks mirror the capability approach, showing clearly that the pandemic's impacts would have been extremely devastating without this active citizenry response. Interestingly, this approach has helped South Africa maintain some semblance of equilibrium, through a strengthened nexus between the state and its citizens.

Therefore, it is safe to conclude that South Africa has the potential to see an effective recovery from COVID-19 because the country used a capability approach to human development in responding to the plight of the COVID-19 pandemic. The nation's residents are left with the hope of a renewed, and inclusive, South Africa, a land of opportunity, the South Africa that was initially envisioned, one with excellent leadership, equality, a country free of corruption, and one that continues to build on human capabilities and a strengthened partnership between the state and its citizens.

References

African Development Bank (AFDB). (2020). *Africa's Economic Performance and Outlook Amid Covid-19. Abidjan, Côte d'Ivoire*. Retrieved from: https://www.afdb.org/sites/default/files/documents/publications/afdb20-04_aeo_supplement_full_report_for_web_0705.pdf

Anand, P., Ferrer, B., Gao, Q., Nogales, R., & Unterhalter, E. (2020). COVID-19 as a capability crisis: Using the capability framework to understand policy challenges. *Journal of Human Development and Capabilities, 21*(3), 293–299.

Bhorat, H., & Köhler. T. (2020). *Lockdown economics in South Africa: Social assistance and the Ramaphosa Stimulus Package*. https://www.brookings.edu/blog/africa-in-focus/2020/11/20/lockdown-economics-in-south-africa-social-assistance-and-the-ramaphosa-stimulus-package/

Bhorat, K., Oosthuizen, S., Steenkamp, F., & Thornton, A. (2020). *The economics of Covid-19 in South Africa: Early impressions*. Development policy research unit working paper 202004. DPRU, University of Cape Town.

Buthelezi, L. (2021). *SA needs to discuss the viability of a basic income grant, says Ramaphosa*. https://www.news24.com/fin24/economy/sa-needs-to-discuss-the-viability-of-a-basic-income-grant-says-ramaphosa-20210108

Council for Medical Schemes (CMS). (2016). *Annual report 2015/2016*, Pretoria, South Africa.

Den Braber, C. (2013). The introduction of the capability approach in social work accross a neoliberal Europe. *Journal of Social Intervention, 22*(4), 61–77.

Government Communications and Information Systems (GCIS). (2020). *The South African Reconstruction and Recovery Plan*. https://www.gov.za/sites/default/files/gcis_document/202010/south-african-economic-reconstruction-and-recovery-plan.pdf

Health Systems Trust. (1995a). *South African health review (SAHR) 1996*, Durban, South Africa.

Health Systems Trust. (1995b). *South African health review (SAHR) 2019*, Durban, South Africa.

Health Systems Trust. (2019). *South African health review (SAHR) 2019*, Durban, South Africa.

Hogan, D. R., Stevens, G. A., Hosseinpoor, A. R., & Boerma, T. (2018). Monitoring universal health coverage within the sustainable development goals: Development and baseline data for an index of essential health services. *Lancet Global Health, 6*(2), 152–168.

Mbeki, T. (1998). *Statement of the Deputy President at the opening of the debate in the National Assembly, on "Reconciliation and Nation Building"*. http://www.sahistory.org.za/archive/statement-deputy-president-thabo-mbekiopening-debate-national-assembly-reconciliation-and-n

McIntyre, D., Bloom, G., Doherty, J., & Brijal, P. (1995). *Health expenditure and finance in South Africa*. Health Systems Trust and World Bank.

Msomi, N. (2020). Covid 19: Healthcare workers on the frontline under stress, survey shows. [blog] *health-E-News*.

National Department of Health. (2011). *Human resources for health South Africa: HRH Strategy for the Health Sector 2012/13–2016/17*. http://www.gov.za/sites/www.gov.za/files/hrh_strategy_0.pdf

National Department of Health. (2015). *National Health Insurance for South Africa: Towards Universal Health Coverage* (White Paper No. 40). https://www.health-e.org.za/wpcontent/uploads/2015/12/National-Health-InsuranceforSouth-Africa-White-Paper.pdf

National Planning Commission (NPC). (2011). *National development plan: Vision for 2030*. NPC.

Orthofer, A. (2016). *Wealth inequality in South Africa: Evidence from survey and tax data*. Working paper 15.

Osmani, S. R. (2021). Coping with Covid-19 from the capability perspective: A view from a developing country. *Journal of Human Development and Capabilities*. https://doi.org/10.1080/19452829.2020.1862974.

Perper, R. (2018). *Labor attrition between South Africa's public and private health sectors: A mixed methods case study of KwaZulu-Natal dietitians*. Duke University.

Republic of South Africa (RSA). (1996). *The constitution of the Republic of South Africa*. Government Printer.

Robeyns, I. (2005). The capability approach: A theoretical survey. *Journal of Human Development and Capabilities, 6*(1), 93–117.

Sen, A. (1999). *Development as freedom* (1st ed.). Oxford University Press.

South African Government (SAGov). (2020c). *The South African reconstruction and recovery plan*. https://www.gov.za/sites/default/files/gcis_document/202010/south-african-economic-reconstruction-and-recovery-plan.pdf

Statistics South Africa (StatsSA). (2014). *Poverty trends in South Africa: An examination of absolute poverty between 2006 and 2011*. StatsSA.

Statistics South Africa (StatsSA). (2017). *South African general household survey 2016: Statistical release*. StatsSA.

United Nations Development Programme (UNDP). (2014). *Sustaining Human Progress: Reducing vulnerabilities and building Resillience*. Retrieved from: https://www.undp.org/publications/human-development-report-2014

United Nations Development Programme (UNDP). (2020). *Broken societies put people and planet on collision course*. Human Development Report Office. Retrieved from: http://hdr.undp.org/sites/default/files/2020_global_press_release_en.pdf

Van Rensburg, H. C. (2014). South Africa's protracted struggle for equal distribution and equitable access – Still not there. *Human Resources for Health, 12*(26), 1–16. https://doi.org/10.1186/1478-4491-12-26

Wadee, H., Gilson, L., Thiede, M., Okoafor, O., & McIntyre, D. (2003). *Healthcare inequity in South Africa and the public/private mix*. United Nations research Institute for Social Development (UNRSID).

World Bank. (2020). *Covid 19 to plunge global economy into worst recession since World War II*. https://www.worldbank.org/en/news/press-release/2020/06/08/covid-19-to-plunge-global-economy-into-worst-recession-since-world-war-ii

World Inequality Database (WID). (2020). *The distributional impact of the pandemic in the UK*. https://wid.world/fr/news-article/the-distributional-impact-of-thepandemic/

Worldometer. (2021). *Covid-19 coronavirus pandemic*. https://www.worldometers.info/coronavirus/

9 The Exposition of the Stark Realities of an Unequal Society Based on the COVID-19 Pandemic

Veronica Nemutandani and Thabisa Matsea

9.1 Introduction

The state of inequality in South Africa is widely documented. Although South Africa is regarded as a middle-income country in terms of Gross Domestic Product (GDP), its social indicators are not far from those of the low-income countries, reflecting the unequal distribution of resources and opportunities (Servaas van der Berg, 2010; World Bank, 2016). The level of inequality in the country is ascribed to the history of colonialism and apartheid, which are regarded as a crime to humanity. South Africa acquired democracy in 1994, and has made efforts to address inequality and the related challenges. The country has since made progress in reducing poverty, but very little has changed in terms of inequality and the improvement of the quality of life for most citizens: this is attributable to the high inequality rate that acts as a barrier to poverty reduction (David et al., 2018). For instance, although whites constitute the minority of the South African population, they own a large chunk of the existing land whereas most of the black people live below the poverty line as they do not own land.

V. Nemutandani (✉) · T. Matsea
Faculty of Humanities, Social Sciences and Education, Department of Social Work, University of Venda, Thohoyandou, South Africa
e-mail: veronica.nemutandani@univen.ac.za; Thabisa.matsea@univen.ac.za

With the outbreak of COVID-19, it has become clear that inequality requires immediate attention. The implementation of lockdown, which resulted in the halting of economic activities, exposed the dire situation of the existing inequalities. Many businesses could not survive the lockdown, causing job cuts that saw many people losing jobs and increasing the already high levels of unemployment. This situation, brought by COVID-19 shows that the pandemic will continue to wreak havoc long after its nonexistence, which will be to the detriment of the poorest people. It is important to note that the current situation of inequality is not conducive to the general well-being of individuals, families, groups, and communities. This situation will exacerbate the current social ills that have a negative impact not only on the population but also on the government's efforts to improve the quality of life for all. As such, there is a need to put in place efforts to mitigate the consequences of inequality on vulnerable populations.

Given that existing efforts to promote inequality have failed to address the challenges, it is important to adopt strategies that can facilitate meaningful social development processes. These strategies should embrace social inclusion and strive toward creating a just society with equal opportunities that will contribute to the improved social functioning of the society. These needs challenge the social work profession as ambassadors of social justice because they should insti-

M. C. S. Gonçalves et al. (eds.), *The Coronavirus Crisis and Challenges to Social Development*,
https://doi.org/10.1007/978-3-030-84678-7_9

gate with interventions to help the vulnerable populations and people in distress. This goal can be achieved through promoting democratic values and fundamental rights, social inclusion, nondiscrimination, and active citizenship. This chapter discusses current inequalities in South Africa that are persistent despite various measures put in place to counteract the problem. Moreover, this chapter brings to the fore the inequalities in South Africa that are proving to be turbulent with the emergence of COVID-19. This chapter is divided into three parts. Part one provides a contextual reality of inequality in South Africa. Part two outlines the interaction of the COVID-19 pandemic with the existing inequalities. Finally, part three provides social work response to inequality.

9.2 Background on Inequality in South Africa

The history of South Africa cannot be overlooked when discussing inequality and related issues. The country has a long history of inequality from the discriminatory practices of colonialism and apartheid that has resulted in the racially based poor quality of life. In this scenario, the black population is suffering the greatest even though they are the majority. The two past regimes prohibited the free interaction of people across race lines, hence forcing racial groups to live in segregated areas (Noyoo, 2020). According to Pillay (2017), whiteness as the superior pigmentation and population group was affirmed. This attitude was then imposed on the black masses to oppress and dehumanize black people, which led to black people believing that they were inferior. The apartheid policies were designed in such a way that they catered to the needs of the whites. The economy was also monopolized and manipulated to sustain white people to the detriment of the well-being of the black peoples.

Since the emergence of democracy in 1994, the South African government has made efforts to redress the ills of the past. However, the country is still grappling with inequality despite these efforts and commitment to equality. Mayosi and Benatar (2014) argue that, although there have been various policy interventions targeting reductions in socioeconomic inequalities, nothing has changed. Changes in the political landscape did not have any effect as many forms of inequalities persist and contribute to various challenges that the majority of the population experience. The study by Hodgson (2012) regarded rising inequality as a key challenge that has adverse effects on economic development and sociopolitical stability in South Africa. As such, this results in the undermining of the reconciliation progress made since 1994 because privileges are still drawn along racial lines. In South Africa, the gap between rich and poor is wider than in any other country with the highest concentration of resources in certain races. For example, the top 1% of South African earners take home almost 20% of all income in the country: the top 10% of earners take home 65% of the available income, whereas the remaining 90% of South African earners get only 35% of total income (World Inequality Database, 2018). To date, previously disadvantaged South Africans, who have limited or no access to land, hold fewer assets, earn lower wages, and are still more likely to be unemployed. The levels of poverty remain high with one in ten South Africans living in informal settlements, where living conditions are abysmal and forced evictions are frequent. Patterns of inequalities in educational opportunities and outcomes in South Africa persist amongst the previously disadvantaged (World Bank, 2018).

9.3 COVID-19 and Inequality in South Africa

No country in the world has been spared by the current coronavirus pandemic. The World Health Organization (WHO) declared the outbreak of this pandemic to be the sixth public health emergency of international concern because it continues to spread and results in large numbers of fatalities (WHO, 2020). These numbers are increasing daily. It is believed that COVID-19 is more likely to cause greater human suffering when compared to similar diseases and their consequences (Yoo, 2020). Since its initial outbreak in China, the COVID-19 pandemic has spread rapidly around the world, forcing many countries to adopt unconventional strategies to curb and prevent the spread of the virus (Chakraborty & Maity, 2020). As did other countries in the world, South Africa implemented national lockdown strategies that resulted in the halt of many activities because it restricted the movement of people: people were only allowed to leave home to get essential services such as food and medical assistance. Although the implementation of lockdown proved effective in arresting the spread of the virus, unprecedented challenges emerged that caused major disruptions in the economic, social, political, and environmental structures (Chakraborty & Maity, 2020). The next part examines how efforts made to flatten the curve of COVID-19 interact with the existing inequalities.

9.3.1 Challenges in the Health Sector

The COVID-19 pandemic has generated devastating socioeconomic crises in many countries. It has proved to be not only the greatest threat to global public health of the century, as it is currently, but also a determinant of the inequity and deficiency of social advancement because it highlights the deep-rooted inequality that exists in the global society and within countries (Chakraborty & Maity, 2020). Although certainly no country was prepared for the devastating effects of the pandemic, its rapid spread has exposed the lack of resources of healthcare systems to cope with the pandemic even in high-income countries. Both low- and middle-income countries, including South Africa, are hard hit by the pandemic effects given that their healthcare systems are already under-resourced and overburdened.

In South Africa, the healthcare system is characterized by inequalities (Mayosi & Benatar, 2014). South African health services are delivered in both private and public sector components, and there is a huge gap between the two components in terms of resource allocation. The private health systems tend to be well resourced with full staff complements and well-equipped facilities, but at a high cost, which is a barrier to access for many people. On the other hand, although the public health sector appears comprehensive with primary, secondary, and tertiary healthcare levels to ensure better health for all, this component is often characterized by a lack of resources including staff and equipment, with long waiting times, old facilities, poor disease control and prevention practices, and poor quality of care, combined with unavailability of specialized services especially at the primary health level (Young, 2016; Burger & Christian, 2020; Matsea et al., 2018).

Healthcare in South Africa is characterized by spatial inequalities with clear disparities between rural and urban areas. Evidence shows that although people in rural areas depend on public access, unavailability and poor health service delivery persist in South Africa (Oloyede, 2017). As healthcare in rural areas is resource constrained, the issues of spatial inequalities spark fear regarding the impact that the pandemic would have on these resources. Surprisingly, COVID-19 exposed the preexisting spatial inequalities within cities as it widened the gap between suburbs, townships, and informal settlements. Given that coronavirus spreads through human contact, Harrisberg (2020) observes that townships, which are usually areas with high densities, are hard hit by a coronavirus and have become hotspots with a high mortality rate, whereas rural areas have reported relatively low numbers of cases. However, this should not suggest complacency in rural areas as health prospects are limited, and many people have chronic conditions that make them vulnerable to COVID-19 which have a devastating impact on the rural healthcare services.

The pandemic has imposed unprecedented health challenges on individuals and countries globally. Its unprecedented nature has affected the general physical and psychological health of individuals. In addition to physical illnesses, many people have experienced negative psychological reactions such as trauma, shock, fear, existential anxiety, and grief, all reflected by the increase in hospitalizations and heightened use of mental health services (Pawar, 2020). The rapid spread of the virus and the increased social and psychological problems ascribed to it have put healthcare and other systems under pressure. Thus, ethical and practice mandates have been generally compromised as a priority has been put on responding to COVID-19 cases while unintentionally denying other people the right to healthcare and other services (Pawar, 2020). Similar occurrences have also been reported in South Africa. A decline in the number of patients with chronic illnesses in many South African healthcare facilities has been reported as people have avoided seeking medical care for fear of contracting COVID-19, with significant changes in their daily lives caused by continuous lockdown, forced quarantine, and self-isolation, as well as restricted access to psychosocial support, which lead to mental health problems such as anxiety, depression, and acute panic (Mbunge, 2020).

Continued lockdown can present overwhelming effects on the already inadequate South African healthcare system long after COVID-19. As the country is grappling with the burden of communicable and noncommunicable diseases such as HIV and AIDS, and hypertension as well as diabetes (Nyalusu & Pandya, 2020), the lengthened lockdown could result in a resurgence of these disease and other comorbidities resulting from reduced physical activities (Mbunge, 2020). Furthermore, the emergence of COVID-19, which shifted the services providers focus from basic essential services to measures to curb the spread of the virus (Nyalusu & Pandya, 2020), has the potential to worsen the existing gaps in healthcare and exacerbate the risks of the burden of disease.

9.3.2 COVID-19 Exposing the Impact of the Divide in the Education System

COVID-19 is widening the inequality gap in education. It is estimated that, in 2018, 258 million children globally were not in school and Sub-Saharan Africa accounts for 31% of this number (UNESCO, 2020). From the onset of the pandemic, many countries including South Africa opted to close schools and other places of learning as a measure to contain the virus. To date, South African children have lost more than 25% of the normal school days (Van der Berg & Spaull, 2020): the extended school closures may increase the number of children who are not in school. In an attempt to save the academic year, strategies were adopted to ensure that teaching and learning continue. As such, many schools opted to use online platforms for this purpose, which has revealed divides in digital-based learning and inequalities that are a real threat to education. For instance, it has been reported that more than 75% of children in South Africa are from poor families and they attend poorly performing schools that offer poor-quality education (Spaull, 2015).

Therefore, adopting online teaching and learning meant that learners from poor families were left behind, as many did not have the relevant devices whereas those who managed to get their hands on such gadgets struggled with connectivity to a poor network and securing data (UNESCO, 2020). Online teaching and learning were not only affecting learners but equally so their teachers, causing teaching and learning to come to a complete stop in most disadvantaged schools while it continued in privileged schools. As schools shifted to online learning, Dube (2020) observed that this appeared to favor urban and privileged learners because many rural learners were excluded from schooling as they could not access online resources for lack of infrastructure, or the unavailability of electricity and electronic devices, and also the lack of qualified teachers who can assist with online learning. This consequence has the potential to worsen the existing education crisis while also widening inequality in South Africa.

Given that many children were already struggling to keep up with their curriculum, missing out on months of classes proved to be a disadvantage for low-achieving learners who need continued support. Because South Africa has a high rate of functional illiteracy (Chokwe, 2016), many children whose parents or older siblings are not educated cannot provide the necessary support to help children master critical skills: this has put these children at a disadvantage and high risk of performing far below their potential, thereby denying them the opportunity to enter university. Thus, they could feel discouraged, and their learning time is replaced by noneducational activities, thereby increasing the risk of repeating grades which may result in dropping out of school (UNESCO, 2020).

9.3.3 The Effects of the Business Shutdown on the Vulnerable Population

It is undeniable that coronavirus has indiscriminately spread and affected the population all over the world. However, its impact has been discriminately biased on vulnerable populations such as poor people, immigrants as well as elderly people. Given the structural and socioeconomic discrimination that the vulnerable populations constantly experience, this group's capacity to cope with the pandemic has weakened (Pawar, 2020). The COVID-19 pandemic and the implemented mitigation measures have impacted the general population, especially the vulnerable groups and those involved in the informal labor market, as it poses a threat to food security and exacerbates the food crisis that existed long before lockdown (Seekings, 2020; United Nations, 2020). This, in turn, increases the existing income inequality: a growing body of evidence indicates the correlation between high levels of income inequality and poverty. Income inequality and poverty have a direct and indirect impact on each other. Income inequality hinders efforts for poverty reduction as it slows the pace at which growth facilitates poverty reduction, as occurs in South Africa (Bhorat et al., 2015; Dabbla-Norris et al., 2015).

In South Africa, the implementation of lockdown resulted in the shutdown of sections of the economy. As such, nonessential suppliers were closed, but grocery stores, pharmaceutical retail, and banks remained operational for essential supplies. The lockdown had a direct and severe impact on people employed in industries that shut down and those involved in the informal labor market. This impact was concentrated on certain racial groups and varied according to age and gender. In South Africa, the lockdown affected black Africans as unemployment is prevalent among this racial group, with the majority concentrated in unskilled and low-paying jobs (Dludla, 2020). Although there has been an increase in the participation of women in the labor market, they are more likely to experience social responsibilities while men remain active and consistently participate in the labor market. Furthermore, unemployment rates are high among South African youth (Bhorat et al., 2015). A survey conducted by the International Labour Organization (ILO) (2020) found that more than one in six young people had stopped working since the beginning of the pandemic while those who remained employed experienced a 23% cut in working hours: salary cuts came with the decreased working hours.

As ILO (2018) observed, many people in most African countries, including South Africa, live from hand to mouth as they are either involved in the informal economy or doing low-paying jobs. Therefore, the halting of economic activities meant that many people lost income and became unable to meet their basic needs and those of their dependents.

The issues raised here are crucial because they highlight the intensity of inequality as exposed by COVID-19. These issues point out the more intense challenges that can erupt should the issue of inequality be left unattended. Therefore, this calls for professional interventions to provide sustainable solutions to prevent future challenges. Addressing the COVID-19 impact requires varied approaches for reshaping various systems with the focus on building resilience, reduction of inequalities, and rebuilding communities through the active participation of vulnerable groups. All this challenges a social work profession to take the lead in addressing inequalities as discussed in the following section.

9.4 Socioeconomic COVID-19 Response by Government, Civil Society, Business, and Nongovernmental Organizations (NGOs) in South Africa

Understandably, no one was ready or expected COVID-19 to rapidly take over people's lives as it did. In a literal sense, it caught the South African population unexpectedly. Hence, it created a set of expectations and demands from the vulnerable and affected population, to which the government had to immediately respond to suppress the frustrations and uncertainties about the well-being of the most vulnerable. Lingam and Sapkal (2020) note that the present state of South Africa for the jobless growth agenda, half-hearted social protection measures, and underfunding of healthcare services have widened the socioeconomic and health inequalities of the already struggling masses. The nature of the pandemic demanded a collaborative approach to tackle the challenges created by COVID-19. Hence the South African government called upon the support of NGOs, civil society, and business to come on board as a means of strengthening their partnership in the fight against the pandemic. Most importantly, the partnership was to come up with rapid measures that would serve as safety nets for vulnerable groups.

9.4.1 Civil Society and Ubuntu to Combat COVID-19

The lockdown created an urgency that witnessed individuals and families coming on board to avail their services and whatever they could donate. This by no means meant that some people have abundant resources; for them, this deed meant "sharing the little you have with others." It did not matter what or how little it was. In its relentless endeavors to reach the most vulnerable, civil society demonstrated a strong and emotional sense of Ubuntu. Ubuntu is defined by Mugumbate and Nyanguru (2013) as an African philosophy that emphasizes being human through others. An understood meaning of Ubuntu in its Nguni origin means umuntu ngu muntu nga banye (being self, through others). This demonstration of Ubuntu by civil society happened at a time when society had lost hope in its meaning. The vulnerable groups were and are still seen, to a certain extent, to be the sole responsibility of the government. Families and community members appeared to have transferred a task that they used to effortlessly execute. Gone are the days when families and community members would take care of the vulnerable families within their environment.

Despite its negative and devastating consequences, COVID-19 has succeeded in schooling civil society to revisit past practices of togetherness and taking care of each other. Will ubuntu stand the test of time even after COVID-19? Time will tell.

9.4.2 Business Responding to the Call to Combat COVID-19

The role of business in corporate social responsibility did not go unnoticed. The business community responded to the government call to join in the fight against COVID-19, which has created untold suffering among the most vulnerable. One of the major challenges throughout the pandemic was, first, for businesses to protect their interests against all odds by ensuring that the economy is unharmed or minimally so. Second, business needed to ensure that their employees' livelihoods are protected. The latter was not the case for most businesses as their responsibility to their workers was overtaken by their own economic interests, thus leaving their employees to join the vulnerable masses and adding this responsibility to the already overstretched resources of the state.

However, several businesses fulfilled their role by their strengths and capabilities. Provision of the following from businesses to assist in flattening the curve ranged from healthcare support including field hospitals, masks, and sanitizers; free educational material and online learning;

network availability to support with "work from home"; free online medical screening and consultations; donations to NGOs that work directly with communities to support their work; tracking and tracing people who might have contracted COVID-19; supplying food and hygiene products for the vulnerable groups in different communities and schools; and payment relief from banks for small businesses.

While the spread of COVID-19 continues, businesses are required to adjust to sustainable ways of addressing their challenges, especially in local employment as the hardest hit sector, which will contribute to the livelihoods of the vulnerable people.

9.4.3 NGOs: The Pulse of the Community During the Pandemic

In South Africa, COVID-19 has affected every aspect of society. Unemployment and poverty have increased beyond measure and thus strained the already ailing socioeconomic conditions of the country. Despite the socioeconomic challenges, the NGOs have always been there to support the government in its attempts to address the socioeconomic challenges experienced by the vulnerable communities. These organizations work closely with communities and understand their circumstances and challenge better. They are the "foot soldiers" with whom most government officials work closely.

Some businesses also rely on NGOs through funding to realize their social responsibility intentions. The gift of the givers is just but one example of an NGO that understands the plight of the communities and has adopted a "foot soldier" role throughout their engagements with communities. Understanding the seriousness of the pandemic, the 'Gift of the Givers' (2020) has assisted communities, including hospitals, in the following ways: provision of medical supplies including protective clothing; medical supplies; refurbishment of some hospitals and beds; boreholes in rural communities so that communities may have access of water; and the most needed food parcels.

9.4.4 Social Work Intervention as a Mechanism of Curbing the Effects of COVID-19

Social work as a profession focuses its commitment to social justice for the vulnerable and those in distress from circumstances beyond their control and capabilities. Also, Seafor (2006), in his discussion, referred to social work as a profession that has always directed its focus to poverty and difficulties experienced by the most vulnerable populations. Therefore, the social worker's skills and knowledge would appear to be most appropriate to confront the psychosocial and economic effects of COVID-19. This chapter confirms that most of the inequalities referred to and the effects thereof represent the most vulnerable and poor. This part of the population does not have enough resources or as in some cases does not have the necessary basic resources to satisfy their desired needs, which results in poverty having devastating effects and inhuman experiences on the vulnerable. On 11 May 2020, the Social Development Minister Lindiwe Zulu made a pronouncement on the intervention strategies that her Department of Social Development (DSD) was undertaking to ensure that the livelihoods of the most vulnerable population are protected from the pandemic. Social workers and volunteers were employed to assist in the DSD program in its response to COVID-19. Volunteers assisted the DSD with food distribution; educating families on COVID-19 preventions, verification of applicants for the special COVID-19 Social Relief of Distress Grant; and fast-tracking the process of payment of the grant (Zulu, 2020). The Department has been providing food and nutrition services to combat the growing challenge of malnutrition and hunger among the poor and vulnerable communities (Zulu, 2020). The worst part of this venture occurred when a few corruption cases were reported about food parcels. Some reported cases concerned the recipients themselves and some were government officials responsible for the food and nutrition program. Recipients were reported to be selling food items to shop owners. Although the DSD intervention met with a few challenges, it did, however, lighten the burden on the vulnerable families.

Although the grant was a short-term intervention strategy meant for the most vulnerable and with specific qualifying criteria, nevertheless a few administrative loopholes were detected. The following qualifying criteria were set for the prospective recipients of the grant by SASSA: Applicants to be South African Citizens; Permanent Resident or Refugees registered on the Home Affairs system; Must be above the age of 18; Unemployed; Not receiving any income; Not receiving any social grant; Not receiving any unemployment insurance benefit and does not qualify to receive unemployment insurance benefits; Not receiving a stipend from the National Student Financial Aid Scheme; and Not resident in a government-funded or subsidized institution (Seekings, 2020). The successful applicants received R350 per month, which was to continue until October 2020. This grant came with its share of challenges and complaints from the prospective recipients. These complaints varied from no response for applications received from applicants; delayed payments; and sudden termination of grants in September instead of October. Currently, the social security system has demonstrated that the system is not ready nor designed to work under pressure. The pandemic on the other hand has certainly created learning areas for those in authority that demand a revisit of the configuration of their systems.

What appeared to be the biggest challenge, however, was having to maintain a household on R350. It is of the researchers' view that this amount is another negative on the already stressful population and would be a challenge even to maintain an unemployed family of two. Nevertheless, despite the challenges experienced by the beneficiaries of this grant, it still appears to be "better than nothing" and something to look forward to every month.

Social work also had a crucial role during COVID-19, by providing counseling and identifying vulnerable groups for livelihood intervention; and collaborated with other organizations to deliver food parcels to those in need. It is, however, equally important to mention that the pandemic has also exposed the shortcomings of DSD and challenged its extent of readiness to manage the pandemic. For DSD to effectively deal with the challenges aggravated by the pandemic, it needed a well-resourced, capable, and empowered social work official to render effective social services to individuals, families, and communities in the protection of the most vulnerable. However, DSD's limited essential resources (especially in rural areas) such as infrastructure; transport; telephones; data; and limited exposure to technological knowledge have made it difficult for DSD to effectively ensure that services to individuals and communities in need are delivered by the officials. These challenges meant that limited social interaction imposed by the implementation of lockdown regulations hindered people trying to seek and receive support, requiring social workers to be innovative and introduce strategies that would mitigate the effects of COVID-19. As such, very few social workers used technology to render counseling and related services to those families who were infected and affected by COVID-19. However, this was problematic for those who do not have relevant resources: a "skeleton" staff approach was adopted wherein staff was required to work on a rotational basis to address the challenges confronted by communities.

It is, however, worth noting that although the lockdown measures affected the entire population, the socioeconomic levels and outcomes were entirely dependent on the status and class of the population. This reasoning is supported by the study done by Lingam and Sapkal (2020) stating that, in India, the lockdown forced the informal sector migrant workers to abandon their urban settlements to move back to their villages because of loss of livelihoods. Similarly, in South Africa, those who have lost their jobs in urban areas had to consider going back to rural areas because they understood the cost of living to be manageable in their places of origin. Therefore, the experiences and struggles of the poor and vulnerable during the pandemic proved to have no boundaries.

Faith-based organizations (FBOs) also had a role, especially in soup kitchens, for instance, run by churches, families, and even individuals, which were emerging from the needy communities to fill the gap of the struggling communities. What is quite eminent and commendable from the COVID-19 experience is the strong sense of community togetherness.

9.5 Adversities Versus Coping Mechanisms

Having analyzed the initiatives of NGOs, government, families, and individuals, it is important to note that the pandemic continues to display devastating effects on the vulnerable populations. A study conducted by Devereux (2020) acknowledges that despite the safety nets that have been put in place, several groups remain at risk. The most vulnerable groups mentioned by Devereux include domestic workers; farmworkers; self-employed workers such as guards; and hawkers whose livelihoods depend on daily interactions. The groups mentioned by the author represent most of the struggling population. The question is: How do these vulnerable groups cope with life challenges when they continuously find themselves at the bottom of the safety net? Thus, it is in times such as the COVID-19 pandemic when the inequalities of the population are exposed.

The question is: Is the population equipped or even able to come up with coping mechanisms when every aspect of their lives seems to be pointing downward? It is therefore the researchers' view that one can only think of coping mechanisms when there are tangible options at hand, and that the context people find themselves in is favorable and conducive. Lever (2008) states that people of the low socioeconomic class have less efficient coping mechanisms and lack the social resources to combat stress. Lever further mentions that coping has two primary functions: to grapple with the stress-inducing problem at hand and to regulate the emotions it provokes. Parents or breadwinners in families have lost their jobs; they found themselves unexpectedly, unemployed. What they could provide to their families they no longer could. These families were forced to adjust and adapt to different coping mechanisms. Similarly, some parents and breadwinners died from COVID-19, leaving their children and families in a dire state. With the loss of their loved ones, they are forced to confront the unforeseen and the heartache of having to start from nowhere. The sad reality is that in most circumstances, these families have accepted and adjusted their lifestyles to the situation they are experiencing by regulating the emotions brought about by their struggles. Some of the changes experienced by these families were positive as families searched for alternative ways of survival.

Small business start-ups became famous solutions to those who lost their jobs but had the skills to pursue alternatives. They found themselves selling their services in the form of carpentry, building, painting, including selling scones and sandwiches to community members and offices. A 45-year-old man who worked at a well-established paint shop in Johannesburg relates his story: "*I worked in a paint shop in Johannesburg for 15 years. I have a wife who is unemployed and 5 children who are at home. I was satisfied with the little salary I was earning because my children could eat and go to school. In June 2020, my employer contacted me to tell me that I will not be able to go back to work as he had to close his paint shop. At first, I thought he will call me to tell me that I could come back to work. The second call was to tell me that my severance package is in the bank. Upon checking the amount deposited, I realized that I will not survive beyond three months. I had to quickly look at alternative ways to keep my family's survival. I erected a shack on my site that would serve as a paint shop and all the necessary equipment to start my paint shop. "Mixing paint is what I knew best and could not think of anything else. Presently, I have mixed paint and painted a lot of houses in my community and beyond. I am a well-known painter and the rest is history.*" He went on to say "Thank you, COVID." Examples of such initiatives became the norm. On the flip side of the coin, COVID-19 proved to have altered the mindset of the working citizens who found themselves unemployed.

9.6 Conclusion

Undoubtedly, COVID-19 has created a negative socioeconomic impact, especially among the vulnerable South African population, and therefore highlighted several challenges. The already poor and vulnerable South African population found themselves in a wanting situation with fears of having to cope with yet another incapacitating effect of their well-being.

The nature of the estimated effects of COVID-19 on the South African population left government, business, and some NGOs with no choice but to put in place immediate mechanisms to reduce the effects of the pandemic on the vulnerable population. The lockdown imposed by the government on 15 March 2020 served as a mechanism to curb the spread of the pandemic. Although this was an important intervention strategy to flatten the curve of the COVID-19 pandemic, it exacerbated the plight of the vulnerable population subject to extreme conditions such as job losses and reduced income and poverty, leaving the most vulnerable in a compromised condition.

The devastating disorder created by COVID-19 caused a rapid decline in people's livelihoods. The feasibility of providing adequate much-needed services during trying times exposed the vulnerability of the poorest population in unmeasurable terms. These are most of the people who, if working, would have experienced a salary cut or lost their jobs, and if they are lucky, will at least have child support grants as a source of income on which to solely depend.

It is important to note that COVID-19 has also challenged the social work profession to rethink its role and its effectiveness, especially in the current turmoil in which it finds itself. The social work profession has been and is still vocal on matters of the transformation of historical and structural inequalities, social justice, and decolonization of the curriculum that addresses its sociocultural setting. The profession needs to become relevant to its indigenous context so that it can devise indigenous methods to indigenous challenges, which ultimately result in tangible solutions to the challenges faced by the population it serves.

References

Bhorat, H., Naidoo, K., Oosthuizen, M., & Pillay, K. (2015). *Demographic, employment, and wage trends in South Africa*. UNU-WIDER.

Burger, R., & Christian, C. (2020). Access to health care in post-apartheid South Africa: Availability, affordability, acceptability. *Health Economic Policy Law, 15*, 43–55. https://doi.org/10.1017/S1744133118000300

Chakraborty, I., & Maity, P. (2020). COVID-19 outbreak: Migration, effects on society, global environment, and prevention. *Science of the Total Environment, 782*(2020), 138882. https://doi.org/10.1016/j.scitotenv.2020.138882

Chokwe, J. M. (2016). The acquisition of academic writing skills model for English second language students: From elementary to tertiary education. *Journal of Educational Studies, 15*(2), 136–161.

Dabbla-Norris, E., Kochhar, K., Ricka, F., Suphaphiphat, N., & Tsounta, E. (2015). *Causes, consequences of income inequality: A global perspective*. International Monetary Fund. https://www.imf.org/external/pubs/ft/sdn/2015/sdn1513.pdf

David, A., Guilbert, N., Hino, H., Leibbrandt, M., Potgieter, E., & Shifa, M. (2018). *Social cohesion and inequality in South Africa*. Cape Town.

Devereux, S. (2020). *Social protection responses to the COVID-19 lockdown in South Africa: Research fellow*. Institute of Development Studies, University of Sussex.

Dludla, S. (2020). *The unemployment rate in SA is at the lowest ever since the survey began*. https://www.iol.co.za/business-report/economy/unemployment-rate-in-sa-is-at-lowest-ever-since-survey-began-3c99ad18-e1fb-4535-8dc6-c20907049cc4

Dube, B. (2020). Rural online learning in the context of COVID-19 in South Africa: Evoking an inclusive education approach. *Multidisciplinary Journal of Educational Research, 10*(2), 1–24. https://doi.org/10.4471/remie.2020.5607

Gift of the givers. (2020). *Project report – Covid-19*. www.giftofthegivers.org

Harrisberg, K. (2020). *Coronavirus exposes the 'brutal inequality' of South African townships*. Thompson Reuters Foundation News. https://news.trust.org/item/20200612142951-tx2r5/

Hodgson, A. (2012). *South Africa – The most unequal income distribution in the world*. Euro-Monitor International.

International Labour Office (ILO). (2018). *Women and men in the informal economy: A statistical picture* (3rd ed.). Author.

International Labour Office (ILO). (2020). *Youth & COVID-19: Impacts on jobs, education, rights, and mental well-being*. ILO.

Lever, J. P. (2008). Poverty, stressful life events, and coping strategies. *The Spanish Journal of Psychology, 11*(1), 228–249.

Lingam, L., & Sapkal, R. S. (2020). COVID-19, physical distancing and social inequalities: Are we all really in this together. *The International Journal of*

Community and Social Development. https://doi.org/10.1177/2516602620937932
Matsea, T., Ryke, E., & Weyers, M. (2018). Assessing mental health services in a rural setting: Service providers' perspective. *International Journal of Mental Health, 47*(1), 26–49. https://doi.org/10.1080/00207411.2017.1377805
Mayosi, B. M., & Benatar, S. R. (2014). Health and health care in South Africa—20 years after Mandela. *New England Journal of Medicine, 371*(14), 1344–1353.
Mbunge, E. (2020). Effects of COVID-19 in south African health system and society: An explanatory study. *Diabetes & Metabolic Syndrome: Clinical Research & Reviews, 14*, 1809–1814.
Mugumbate, J., & Nyanguru, A. (2013). Exploring African philosophy: The value of Ubuntu in social work. Faculty of Social Sciences, Paper 3266. https://ro.uow.edu.au/sspapers/3266
Noyoo, N. (2020). Resurgent racism in post-apartheid South Africa and the need to promote healthy relationships. In N. Noyoo (Ed.), *Promoting healthy human relationships in post-apartheid South Africa: Social work and social development perspectives* (pp. 21–33). Springer. https://doi.org/10.1007/978-3-030-50139-6
Nyalusu, J., & Pandya, H. (2020). The effects of coronavirus disease 2019 pandemic on the south African health system: A call to maintain essential health services. *African Journal of Primary Health Care & Family Medicine, 12*(1), 1–5. https://doi.org/10.4102/phcfm.v12i1.2480
Oloyede, O. (2017). Rural-urban disparities in health and health care in Africa: Cultural competence, lay-beliefs in narratives of diabetes among the rural poor in the Eastern Cape Province of South Africa. *African Sociological Review, 21*(2), 36–57.
Pawar, M. (2020). The global impact of and responses to the COVID-19 pandemic. *The International Journal of Community and Social Development, 2*(2), 111–120.
Pillay, J. (2017). Racism and xenophobia: The role of the Church in South Africa. Economy life in its fullness. *Verbum et Ecclesia, 38*(3), 3–17. https://doi.org/10.4102/ve.v38i3.1655
Seafor, B. W. (2006). *Techniques and guidelines for social work practice, 7/e*. Allan and Baker Pearson.
Seekings, J. (2020). SASSA's big test: When will the emergency COVID-19 social grant be paid? *GroundUp*. https://www.groundup.org.za/article/sassas-big-test-when-will-the-emergency-covid-19-social-grant-be-paid/
Servaas van der Berg, (2010). Current poverty and income distribution in the context of South African history, Working Papers 22/2010, Stellenbosch University, Department of Economics.
Spaull, N. (2015). Schooling in South Africa: How low-quality education becomes a poverty trap. *South African Child Gauge, 12*, 34–41.
UNESCO. (2020). *Policy Brief: Education during COVID-19 and beyond*. https://www.un.org/development/desa/dspd/wp-content/uploads/sites/22/2020/08/sg_policy_brief_covid-19_and_education_august_2020.pdf
United Nations. (2020). *Policy Brief: The impact of COVID-19 on food security and nutrition*. https://www.un.org/sites/un2.un.org/files/sg_policy_brief_on_covid_impact_on_food_security.pdf.
Van Der Berg, S., & Spaull, N. (2020). *Counting the cost. COVID-19 school closures in South Africa and its impact on children. Research on socioeconomic policy (RESEP)*. Stellenbosch University.
WHO. (2020). *WHO coronavirus disease (COVID-19) dashboard*. https://covid19.who.int/
World Bank. (2016). *South Africa overview*. https://www.worldbank.org/en/country/southafrica
World Bank. (2018). *Overcoming poverty and inequality in South Africa: An assessment of drivers, constraints and opportunities*. The World Bank.
World Inequality Database. (2018). *Where are you in the income distribution?* https://wid.world/
Yoo, J. H. (2020). The fight against the 2019-nCoV outbreak: An arduous march has just begun. *Journal of Korean Medical Science*, 35–56. https://doi.org/10.3346/jkms.2020.35.56
Young, M. (2016). *Private vs. public healthcare in South Africa*. Scholar works at Western Michigan University (WMU).
Zulu, L. (2020). *Social development response to Covid 19 for level 4 risk-adjusted approach*. Department of Social Development.

The COVID-19 Crisis: Impact of Social Attitudes and Representations on Social Development in Sub-Saharan Africa

10

Etienne Serupia Semuhoza
and Alexandre Hakizamungu

10.1 Introduction

The context of the COVID-19 pandemic has spread dramatically around the world with its procession of thousands of victims. Among these social categories largely affected by COVID-19 are included Africans. Black African attitudes and representations of COVID-19 expose them to the risk of contagion from it. However, to be effective, the fight against this pandemic will have to be part of an inclusive holistic approach of "One Health," which integrates human, animal, and environmental health (eco-health).

With regard to "One Health," state policies to fight COVID-19 are revealing sociological paradoxes: the science/social representations and culture dialectic, without which the most technically valid fight lacks a solid foundation. This policy cannot leave indifferent social science specialists whose mission is to enlighten various factors involved with financial and material reinforcements in the fight against COVID-19, and the contribution of scientific truths (biology–culture system) with social attitudes and representations (biology/culture dualism) conveyed by standard health control policies, inadequate with the historical contexts of Africans whose cultural schemes are sometimes and not always in contradiction (sociological paradoxes) with state health logics.

This study used a qualitative approach to better understand this complex reality of social attitudes and representations about COVID-19. Our strategy was to use a purposive sample because social processes have a logic and consistency that random sampling would not perceive. So, a small number of people were contacted for interviews in addition to the online questions, with the goal to ask if there was a significant link between the perception of COVID-19 by black Africans and the acceptance of the barrier measures enacted by governments. Respondents to our questionnaire were people in our social network to whom a questionnaire was sent via emails, with an additional few interviews from the same group for data triangulation purposes. The data presented in this chapter are a small extraction from the large study by only considering those focusing only on social attitudes and representations. Other aspects from the survey will be considered for other papers to follow.

The objective was to assess the influence of culture in the response to the pandemic. Would certain cultural practices expose them to easy contamination from COVID-19? Do the populations believe that this virus can be defeated by

E. S. Semuhoza (✉) · A. Hakizamungu
School of Governance, Department of Social Sciences, University of Rwanda, Kigali, Rwanda
e-mail: sserupia@gmail.com; alexahakiza@yahoo.fr

M. C. S. Gonçalves et al. (eds.), *The Coronavirus Crisis and Challenges to Social Development*,
https://doi.org/10.1007/978-3-030-84678-7_10

traditional therapy? Do they think that by avoiding greeting their neighbors or wearing a face mask they are reducing the spread of the virus? This is the reason we bring up the anthropology of cultural causation. Hence, the initial hypothesis of the research states that there is a link between the representations of black Africans and the observance of the barrier measures of their governments. Are they guided by patriotism, or by accommodation? In short, what is the weight of social representations?

For Africans, the COVID-19 pandemic is more than a threat that impacts the heart of society, the very essence of the black African who is socially in general view, anchored in the values of solidarity, proximity, and sharing. This pandemic, brutally imposing new standards of life (social distancing, confinement, etc.), leads to a disruption of social, economic, and cultural links in everyday sociability (UNESCO, 2020).

Social attitudes and representations are indeed the basis of our social and psychic life. These are the ones to which we most easily and spontaneously appeal, to find our way around our physical and human environment. The interface of the psychological, sociological, social attitudes, and representations is rooted in the heart of the social system, with a determining role in the social and mental life of humans, including thoughts, feelings, action plans, and relational references.

However, the theme on the COVID-19 crisis and challenges to social development has been for a few months (and is still today) a subject that has captured the attention of practitioners and researchers, considering the abundance and importance of the work and reports devoted to it. The growing enthusiasm for this theme has revealed a vast field of investigation and reflection, both theoretically and empirically.

This psycho-anthropological research work is part of a holistic approach whose main interest is to explore and try to understand the representations of COVID-19 in black Africans. Representations are generally a set of values, conceptions, and beliefs conceived by a group, put in common, and transmitted during interactions. Thus, we understand that health is a social fact, a fact of culture, and therefore a built-up community because it is the group to which it belongs that defines its representation to the world surrounding it as well as what we can designate as being normal or pathological by its subjects. The group can then offer specific therapies related to its environment. Since its outbreak in China in the city of Wuhan in December 2019, the COVID-19 pandemic, whose causal agent is SARS-COV-2 of animal origin (Xiaolu et al., 2020), has already killed more than 1,711,661 persons (Worldometer on December 22, 2020) worldwide and 59,570 persons in Africa (Xiaolu et al., 2020).

Despite these appalling figures, we observe that the COVID-19 pandemic has been accompanied in Africa by various attitudes and cultural presentations and imaginary contractions of others (Moscovici, 1986a, b, Jodelet, 1989).

This chapter has made it possible to better understand the social representations of Africans and their attitudes on COVID-19. Social representations of COVID-19 find their roots in the information received about this pandemic, whereas the analysis of attitudes reveals that their content fits into their semantic space. This study suggests integrating the sociological and psychosocial approach to understand the social character of the attitudes and social representations of COVID-19 shared by Africans, essentially referring to a conspiracy or an imported disease. First, in this chapter, we consider the theoretical and conceptual aspects necessary for the representation.

The objective in the following part is to show that attitudes and social representations constitute closely correlated variables, in the sense that it is within the latter that evaluations of the individual or group of individuals express in regard the formation of social phenomena. The hypothesis pursued is that attitudes and social representations shape cognitively those variables that allow the expression of spontaneous evaluations through the attitudes expressed.

Finally, understanding the attitudes and social representations of populations in the context of the current coronavirus pandemic is a major challenge. It is on the basis of this analysis of the perception of this pandemic, and its consequences on social development, that the study could inform the choices of public decision makers to curb this pandemic.

10.2 Social Attitudes and Representations of Health and COVID-19

10.2.1 Concept of Attitude

In 1935, Allport, quoted by Cerclé and Somat (2002), after having analyzed more than a hundred definitions of attitude, concluded that most authors agreed on an idea of "predisposition to respond to a social object, and that this predisposition could be learned." In 1955, Cerclé and Somat (2002), showing the convergence of several definitions, indicated much the same characteristic.

Attitude as a predisposition is both a response to the stimulus and a stimulus to the observable response. Cerclé and Somat provide a comprehensive explanation of the structure of variables: "independent, intervening and dependent variables." Attitude can manifest itself verbally, that is, as an opinion, or nonverbally, in the form of behavior. Attitude is this hidden reality that must be captured through opinions or other forms of empirical responses.

Cerclé and Somat indicate that it is not always easy to measure the attitude you want to achieve. When it comes to measuring change, either the affective component or the cognitive component is used. These last statements indicate that it is possible to retain the affective component to measure a change in attitude. There is also research that supports that one can separate the emotional component from the cognitive and behavioral component for the evaluation of a change of attitude; this is explained by the great correlation among these three components.

Despite the spread of the pandemic, a large part of black Africans in both urban and rural areas seemed to have great difficulty in changing their attitudes because their representations indicate a low perception of risk. If the popular discourse at the start of the pandemic referred to religious beliefs that present black Africa as a part of the continent protected by great men of God, then this part of the continent will be transformed, as systematized by one interviewed religious leader:

> The coronavirus is nothing other than a sanction from God in the face of the depravity of morals, the violation of prohibitions, homosexuality, debauchery, many sins, prohibitions .... When God sanctions, he spares no one! We are sent to earth by God to worship him by respecting his prescriptions while avoiding his prohibitions. The only solution we have is prayer and offering.

Popular attitudes and perceptions of COVID-19 combine social representations, values, beliefs, social influences, but also common social practices which, in turn, may increase the level of risk. It is, on the one hand, appreciable and ambient sociability through a strong mobility of the individuals, the primacy to the physical contacts in case of interaction, the proximity of people ... On the other hand, the preponderance of the informal economy that mobilizes a large number of people around income-generating activities, which predispose them to live from day to day in a resourceful economy without the capacity to save, to face the risks of the pandemic has raised lively debates on the applicability of the measures of confinement in a context of precariousness.

Since the onset of the health crisis, containment has emerged as an emergency measure. It has imposed itself as the only measure to face the pandemic. It is important to note that this confinement, which lasted several months, had and will have very important repercussions both economically and socially. This crisis shows, once again, how the economies are very interdependent, vulnerable, and not prepared to face a health shock of this kind. In Sub-Saharan Africa, seven countries have chosen not to impose lockdown: Benin, Burundi, Cameroon, Djibouti, Central African Republic, and Tanzania.

The size of the informal sector has made confinement difficult for those who have to go out every day to earn a living, which explains why some countries have chosen not to take the social risk of confinement.

10.2.2 Concept of Social Representations

This research work is part of a holistic approach whose main objective is to explore and try to understand the representations of COVID-19 among black Africans. Representations are generally a set of values, conceptions, and beliefs conceived by a group, brought together and transmitted through interactions. Thus, the representations of the populations can constitute an obstacle to their assumption of responsibility. Health is a social fact, a fact of culture, and therefore it is embedded in the community because it is the group to which it belongs tthat defines its representation of the world surrounding it as well as what can be designated as a normal or pathological state of health by its subjects. That world can then offer specific therapies related to his environment. Another respondent of our interviewees told us the following: "I think we have always treated everything you say with our natural products. You can treat a cough here, you know. The lungs have their medicine here; headaches and fever are fought every day by the ekuk. Even little children know it [...] what do Whites even want to show?"

In fact, the traditional medicine that this informant evokes and which is advocated by the local populations is a set of know-how reflecting the beliefs and endogenous cultural experiences of the cultures of African origin whose function is to prevent, to cure, to maintain psychic and physical health order and therefore well-being. Seen from the outside, these representations may appear inconsistent or irrational. That said, the interweaving of disease and related care in our lives constitutes, for the developmental psychosociologist, the revelation of the cultural fabric of our African society.

> [...] Also, anthropology thus makes it possible to unveil the logics and norms that characterize daily life, everyday experience, daily practices, by questioning the social links of the dynamics of local communities [...] (Mbonji, 2017, author translation).

Addressing the question of the cultural hypothesis of the social representations of COVID-19 would therefore amount to analyzing the cultural aspects that surround Africans in the face of the pandemic. For example, two of the many barrier gestures in this case, the greeting and the wearing of the face mask, catch our attention. The theory of social representations is of fundamental importance for the study and understanding of social phenomena in the social sciences and in particular by researchers in social psychology. Moscovici (1986a, b) defined social representations as a system of values, ideas, and practices with a dual function. The first function is to establish an order that will allow individuals to orient themselves in their physical and social world to control it. The second is to allow communication to take place among the members of a community by facilitating a code for social exchange and a code for naming and classifying, unambiguously, the different aspects of their world and their individual history and of the group.

Social representations allow us to classify, compare, and interpret cognitive elements, and to objectify them as parts of our social environment. Social representations are formed by the need of individuals to change what is "unknown" into "familiar." We would say, therefore, that social representations bind the mental world of the subject because they relate to the sentimental and imaginary element to the social world, to external reality, given that they are created at the collective level and that they reflect the sociocultural framework in which they are integrated (Moscovici, 1996).

The peripheral elements of the representation are organized around the central core. These elements are hierarchical and have an important role in the realization of the meaning of a representation. The peripheral elements perform three functions:

1. The function of concretization: they assimilate the elements of the situation in which the representation is produced and allow its composition through concrete terms, directly understandable and transmissible.
2. The regulation procedure: to not cast doubt on the bases of representation, new information

can be assimilated either by giving it a minor importance, or by interpreting it again in accordance with the central meaning.
3. The defense function: as the central core of any representation resists change, the peripheral system functions as a defense system. Contradictions can appear and be accepted in the peripheral system.

According to Flament (1994), the peripheral system undertakes the junction between the central core and social practices. Under normal conditions, everyone does what they think. There is, therefore, a correspondence between the symbolic world and social practices. Thus, in this case, the forms of conduct constitute the externalization of the central core through applied social practice.

However, there are many situations in which the subject does not react as expected, believing that he or she is under particular conditions justifying specific behaviors. The specificity or rarity of these conditions therefore allows the individual to act even in complete opposition to representation (Katerelos, 1996). However, more than a means of interpreting the world for the individual or the group, social representations also have a determining role in the configuration of the behavior of the individual. We can, therefore, assume that behavior depends on the altered image of reality and that this guides the practices to be adopted. According to Abric (1994), representation is a "guide to action" that directs actions and social relationships. This function of social representations is the "orientation function," to use Abric's term. The latter is seen as the cultural dimension of representation, because it determines what is fair, acceptable, or unacceptable in a given social context.

What do anthropological and social development studies teach about the possibilities of combating social representations, rumors, and improving the level of information of the population during an epidemic period? The situations can be diverse according to the epidemics: some pathologies are not sufficiently "taken seriously" nor considered by the populations (from the point of view of the doctors). In contrast, during the Ebola epidemic, fear of the disease elicited over-reactions (Atlani-Duault & Kendall, 2009). During this COVID-19 epidemic, the contextualized analysis of health messages showed that they were ineffective in stemming social representations and rumors and had little favorable effect on perceptions about the coronavirus (Dingwall et al., 2013). In addition, they generated mistrust of the populations vis-à-vis healthcare systems—especially when they claimed that the virus does not kill Africans.

Low adherence to prevention recommendations is therefore a multifactorial phenomenon that takes into account the context of doubt, mistrust, and denial to which must be added the absence of a framework adapted to the optimal application of physical distancing, especially in its social aspect. Indeed, in the social and cultural context, it is difficult to express reservations about acts of decorum (shaking hands and hugs) and spontaneous solidarity during social events.

10.2.3 Attitudes and Social Representations in the Study of Coronavirus

Knowledge of the social representations and management of COVID-19 is an important element for any public health policy. However, surprising as it may seem, there has not yet been a significant scientific study in Africa on this important subject. Coronavirus is not only a disease of the individual body; it is, moreover, a social disease which links the intuition of the biological world to that of the social world, because we are called to define it, to interpret it, and to situate ourselves in relationship to it, to manage the present but also to plan for the future.

In the process of interpreting the 'unexplicable,' people appeal to previous representations of the events associated with it, developing a representation, in which images and information are found amalgamated with opinions, beliefs, stereotypes, archetypes, values, and social rules. COVID-19 has been interpreted on the basis of preexisting beliefs and opinions concerning members of the so-called risk groups (the elderly, the sick, etc.). It thus has been linked to preexisting stigmata (Agnissan and Ehouma, 2020), by acquiring a psychosocial functionality through the archetypal forms of the antithetical pair "innocent"/"guilty."

When it comes to the transmission of COVID-19, it is very important to study the social representations that apply to it, because they are revealing how the individual perceives the risk of COVID-19 and copes with this. When information remains a critical subject, the existence of valid information does not contribute to change in behavior if public representations regarding COVID-19 are not questioned beforehand (Agnissan & Ehouma, 2020).

The COVID-19 study should focus on studying the level of knowledge about modes of transmission and the degree to which individual behavior has changed to avoid possible infection. From the onset of coronavirus and during the first months, the emerging concern of an urgent nature for public health professionals was the dissemination of medical knowledge, knowledge appropriate to the prevention of transmission of COVID-19. The dominant conviction was that the "right" knowledge would lead to behavior change and to control the rapid spread of the disease.

Addressing the question of the cultural and social representations of COVID-19 would therefore amount to analyzing the precisely cultural aspects of black Africans faced with the pandemic. For example, two of the many barriers in this case, the greeting and the wearing of a face mask, caught our attention. Africans see the greeting as a mark of acceptance of the other, a sign of tolerance, a highly symbolic act loaded with meaning and therefore a cultural code. However, with the arrival of the coronavirus pandemic, these expressions of the body and social identity are presented as factors of epimerization. Will the decline of bodies through claimed social distancing now become acculturated as a customary neo-practice?

Acceptance of the imported and imposed face mask culture poses problems: in most African countries the authorities had hesitated to move to total containment and the wearing of compulsory masks in public places (Kofi, 2020). Fortunately, among the African countries, Algeria, Rwanda, Tunisia, and Morocco were cited as models; by allowing these masks to be accessible in pharmacies, the measures taken by the government were consistent with their means. In these countries, social distancing measures are respected. So, it has appeared as the civilizing action of the face mask.

Wearing a mask, in fact, marks one of the cultural differences between Africa and Asia; hence, a certain ethnocentrism perception in the discourse of Africans. Note that a mask is not just a piece of cloth that covers the face; it is an object that has a history and symbolism in various cultures. From an anthropological point of view, it does not only serve to hide the face, it transforms it. It is observed in some people such as the Dogons (2020) of West Africa. Asians purposefully wear masks on the streets as they do not want to infect their compatriots. For Agnissan and Ehouma (2020), the first medical masks appeared in China at the start of the twentieth century during the plague pandemic; hence, its social and cultural function.

The mask is a functional and ubiquitous "object" in traditional African society; it fulfills social, religious or recreational functions. There is a brotherhood mask that plays a major role in the initiation of young boys. As for the playful function of the mask, it is found during celebrations, parties, and games. In conclusion, Agnissan et al. (2020) asserts that for Africans in general, the individual who voluntarily shapes his face by the mask hides part of his real identity. Masks protect our privacy and even our personality. It is a second face, another me.

As the COVID-19 pandemic spreads across Africa, there is a collective fear and a resurgence of traditional medicine. Some Africans believe they are protecting themselves from COVID-19 by eating garlic and ginger and drinking concoctions of bark from certain trees. The hard situation the world is currently experiencing shows without doubt that medicine needs new drugs.

Talking about traditional African medicine means recognizing that the latter does not enjoy prior recognition. If the fundamental data of this medicine are recognized by all African social layers, obviously thanks to its successes and the many cases of cure that they offer to its patients with its curative capacities on several diseases, the fact remains that African colonial history, written by the West and marred by many prejudices, totally disconnected it from its ancestral environment to expose it to the inexplicable criticisms of cruel globalization.

Cultural relativity is the domain of anthropology. It is the basis for the development of cultural heritage: belief systems, social representations, and practical values about the disease that are unique models of each society. When the pandemic alert was given, much research documented the forms of transmission, or even representations of body contact. Hence, the proscription of all contact by the distancing and total confinement of individuals appears as attitudes contrary to African culture. It can be argued that our communities would be more united, for reasons that can be described as cultural linked to belief systems.

10.3 Cultural Representations and Practices

10.3.1 Cultural Dimension

10.3.1.1 The Ethnography of Greeting in Africa

Africans see the greeting as a mark of acceptance of the other, a sign of tolerance, a highly symbolic act loaded with meaning and therefore a cultural code. However, with the arrival of the coronavirus pandemic, these expressions of the body and social identity are presented as factors of epidemization. Is the decline of bodies through the proclaimed social distancing now going to be inculturated as a customary neo-practice?

> *Coming into contact with others and greeting a loved one is a symbolic act of living together that is of capital importance. The greeting is no longer an optional act, but a gesture backed by a socio-cultural ethic, as is the face mask which has long been adopted in Asian countries. Moreover, this last practice seems to be a social fact linked to their continent where it draws its historical origins. It is a way of life relating to a culture of restrictive hygiene and respect for order since the SARS (*Severe Acute Respiratory Syndrome*) epidemic in the early 21st century in Asia* (Edongo Ntede, 2020, translation).

10.3.1.2 Wearing a Face Mask

Wearing a mask marks one of the cultural differences between Africa and the rest of the continents. Hence, a certain ethnocentrism perception in the discourse of Africans. After all, a mask is not just a piece of cloth that covers the face. It is an object that has a history and symbolism in various cultures. From an anthropological point of view, it does not only serve to hide the face, it transforms it. For Zang Ndong (2017), the first medical masks appeared in China at the start of the twentieth century during the plague pandemic: hence its social and cultural function.

The mask is therefore a functional and omnipresent "object" in traditional African society. It fulfills social, religious, or recreational functions. As for the playful function of the Mask, the author focuses on her perceptions during celebrations, parties, and games. In conclusion, Zang Ndong (2017) argues that for Africans, in general, the individual who voluntarily shapes their face with the mask is concealing part of their real identity: masks protect our privacy and even our personality.

10.3.1.3 The Endogenous Approach to Diseases in Africa

As the COVID-19 pandemic spreads in Africa, we are seeing collective fear and a resurgence of traditional medicine. This is the case with a remedy based on medicinal plants (herbal tea) called Covid-organics, by the Malagasy or Beti of Cameroon who believe they are protecting themselves from COVID-19 by eating garlic and ginger and drinking decoctions of bark of the "ekuk tree." Could not the local culture have an influence on the perception and representations of the disease?

Cultural relativity is the domain of anthropology. It is the basis for the development of cultural heritage: belief systems, representations, and practical values about the disease that are unique models of each society. When the pandemic alert was given, much research documented the forms of transmission, or representations of body contact. Hence, the proscription of all contact by the distancing and total confinement of individuals are the attitudes contrary to African culture. It can be argued that our communities would be more united, for reasons that can be described as cultural related to belief systems.

This approach, which is an overt culturalism, would border on ethnocentrism and would undoubtedly be widely criticized. Instead of wanting to weaken it, cannot public policies clearly take a position on an epidemiological approach or a model to fight against the spread of COVID-19 such as mass immunization, massive screening, and taking into account cultural factors? These representations certainly have a socioeconomic impact or impact on the continent.

10.3.2 The Impact on the Informal Economy

The COVID-19 crisis has brought about the shutdown of almost all economic activity. With a total loss of workers' incomes, the informal sector has suffered the full brunt of the consequences of confinement in all countries of the world. In addition, the living conditions of the population living in this sector, such as poverty and density in marginalized neighborhoods, expose them to more risk of contamination by the virus. A health crisis that leads to an economic crisis which in turn worsens the health crisis: in this vicious circle, resilience loses its "effectiveness."

In sub-Saharan Africa for example, and in the past, the repercussions of an economic crisis in the world resulted in a drop in the incomes of raw materials, tourist resources, and financial transfers from migrants to their countries. Declines in the demand for labor and the demand for consumer and investment goods follow. The informal sector played the role of regulator on the two markets, the labor market and the market for goods and services. Governments react with the usual stimulus policies and rely on foreign aid. The nature of this COVID-19 crisis has neutralized the resilient responses of the informal sector. On the one hand, this resilience confirmed the interactions between formal and informal and the porosity of the borders between the two sectors. On the other hand, it is itself confirmed by the proven underestimation of the main economic aggregates (GDP and household income) in the absence of consideration of the informal sector. This "resilience trap" of the informal sector has pushed the governments of the various countries to set up operations to support the various sectors of the economy and in particular the informal sector.

10.3.3 Social Inequalities in Relationship to COVID-19

The scientific literature has already highlighted the presence of social inequalities in past epidemics. This phenomenon results from three factors, often cumulative: inequalities in the risk of exposure, differentiated vulnerability to the disease, and differences in care. In fact, the public debate in Africa quickly highlighted that the inequalities caused by COVID-19 are socially very marked. In addition to health inequalities in the face of the pandemic has been added a second phenomenon, just as striking: social inequalities in the face of confinement.

The coronavirus pandemic is hitting an Africa already deeply marked by inequality. Country after country, the pandemic has exacerbated and amplified these inequalities. Poorer people have more problems isolating and protecting themselves. They are more likely to have preexisting health problems, and are therefore candidates for dying. With their inability to combat inequalities, the majority of African countries have found themselves much more vulnerable to the health and economic impacts of the disease; most were not prepared at all. The response to the coronavirus crisis is very revealing of a government's commitment to reducing inequalities.

Before the pandemic, many of these African countries were able to reduce poverty and increase life expectancy, but they struggled to reduce income inequalities. At the same time, a large part of the youth of these countries has remained permanently immersed in inactivity, that is to say without employment, education, or training; inequalities in education are considerable; and much remains to be done to improve the economic prospects of women. COVID-19 is likely to deepen these inequalities even further than previous crises, as measures taken to stem the epidemic disproportionately affect precarious workers and women.

After the entry into force of the lockdown characterized by the closure of schools, colleges, and universities in most African countries, governments have adopted virtual work, distance education. However, it is common knowledge that access to the internet and social networks is not the most widely shared condition in the world. The result is that the haves welcome these measures to digitize work and school, while the poor, the majority of whom are in the hinterland, believe that their children's future is in jeopardy.

10.4 Conclusion

The aim of this research was to describe the attitudes and social representations of COVID-19 as they are culturally constructed and shared among Africans in relationship to cultural factors. Decision makers must therefore adopt a plural approach to the pandemic and its representations. Thus, a valued partnership between biomedicine and traditionalists could ensure the manufacture of drugs adapted to the African cultural context. By concluding this nonexhaustive reflection on the cultural dimension of COVID-19, a host of questions arises in our minds: How, for example, to manage the thousands of people who crowd together in the slums of our megalopolises? Can they only respect social distancing? How can we stem the water shortages in our capitals? Ultimately, the response to COVID-19 must be community based. The government should also bring in social science experts who can help raise awareness. To inform citizens, you have to know which community you are addressing and what is its specificity.

References

Abric, J. C. (1994). *Pratiques sociales et représentations*. Presses Universitaires de France.

Agnissan, A. A., & Ehouma, K. L. (2020). Le Covid-19: attaque planétaire, réponses africaines. *Vigieafrique, 3*(2).

Atlani-Duault, L., & Kendall, C. (2009). Influenza, anthropology, and global uncertainties. *Medical Anthropology, 28*(3), 207–211.

Cerclé, A., & Somat, A. (2002). *Psychologie Sociale*. Dunod.

Dingwall, R., Hoffman, L. M., & Staniland, K. (2013). *Pandemics and emerging infectious diseases: The sociological agenda*. Foundation for the Sociology of Health & Illness, Wiley.

Edongo Ntede, P. F. (2020) *Représentations, Pratiques Culturelles et Propagation Spatio-Temporelle Du Covid 19: Contribution à une anthropologie de la causalité culturelle au Cameroun*. https://nkafu.org/representations-pratiques-culturelles-et-propagation-spatio-temporelle-du-covid-19/

Flament, C. (1994). Structure, dynamique et transformation des représentations sociales. In J. C. Abric (Ed.), *Pratiques sociales et représentations* (pp. 37–57). Presses Universitaires de France.

Jodelet, D. (1989). *Les représentations sociales*. Presses Universitaire de France.

Katerelos, G. (1996). *Dynamique des représentations sociales*. Odysseas.

Kofi, S. (2020). *Pandémie de la Covid-19: impact des mesures de restrictions en Afrique de l'ouest*. Recherche et Développement, CERFAM.

Mbonji, E. (2017). *Santé, maladies et médecine africaine – Plaidoyer pour l'autre tradipratique*. Coédition NENA/Presses universitaires de Yaoundé.

Moscovici, S. (1984). The phenomenon of Social Representations in 'Social Representations", Cambridge, University Press.

Moscovici, S. (1986a). L'ère des représentations sociales. In W. Doise & A. Palmonari (Eds.), *l Etude des représentations sociales* (pp. 34–80). Delachaux et Niestlé.

Moscovici, S. (1986b). Notes towards a description of social representations. *European Journal of Social Psychology, 18*(3), 211.

Moscovici, S. (1996). Introduction. In C. Herzlich (Ed.), *Sante et maladie, analyse d'une représentation sociale* (p. 11). Editions de l'Ecole des Hautes Etudes en Sciences Sociales.

UNESCO (2020). *Imaginer le monde à venir: Comment l'Afrique perçoit-elle la crise de la Covid-19 et ses conséquences futures?* https://fr.unesco.org/covid19/aftermath-africa

Worldometer. (2020). *Coronavirus pandemic*. https://www.worldometer.info/coronavirus

Xiaolu, T., et al. (2020). On the origin and continuing evolution of SARS-CoV-2. *National Science Review, 7*(6), 1012–1023. https://doi.org/10.1093/nsr/nwaa036

Zang Ndong, P. (2017). *Écriture et masque. approche sémiotique et poétique*. Thèse de doctorat en Sciences du langage, Université de Limoges. https://tel.archives-ouvertes.fr/tel-01709685/document

11 Knowledge, Adherence, and the Lived Experiences of Refugees in COVID-19

Gloria Seruwagi, Catherine Nakidde, Eric Awich Ochen, Betty Okot, Stephen Lawoko, Joshua Kayiwa, Dunstan Ddamulira, Andrew Masaba, Brian Luswata, Johnmary Ssekatte, and Denis Muhangi

11.1 Introduction and Background

This chapter presents the qualitative findings from a study (REFLECT[1]) conducted on adherence to COVID-19 preventive measures among multinational refugees in three hosting districts and 13 settlements of refugees in Uganda.

Uganda is among the world's top three refugee-hosting nations, hosting more than 1.4 million refugees, and its open-door approach has been internationally acclaimed as "*the world's most compassionate*" refugee policy.[2] As part of the Uganda government response to COVID-19, a number of guidelines and directives were announced from March 2020, including regular hand-washing; social distancing; quarantining of all entrants from outside the country; isolation of suspected cases and contacts; night curfew; closure of schools, bars, gyms, salons, malls, churches, business premises, football pitches, and sports centers; stay-at-home measures that eventually became a total lockdown; wearing of personal protective equipment, especially face

[1] **REF**ugee **L**ived **E**xperiences, **C**ompliance and **T**hinking (REFLECT) in COVID-19.

[2] https://www.theguardian.com/global-development/2017/apr/03/uganda-at-breaking-point-bidi-bidi-becomes-worlds-largest-refugee-camp-south-sudan

G. Seruwagi (✉)
Centre for Health and Social Economic Improvement (CHASE-i), Department of Social Work and Social Administration, Makerere University, Kampala, Uganda

Makerere University School of Public Health (MakSPH), Kampala, Uganda
e-mail: gloria.seruwagi@mak.ac.ug

C. Nakidde · B. Okot
Centre for Health and Social Economic Improvement (CHASE-i), Kampala, Uganda

E. A. Ochen · D. Muhangi
Department of Social Work and Social Administration, Makerere University, Kampala, Uganda

S. Lawoko
Department of Public Health, Faculty of Medicine, Gulu University, Gulu, Uganda

J. Kayiwa · B. Luswata
Ministry of Health (MoH), Kampala, Uganda

D. Ddamulira
Agency for Cooperation in Research and Development (ACORD), Kampala, Uganda

A. Masaba
The Lutheran World Federation (LWF), Kampala, Uganda

J. Ssekatte
National Association of Social Workers of Uganda (NASWU), Bunga, Uganda

M. C. S. Gonçalves et al. (eds.), *The Coronavirus Crisis and Challenges to Social Development*, https://doi.org/10.1007/978-3-030-84678-7_11

masks; use of sanitizers and frequent handwashing with soap. A vibrant communication strategy was also implemented throughout the country, including in refugee settlements, to spread awareness on these preventive measures and bring about the required behavioural changes to minimise the risk of COVID-19 spread.

11.1.1 Rationale for This Research

Whereas all people, refugee or non-refugees, were affected by the COVID-19 pandemic, refugee populations have heightened vulnerability for different reasons. First, they are in a foreign country with limited social networks, livelihoods or other resources to draw from to survive through a pandemic like COVID-19. As foreigners and minority groups, refugee communities were stigmatized because the Coronavirus is known to have originated from outside the country, and was initially brought in by travelers from other countries. Other aspects of vulnerability were factors such as language barriers and lack of identification documents. Moreover, most COVID-19 information and support were only available in English and some local Ugandan languages which most refugees did not understand. Most refugee communities tend to be closed in with limited information sharing. And, the nature of Ugandan refugee settlements—consisting mainly of crowded housing units—was likely to make implementation of some COVID-19 guidelines difficult (e.g., social distancing), while poor access to safe water and sanitation facilities was likely to limit the feasibility of preventive measures like rigorous handwashing with soap.

Although all refugees have no doubt been affected by COVID-19, there were differences in contextual and other socioeconomic dynamics that determined their response to the COVID-19 threat. Contextual specificities are known to have a bearing on the dissemination of lifesaving information or enforcement of government directives and guidelines in different settings. For example; our study's urban refugee community of focus was located in Kisenyi, which is in Metropolitan Kampala, the epicenter of COVID-19 activities. It was clear that this proximity put urban refugees at a comparative advantage—in terms of information flow, reception of relief and outreach services or resulting behavioural change—when compared to their rural settlement counterparts. The other difference is that the Kisenyi refugee community is not an exclusive refugee settlement but is instead largely integrated in Kampala's city life, with people having jobs in the city and freely interacting with other Kampala residents. We were cognisant of the fact that this level of integration may create more exposure or resilience in the face of COVID-19; however, we did not know in what ways. On the other hand, the rural settlement refugee communities are organised largely into nationalities of origin, with each community practising their sociocultural norms: south Sudanese, Congolese, Burundians, and others. Against this backdrop, our study sought to establish whether these contextual differences have a bearing on refugee people's response to the government guidelines, how they had experienced implementation, and whether existing social norms and practices had been a facilitator or hindrance to understanding of COVID-19 prevention measures and compliance to them. At the time we conducted this study, nearly all information readily available was on stable (non-conflict) populations, and even among these populations the effect of these COVID-19 government measures had not been fully measured or explained.

Objectives. This research therefore sought to assess the COVID-19 situation in Uganda's humanitarian settings; to engage the refugee population on their understanding of the COVID-19 risk, their changing lifestyle, and how they were coping using existing support systems or resources.

The study's major aim was to establish the extent to which refugee communities were aware of COVID-19 prevention measures issued by the government of Uganda, and the extent to which they had adhered to these measures in both urban and rural settings.

Specific Objectives

1. To assess knowledge or awareness of COVID-19 and local perception of risk in urban and rural refugee settings[3]
2. To identify local pre–post COVID attitudes and practices relating to health and social norms[4]
3. To explore implementers' interpretation and enforcement of COVID-19 guidelines
4. To determine the feasibility of, and adherence to, COVID-19 preventive measures[5]
5. To identify community resources and assess their efficacy in the COVID-19 response[6]
6. To compare urban and rural refugees in line with Objectives 1–5

11.2 Methods

The study was cross-sectional and a mixed method, using both quantitative and qualitative approaches. The study's primary population were refugees in 11 different (urban, rural, multi-national) settlements and members of their respective host communities. The specific target groups included men, women, youth, elders, local leaders, persons with disabilities, frontline implementers, and law enforcers. The secondary study population comprised key stakeholders from government ministries, departments, and agencies (MDAs) involved in the refugee response such as the Ministry of Health (MoH), Office of the Prime Minister (OPM), NGOs, district local governments, and international agencies such as UNHCR. A total of 115 key informant interviews (KIIs) (Adjumani 47, Kyaka 40, and Kisenyi 28) were conducted across the three study sites, and 34 FGDs (Adjumani 11, Kyaka 13, and Kisenyi 10) were conducted, with a total number of 319 study participants for just the qualitative arm of the study (the overall study participant sample size, including the quantitative arm, was 2093). Methods of data collection included personal interviews (IDI, which also included child-centred interviews), key informant interviews (KIIs), focus group discussions (FGDs), observations, and document review. The qualitative data were analysed thematically.

In terms of data management and processes, qualitative interviews were audio-recorded, transcribed, and coded. Interview summaries produced by interviewers were initially used to capture the main highlights from each interview. Subsequently, following the completion of data collection, data matrices were used to map out responses from different participants across key themes and sub-themes aligning to study objectives. Data were analysed along major themes such as knowledge, beliefs, practices, coping mechanisms, levels and nature of enforcement of guidelines, feasibility of promoted measures, and community resources. Texts that could potentially be used as quotations were also identified and labelled.

The research protocol and all project tools were submitted to the Makerere University School of Public Health Institutional Review Board (MakSPH IRB). Upon approval, the proposal was then submitted to the Uganda National Council of Science and Technology (UNCST) and the Ministry of Health (MoH), as required, for ethical and administrative clearance, respectively. Approval was also sought from the Uganda Office of the Prime Minister (OPM), which oversees refugee affairs and Kampala Capital City Authority (KCCA) before the study commenced. We sought oral and written consent from all study participants, assuring them of anonymity and confidentiality. We adhered to all standard ethical principles including privacy, voluntary participation, and *doing no harm* to study participants. In addition to these, the study team adhered to the COVID-19 standard operating procedures (SOPs) as issued by the MakSPH-IRB, Ministry of Health, and UNCST. The study leadership operationalised these SOPs by developing further guidelines tailored to our study contexts and

[3]Including the infodemic challenge - excessive information, myths, and fears.

[4]Including, e.g., WASH, health-seeking behaviour, community cohesion practices.

[5]Including local interpretations, experiences, innovations, improvisations, and explanatory factors.

[6]Including access to water, soa,p and active engagement with community leadership.

different refugee settlements, in consultation with sub-national and settlement-level leaders.

11.2.1 Key Findings

11.2.1.1 Knowledge and Awareness of COVID-19

This study found a high level of knowledge and awareness of COVID-19, its signs and symptoms, how it is spread, and how it can be prevented. In a focus group discussion (FGD), adolescent girls in the Nyumanzi refugee settlement in Adjumani demonstrated awareness of COVID-19 severity: being a killer disease, spread through "*cough and sneeze droplets, and close bodily contacts such as hugs and handshakes.*" Despite expressing anxiety about the disease, they explained how they are informed about appropriate protection and prevention to reduce its spread in the community. The most commonly identified manifestations of COVID-19 were fever (high temperatures), cough (dry), running nose, sneezing, and general body infirmity, and this was true for all three study sites (Adjumani, Kisenyi, and Kyaka). Most study participants were also aware of how COVID-19 is transmitted and how to avoid it, as shown in the following excerpts:

> *It is a deadly disease that can be transmitted from person to person. The signs and symptoms of corona are headache, high fever and coughing. Elderly people and children are the ones at a high risk. To prevent ourselves from getting corona, practice: social distance, avoid being in crowded places, wear masks, wash your hands for 20 seconds, self-quarantining* (IDI, Nyumanzi Settlement, Adjumani)

> *Washing hands regularly, wearing masks, social distancing, avoiding crowded places, good personal hygiene, and self-isolation/quarantine in case one suspects self* (IDI, Kisenyi)

However, there was a small minority section of refugees who generally unfamiliar with the signs and symptoms of COVID-19, indicating a negligible knowledge gap.

Overall, there were high levels of knowledge and awareness; however, although the majority of the refugee community members are well informed about COVID-19, up to 40% were found to have knowledge gaps on the nature, transmission, symptoms, and dangers. Additionally, a large number of refugees (between 1 and 40%) were found to have adopted at least one risk behaviour likely to lead to transmission of COVID-19, including behaviours related to hygiene, congestion, and physical and social activity. A wide knowledge gap was found among children and adolescents, with up to 75% not being fully knowledgeable on causes, transmission, risk/protective factors, and management of COVID-19. Moreover, there was no targeted information for different age groups or even disadvantaged groups such as the elderly or those with disabilities.

These findings reiterate not only a level of informed awareness about how COVID-19 presents in a patient, but also suggests that people are informed that age could be a risk factor from the various physical vulnerabilities known to impact the health of older persons. Some of the younger and middle-aged people could be using this argument to not adhere to the guidelines, dismissing the COVID-19 risk as only a threat to the elderly:

> *The people in both hosting and refugee communities know that COVID-19 is in the community, how it is transmitted, signs and symptoms, and they know the preventive measures. …but there is inadequate behavior change in the community because some people think the disease is only for the elderly* (KII, Health Educator)

Equally, the knowledge about hand-washing as a COVID-19 prevention measure was seemingly well understood, but also applied differently, as shown in later sections of this chapter. Again, this was happening despite the recognisably sound knowledge of the importance of hand-washing in COVID-19 prevention. Social distancing is yet another well recognised prevention measure. However, practising social distancing seemed to be quite difficult in the study contexts, especially when refugees are in living and working contexts that are largely crowded.

Refugee communities were found to have several myths and falsehoods around COVID-19. For example, that Africans have immunity against

COVID-19; that COVID-19 is not real and is instead a fabrication of scientists and politicians; and that their religious faith will protect them against the virus. These perceptions were mostly driven by the fact that Uganda took long to register a COVID-19 case or death and refugees had not witnessed a COVID-19 death of somebody they knew well or close to them. The myths and falsehoods are further discussed in the next section.

Major sources of information on COVID-19 were reported to include mainstream sources such as television and radio. However, an increasing use of social media and international TV channels was also found to act as a key information source. Social media and the diaspora were reported as a double-edged sword and key knowledge agents among refugee communities, leading to both compliance and noncompliance to preventive guidelines. Local and grassroots agents such as community leaders and self-help groups and associations were also proactively involved in the translating and dissemination of COVID-19 information.

Study findings also show that the information coming through the various sources was not accessible to all, especially because of the coverage and language of the media used. The challenges of accessing information technology/equipment and language barriers affect refugees because many do not have televisions or radios or understand the local languages used in preventive measure. Members of the refugee community receiving this information often do not understand it because the majority do not speak English, Luganda, or Kiswahili, the main languages used by the Ministry of Health (MOH) to disseminate information about COVID-19, as seen next:

> *It's not easy to get this information because some people do not have TVs or radios and neither do they have smart phones. Moreover, the messages are in different languages from those the refugees know so they miss out on a lot of information* (KII, religious leader, Kisenyi)

Differences were also cited in access to information by refugees of different nationalities. As most Congolese, Rwandese, Sudanese, Eritreans, and Ethiopians understand either Kiswahili or English, they are more likely to benefit from messages delivered through these languages. The Somalis, on the other hand, rarely understand Kiswahili and English. So, for them to access information, the messages would have to be in their language.

This study found that most refugees get information *on-the-go*. However, some refugees are isolated from the rest of the host communities, which complicates their access to lifesaving information. Hence, those who are not very mobile, such as people with disabilities and the elderly, are inadvertently at a disadvantage. Although they are a useful source of information, the use of public radios that only service designated areas instead of the entire community was identified as one of the major media options that had coverage pitfalls, which made them a barrier to information access. In addition, some population groups were not targeted by available information sources; for example, as children mostly do not listen to the radio; they are less likely to get information from such a source. Furthermore, the public address messaging via roving megaphones were also said to have been less effective because the vehicles only drive through the main roads in the process, leaving out remote communities.

11.2.1.2 COVID-Related Myths and Perceptions

The study found that there were initial misconceptions and myths about the existence, severity, and nature (biology) of the coronavirus. At the time of the study however, the level of public awareness that COVID-19 is a real and dangerous virus was higher. Before COVID-19 reached Uganda, many dismissed it as a simple disease attacking only international travellers while others took it as '*just a rumour*' or a disease about which little was known, as one respondent expressed:

> *When COVID had just come, just like everyone in Uganda, we thought it was just a rumour and it was not in Uganda. We thought it was a manufactured disease and that it will not reach Uganda, it would stay there. That was our suspicion. We did*

not have any fears on COVID-19 (FGD, Kyaka Refugee Settlement)

The major myths circulated about COVID-19 included labelling as a "manufactured" disease that kills instantly but would never reach Uganda or kill Ugandans. Another myth was about the white race being more susceptible to COVID-19 than people of color led to risky behaviour and noncompliance with existing COVID-19 SOPs. However, when COVID-19 later broke out in Uganda, the president instituted a lockdown, and many began to get ill or test positive for the virus: this was a turning point that forced people to take the disease more seriously as it emerged from the FGD perspective below:

People started hearing about COVID as news. It was not very serious and we did not even know what it was about. We thought it was a simple disease and it was only attacking people who travel in planes. But it kept on coming nearer and nearer until it reached Uganda and that is when we saw the president putting the lockdown, people falling sick, testing positive and so it became very serious (FGD, Kyaka Refugee Settlement)

Based on the initial misconception that COVID-19 was a 'joke,' many people adamantly refused to mask. They later took to masking when it became compulsory in most public places where the refugees sought services such as health facilities, reception centres, and food distribution points. In the villages and homes, it was very rare to see anyone in a mask. However, this requirement compelled some refugees to share masks (as a necessity) in situations where it was obligatory to wear a mask to access services:

When you go deep into the community, these people are not adhering to the guidelines for sure. But when they come to the base camp for services or they want to enter the office of OPM or they want to go to the health facility that is when someone remembers to come with a mask. But at their homes, these things are not there (KII, Kyaka II)

Because Uganda took long to register the first cases of COVID-19 infection and deaths; for many this was taken as a confirmation of the then prevailing idea that there was no COVID-19 in the country. The low death rates, however, caused many to believe that there was no COVID-19 in Uganda, which was especially compounded by the fact that many of the respondents had not witnessed any COVID-19 deaths in their communities. These sentiments were dangerous by their potential to sway people who would otherwise comply not to take the preventive measures seriously. The general community perspective was that people would only be convinced that COVID-19 exists if they got it or had a patient in the family. This view persisted despite some study sites like Kisenyi having recorded two COVID-19 deaths of elderly persons with underlying conditions (co-morbidities) by the time of the study; these were largely attributed to age. Deaths were also reported in Kyaka II at the time of data collection in Adjumani; there were many cases in the quarantine centre while most of their positive cases were being referred to either Arua or Gulu Referral Hospitals for treatment.

Regardless of this awareness, findings still showed that the community was not convinced that COVID-19 actually kills black people. The comparatively high death rates reported in countries such as the United States of America (U.S.), Spain, Italy, Brazil, and the United Kingdom while there was no or minimal COVID-19 deaths in Uganda seemed to fuel the belief that the virus does not kill people of colour. The media reported death rates, however, did not give the actual demographics behind the numbers, so it was difficult to associate it with the black, white, or any other race:

But there is ignorance in Africa. Some people believe that it doesn't kill black people but white people (CPC/RWC,[7] Nyumanzi Settlement, Adjumani)

Considering that "*at the beginning, the disease was not killing people and actually in the community they haven't seen any death thus, … people are getting more relaxed in putting guidelines into practice*" (DHE,[8] Adjumani). The growing negligence and complacency are

[7]Child Protection Committee/Refugee Welfare Committee.

[8]District Health Educator.

probably because people were not dying in large numbers in Uganda.

Some perspectives also indicated that COVID-19 management procedures had been politicised and monetised, which greatly impacted adherence levels. There were references to politics of COVID-19, drawn from presumed roles of superpowers such as Russia and the U.S. in the 'invention' and spread of the virus. This perspective can be linked to the various stories that were circulating on social media at the height of the pandemic. However, the political leadership of the Ugandan President and Ministry of Health in promptly instituting measures to slow down the spread of the disease was highlighted despite the sentiments that the President was probably drawing political capital from the pandemic.

Under the circumstances, it is clear that the refugee community was not doing enough to protect itself and myths were significantly contributing to this laxity.

11.2.1.3 Compliance to Preventive Guidelines and Standard Operating Procedures (SOPs)

A wide disconnect was found between the high knowledge levels and levels of compliance with the recommended COVID-19 preventive measures. Most refugee persons were not fully complying with government measures despite their knowledge. Compliance levels declined over time (between March/April 2020 when lockdown was announced and July/August 2020 when it was lifted), unfortunately coinciding with increasing number of COVID-19 cases and deaths. Enforcement of guidelines was also found to be on the decline, although the declining trend was not as steep as the observed noncompliance. Inappropriate use of masks was found in some of the study sites: including sharing of masks, and only wearing them when the refugees met the police or other enforcement authorities such as settlement leaders from OPM or UNHCR. Handwashing with soap was found to be the most feasible guideline with consistent adherence. However, it was mostly observed between March 2020 and May 2020, and the practice also significantly declined after the government lifted some of the restrictions including lockdown.

The reasons for low compliance are diverse. First, some of the COVID-19 preventive measures such as physical distancing are not feasible in refugee settings such as congested workplaces and residential houses. Others, such as sanitising, are considered a luxury by most refugees who could not access or afford them; other refugee communities such as the predominantly Muslim Somalis did not use sanitizers because of the alcoholic content. In addition, the study findings revealed that the low level of adherence could also partly be explained by the "survivor" lifestyle of the refugees who felt that they had gone through harder situations than COVID-19, for example, war, torture, rape, or hunger.

Culture and deeply entrenched sociocultural norms such as eating together, shaking hands, and hug greetings remain a key barrier to compliance among refugee communities. Sociocultural norms have a strong bearing on behaviour; during the COVID-19 era, some local lifestyles and norms changed while others remained the same. Hence some people maintained their routines during the lockdown days, including visiting and/or hosting, meeting for prayers, child naming, traditional marriages, rites of passage for girls, funerals, and cross-border movements, especially among those in Adjumani.

> *The Somali community practices a lot of hand shaking and hugging in case it has been long since the individuals last met.... We also shake hands in the morning with neighbours as a sign of respect. When you find a young child you have to place your hand on their head and also carry them. We do visit one another a lot and also eat together. For example, you can find two households that eat on the same plate because of culture* (KII, Kisenyi)

> *People's cultures are very strong. People are still greeting while shaking hands because they believe it is a spirit of brotherhood. However, this comes with a problem of continuous spread of the disease because people have not yet adopted the practice of using sanitizers and sometimes they forget to wash their hands. At times there is no water and soap at the washing facility. People are still eating from one plate because it is a spirit of togetherness* (KII, Religious Leader, Adjumani)

Eating together as a family, even from one huge plate, was cross-cutting in the three study sites as were sneak visits, hosting, and socialising. Youth social gatherings over games of cards and children playing or gathering in large groups were also common sights in all three study sites.

The most common explanatory factor for nonadherence was related to livelihoods and the need to make a living. It did not make sense to stay home and socially distance, for example, when people did not have food to eat. So, they got out and went to work—in host community gardens or at their market stalls. By doing so, they were breaking rules and contravening directives; however, a corrupt environment and enforcement fatigue enabled refugee communities to continue looking for money while contravening the COVID-19 preventive measures:

> *You want us to stay here* [home] *and just look at each other with nothing to eat? It is very stressful. We have to go and look for what to eat. Most people here already lost their small businesses and can no longer work, yet we are getting little food rations… so things are really difficult. We shall not wait for hunger to first kill us* (IDI, Kyaka II)

The livelihoods and food security factor was very serious and exacerbated by the declining rations given out by the World Food Programme during COVID-19 as implementing partner agencies also struggled to allocate their limited resources to intervene in refugee settlements. Relating this to perceptions, attitudes, and reported needs, most refugees were more worried about hunger than COVID-19; therefore, nonadherence to preventive guidelines was inevitable in the pursuit of food and income.

Other reasons for nonadherence to SOPs included the lack of masks, masks being uncomfortable to wear, and the observed noncompliant behaviour of leaders (especially politicians canvassing for votes as the political season, complete with campaigns and elections, coincided with the pandemic outbreak).

11.2.1.4 Implementers' Interpretation and Enforcement Experiences

A number of stakeholders were involved in implementing the guidelines and directives to prevent further COVID-19 spread, including the police and local leaders. In addition, front-line service implementers including civil society organisations (CSOs), local governments, refugee settlement staff, and OPM staff also have key roles in sensitising the refugee populations about COVID-19, interpreting the guidelines and operationalizing them in the local contexts. They had been active in explaining to the population what COVID-19 is, how it spreads, how it can be prevented, and other attendant information, as various key informants explained:

> *We have been carrying out sensitization about COVID-19, telling them that it's a virus, this is how it came into the world so they know it's a virus that affects people and kills people and it's deadly and you need to take precautions about* (OPM[9] official, Kyaka II)

> *There are people who have been sneaking from South Sudan using porous border points. We have been able to report and they are quarantined. These ones who have been running away they have been got and brought back by police. And it is our office that facilitates the police* (OPM official, Adjumani)

> *When someone came from South Sudan to this block and when I heard because the community alerted me and told me where he was staying. I took the case to police who told the Ministry of Health officials who came to the ground and they took him to the quarantine center* (Local leader, Ayilo, Adjumani)

Lessons Learnt

A number of lessons were learnt in the COVID-19 pandemic era, including the following:

[9] Office of the Prime Minister—oversees refugee affairs in Uganda.

1. Implementation and enforcement of COVID-19 containment measures is multi-actor and multi-sectoral, and can only succeed as a result of joint effort.
2. As enforcement and compliance fatigue set in, there is need to draw upon the community's own vigilance and norm change to attain desired behavioural changes for COVID-19 prevention.
3. Divergence between the knowledge of COVID-19 prevention and compliance with recommended measures and guidelines. Many members of the refugee communities had maintained their routines and lifestyles, including the risky ones with close contact and high potential for disease spread.
4. Some of the recommended COVID-19 prevention measures such as social distancing were not adhered to because they are dictated by structural factors and are not feasible in the local humanitarian context. Alternatives to social distancing must be emphasised.
5. There are declining levels of compliance amidst a heightening epidemic, signalling increased risk of exposure to infection for many people.
6. Inappropriate use of masks suggests low levels of adoption of a new behaviour, much more than just a gap in prevention knowledge. Issues of feasibility must be addressed and practicable measures found.
7. Government and other actors should support refugee communities to implement recommended measures by supplying basics such as soap, hand-washing facilities, and masks.
8. Communication campaigns on COVID-19 should emphasise individual responsibility and the benefits of adherence.

Overall, the government's directives and guidelines for the prevention of COVID-19 spread were correctly interpreted. Implementation and enforcement of COVID-19 containment measures were multi-actor and multi-sectoral and had largely succeeded as a result of this joint effort. In some cases, the community structures had innovated coping mechanisms to allow the people respond to the COVID containment measures. Such mechanisms include controlling access to water points under supervision of the Water Use Committees (WUC) and installing hand-washing facilities at the household level. NGOs and international agencies had supported the response by distributing soap, hand-washing facilities, face masks, and other relief items. In Kisenyi, the National Water and Sewerage Corporation installed public hand-washing points.

However, the implementation and enforcement from the government's side was largely top down and relied more on security and law enforcement while it marginalised grassroots participation. Study findings showed that in some cases, especially in the urban Kisenyi, refugee persons were a target of harassment and extortion by law enforcers, who took advantage of the situation to extort money, hence heightening the vulnerability and abuse of the refugee's rights. Eventually, enforcement fatigue set in, and by the time of the study, little was being done to enforce compliance, except at institutional premises such as health facilities and public offices where hand-washing and wearing of face masks was still a requirement.

11.2.1.5 Community Resources, Systems, and Their Contribution in the COVID-19 Era

The COVID-19 pandemic resulted in several negative outcomes that included food shortages, loss of jobs, and closures and losses in people's businesses. COVID-19 came with demands for policy change and a necessity for behavioural changes if refugee communities were to successfully control the spread of this virus in their settlements. There are a number of community resources and systems that were reported as essential in the COVID-19 response in the refugee settlements of Kisenyi, Kyaka, and Adjumani. These resources had eased or had the potential to ease the process of adapting to these changes that arose as a result of COVID. They can be categorised into resources from NGOs, resources from government, local leadership, and community structures, the healthcare system, community members, and water systems.

A wide range of community resources and systems exists in refugee communities. The study found that these had been used to disseminate COVID-19 prevention information, support adherence to recommended measures, and support those affected. These resources include grassroots structures such as local leaders amongst both the refugees and host populations; community agents such as Village Health Teams (VHTs) and Local Defense Units (LDUs); and religious and cultural leaders and social services. There was also a level of social capital in the form of associations, such as that found among the Somali community in Kisenyi, which had been instrumental during the COVID-19 period, for example, through translating information into their local language and distributing relief items and personal protective equipment (PPE). These various resources provide an opportunity to change or complement the mainstream top-down response to COVID-19 and leverage them to deploy a more participatory and community-based response to the epidemic. However, the resources in the form of human resources (such as local leaders or VHTs) need information, training, and supervision to effectively support their communities.

11.3 Conclusion

Overall, study findings show that the high level of knowledge on COVID-19 does not match with the low and steadily declining levels of adherence to preventive guidelines. Adherence to preventive measures and SOPs drastically dropped after July 2020 (compared to the period between March 2020 and July 2020), when some restrictions, including lockdown, were lifted. Recommended practices have not been fully adopted to become a 'new normal.' Moreover, some COVID-19 prevention measures such as hand-washing are more feasible than others, such as practising physical distancing, which is impossible in crowded refugee settings. To some extent, it seems that measures may be more feasible if they resonate with preexisting sociocultural norms. Hence, despite the high levels of knowledge and awareness, the local perceptions, myths, fatigue, social pressure, low incomes, and other contextual factors are not entirely favourable for behaviour change. The findings show that the COVID-19 challenge had rallied together different actors for complementary and collaborative roles to address not only COVID-19 prevention but also mitigation of its offshoot effects.

The findings further show a decline in both enforcement of and compliance with COVID-19 preventive measures. The decline in compliance levels is a function of diverse and complex mix of factors including cultural norms, religious beliefs, and lack of personal commitment, as well as structural factors such as the crowded and impoverished nature of refugee settlements. On the other hand, it also seems plausible to argue that Uganda has become a victim of its early success, having managed to successfully delay the onset of COVID-19 in the country. With increasing community transmission and an extremely fragile healthcare system, there is need to reverse the country's initial top-down response to COVID-19 and promote a more participatory, community-led response to the pandemic.

Exclusion of refugees was believed to be the key explanatory factor for why they are among the most vulnerable to the COVID-19 pandemic.[10] To ensure refugee inclusivity, involvement, and access to accurate and relevant information in appropriate languages, government and other stakeholders should ensure COVID-19 messages are translated to refugee languages.[11] This action will, in turn, lead to full participation of refugees in national preparedness plans and prevention and response measures to the COVID-19 pandemic. Only an all-inclusive approach[12] to public

[10] Truelove, S., Abrahim, O., Altare, C., Lauer, S. A., Grantz, K. H., Azman, A. S., & Spiegel, P. (2020). The potential impact of COVID-19 in refugee camps in Bangladesh and beyond: a modeling study. *PLoS medicine*, 17(6), e1003144.

[11] Hargreaves, S., Zenner, D., Wickramage, K., Deal, A., & Hayward, S. E. (2020). Targeting COVID-19 interventions towards migrants in humanitarian settings. *The Lancet. Infectious Diseases*, 20(6), 645.

[12] Inter-Agency Standing Committee (IASC). (2020). Interim guidance: scaling-up COVID-19 outbreak readi-

health with meaningful community involvement and socioeconomic response will suppress the virus, restart the economy, and keep Uganda on track to attain its global (e.g., SDG) and national targets.

11.4 Recommendations

Government and key stakeholder actors should undertake these actions:

1. Address the drivers of noncompliance to COVID-19 guidelines in refugee communities. These drivers extend beyond the health sector and include culture, politics, livelihoods, noncompliant leadership examples, and the infodemic challenge.
2. Adopt content and age-appropriate messaging to reach children, youths, and marginalised groups such as those living with disabilities and co-morbidities, and the elderly. Adopt the "*leave no one behind*" message for COVID-19 prevention.
3. Use multiple channels including mobile vans and *bodabodas* (motorcycles) fitted with public address systems and door-to-door approaches to penetrate villages and settlements to reach remote and vulnerable populations with the message of behavioural change, not just awareness. Stakeholders should facilitate and expand communication on radios by lobbying all radio stations provide free airtime of at least 2 h a week for partners to speak about COVID-19.
4. Leverage the agency of cultural structures, resources, and leaders to increase local acceptance of the COVID-19 preventive measures and minimise spread.
5. As the dynamics of the pandemic continue to evolve, there is need for government and other actors to keep the implementers and enforcers informed, trained, and equipped to adjust their actions to suit the changing implementation needs.
6. As enforcement and compliance fatigue set in, draw upon the community's own vigilance and norm change to attain desired behavioural changes for COVID-19 prevention.
7. Support refugee communities with regular supplies of basic items such as food, face masks, hand-washing containers, soap, and hand sanitizers, which will go a long way in supporting sustained adherence.
8. Amidst the declining levels of compliance to recommended COVID-19 containment measures, continue to provide behaviour change communication to refugee communities, with emphasis on taking individual responsibility to prevent the spread of coronavirus and mitigate the effects of COVID-19. This step calls for reversing the current top-down response to COVID-19 and promoting a more participatory and community-based and -led response to the epidemic.
9. Government should restore people's trust and confidence in its leadership to deal with the epidemic by ensuring consistency in its messaging, and effectively managing of COVID response processes including testing, communicating test results, treatment services, management of burials of COVID-19 deaths, spending, and accountability. Government officials, for instance, should avoid contradictory messages and abuse of SOPs as their conduct misled the public to assume the disease is not deadly.
10. Strengthen measures to curb stigmatisation of refugee populations, as well as harassment and victimisation by law enforcement officials. Protection mechanisms for vulnerable groups should be strengthened to match and address their heightened vulnerability in the era of COVID-19.

Uganda's COVID-19 trend is steadily moving towards "peaking" with high levels of community transmissions. The health system is fragile and overwhelmed to address increasing cases; therefore, any reversal of the epidemic, or flattening the curve when required, is going to rely heavily on its community systems and individual responsibility. As noted from the beginning, the

ness and response operations in humanitarian situations, including camps and camp-like settings.

country is a top refugee-hosting nation globally which also miraculously managed to keep a steady grip on new COVID-19 infections even at the peak of its intense political season that coincided with the pandemic outbreak. Uganda must now consolidate its largely successful awareness campaign on COVID-19 to ensure that the barriers to noncompliance and increasing risk to COVID-19 infection are addressed and the required behavioural shifts attained among both its refugee and its host populations.

11.5 Implications for Social Work Practice

A notable gap in Uganda's COVID response was the underutilisation of the social work professions, in spite of known negative experiences usually associated with vulnerable communities such as refugees. In times of pandemics and other adversity, the likelihood of increased deprivation and violation of human rights is usually high. Increased rates of unemployment and loss of livelihoods, food insecurity, and all forms of violence (domestic, violence against children, violence against women, and sexual violence leading to unwanted pregnancies, including among teenagers) were reported.

Although the need for mental health and psychosocial support was recognised from the onset and some interventions put in place, implementation was largely skewed to the clinical, and social workers were not categorised as "essential workers" allowed to move or continue providing services. Yet community support systems broke down during the pandemic and the need for social work intervention was high. This lack of engaging and working with social workers to address societal challenges was a missed opportunity whose effects continue to be seen. However, lessons can be learnt, especially with several countries experiencing second waves of COVID-19, and alongside community-led solutions to prevention, the social work profession should be actively engaged for better outcomes in emergencies.

References

Alzoubi, H., Alnawaiseh, N., Asma'a Al-Mnayyis, M. A., Lubada, A. A., & Al-Shagahin, H. (2020). COVID-19-knowledge, attitude and practice among medical and non-medical university students in Jordan. *Journal of Pure and Applied Microbiology, 14*(1), 17–24.

Anguyo, I., & Storer, L. (2020). *In times of Covid-19 Kampala has become 'un-Ugandan'*. [Blog post]. https://blogs.lse.ac.uk/africaatlse/2020/04/09/kampala-epidemic-un-ugandan-society-in-times-covid-19/

Ariaka, R. (2020) We are sorry for beating people – Police. *The New Vision*. https://www.newvision.co.ug/new_vision/news/1517160/sorry-beating-people-police

Bikbov, B., & Bikbov, A. (2020). Communication on COVID-19 to community–measures to prevent a second wave of epidemic.

Burti, L., & Mosher, L. R. (2003). Attitudes, values and beliefs of mental health workers. *Epidemiology and Psychiatric Sciences, 12*(4), 227–231.

Chen, Y., Jin, Y. L., Zhu, L. J., Fang, Z. M., Wu, N., Du, M. X., et al. (2020). The network investigation on knowledge, attitude and practice about COVID-19 of the residents in Anhui Province. *Journal of Preventive Medicine, 54*(4), 367–373.

East African. (2020). *Uganda police shoot 2 for violating movement ban*. https://www.theeastafrican.co.ke/news/ea/Uganda-police-shoot-2-for-violating-movement-ban/4552908-5506106-6us1wnz/index.html

Favas, C., Abdelmagid, N., Checchi, F., Garry, S., Jarrett, P., Ratnayake, R., & Warsame, A. (2020). *Guidance for the prevention of COVID-19 infections among high-risk individuals in camps and camp-like settings*. Health in Humanitarian Crises Centre and London School of Hygiene and Tropical Medicine.

Hanafiah, K., & Wan, C. D. (2020). Public knowledge, perception and communication behavior surrounding COVID-19 in Malaysia.

Hargreaves, S., Zenner, D., Wickramage, K., Deal, A., & Hayward, S. E. (2020). Targeting COVID-19 interventions towards migrants in humanitarian settings. *The Lancet. Infectious Diseases, 20*(6), 645.

Hughes, G. D., Puoane, T., & Bradley, H. (2006). Ability to manage diabetes—Community health workers' knowledge, attitudes and beliefs. *Journal of Endocrinology, Metabolism and Diabetes of South Africa, 11*(1), 10–14.

Inter-Agency Standing Committee (IASC). (2020). Interim guidance: scaling-up COVID-19 outbreak readiness and response operations in humanitarian situations, including camps and camp-like settings.

Kluge, H. H. P., Jakab, Z., Bartovic, J., D'Anna, V., & Severoni, S. (2020). Refugee and migrant health in the COVID-19 response. *Lancet, 6736*(20), 1237–1239.

Kreuter, M. W., & McClure, S. M. (2004). The role of culture in health communication. *Annual Review of Public Health, 25*, 439–455.

Lamunu, M., Lutwama, J. J., Kamugisha, J., Opio, A., Nambooze, J., Ndayimirije, N., & Okware, S. (2004). Containing a haemorrhagic fever epidemic: The Ebola experience in Uganda (October 2000–January 2001). *International Journal of Infectious Diseases, 8*(1), 27–37.

Leter, D., & Gatkuoth, G. (2020). Fears in Uganda over coronavirus outbreak in refugee settlements. [News report]. *Aljazeera*. https://www.aljazeera.com/news/2020/04/fears-uganda-coronavirus-outbreak-refugee-settlements-200406145749564.html

Mathieu, E., & Sodahlon, Y. (2017). Epidemic investigation. *International Encyclopedia of Public Health, 2017*, 518.

Medscape. (2020). *In memoriam: Healthcare workers who have died of COVID-19*. https://www.medscape.com/viewarticle/927976

Ministry of Health Uganda. (2020, 10 April). *MoH Uganda: COVID-19 information portal*

Monteith, W., & Lwasa, S. (2017). The participation of urban displaced populations in (in) formal markets: Contrasting experiences in Kampala, Uganda. *Environment and Urbanization, 29*(2), 383–402.

Musinguzi, G., & Asamoah, B. O. (2020). The science of social distancing and total lock down: does it work? Whom does it benefit? *Electronic Journal of General Medicine, 17*(6), em230. https://doi.org/10.29333/ejgm/7895

Musoke, S. (2020). *Covid-19: Let's not leave urban refugees behind*. https://www.monitor.co.ug/OpEd/Commentary/Covid19-Let-s-not-leave-urban-refugees-behind/689364-5522472-8khto4/index.html

Mwenyango, H., & Palattiyil, G. (2019). Health needs and challenges of women and children in Uganda's refugee settlements: Conceptualising a role for social work. *International Social Work, 62*(6), 1535–1547.

Olum, R., & Bongomin, F. (2020). Uganda's first 100 COVID-19 cases: Trends and lessons. *International Journal of Infectious Diseases, 96*, 517–518.

San Lau, L., Samari, G., Moresky, R. T., Casey, S. E., Kachur, S. P., Roberts, L. F., & Zard, M. (2020). COVID-19 in humanitarian settings and lessons learned from past epidemics. *Nature Medicine, 26*, 647–648.

Sengwana, M. J., & Puoane, T. (2004). Knowledge, beliefs and attitudes of community health workers about hypertension in the Cape Peninsula, South Africa. *Curationis, 27*(1), 65–71.

Tarwirei, F., Chirenje, Z. M. & Rusakaniko, S. (2003). *Cancer of the cervix: Knowledge, beliefs and screening behaviours of health workers in Mudzi District in Mashonaland East Province, Zimbabwe*.

Thomas, S. B., Fine, M. J., & Ibrahim, S. A. (n.d.). Health disparities: the importance of culture and health Communication.

Truelove, S., Abrahim, O., Altare, C., Lauer, S. A., Grantz, K. H., Azman, A. S., & Spiegel, P. (2020). The potential impact of COVID-19 in refugee camps in Bangladesh and beyond: A modeling study. *PLoS Medicine, 17*(6), e1003144.

Williams, R. E., Black, C. L., Kim, H. Y., Andrews, E. B. Mangel, A. W., Buda, J. J., & Cook, S. F. (2006) Determinants of healthcare-seeking behaviour among subjects with irritable bowel syndrome. *Alimentary Pharmacology & Therapeutics, 23*(11), 1667–1675.

Woodward, A., & Kawachi, I. (2000). Why reduce health inequalities? *Journal of Epidemiology & Community Health, 54*(12), 923–929.

World Health Organization. (2020). *Rational use of personal protective equipment (PPE) for coronavirus disease (COVID-19): interim guidance*, 19 March 2020 (No. WHO/2019-nCoV/IPC PPE_use/2020.2). World Health Organization.

Zhong, B. L., Luo, W., Li, H. M., Zhang, Q. Q., Liu, X. G., Li, W. T., & Li, Y. (2020). Knowledge, attitudes, and practices towards COVID-19 among Chinese residents during the rapid rise period of the COVID-19 outbreak: A quick online cross-sectional survey. *International Journal of Biological Sciences, 16*(10), 1745.

12 The Impact of COVID-19 Among the Vulnerable Population of Children and Youth in Lesotho: The Circle of Courage Perspective

Katiso Samuel Sehlabane
and Thandie Keromamang Hlabana

12.1 Introduction

The COVID-19 pandemic, as the greatest global challenge since World War II, is facing the world today, with all countries reporting rapid infections and deaths. Relative to other regions, Africa was slow in recording COVID-19 cases. The first cases of COVID-19 were recorded on 28 January in Sub-Saharan African countries and on 14 February 2020 in Egypt. For a while, Lesotho seemed to have been spared from the pandemic. It was only on 13 May 2020 that the first case of COVID-19 was recorded in the country, making it the last country in Africa to report a first COVID-19 case, 2020). In the first wave of the pandemic, the spread of the disease in Lesotho had been slower than the observed exponential spread in other regions such as Europe, Asia, and the Americas. By June 2021, official records indicated 11,168 cumulative COVID-19 cases, with 329 deaths in the 2.2 million population (National COVID-19 Secretariat (NACOSEC), 2021). These cases were dominated by youth and the elderly.

Medical literature suggests that children have minimal susceptibility to COVID-19 infections and deaths (WHO, 2020). However, the epidemic has brought a myriad of development and well-being impacts on children that include psychosocial impacts. For example, Ghosh et al. (2020) indicated that being quarantined in homes and institutions imposes a psychological burden on children. Moreover, Nearchou et al. (2020) conducted a systematic study that highlighted depression and anxiety among young people. Others have shown socioeconomic impacts such as poverty, malnutrition, school dropout, child abuse and child labour, early marriage, teen pregnancies, and the risk of other diseases because of the lack of immunisation (UNICEF, 2021).

Like many countries in Africa, Lesotho faces significant development challenges and persistent poverty. The government's response to COVID-19 was swift. Before the recording of the first case, a National Emergency Command Center (NECC) was established under the leadership of a cabinet sub-committee and the Ministry of Health. With the advice of the NECC, the government shut down all schools from 19 March 2020, and from 29 March 2020, a compulsory lockdown of all nonessential services was declared for 6 weeks. The Ministry of Education and Training as well as the Ministry of Social Development were tasked to respond to children's needs during the pandemic. The Ministry of Education focused on children's continued education and nutrition, while the Ministry of Social Development focused on social protection through Child Grants to households with vulnerable children. Despite direct COVID-19 impact,

K. S. Sehlabane · T. K. Hlabana (✉)
Department of Sociology and Social Work, National University of Lesotho, Maseru, Lesotho
e-mail: sehlabanek@gmail.com; tk.hlabana@nul.ls

M. C. S. Gonçalves et al. (eds.), *The Coronavirus Crisis and Challenges to Social Development*,
https://doi.org/10.1007/978-3-030-84678-7_12

the youth were neglected. Social protection interventions often target children and the elderly, leaving the youth to only benefit indirectly (Ansell et al., 2018). Lesotho's national response to COVID-19 has been no different as there was no intervention targeted at young people.

12.2 The Situation of Children and Youth in Lesotho

Children in Lesotho are defined as all persons below the age of 18 years (UNICEF, 2021). They represent 765,614 of the population (Bureau of Statistics/BOS, 2018). According to the 2016 population and housing census, 210,712 children (28%) in Lesotho are orphaned and many are vulnerable (BOS, 2018). HIV/AIDS have caused 68% of the orphans and vulnerable children. Although children in Lesotho do not represent a high-risk group for direct COVID-19 morbidity and fatality, there are some far-reaching secondary impacts. For example, between March 2020 and April 2021, the majority of children have been out of school because the public schools were closed, resulting in loss of learning that might not be recovered after the epidemic COVID. Furthermore, the Ministry of Education and Training (2020) reported an increase in school dropouts among children who were recalled to sit for exit examinations. Moreover, schools do not only offer a learning environment for children: they also provide protection from violence and exploitation, as well as food security through schooling feeding schemes for many vulnerable children. Teachers and peers are also an important social support for children. This social support is critical for promoting positive academic performance and psychosocial outcomes for children. In addition, as parents and guardians lost their jobs and livelihoods because of the economic shutdown, many children were left at wits' end. It is, therefore, evident that the epidemic magnified the vulnerability of children in Lesotho.

The youth were highly affected by the epidemic. Youth are defined as persons between 15 and 35 years of age (Ministry of Gender and Youth, Sports and Recreation, 2014). The Lesotho Bureau of Statistics (BOS) (2019) reported 38.9% of the population as youth. This youth bulge is defined as a demographic dividend that can be harnessed for economic growth (United Nations Population Fund, 2018). However, young people are subjected to many developmental challenges. For example, Hapazari (2019) affirmed that most of the youth in Lesotho are educated but unemployed. In 2020, the estimated youth unemployment rate in Lesotho was at 32.8% (Plecher, 2020). In addition, young people in the country have the highest HIV prevalence of 35% (International Center for Care and Treatment Program, 2017). Moreover, COVID-19 has affected young people directly, as more cases were found within this age group (NACOSEC, 2020). Indirectly, young people have been pushed into education disruption and unemployment, leading to increased poverty, distress, and vulnerability to HIV. Thus, COVID-19 has been a great illuminator of the developmental challenges of youth and children in Lesotho.

12.3 Circle of Courage

This chapter relies on the Circle of Courage (CoC) as a conceptual framework for understanding the impact of COVID-19 on the development of children and youth in Lesotho. CoC was coined by Brendtro, Bockern, and Brokenleg in 1988 as a psychological framework (Dyke et al., 2019) and was developed with a focus on Native American children's development principles. Van Bockern and McDonald (2012) recognise that the CoC's shared human needs emanate from the traditions and practices of cultures that deeply valued children and afforded them due respect and dignity. In addition, Brendtro et al. (2005, 2012) in Dyke et al. (2019) assert that all children and youth have a need to be unlocked so as to enjoy the common developmental needs of belonging, mastery, independence, and generosity. For example, for children to develop a sense of belonging, charity, and acceptance, they need to build relationships of trust with their adult carers and optimistic peers (Brendtro et al., 2019 in

Reyneke, 2020). Belonging is, therefore, the ability to meaningfully relate and connect with others. On the other hand, mastery provides a platform for young people (children inclusive) to learn new skills and opportunities to practice them (Sapp et al., 2004). Mastery places endless opportunities to achieve and be successful while similarly availing at disposal the necessary assistance to achieve. Lotter (2005) additionally defines independence as the ability to exercise inner control and self-discipline. Persons with no sense of autonomy come to see themselves as powerless in the world where others control their destiny (Douglas, 2007). Lastly, generosity consists of contributing to others. Children who are exposed to nurturing environment do, in return, show care to others, thereby forming the basis of empathy and compassion (Dyke et al., 2019). In a nutshell, the circle of courage has been preferred for this chapter for its concern and holistic view on the needs of children and youth. Its quadrants make it more suited at this time when the world, including Lesotho, is battling the universal pandemic of COVID-19. The following analysis employs the CoC to show the impact of COVID-19 on the vulnerable populations of children and youth in Lesotho.

12.4 Sense of Belonging: COVID-19 Impact Analysis on Children and Youth in Lesotho

The national lockdown in Lesotho took effect after a gravely short notice and was hastily implemented. At a glance, many wondered about the country's preparedness to implement a complete shutdown. It was believed that the then lockdown held no basis because the mountain kingdom, as Lesotho is affectionately called, had not recorded a single case of COVID-19 at that time. A bystander's thoughts may then be justifiable and prove valid on account of loss of livelihoods from an invisible virus amid increases in hunger and poverty, as well as domestic violence (UNFPA Lesotho, 2020).

Amid COVID-19, the children's home environments became insecure. Increased domestic violence was a consequence of unusual and prolonged confinement for which family members were neither prepared nor accustomed to experiencing. Some of these couples experiencing the said contentions are within the youth population group. As it is commonly accepted and perhaps globally, that the young men who are cohabiting or even married would usually prefer to get a "temporary relief" from their partners, but a prolonged stay with their male buddies where they would merrily share in socially rewarded male activities such as sporting events (predominantly soccer), male clubs, and associations that are in most cases glorified with alcoholic beverages. These tendencies tend to be greatly rewarded in patriarchal societies such as ours (Basotho). Similar gestures are interpretable in part as men's manner of creating a room for their spouses or partners to carry out their socially prescribed roles such as housekeeping, cooking, assisting children with schoolwork, and grocery shopping without interruption while they (the men) would barely have anything to do with similar tasks.

Much of these divided specialties are devisable over the weekend; 2 days' relief from what one would call a full 5 days of commitment to the employers' dictates for some, while for some a weekend is one to two days of relief from merchandising indigenously or even exotically with the purpose of making ends meet. Thus, before the lockdown restrictions, some young couples would infrequently if ever, and in rare cases, spare time to know each other's interests, hobbies, dreams, and/or personal values. It is unlikely then that a sense of belonging among the partners may fully blossom. The victims are in most cases women who frequently are desirous to spend quality time with their men, which explicitly explains why many couples were at loggerheads given the familial and binding confinement imposed through the lockdown restrictions, thereby perpetrating domestic violence and abuse. The initial lockdown, the practice which from all angles was foreign to the Basotho manner of conduct, was introduced to be a temporary measure. With several extensions, however, in totality it lasted for a period close to 2 months.

The common adage goes that when two elephants fight the repercussions are unfortunately felt by the grass. The diverse instabilities that were experienced at household level during the full lockdown effect might have had devastating consequences on the lives and livelihoods of children. It is from all angles unquestionable that children's tranquil disposition is to a large extent linked to that of their parents. Hence, a lack thereof in any way will equally affect them. Research has on several occasions revealed that consequences of gender-based violence may not only negatively impact on children in their childhood but when they may marry, thereby producing long-term undesirable effects, even in their later life. Secondary or indirect victims of gender-based or domestic violence (in this case, immediate children) may internally harbour long-term scars resulting from these misdemeanours, or even if not, they may turn into perpetrators of violence themselves, unless a meaningful intervention is availed to them (UNFPA, 2020).

Another group of children and youth who have suffered a great blow from the lockdowns, as a strategy to curb the spread of COVID-19, are children and youth on and off the street. These are individuals who are grappling to court any welcome sense of belonging because varying predicaments have pushed them onto the street. Some of them would, now accustomed to the street as their home, eventually and fortunately manage to generate just about enough capital to engage in petty but significant trade with the multitudes who are carrying on with their daily errands. This then was a guaranteed avenue which generated means of sustenance for them, especially from compassionate others. Meanwhile, the better-off traders would philanthropically extend a hand to other street children who are hopeless beyond setting up a trade of whatever calibre. These acts of kindness generate a ray of hope and inversely some sense of belonging to this vulnerable population (Patel, 2007). The effects of the abrupt and continuous lockdowns, which overwhelmed these compassionate philanthropists, can only be lamentably thought and never equalled on children and youth on and off the street. Their agony can with greater speculation be guessed, particularly when the government had no single intervention strategy implemented, at least not until many months were past, on how they would sustain these vulnerable groups until lockdown restrictions were lifted, or prudently, until all the successional waves of COVID-19 are over.

Children and youth who were yet again and somehow at stake after the outbreak of the coronavirus pandemic in Lesotho are children in residential care and homes. These centres of care are usually burdened with increased numbers of children who are in need of residence or abode. The majority of these facilities legally accommodate children between the ages of 0 and 18 years; even though some may rarely go beyond the age of 21 years. Overcrowding would therefore be an issue of concern, perhaps not only to immediate caregivers in these residences but also to some social workers, especially given the manner of contact and spread of COVID-19 in such concentrated places as residential facilities. It later became apparent, however, that the immediate lockdown would work to the advantage of such facilities if all children would carefully remain quarantined and contained within these facilities and if care was taken that not a single positive COVID-19 case was recorded among them. Hence, their need for belonging was kept intact.

In a conclusive reflection on the circle of courage quadrant of belonging and how it has impacted the lives of vulnerable population of children and youth in Lesotho, particularly during the COVID-19 era, it may be the case that the majority of these groups have been negatively affected. The shortage or rather the absolute absence of impact mitigation measures from key stakeholders in children and youth affairs, in the authors' views, further exacerbated their predicament. Contrarily, it can also be speculated and possibly with precision that some couples or partners or even families were for the first time graced by the nationally imposed lockdown to have a sense of family reunion and share in the ever-desired and longed-for moments with each other, thereby fulfilling the family's sense of belonging.

12.5 Mastery: COVID-19 Impact Analysis on Children and Youth in Lesotho

Principally, mastery lays a foundation on knowledge acquisition and dissemination. The art of mastery has on many accounts been compromised in Lesotho as a result of the COVID-19 pandemic. The reflection on the foregoing quadrant of belonging has revealed, without hesitation, the unfathomable quakes that have destabilised the familial tranquillity throughout the COVID-19 reign. It is, in light of the earlier deliberations, clear and again sensible that a peaceful and equally permitting environment, one which is void of offences and parental chaos, determines highly the fruitful or desirable manner in which even their children can and will grasp any educational content. In contrast, an environment that is violent or full of abuse can prove to be a barrier or an impediment to desired learning for youth and children.

The educational institutions at all levels were greatly perturbed. Schools at all levels usually house large numbers of students who are many times constituted of both day scholars and boarders, the latter residing in schools' student-friendly facilities meant to accommodate those who come from a distant home. The overall head counts, therefore, within each educational institution, as constituted by the aforementioned categories, would prove a syndicate of quicker communication of the coronavirus, be it one among the mob (peers) who became infected. The government of Lesotho, in June 2020, adopted the SIR model to manage the spread of the COVID-19 pandemic. This model outlines different levels of risk determination and mitigation measures for social activities. About five levels were identified, ranging from low cases to high community transmissions. Citadels of knowledge dissemination, the schools, were here identified as a super spreader group and were granted a chance to remain operational only on the first two levels of risk determination, low and sporadic levels. At the low cases level, schools remained utterly functional with no restrictions whereas the sporadic level restricted schools' operations to external classes of standard 7 and form E. Tertiary institutions were as well at liberty to remain operational but only on the ground that they would exercise and put into full effect the prescribed national and WHO precautionary regulations against COVID-19.

At the heart of such crucial decisions lay the government's will to rescue the nationals from the scourge of the deadly coronavirus. Some members of the public would not however care to bend to these regulations without raising a roar. Free primary education in Lesotho brought with it the introduction of free meals for all pupils, which particularly proved beneficial to vulnerable children coming from the poorest of households. Hence, this formed the basis of the lamenter's argument on how such children would survive. The World Bank (2020) indicates that the Nominal Gross Domestic Product of Lesotho amounts to \$1.299. The World Bank carries on showing that unemployment remained high at 23.6% in 2018, coupled with inequality and poverty levels. This finding then evidently reveals that unless appropriate intervention measures were designed specifically for and targeting the identified vulnerable children and others in similar predicament, the lockdown would definitely make it difficult for them to survive. The other cohort lamented over their tuition, which was not refunded even with the immediate halt in class attendance by their children: these assumably were majorly parents and/or guardians of pupils in private primary schools and of course high schools because all public primary schools are free of tuition fees. The final category to express dissatisfaction were those who vividly could foresee a year or perhaps two passing by without their children attaining the ever-needed education, and needed more so in a competitively growing world.

To mitigate the impact of COVID-19 on mastery, several avenues were suggested and some were implemented. COVID-19 therefore provided a platform for newer experiences that are likely to feature under the concept of the "new normal" manner of conduct emergent during this pandemic outbreak. The new venture, in fact, which possibly came about as the last resort to enable educational knowledge dissemination amid COVID-19, was through online teaching and learning. Although this option might have encountered few if any hurdles in developed countries, perhaps because of abundance of resources to facilitate this exercise and again because it was practically operational pre-COVID-19 era, there is no doubt on the opposite end that it came with unequalled and perhaps unexpected challenges in developing countries such as Lesotho. Precisely, the challenges were not only felt by the few primary and secondary schools that attempted this new venture but, as one would say, were multiplied in institutions of higher learning. Shortage of basic resources needed to drive this initiative and lack of necessary knowledge to use this avenue might have been the prime challenges. This, at the National University of Lesotho, resulted in students boycotting classes while lecturers, on the other hand, outlined in detail their challenges over the THUTO portal, an avenue created to facilitate online teaching and learning. One would say that this was a way to express their frustrations. When immediate solutions seemed to be farfetched, some lecturers resorted to other social media platforms and in particular, WhatsApp, to ease their teaching burdens. WhatsApp groups were therefore created and served as convenient avenues of knowledge dissemination.

Blended teaching, which is a combination of both physical and online teaching, was also suggested and tried, even though it could not produce desired results because large numbers would still remain at risk, if ever they were to meet physically. The method, however, benefitted the Faculty of Science and Technology (FoST) where the sizes of student bodies are manageable. A one-on-one talk with one of the university's psychologists revealed that the frustrations of online teaching and learning at the National University of Lesotho resulted in about three suicidal cases of students; the souls who would otherwise contribute to the country's economic development after completing their studies. On 29 January 2020, the National University of Lesotho had lost about four lecturers, with three being confirmed COVID-19 cases. This loss again impacted negatively on young students as they would have to wait until the replacements for such lecturers materialised. Building rapport with the replacement lecturers may again cost students time.

The need for mastery on children and youth has therefore been greatly challenged, especially among the vulnerable population of children and youth. The prevalent conditions make it difficult for anyone to calmly and eagerly maintain a zeal for acquisition of knowledge, be it academic, cultural, or social. The COVID-19 era has however provided a platform for nations, including Lesotho, to employ newer modes of knowledge dissemination using technology. For some this is altogether a new venture, which emerged with tumult, but we can on the bright side anticipate that online teaching and learning shall in the sooner future be preferred, with all challenges addressed. It may perhaps be desired even over physical lectures post-COVID-19.

12.6 Independence: COVID-19 Impact Analysis on Children and Youth in Lesotho

When an already shaky country is scourged on all sides by a pandemic as fatal as COVID-19, a sense of independence becomes but a mirage. Independence is a fundamental value in society that accords liberty to choose how to live one's life within one's inherent capacities and means, consistent with one's personal values and preferences (Turnbull & Turnbull, 1985). Independence entails one's position of satisfactory ownership of necessities of life, which eventually lead to total autonomy to do as one pleases. Thus, independence cannot exist in a state of chaos and instability. Right at the beginning of the epidemic, the then ruling government was toppled and a new government rose to power and restructured with the aim of responding to the epidemic. The National Emergency Command Center was dismantled and the National COVID-19 Secretariat was established. This transition left the society, as well as the donor community, confused. As a country, Lesotho is down on its knees economically, and COVID-19 and political instability exacerbated this situation as the economy spiralled even further downwards to its toes, or in the worst of cases to its underfoot. The World Bank (2020) reported an unemployment rate of 23.6% in 2018. This high unemployment rate undoubtedly compromises economic and other forms of independence among vulnerable populations of children (as dependents) and the youth as economic drivers. Uncertainty and confusion/panic brought by the epidemic amidst political and economic instability threatened children's and youth's sense of independence. Factors that lead to high unemployment rate relate to political instability, government's negligence, and corruption. On her YouTube channel, Nthakoana Ngatane, a local and international journalist, premiered a video entitled "my land my people" in May 2019. Presenting her concerns in the video, Nthakoana was moved to mobilise those who cared to challenge the government over neglecting their responsibility of job creation. while rather bickering over the non-essentials, or alternatively devoting to matters of personal aggrandisement

Social work in Lesotho constitutes a growing profession, which although having gained some ground-breaking recognition is yet to reach exponential levels. The Ministry of Social Development remains the greatest employer of social workers. It would therefore become a challenge for the ministry and inversely the profession that is less endowed with both in kind and fiscal resources to meet children and youth's needs holistically using the circle of courage, particularly during the COVID-19 era. The absence of social workers' national counsel in Lesotho also makes it difficult to keep the politicians to their word. It is one of the social workers' many roles to stand in the gap and advocate for the vulnerable groups that are being exploited or mistreated. Patel (2007) quotes Kirst-Ashman, who explains that an advocate role is one in which social workers speak out on behalf of clients to promote fair and equal treatment or gain needful resources. This goal of course cannot be easily achieved unless social workers unanimously stand up to confront governmental compromises that put the welfare of the citizens at risk. Social workers should, however, do this in the best interests of the citizens and not for personal aggrandisement. The social workers' counsel would be a good avenue to ensure this.

Children's and youth s social independence (free or unrestricted gatherings) has also been compromised during the several lockdown restrictions that were imposed as a strategy to curb the spread of COVID-19. Imposition of the lockdown restrictions implied that people could not travel as freely and as frequently as they would please. Detrimental to some students who are schooling far from home, this would mean that if lockdown restrictions took effect before they reached their homes, they would be forced to remain within their distant abodes until the lockdown restrictions were lifted. Movements under the hard lockdown were only permitted to essential services providers and seekers, with the former granted permits of approval that they were indeed in essential services provision. The criteria of granting permits to the latter, however, were unclear.

Students' travel to their homes during the lockdown would therefore remain complicated, especially with unknown criteria of whether they qualified for permits. According to Koprowska (2008), human beings are social species who desire to be in the company of others for maintenance of their physical and psychological wellbeing. Koprowska's statement makes us understand that social isolation, and for a length of time beyond acceptable limits, may affect an individual both physically and psychologically. Perhaps this has been the case with all children and youth who for a length of time were isolated without meeting with their families and friends. Children, especially those in their early childhood, become highly restless once they are confined in one setting without meeting with their peers to play. Imposed social isolation again sabotaged young people whose lives gloat with frequent attendance to parties and other such places of merriment. Closure of bars, clubs, and other recreational facilities such as sporting fields may have been as a splash of cold water on youth who frequently visit such sites. Meanwhile, the inability to perform anything while remaining indoors may be daunting by itself.

Contrary to the earlier narrative, a personal interaction and conversation with some young people after the first phase of lockdown revealed that the lockdown was actually a time to rid or separate themselves from the mob (their peers) and to sober up. Some of these young people therefore secured an incredible spot away from their influential peers who at times may not advise them alright. While aloof, they seized the opportunity to rework and reshape their lives as they would independently wish. Some young people who often times prefer to channel or shape their lives according to the mob's consensus may lose a sense of individual or independent purpose of existence in their lives. This, on the other hand, is a true reflection that lockdown was to some extent beneficial.

12.7 Generosity: COVID-19 Impact Analysis on Children and Youth in Lesotho

Generosity is an important aspect of social cohesion and solidarity. It is often expressed as a gesture of reciprocity. People who show themselves as generous are likely to have been recipients of generous acts themselves (Swanzen & Jonker, 2020). The acts of kindness and/or expression of the spirit of ubuntu (solidarity) are critical at a time of crisis and uncertainty. Which would particularly hold the greatest of values to children who are helplessly dependent on their parents or caregivers. With loss of jobs and livelihoods caused by COVID-19, many children and youth experienced heightened vulnerability and depended on others' generosity. Although the government of Lesotho increased child grants beneficiaries, there was no direct support to the youth. In addition, with school closure, vulnerable children's nutrition was compromised as many depend on school feeding schemes. Consequently, many children and young people were forced to rely on the generosity of others.

As the strikes unfolded at the National University of Lesotho, because of coronavirus-related complications that eventually led to the university's temporary closure, some of the students could be seen stranded shortly after closure of the university, short of transport fare to their homes. Perhaps their Good Samaritan co-students generously came to their rescue.

In Lesotho, as with many other countries in Africa and beyond, no one person could really and fully with precision anticipate when the next lockdown would be. This uncertainty would more specifically be detrimental to the informal traders who would buy commodities in bulk for resale, only for lockdown to be called into full effect hastily once coronavirus infection cases escalated sharply. As previously indicated, some of these street sellers are diploma and degree holders who have been compelled to street trade given the heat of high unemployment in the country. As news broke that lockdown was about to be imposed then, to rescue the situation, the locals, including the youth who have the wherewithal, would in unison make it a point to generously clear the sales commodities of the street sellers lest they perish during the lockdown or become waste. A rapid assessment of the socioeconomic impact of COVID-19 in Lesotho conducted by Hlabana in 2020 further reveals that amidst the precarity of sustainable economic opportunities during the lockdown, some of the youth lost their jobs because most of them run informal businesses. These trying times have in part forced the natives to retrieve some of the forsaken indigenous informal means of ensuring welfare in the society. The traditional distribution of welfare model prescribes that the family, either nuclear or extended, has the responsibility of filling the gap or providing for its members in the event that their source of livelihood collapses. This attitude also transpired to rescue the youth from their lack of self-sustenance predicament emanating from the lockdowns. It was again time for family to take care of its own, at times before extending a hand outside familial setup.

12.8 Conclusion/Building Circle of Courage Through Resilience

COVID-19 is clearly exacerbating existing vulnerabilities among children and youth in Lesotho. This chapter has highlighted how this epidemic is threatening positive development of these population groups in the country. However, in wrapping up this chapter, we want to show that this challenge can be turned into an opportunity. For example, research has highlighted the importance of family processes in buffering against risks among children and youth in South Africa (van Brenda and Theron, 2018). A recent study on COVID-19 has also supported the role of families during social disruption (Masten & Motti-Stefanidi, 2020). A similar role of families has been observed in Lesotho. Families have been sources of resilience during this pandemic as they are forced to assume more responsibility for children and youth. For example, the family is forced to assume more belonging for children and youth during the pandemic through lockdowns and home isolation and quarantine as they became the only source of spaces and contacts belonging. As a result, there has been more bonding within families and households. However, family poverty and instability threatened achievement of this quadrant for many children and youth. Thus, it is important to target and support vulnerable families and households during the pandemic. Although the Ministry of Social Development provided food parcels and child grants to vulnerable households with children, the youth were not a target. Moreover, provision of psychosocial support was not considered, undermining social work in Lesotho.

In addition, homes have been turned into classrooms as children and young people still in school are forced to study from home. While skill development has been relegated to schools, parents and guardians are now forced to play a pivotal role in the learning and imparting of knowledge and skills to children. Thus, the mastery quadrant is now family centred, elevating the role of the family in society, a role that sometimes caused a barrier between children and parents, as schools were seen as superior to the family knowledge. The reliance on schools and teachers for knowledge and guidance took away some independence from children and youth. With schools closed for almost a year, pupils have been forced to be independent learners and thinkers. Young people have been challenged to be innovative and find alternative livelihood strategies. For example, cross-border traders are now using technology to find and import goods, whereas vegetable and fruit street vendors have turned to local producers to buy goods instead of relying on South African produce: this has stimulated local production. There is the adage that "charity begins at home." Long-term lockdown meant that family members had to rely on each other more for support and courage during uncertainty. Therefore, the resilience of youth and children in Lesotho highlight hopes for the circle of courage and positive development.

References

(2020) *Polihali Dam-Bitter Sweet* (N. Ngatane, Interviewer).

Ansell, N., van Blerk, L., Robson, E., Hajdu, F., Mwathunga, E., Hlabana, T., et al. (2018). *Social cash transfers, generational relations and youth poverty trajectories in Lesotho and Malawi*. www.cashtransfers-youth.net

Brendtro, L. K., Brokenleg, M., & Van Bockern, S. (2005). The circle of courage and positive psychology. *Reclaiming Children and Youth, 14*(3), 130–136.

Bureau of Statistics. (2018). *Lesotho Population and Housing Census Report* Maseru: Bureau of Statistics

Bureau of Statisctics. (2019). *Labour Force Survey Report*. Maseru: Bureau of Statistics (BOS).

Douglas, V. (2007). *What makes a school a learning organisation? A guide for policy makers, school leaders and teachers. Celebrating in the learning organisation*. OECD.

Dyke, G., Carelse, S., Lombard, A., Mbezi, P., Rasool, S., & Schenck, R. (2019). *Circle of Courage.Theories of decolonial social work practice in South Africa*. Oxford University Press.

Ghosh, R., Chatterjee, S., & Dubey, S. (2020). Impact of COVID-19 on children: Special focus on the psychosocial aspect. *Minerva Pediatrics, 72*(3), 226–235.

Hapazari, J. (2019). Challenges *Faced by Unemployed People in Lesotho. A case of Manonyane Rural Community*. South African Reveiw of Sociology, 50(1), 65-82.

Koprowska, J. (2008). *Communication and interpersonal skills in social work*. en.bookfi.net

Lotter, C. B. (2005). Circles of courage: *Music therapy with adolescents in conflict with the law at a community based setting*. Thesis submitted to the University of Pretoria.

Masten, A., & Motti-Stefanidi, F. (2020). Multisystem resilience for children and youth in disaster: Reflections in the context of COVID-19. *Adversity and Resilience Science*, 1–12.

My Land My People. (2019). www.youtube.com/watch?v=nzJQH0uBeoQ&t=5s

Ministry of Gender, Y. a (2017). *Lesotho National Youth Policy*. Maseru: Ministry of Gender, Youth Sports and Recreation.

Ministry of Training and Education. (2020). *Education Sector Response Plan for the Novel Coronavirus (COVID-19)*. Maseru: Ministry of Education and Training.

NACOSEC. (2021). *Situational Analysis: COVID-19 Epidemiology in Lesotho*. Maseru: National COVID-19 Secretariat (NACOSEC).

Nearchou, F., Flinn, C., Niland, R., Subramaniam, S., & Hennessy, E. (2020). Exploring the impact of COVID-19 on mental health outcomes in children and adolescents: A systematic review. *International Journal of Environmental Research and Public Health, 17*(22). (22).

Patel, L. (2007). *Social welfare and social development in South Africa* (2nd printing). Oxford University Press.

Reyneke, R. (2020). Increasing resilience, lowering risk: Teachers' use of the circle of courage in the classroom. *Perspectives in Education, 38*(1), 144–162.

Sapp, D., Horn-Loiben, T., Nicholas, A., & Franklin, T. (2004). *Circle of courage: Involve to evolve*. Presented at Hand in Hand 2004 (pp. 1–18). North American Association of Christians in Social Work (NACSW)

Swanzen, R., & Jonker, G. (2020). COVID-19 and alternative care in South Africa: Children's responses to the pandemic. A case study from a child and Youth Care Center in Mogale City. *Institutionalised Children Explorations and Beyond, 8*(1), 51–64.

Turnbull, A. P., & Turnbull, R. H. (1985). Developing independence. *Journal of Adolescent Health Care, 6*, 108–119.

UNFPA. (2020). *Gender-based violence*. https://www.unfpa.org/gender-based-violence

UNFPA Lesotho. (2020). COVID-19 *Lockdown exacerbates gender-based violence cases in Lesotho*. https://lesotho.unfpa.org/en/news/COVID-19-lock-down-exacerbates-gender-based-violence-cases-lesotho

UNICEF. (2021). *Humanitarian action for children*. UNICEF in Emergencies. https://www.unicef.org/appeals

UN. (2018). *Youth and the 2030 Agenda for Sustainable Development*. Retreived February 13, 2021, from United Nations Populations Fund: http://www.un.org/development/desa/youth/wp content/uploads/sites/21/2018/12/WorldYouthReport-2030Agenda.pdf

UNAIDS. (2021). *Report for Joint Review of HIV/Tuberculosis and Hepatitis Programmes*. Retreived December 2020, 9, from UNAIDS Country Report: LSO_2018_countryreport:pdf(unaids.org).

Van, B., & McDonald, T. (2012). *Creating Circle of Courage Schools. Reclaiming Children and Youth*, 20(4), 13-17.

Van, B., & Theron, L. (2018). *A Critical Review of South African Child and Youth Resilience Studies 2009-2017*. Children and Youth Services Review, 91, 237-247.

Van Breda, A. (2018). A critical review of south African child and youth resilience studies, 2009–2017. *Children and Youth Services Review, 91*, 1–28.

WHO. (2020, 29 June). *Archived: WHO Timeline-COVID-19*. https://www.who.int/news/item/27-04-2020-who-timeline-COVID-19

World Bank. (2020). *The World Bank in Lesotho*. The World Bank IBRD.IDA. www.worldbank.org/en/country/lesotho/overview

13 Analysing the Situation of Migrants and Social Work Interventions in South Africa During the Coronavirus (COVID-19) Pandemic

Nomcebo Dlamini, Thabisa Matsea, and Ndangwa Noyoo

13.1 Introduction

Migrants are a transient population group. They move from their countries of birth to other societies across the globe, in response to various 'push and pull' factors. The former are basically negative drivers and perceived incentives that trigger migrations across the globe. According to the United Nations High Commission for Refugees (UNHCR) (2020), by the end of 2013, more than 232 million people globally were estimated to be migrants, of whom 19 million were projected to be in Africa. According to Mukumbang et al. (2020), close to two million foreign-born migrants of working age (15–64 years) were living in South Africa in 2017. Nevertheless, when discussing vulnerable groups such as migrants, it is important that we know who they are. Hence, it is crucial to define them appropriately. However, definitions of migrants vary as there are different interpretations and perspectives about this group. The United Nations (2020) explains that although there is no formal legal definition of an international migrant, most experts agree that such an individual is someone who changes his or her country of usual residence, irrespective of the reason for migration or legal status. Generally, a distinction is made between short-term or temporary migration, covering movements with a duration between 3 and 12 months; and long-term or permanent migration as well as referring to a change of country of residence for a duration of 1 year or more (United Nations, 2020). Furthermore, the International Organisation for Migration (IOM) (2020) asserts that migrants include a number of well-defined legal categories of people, such as migrant workers; persons whose particular types of movements are legally defined, for instance, smuggled migrants; as well as those whose status or means of movement are not specifically defined under international law, for example, international students. Their transient nature causes this group to be prone to various vulnerabilities and insecurities.

According to the IOM (2020, p. 1), South Africa is the preferred destination for various categories of migrants and faces a host of migration-related challenges, encompassing, inter alia:

N. Dlamini (✉)
Faculty of Humanities, Community Development Unit, University of the Free State, Phuthaditjhaba, South Africa
e-mail: dlaminin@ufs.ac.za

T. Matsea
Faculty of Humanities, Social Sciences and Education, Department of Social Work, University of Venda, Thohoyandou, South Africa

N. Noyoo
Department of Social Development, University of Cape Town, Cape Town, South Africa

M. C. S. Gonçalves et al. (eds.), *The Coronavirus Crisis and Challenges to Social Development*, https://doi.org/10.1007/978-3-030-84678-7_13

increased prevalence of irregular migration, including women and unaccompanied minors; inadequate migration management policies and border management processes; rising xenophobic sentiments that in some cases turn into actual violence against migrants; high prevalence of communicable diseases such as HIV and AIDS, and tuberculosis; and continued brain drain from the emigration of skilled nationals. Therefore, the onset of the COVID-19 pandemic only compounded the migrants' already dire situation in South Africa. Taking the aforementioned issues into critical account, the purpose of this chapter is to shed light on the plight of migrants in South Africa during the COVID-19 pandemic from a social work perspective. In this regard, the chapter closely examines the roles of social workers during this global health crisis and also proposes other roles in which they could meet the needs of migrants during the COVID-19 health crisis. It is important to do this because the COVID-19 pandemic has profoundly disrupted many people's lives and the welfare of families all over the world and in South Africa. Even the citizens of South Africa are struggling, with many of them losing their jobs and livelihoods. Many have also lost their lives or are gravely ill from the pandemic. In the same vein, many couples have divorced during this period (Daniel, 2020), and suicide rates have also increased during the lockdown because of the pandemic (Mkhize, 2020 cited in the South African Broadcasting Corporation (SABC), 2020). If the citizens of the country are suffering in this manner because of COVID-19, what more of migrants and other 'outsiders' such as refugees and asylum seekers?

It is therefore critical that professions such as social work alleviate the harsh living circumstances of migrants during this pandemic. Social workers are professionals who are trained to solve people's problems or offer solutions towards making the lives of people and communities better. Therefore, it is important to ascertain how social workers are responding to COVID-19's devastating and negative psychosocial impacts. Before delving into the reasons why social work should be among those leading the charge against human misery during the pandemic and why it should focus on migrants and other transient populations, this chapter first provides a backdrop to COVID-19 in South Africa. Then, it highlights the situation of migrants during the national lockdown. It then discusses broadly how the profession works with migrants and specifically how social workers have engaged with migrants in South Africa, before and during the pandemic. Thereafter, the chapter makes proposals for social work interventions with migrants in a post-COVID-19 era in South Africa.

13.2 COVID-19 in South Africa: A Backdrop

It is not an exaggeration to assert that COVID-19 has disrupted the lives of millions of South Africans and compounded social ills that already existed in the country before it reached the country's shores. In a space of 10 months South Africa has practically been turned upside down by the pandemic. This chapter is being finalised exactly 1 year after the pandemic exploded around the world, after it was first reported in China in late 2019. It is also a year later after the World Health Organization (WHO) declared COVID-19 a public health emergency. South Africa experienced the first wave in mid-July 2020, and the second wave in January 2021, when COVID-19 spread faster and was more virulent than the first wave. After the first wave, it seems many people became relaxed and careless, and stopped adhering to the COVID-19 protocols of washing hands and sanitizing, maintaining social distancing, and wearing of masks. South Africa has now 1,613,728 identified positive cases, with 1,523,359.232 recoveries and 55,210 deaths according to the Republic of South Africa (RSA) (2021). South Africa is the worst COVID-19-affected country in Africa.

The first case of COVID-19 was identified in South Africa on 5 March 2020 after the authorities traced it to KwaZulu-Natal province. It was discovered that this case was imported from Europe, after the infected person who had travelled to Italy with 11 other people returned to South Africa. Immediately thereafter, COVID-19 cases were identified in the Free State province. After this, the big metropoles of Johannesburg and Cape Town starting having COVID-19 infections. As the infections began to rise, the government decisively swung into action, with the president of the country, Cyril Ramaphosa, declaring a state of national disaster on 23 March 2020. In the same breath, a mandatory national lockdown was announced. The lockdown commenced on 26 March 2020 and was meant to decrease and control the rate of new infections. Inadvertently, the lockdown negatively impacted the well-being and livelihoods of all citizens and residents of South Africa. Although well intentioned, the lockdown disrupted all social and economic activities. Migrants faced exponential challenges during the lockdown because their living conditions were already precarious.

13.3 Living Conditions of Migrants During the Lockdown

It is important to note that before COVID-19, millions of citizens were already suffering from high levels of poverty and unemployment (The World Bank, 2018; Strauss et al., 2020). In addition, before the lockdown containment measures, migrants had relatively weakened social support structures, bleak socioeconomic prospects, unequal access to healthcare and various social services; precarious housing conditions, tenuous living and working conditions, and higher risks of exploitation and abuse. Many migrants found themselves suddenly jobless, being evicted from their homes, hungry, insecure, and trapped in dormitories or camps where adequate physical distancing is impossible to observe (Mukumbang et al., 2020, p. 3). According to Garba (2020) the South African state's response to the COVID-19 crisis ignores the full range of vulnerability and its dynamics. This attitude is especially true for migrants, who face grave vulnerability in that they are confronted with issues of political and social marginalisation and a lack of socioeconomic resources afforded primarily to citizens. It is also not based on the structure of the society and local economies in townships and inner-city neighbourhoods. The former author further argues that the state was only able to adopt an exclusionary citizenship-based criterion, that excluded small enterprises whose employees, customers, and creditors were made up of locals and migrants, by categorising the vulnerable into those deserving of social support and the undeserving. Indeed, when it came to migrants, government interventions seemed to have had some embedded barriers leading to exclusion as Mukumbang et al. (2020, p. 4) report:

> The South African government also embarked on providing food parcels to those who are threatened by food insecurity. During these food distribution campaigns, it has been observed that foreign-born migrants form a significant number of attendees. Similar to accessing the Social Relief of Distress grant of R350 ($20) and receiving [Unemployment Insurance Fund] UIF payments, a South African national Identity Document (ID) or special permit is required to receive food parcels, which foreign-born migrants are unlikely to possess. In this way, asylum seekers, refugees, and undocumented migrants are excluded from the government's food relief programmes.

As many migrants could not eke out a living or ply their trade during the lockdown, their ability to earn an income was severely diminished, so that they could not meet the needs of their families. According to Statistics South Africa (StatsSA) (2020), more than 20% of migrants who participated in its survey on mobility and migration during the lockdown indicated that they did not send remittances during the lockdown because they could not afford to send any money. Also, the results show that, generally, migrant respondents were more vulnerable than nonmigrant respondents. A much higher percentage of migrant respondents (22.5%) were unemployed as compared to nonmigrants (9%). Findings from the report underscores the important role of mobility and migration on the South African economy during the national lockdown.

It is noteworthy that many undocumented individuals constitute a large number of migrants in South Africa, and as a consequence they earn their living mainly in the informal sector. They operate retail kiosks (locally called spaza shops) and hawk goods (Garba, 2020). The national lockdown in South Africa has led to a situation where many migrant-owned small businesses have either collapsed or are on the verge of bankruptcy. Many working-class migrants have lost jobs and are unable to meet their needs and provide basic necessities for their families. Many who sell items on the sidewalks of streets and traffic intersections have all but subsisted on their capital and are therefore without any means of livelihood (Garba, 2020, p. 1). Despite these challenges, migrants have also proved to be resilient and have tried to survive the harsh effects of the pandemic by tapping into their indigenous knowledge systems (IKS) and indigenous social security systems. In their research on migrants during the lockdown, Chekero and Ogude (2020) discovered that Zimbabwean migrants relied on 'money rotating and grocery savings groups.' Membership to these groups is based on preexisting relationships or other common ties such as coming from the same area or working for the same company. These groups use money to buy food and other essentials. Also, members are able to secure interest-free loans from the groups. Members can lend money to other trusted nonmembers as a way of opening networks and opportunities for easy access to other services and opportunities in return.

13.4 Xenophobia During a Pandemic

It seems whenever South Africans face national stress or challenges, there is an increase in xenophobia and xenophobic violence. Xenophobia and xenophobic violence seem to be mainly targeted at migrants, refugees, and asylum seekers from mainly Sub-Saharan African countries (Chagunda, 2020; Egwu, 2021; Noyoo et al., 2021; Noyoo, 2018). A report by Human Rights Watch which documents xenophobic harassment and attacks by South Africans, including government and law enforcement officials, between March 2019 and March 2020, based on interviews with 51 people in the Western Cape, Gauteng, and KwaZulu-Natal provinces, is instructive to this discussion as it shows how xenophobia is nuanced during the pandemic:

> In that period, mobs of angry rioters throughout South Africa have attacked and harassed non-nationals, blaming them for unemployment, crime, neglect by the government, among other things. In September 2019 in Western Cape, Gauteng, and KwaZulu-Natal, hundreds of people believed to be South African organised a national shutdown, blocking roads and highways; closing taxi ranks, schools, and businesses; and chanting for all foreigners to leave. The shutdown turned violent with mobs looting and torching homes, shops, and malls owned or rented by non-nationals. The government has said 12 people, 10 of whom were South Africans, died during the September 2019 unrest. However, Human Rights Watch's research, based on interviews with shop owners, community leaders, teachers, students, truck drivers, lawyers, civil society organisations, academic scholars, and credible media reports, indicates a higher number of fatalities for both foreigners and South Africans (Human Rights Watch, 2020, p. 2).

Furthermore, the pandemic has led to increased narrow nationalism across South Africa, which has expressed itself in government circles and translated into policy ambivalence. Eyewitness News (2020) reports that the government's policy ambiguities have been laid bare by the coronavirus pandemic. For instance, during the lockdown, South Africa's Finance Minister Tito Mboweni called for locals to be favoured for jobs when the country emerged from the health crisis. "The proportion of South Africans working in a restaurant must be greater than that of non-South Africans," he declared. There are also disturbing accounts which note that anti-migrant sentiments have even been taken up by the former freedom fighters of the Umkhonto we Sizwe (MK) military wing of the African National Congress (ANC). Now operating under the banner of the Umkhonto we Sizwe Military Veterans Association (MKMVA), it seems the military veterans had struck an alliance with unemployed graduates, truck drivers, hawkers, and saloon workers in the city of Durban. These groups also joined them in "taking back" Durban in early November 2020. The MKMVA unfortunately has been displaying xenophobic tendencies of late. The puzzling case of the MKVA antimigrant and xenophobic sentiments needs some dissecting:

these are individuals who had fled into exile during the liberation struggle to other African countries. These countries, with their meagre resources, welcomed them and treated them well and with dignity. Given apartheid South Africa's scorched earth policy, its security forces and death squads continuously carried out cross-border raids and killed many citizens of these African countries, as they hunted down MK combatants. Despite such harsh reprisals from the apartheid regime, meted out to the countries harbouring the freedom fighters, people in these countries did not harass or blame the MK combatants for the difficulties they were facing.

Xenophobia that is directed at migrants has only gone to make their lives extremely precarious, during the COVID-19 pandemic. This dangerous trend continues to amplify itself even after the government has made some effort to eradicate it. For example, in March 2019, the South African government launched its National Action Plan to Combat Racism, Racial Discrimination, Xenophobia, and Related Intolerance (NAP). Among the actions the NAP identifies to be taken to combat xenophobia are creating mechanisms to ensure that foreigners receive services they are entitled to, facilitating their integration, and embracing a humane and dignified approach to managing migrants, refugees, and asylum seekers (Human Rights Watch, 2020). However, such intentions are failing to percolate down to the mass of the people who are engaged in xenophobia and xenophobic violence. During this health crisis:

> The South African response in dealing with the Corona pandemic needs to speak to the realities of all people living in the country, including migrant and refugee communities. Reflecting on this in light of ongoing research on the political stakes of migration governance, we find that the virus response shows little change in the government agenda when it comes to dealing with refugees and other migrants. ...The temporary stay on renewing asylum seekers permits counts as a perfunctory exception. (Zanker & Moyo, 2020, p. 1).

The next section casts some light on social work and how it engages with migrants.

13.5 Social Workers Working with Migrants

When examining the connection between social work and migrants, it is important to first locate it in the historical origins and mission of the profession. A historical perspective and appreciation of the profession's early roots and subsequent development of social work is an important first step in critically understanding the current role of social work, its challenges and contradictions, and provide a useful foundation for critically exploring these issues. The history of social work shows that it is a product of political, social, and economic forces within society (Finch & Parker, 2020). Social workers engage with people who are vulnerable and who are struggling in some way to participate fully in society. Social workers walk that tightrope between supporting and advocating on behalf of the marginalised individual, whilst being employed by the social, economic, and political environment that may have contributed to their marginalisation (Horner, 2012). However, this history of social work is context specific as it is derived from a Western context and is nuanced differently in the developing world particularly in Africa. Therefore, social work in Africa was exported to the continent during colonial rule. In this regard, Noyoo and Kleibl (2020) argue that contemporary social work in Africa needs to be viewed through the prism of decolonisation. What is worth noting, when it comes to Africa, is that colonialism supplanted, and at times erased, the indigenous forms of social care that responded to and met the needs of indigenous populations in precolonial times. As a result, Noyoo argues that IKS should be reestablished as a means of reifying some of the erased African values and then remodifying them in an indigenised form of social work (2020, p. 265). As the latter part of this chapter shows, this standpoint is not far fetched, as many South Africans and migrants fell back on these indigenous forms of care and bonds of social solidarity to protect themselves from the ravages of COVID-19.

It is worth underscoring the point that the pandemic can be likened to a national and global disaster. To this end, it can be noted that social workers have long been engaged in disaster management (Nikku, 2015). Social workers are among the frontline workers who provide primary services to destitute groups such as migrants in states of disaster (Diaconu et al., 2016). Given their effectiveness in trauma stress management, social workers also provide services during and after natural disasters to improve the general well-being of affected populations (Bourassa, 2009). Based on their understanding of the person-in-environment, social workers draw on various methods and skills to intervene at different levels of society with the aim to assist those in need (Reichert, 2011). For social work, migration raises many issues from the practical—how to work with individuals, families, groups, and different cultures often displaced in traumatic circumstances—to the theoretical values and philosophies (Ibrahim, 2016). Social workers are thus not only well trained but well disposed to help marginalised and displaced populations such as migrants:

> Immigration continues to be central to social work services because immigrants are vulnerable to all types of substandard living conditions and abuses, including child-labour, prostitution and human trafficking. Furthermore, 'social workers are in a good position to foster deliberation by presenting more positive points of view on the immigration phenomenon', particularly in the area of immigration policy. (Ibrahim, 2016, pp. 95–96).

In South Africa, Roestenburg (2013) observes that migration is an often-neglected practise area for social workers. He advises that at the micro level social work should have an important role in, among other areas, helping migrants to settle in the new country: from reception and documentation, to housing and employment-related issues. Trauma counselling is another area requiring development, as is evidenced by the relatively large population of traumatised migrants in the country from xenophobic attacks, and other forms of violence and societal abuse.

13.6 Social Work Interventions Amidst the COVID-19 Pandemic

Since 2019, social workers have been feverishly dealing with social problems and other ills that have been compounded by COVID-19 such as hunger and food insecurity, gender-based violence, and child abuse. Social workers have been providing psychosocial support to individuals, families, groups, and communities. Also, social workers responded to the pandemic by providing food parcels, food vouchers, and grants for rentals and daily expenses as well as shelter. When it came to migrants, provision of the material assistance was based on the set criteria, such as documentation to prove their migrant status in South Africa. Those who did not meet the criteria found themselves in a difficult situation. However, it must be noted that social workers are human beings who experience the same pain, sorrow, and fear as everyone. They were in the forefront of intervention, while they themselves and their families needed the very intervention. The Registrar of the South African Council for Social Service Professions (SACSSP), Langi Malamba, captures this dire issue quite poignantly:

> Being thrust in the forefront of the COVID-19 pandemic means a lot of social service practitioners harboured a lot of the fear and pain. The way we conduct our business and offer interventions can never be the same again. We cannot revert to the former 'normal' that we used to know because many great opportunities have been created where the global village is far reachable than before. The challenges of offering supervision to social service practitioners in outlying communities can be mitigated by having interactive supervision using secure virtual platforms. A good number of essential service workers were lost to COVID-19 and we must never forget or take their deaths in vain. We need to forge forward with more vigour and conscientiousness… (SACSSP, 2020, p. 1).

Indeed, many social workers lost their lives (as did other essential workers) during the pandemic. However, they continue to fight for the marginalised and vulnerable people as well as communities, despite such dangers. There seems to be less work being undertaken with migrants in South Africa. In fact, it can be argued that the

COVID-19 pandemic has exposed the minimal roles and responsibilities that social work plays, broadly in the area of migration, and specifically with migrants, and with similar populations such as refugees and asylum seekers in South Africa (Blaauw et al., 2017; Roestenburg, 2013). There is thus a need for general reorientation of social work in South Africa.

13.7 Social Work and Migrants in a Post-COVID South Africa: A Call to Action

One of the key issues to emerge during the COVID-19 pandemic is that social work is fulfilling minimal roles and responsibilities in the area of migration, as was also the case before the pandemic (Blaauw et al., 2017; Roestenburg, 2013). Also, during the COVID-19 pandemic many human rights issues came to the fore and it was discovered during the lockdown that many migrants experienced human rights abuses (Garba, 2020; Mukumbang et al., 2020; Ndlovu, 2020), with minimal interventions from social workers on behalf of migrants. There is thus a need to strengthen the role of social work in human rights-related matters and especially related to the rights of migrants: this should be the case as we prepare for a post-COVID South Africa. Apart from human rights, two issues were also sharply brought into focus: the need to build the migrants' resilience and also enhance indigenous social work practise in South Africa, especially when it came to the plight of migrants.

13.7.1 Human Rights, Social Work, and Migrants

The social work profession has its values aligned with the concept of human rights. Therefore, social workers have an ethical obligation to advocate for social justice and social inclusion of marginalised groups such as migrants and promote social change to enhance their well-being (Bourassa, 2009; Kafula, 2016). The Bill of Rights included in the *Constitution of the Republic of South Africa* enshrines the rights of all people in the country and affirms the democratic values of human dignity, equality and freedom. The Constitution recognises a range of rights and gives meaningful protection to socio-economic rights including rights to housing, healthcare, food, and water, as well as social security and assistance (Trilsch, 2009). Although the Constitution makes provision for human rights, the rights of migrants are not always realised. The implementation of the national lockdown, which many saw as a violation of human rights, posed a threat to the socioeconomic rights of many marginalised people, especially migrants. Since most migrants are engaged in low-cost labour and temporary employment (Kavuro, 2015), the lockdown meant that they had diminished sources of income and this situation consequently threatened their livelihoods. The former situation was also exacerbated by the fact that most migrants did not qualify for government assistance or received limited social protection. During the lockdown the government's relief measures did not extend to them (Dafuleya, 2020; Kavuro, 2020).

13.7.2 Building Migrants' Resilience

Building resilience is crucial in dealing with the pandemic's devastating effects. Resilience is the ability of individuals, families, and communities to overcome crises, and social workers can help migrants to adapt positively in these difficult times (Walsh, 2016).

The unprecedented nature of COVID-19 challenged people's ability to cope with the crises it induced as many experienced fear resulting from uncertainties about the future or experienced pain from a range of losses, especially after losing their loved ones, or anxiety caused by isolation stemming from social distancing (Davis, 2020). Many migrants have yet to manage the traumatic stressors of displacement, and postmigration challenges including lack of resources, family separation, social isolation, and discrimination, as well as socioeconomic factors (Li et al., 2016). The outbreak of COVID-19 increases the vulnerability of the already vulnerable migrants in terms of job losses as this group is overrepresented among temporary contracts employment (OECD, 2020). The issue of job loss contributes to lack of material resources and exacerbates food security challenges among these groups as they do not meet the set criteria to receive food parcels provided for relief. Furthermore, as this group is yet to be socially integrated, they have weaker social support structures that can be deployed during difficult times. This lack can result in feelings of uncertainty, fear, and hopelessness, and might retrigger psychological disruptions or evoke emotions that had been supressed, thereby threatening migrants' ability to manage adverse situations (Mukumbang et al., 2020). The seriousness and acuteness of these experiences may be prolonged and have a persistent negative impact on their mental health. This impact requires social workers to help migrants to be prepared to accept the long-term consequences of the pandemic. To reduce the impact of the pandemic, it is important for social workers to minimise risks of exposure to further adversity and build/facilitate the building of renewed resilience of migrants' families and their communities.

13.7.3 Enhancing Indigenous Social Work Practice

When it comes to the well-being of migrants, Chekero and Ogude (2020) intimate that to fully understand and engage with the lived experiences of migrants, fundamental aspects such as conviviality, social relationships, social networks, and individual dispositions that influence people's health and well-being should not be ignored: these are essential in the maintenance of social ties and of migrant ability to support one another in times of crisis. It can be discerned from the aforementioned authors' accounts pertaining to migrants and their indigenous social support systems that the former were crucial in helping migrants in cushioning the harsh effects of COVID-19. Indeed, if it were not for their indigenous forms of social protection, these migrants would have found themselves in even a worse position. As the numbers of migrants increase in the country, it is imperative that South African social workers equip themselves with indigenous social work practise knowledge, skills, and intervention methods. Social work can only be meaningful and effective in South Africa if it provides context-specific and tangible responses to the given social problems. These responses must be related to the sociocultural realities in the country. Owing to the overdependence of social work education and practise on Western models in this country, there is a dire need for research on what we call indigenous and innovative practics models that can effectively respond to the plight of migrants (Twikirize & Spitzer, 2019).

13.8 Conclusion

Migrants are a marginalised population group in South Africa facing multiple challenges. They are faced with overcoming adverse situations such as limited access to adequate housing, with minimal material resources to afford basic needs, while trying to heal from physical and psychological trauma they suffered in their countries of origin. Before the pandemic, these individuals were constantly experiencing exclusion, violence, and death from xenophobic violence (Noyoo et al., 2021). The problems they encountered have been amplified by COVID-19. What remains stark in this scenario is the minimal role of social work, compared to the gravity of intervention needed by immigrants, which goes well beyond the scope of social workers. This chapter analysed the situation of migrants and social work interventions during COVID-19. It argued that social workers should focus on upholding migrants' human rights and aim to build their resilience as a way of helping them assimilate more easily into the South African society. Social workers have been confronted with new realities, and lockdown restrictions that have prohibited them to practise as they normally would, and are. Through revisiting indigenous ways of addressing challenges, migrants have come together and helped each other as a collective of members rather than facing a common challenge in isolation. This finding should serve as a lesson and reminder of how Africans have addressed problems indigenously, and how it is the very IKS that has brought much-needed social relief. For this reason, the chapter proposed that social workers needed to be competent in indigenous social work practise to address migrant challenges during the COVID-19 pandemic.

References

Blaauw, P. F., Schenck, C. J., Pretorius, A. M., & Schoeman, C. H. (2017). All quiet on the social work front: Experiences of Zimbabwean day labourers in South Africa. *International Social Work, 60*(2), 351–365. https://doi.org/10.1177/0020872815594223

Bourassa, J. (2009). Psychosocial interventions and mass populations. *International Social Work, 52*(6), 743–755.

Chagunda, C. (2020). Refugees and asylum seekers from sub-Saharan African countries and the promotion of healthy human relationships. In N. Noyoo (Ed.), *Promoting healthy human relationships in post-apartheid South Africa: Social work and social development perspectives* (pp. 49–66). Springer.

Chekero, T., & Ogude, H. R. (2020). *Convivial networks: How migrants cope with the pandemic in South Africa.* https://www.coronatimes.net/convivial-networks-migrants-pandemic-south-africa/

Dafuleya, G. (2020). Social and emergency assistance ex-ante and during Covid-19 in the SADC region. *The International Journal of Community and Social Development, 2*(2), 251–268.

Daniel, L. (2020). *Divorce is surging in SA - and for many couples, this holiday may be the final straw.* https://www.businessinsider.co.za/sas-divorce-rate-up-30-in-2020-heres-why-its-expected-to-get-even-worse-after-the-holidays-2020-12

Davis, J. A. (2020). *Family resilience in the time of Corona.* https://cfeg.com/insights_research/family-resilience-in-the-time-of-corona/

Diaconu, M., Racovita-Szilagyi, L., & Bryan, B. A. (2016). The social worker's role in the context of forced migration: A global perspective. *Interdisciplinary Journal of Best Practices in Global Development, 2*(2), 1–14.

Egwu, P. (2021). *Pandemic and xenophobia: The plight of migrants in SA.* https://www.msn.com/en-za/news/editorpicks/pandemic-and-xenophobia-the-plight-of-migrants-in-sa/ar-BB1d5oCR?ocid=msedgdhp

Eyewitness News. (2020). *Migrants in SA face hunger, xenophobia during virus lockdown.* https://ewn.co.za/2020/05/27/migrants-in-sa-face-hunger-xenophobia-during-virus-lockdown

Finch, J., & Parker, J. (2020). The history and context of contemporary social work (including global social work). In J. Parker (Ed.), *Introducing social work* (pp. 3–13). Sage.

Garba, N.W.F. (2020). *Covid-19 in South Africa: Whither migrants?* https://africanarguments.org/2020/06/17/covid-19-in-south-africa-whither-migrants/

Horner, N. (2012). *What is social work? Context and perspectives.* 4th ed. London: Sage.

Human Rights Watch. (2020). *"They have robbed me of my life": Xenophobic violence against non-nationals in South Africa.* https://www.hrw.org/sites/default/files/media_2020/09/southafrica0920_web_4.pdf

Ibrahim, K. A. M. A. H. (2016). Social worker roles with refugees. *Egyptian Journal of Social Work 2*(1), 93–107.

International Organisation for Migration (IOM). (2020). *IOM definition of "migrant".* https://www.iom.int/who-is-a-migrant

Kafula, S. C. (2016). The role of social work in peace, human rights, and development in Africa. *Journal of Education and Social Policy, 3*(5), 115–121.

Kavuro, C. (2015). Refugees and asylum seekers: Barriers to accessing South Africa's labour market. *Law, Democracy & Development, 19*, 232–260.

Kavuro, C. (2020). *South Africa excludes refugees and asylum seeker from Covid-19 aid.* https://mg.co.za/coronavirus-essentials/2020-05-29-south-africa-refugees-coronavrus-exclude-law/

Li, S. S., Liddell, B. J., & Nickerson, A. (2016). The relationship between post-migration stress and psychological disorders in refugees and asylum seekers. *Current Psychiatry Reports, 18*, 82. https://doi.org/10.1007/s11920-016-0723-0

Mukumbang, F. C., Ambe, N. A., & Adebiyi, B. O. (2020). Unspoken inequality: How COVID-19 has exacerbated existing vulnerabilities of asylum-seekers, refugees, and undocumented migrants in South Africa. *International Journal for Equity in Health. 19*(141), 1–7.

Ndlovu, S. (2020). *Military vets shut down foreign-run shops in Durban city centre.* https://www.timeslive.co.za/news/south-africa/2020-11-02-military-vets-shut-down-foreign-run-shops-in-durban-city-centre/

Nikku, B. R. (2015). Living through and responding to disasters: Multiple roles for social work. *Social Work Education, 34*(6), 601–606. https://doi.org/10.1080/02615479.2015.1090942

Noyoo, N. (2018). Xenophobia and social welfare in South Africa. In L. Wagner, R. Lutz, C. Rehklau, & F. Ross (Eds.), *Hanbuch Internationale Soziale Arbeit: Dimensionen – Konflikte – Positionen* (pp. 145–158). Beltz, Juventus.

Noyoo, N. (2020). Decolonising social work practice and social work education in post-colonial Africa. In K. Kliebl, R. Lutz, N. Noyoo, B. Bunk, A. Dittmann, & B. Seepamore (Eds.), *The Routledge handbook of post-colonial social work* (pp. 261–268). Routledge.

Noyoo, N., & Kleibl, T. (2020). Introduction: Setting the scene for critical new social work approaches in the neoliberal postcolonial era. In K. Kliebl, R. Lutz, N. Noyoo, B. Bunk, A. Dittmann, & B. Seepamore (Eds.), *The Routledge handbook of post-colonial social work* (pp. 1–8). Routledge.

Noyoo, N., Matsea, T., & Dlamini, N. (2021). Promoting healthy human relationships with sub-Saharan African immigrants in South Africa. In N. Noyoo (Ed.), *Promoting healthy human relationships in post-apartheid South Africa: Social work and social development perspectives* (pp. 67–82). Springer.

OECD. (2020). *OECD employment outlook 2020: Worker security and the COVID-19 crisis*. OECD Publishing. https://doi.org/10.1787/1686c758-en

Reichert, E. (2011). *Social work and human rights: A foundation for policy and practice* (2nd ed.). Columbia University.

Republic of South Africa (RSA). (2021). *COVID-19 corona virus South African resource portal*. https://sacoronavirus.co.za/

Roestenburg, W. (2013). A social work practice perspective on migration. *Social Work/Maatskaplike Werk, 49*(1), 1–21.

South African Broadcasting Corporation (SABC). (2020). *Close to 1,800 people have committed suicide since lockdown started: Mkhize*. https://www.sabcnews.com/sabcnews/close-to-1-800-people-have-committed-suicide-since-lockdown-started-mkhize/

South African Council for Social Service Professions (SACSSP). (2020). *The Bulletin*. https://www.sacssp.co.za/2020/SACSSP%20MONTHLY%20eBULLETIN%20NOVEMBER%202020.pdf

Statistics South Africa (StatsSA). (2020). *Mobility and migration in South Africa during the COVID-19 lockdown*. StatsSA.

Strauss, I., Isaacs, G., Rosenberg, J., & Passoni, P. (2020). *Rapid country assessment: South Africa – The impacts of COVID-19 shock to South Africa's economy and labour market*. ILO Publications.

The World Bank. (2018). *Overcoming poverty and inequality in South Africa: An assessment of drivers, constraints and opportunities*. The World Bank.

Trilsch, M. (2009). What's the use of socio-economic rights in a constitution? Taking a look at the South African experience. *Law and Politics in Africa, Asia and Latin America, 42*(4), 552–575.

Twikirize, J. M., & Spitzer, H. (2019). *Preface. Social work practice in Africa: Indigenous and innovative approaches* (pp. xiii–xiv). Kampala.

United Nations (2020). *Refugees and migrants*. https://refugeesmigrants.un.org/definitions

United Nations High Commission for Refugees (UNHCR). (2020). *Global trends 2012: Displacement: The new 21st century challenge*. United Nations High Commission for Refugees.

Walsh, F. (2016). Family resilience: A developmental systems framework. *European Journal of Developmental Psychology, 13*, 313–324.

Zanker, F. L., & Moyo, K. (2020). The corona virus and migration governance in South Africa: Business as usual? *Africa Spectrum, 55*, 1–13. https://doi.org/10.1177/0002039720925826

Impacts of the COVID-19 Pandemic on International Migration in Brazil: Normative, Economic, and Social Issues

14

Eveline Vieira Brigido,
Roberto Rodolfo Georg Uebel,
and Vítor Eduardo Alessandri Ribeiro

14.1 Introduction

The COVID-19 pandemic hit Brazil dramatically, albeit in delay in comparison to other countries in the world. Declared by the World Health Organization (WHO) on 11 March, the pandemic caused the first death in Brazil on 17 March.

By the middle of April 2021, according to official WHO numbers, the country ranked second worldwide in number of cases and second in number of deaths.[1] Amidst the current-day public health crisis, there has been a significant influx of migrants to Brazil, resulting from a process of immigration shift set forth by the political agenda of the past decade in Brazil.

Currently there are about 2.1 million immigrants, most significantly Venezuelans, but also from other Latin American, Caribbean, and African countries (Brigido et al., 2020). In this scenario, the objective of this chapter is to analyse knowledgeable impacts for immigrants in Brazil during the COVID-19 pandemic, taking the case of Venezuelan immigrants and refugees into special account for being the largest and greatly vulnerable group.

In this sense, the chapter is divided into four sections, in addition to this Introduction and the Final Remarks. The first section is dedicated to normative analysis, that is, a summary of the recent Brazilian immigration legislation, the executive and administrative orders related to COVID-19 in the field of human mobility and border control, as well as their impacts on the migration flows of Venezuelans towards Brazil.

The second section is dedicated to the economic analysis of the impacts of the pandemic on the flow of Venezuelans and on the economic situation in Brazil, a country that was mightily impacted, leaving traces of high indexes of unemployment, decreased income and purchasing power, as well as inflation and the country's economic slowdown. The socioeconomic impacts of the Emergency Aid benefit granted to immigrants are also analysed.

The third section focuses on the social analysis of the Venezuelan immigration issue during the pandemic, with an emphasis on episodes of xenophobic discourses and sentiments exacerbated by the hosting society in Brazil, using the instruments and lenses of social networks.

Finally, the fourth section considers the perspectives for migrations to Brazil in the post-pandemic context, which, even though the country is facing a second wave of COVID-19,

[1]According to data compiled daily by the Coronavirus Resource Center at Johns Hopkins University. Available at: https://coronavirus.jhu.edu/map.html. Accessed on 10 Apr. 2021.

E. V. Brigido · R. R. G. Uebel (✉) · V. E. A. Ribeiro
Escola Superior de Propaganda e Marketing,
Porto Alegre, RS, Brazil
e-mail: roberto.uebel@espm.br

M. C. S. Gonçalves et al. (eds.), *The Coronavirus Crisis and Challenges to Social Development*,
https://doi.org/10.1007/978-3-030-84678-7_14

has the prospect of ending with the provision of vaccines during the year 2021.[2] In this sense, we also discuss in this section the issue of the right of access to health, especially vaccines, by immigrants.

The research is based on qualitative and quantitative analysis, taking on bibliographic references and analysis of legislation over immigration, official statistical data, and large data harvested online.

The aim is to provide a critical view of the economic and social impacts on immigrants resulting from measures adopted by local governments in Brazil during the pandemic.

14.2 Normative Analysis

The pandemic brought several issues to be further regulated with respect to the rights of migrants. In fact, Brazil has quite advanced legislation in terms of migration. The new Migration Law, n. 13,445/17 (Presidência da República, 2017), is based on the protection of human rights, repudiation of any form of discrimination, non-criminalisation of migration, humanitarian reception, and social and labor inclusion of migrants, encompassing the aforementioned points and other rights. Compared with existing international legal framework on migration, it is possible to say that Brazilian legislation is quite advanced in terms of guarantees and foresaw the forms of protection needed.

However, Brazil's current situation in terms of the actual governance of those migration policies has taken a turn otherwise. In 2019, the Ministry of Justice established ordinances facilitating the obtaining of temporary residence in Brazil for Venezuelan, Cuban, Senegalese, Haitian, and Dominican immigrants. However, if they choose temporary residence, they must give up the asylum application. In other words, forced migrants would become economic migrants and could be deported if they do not comply with the requirements set by the Law. Furthermore, Brazil also declared that it would no longer engage or participate in the Global Migration Pact adopted in December 2018.

Therefore, even though Brazilian law is adequate to international humanitarian principles and the main documents related to refugees, the current government's migration policies are moving in the opposite direction. Unfortunately, this weakens the protection of migrants in the Brazilian territory.

These changes in Brazilian migratory governance at the federal level, which set the pace after the inauguration of the Mr. Bolsonaro's presidency in 2019, indicate a tendency to place certain hindrances in relationship to the actual governance in the cause of immigrants, precisely at a time when South America is experiencing its worst migration crisis because of the conflicts in Venezuela. These otherwise uncanny ways of establishing predicaments, so that one edict trespasses the possibility of the maintenance of other guarantees lawfully established to the migrants, make the situation unjustifiably exasperating for them, specially at moments when diffuse xenophobic feelings are increasing amongst certain groups in Brazilian society (Brigido et al., 2020).

With the beginning of the COVID-19 pandemic in early 2020, the situation of such immigrants tended to worsen in Brazil. Beyond the vulnerability in terms of bodily health, there are also stresses related to the immigrants economic and social life (Fernandes & Baeninger, 2020).

In principle, immigrants enjoy a great deal of protection under Brazilian law. Although the Brazilian government has declared that it would not participate in the global pact, Brazil displays a quite advanced legislation providing for many rights guaranteed under Human Rights Treaties. Therefore, in relationship to the pandemic, all basic rights should be guaranteed to immigrants (voluntary, forced, regular, or irregular).

These rights include the right to health. In other words, all migrants who are in Brazilian

[2] Since the second week of January, Brazil has vaccinated around 22.6 million people with the doses of vaccines produced by the Butantan Institute in partnership with the Chinese laboratory Sinovac and produced by the Oswaldo Cruz Foundation, whose vaccines are produced in partnership with the laboratory AstraZeneca and Oxford University. State governors have signed agreements to acquire Sputnik V vaccines from Russia and from the Pfizer laboratory.

territory would have the right to full access of adequate health treatment. In case migrants have been infected with the coronavirus, there are not any forms of restrictions to the right of migrants to the vaccine (see Sect. 14.5).

Although the right to timely treatment must also be guaranteed to undocumented migrants who find themselves in an irregular situation facing the State (Inter-American Court of Human Rights, 2012), there is the risk that those people may refrain from seeking help if misinformed.

In addition to the public health issue, there is evidence that the pandemic has hit immigrants with relationship to their economic means (Fernandes & Baeninger, 2020). To assist the low-income population, the Brazilian government (as well as several other governments) created an emergency support program and included immigrants in this program. "But the problem is irregular immigrants; because they have irregular status, and are undocumented, they find it more difficult to access social welfare benefits" (Brigido et al., 2020; Brigido & Zibetti, 2020, p. 759). Also, the government is not aware of these people, and they are unlikely to come forward to ask for help because they fear deportation or expulsion. Therefore, there are many immigrants in a precarious situation in Brazil that is strongly aggravated by the pandemic.

It is important to mention that the Interamerican Court of Human Rights, in the Declaration of April 9, 2020, points out that economic and social rights must be guaranteed to all persons who are under the jurisdiction of the State. It also notes that because of the need for social isolation, and the impact it generates on personal and family finances, the State must seek ways to provide food, medicines, and other necessities to those people who cannot afford them. Unfortunately, however, the emergency assistance program in Brazil covers only those registered.

In summary, although migrants usually find themselves to be in vulnerable situations in one way or another, those in an irregular documentation situation are more likely to be negatively affected by all the pernicious aspects of the COVID-19 pandemic. "The government should create a program to regularise irregular migrants through the institute of refuge, humanitarian visa or other legal protection." (Brigido & Zibetti, 2020, p. 770). The problem must be faced daily.

In addition to the problems faced by immigrants who are already in Brazilian territory, there is another one: the difficulty faced by those who wish to apply for asylum in Brazil or another form of humanitarian protection.

Like many countries, Brazil also imposed restrictions on the movement of people, especially foreigners. Throughout the year 2020 and at the beginning of 2021, several ordinances were created by the government. At various times, the Brazilian government has restricted the entry of foreigners, mainly by road (or other land means) or by water transport (Brazil, 2021).

Nevertheless, the government has stipulated some exceptions to entry restrictions, not preventing, for example (Brazil, 2021):

(a) Traffic of border residents.
(b) Entry of immigrants with permanent residence.
(c) Entry of immigrants who have family in Brazil (family reunification).
(d) Entry of immigrants who have a National Migration Registration Card.

However, the exceptions do not apply to people from Venezuela. It is clear that the Brazilian government is discriminating against Venezuelans (who are currently facing the second largest migratory crisis).

The only possibility for Venezuelans to enter Brazil would be by air, but all the impediments imposed by the Brazilian government show their unwillingness to receive them. In addition, the main migratory routes are land and sea; that is, allowing only air routes brings even more difficulties.

Finally, it should be noted that based on international documents and the position of the Inter-American Court of Human Rights, migrants arriving at the borders (including land and sea) of countries and requesting refuge must be received, under penalty of violation of the non-refoulement principle. Thus, we understand that the Brazilian Ordinances, by discriminating against

Venezuelans, violate the aforementioned principle. In fact, Brazil could be denounced to the Inter-American Commission on Human Rights and possibly be tried by the Inter-American Court.

14.3 Economic Analysis

The impacts of the COVID-19 pandemic on the socioeconomic arena were observed in the most diverse aspects and segments of society, from large transnational corporations to small family businesses. The sectors of tourism, international logistics, and services were the most affected, because national borders were closed overnight and human mobility was interrupted as measures to physically contain the circulation and transmission of the virus were applied.

Immigrants and asylum seekers were doubly impacted, if we look at it from a sociological and economic perspective, as most of them had their flows and journeys interrupted. According to Sayad (1998), they are, historically, the first groups to suffer from unemployment,[3] social exclusion, and the interruption of economic and social assistance by governments in a scenario of crises and public calamity, such as the one brought by the pandemic.

If, in ordinary times, international migrants already found it difficult to obtain social benefits guaranteed by the hosting and receiving States, as well as facing challenges in accessing governmental assistance and in the implementation of public policies to these groups, the COVID-19 pandemic worsened these conditions, especially in the case of Brazil, which we analyse in this section.

At the end of March 2020, weeks after the WHO's formal declaration of the pandemic, the National Congress of Brazil started to process and discuss the granting of a benefit called "Emergency Aid" in the amount of R$ 600 (about US$ 113 in December 2020 prices) for the population who were unemployed or whose income was interrupted by social isolation and lockdown measures, especially the informal workers.

The benefit, which could be doubled only for single mothers, would also extend to regular immigrants in Brazil as well as to asylum seekers, as in the case of Venezuelans who were mainly concentrated in the state of Roraima, in the northern region of Brazil, bordering to Venezuela and Guyana.

Moreover, the granting and effectiveness of the financial benefit was delayed by the Federal Government and by the bureaucracies required by the intermediary bank, Caixa Econômica Federal (CEF), which prevented many migrants from actually receiving the amount of R$ 600, which would be paid, initially, for only 3 months and which was were extended until December 2020, with no prospect of renewal for the upcoming year despite the lagging effects of the pandemic in Brazil.

In the specific case of immigrants, the nonpossession of documents served as an aggravating factor, because under the authority of the CEF ordination, in the absence of personal documentation they could not open a bank account, nor prove their employment status, and thus did not qualify for financial assistance, resulting apart from that emergency economic relief. This issue made it impossible for thousands of Venezuelans to have access to government assistance and accentuated their situation of social vulnerability in Brazil, which led to the return of many to Venezuela.[4]

[3]On December 1, 2020, the Brazilian Institute of Geography and Statistics released updated data on unemployment in Brazil. In October 2020, the unemployed population was 13.763 million, while the unemployment rate was 14.1%, the highest in the historical series. Available at: https://www.em.com.br/app/noticia/economia/2020/12/01/internas_economia,1216258/taxa-de-desemprego-no-brasil-bate-novo-recorde-na-pandemia.shtml. Accessed on 01 Dec. 2020.

[4]According to projections by the Colombian government, ECLAC and Human Rights Watch, between 100,000 and 130,000 Venezuelans have returned to Venezuela due to the pandemic. Available at: https://exame.com/mundo/pandemia-provoca-retorno-de-100-mil-venezuelanos-ao-pais/ and https://webcache.googleusercontent.com/search?q=cache:3auM-f95dMQJ:https://www.jornaldocomercio.com/_conteudo/internacional/2020/10/760995-

Despite these issues, until October 2020, approximately 149,000 immigrants received the benefit, totaling about R$ 715 million (US $ 138.5 million in prices of December 2020), corresponding to 0.32% of the total available resources. According to Caixa Econômica Federal,[5] the main groups of immigrants that received the financial assistance were Venezuelans, followed by Haitians, Bolivians, and other Latin American, Caribbean, and African migrants.

Another point to be highlighted refers to the impacts on the economic and labor activities of immigrants in Brazil, because many had to interrupt their businesses, especially those dependent on informal and street commerce, and on the foodstuffs as well; for the most part, they did not receive any form of compensation from the Brazilian Federal Government.

It was not uncommon to see immigrants who worked as apps drivers, confectioners, street vendors, general service workers, and small business owners whose income was compromised because of the pandemic in Brazil and had to borrow money from friends, family, and members of their own migratory network.

This situation had a significant impact on international remittances, not only from Venezuelans, but significantly from two other groups, such as Haitians and Senegalese, who sent part of their monthly income to their families in their home countries. After all, it would also have an impact on the tax revenue itself arising from the taxes charged in each international transfer, reflected in the public accounts.

It is worth noting that this set of issues such as the interruption of flows with the border closures, the suspension of employment contracts, the interruption of economic activities, the reduction of financial remittances, and the difficulty of accessing the Emergency Aid benefit triggered a situation of almost social anomie towards immigrants, already in a situation of vulnerability from the xenophobia that emerged with the pandemic, an aspect analysed in the next section.

14.4 Social Analysis

Immigrants and refugees are not vulnerable people by definition but are rather people who are caught in vulnerable situations for whatever reason. Therefore, the proper access to social rights in the receiving country is a must for the migrants to form social bonds and gain adequate conditions to establish themselves and prosper under the new circumstances.

Recent normative advancements are not mirrored in Brazil by substantive measures that could yield incentives towards building material capacity, training human resources, or endowing adequate budgets to face exigencies given by the reception of international migrants. In the current pandemic of COVID-19, the public health crisis sets a deeper note to that tone. There is no such a thing in Brazil as a unified national office for the governance of migration, which not only contributes to the lack of synergy between multiple instances from various levels of government agencies, but also casts shadows on the matters related to the conditions of reception of foreign migration into Brazil.

With regard to the treatment of Venezuelan immigrants in Brazil, the federal government has come together in 2018 with International Organizations and NGOs in an ad hoc operation named Operação Acolhida (Welcome Operation).[6] This humanitarian operation takes on concerted efforts from multiple government agencies (from 11 ministries), military personnel, professionals from the civil society in cooperation with the United Nations High Commissioner for Refugees (UNHCR), the International Organization for Migration (IOM), and the United Nations

movidos-pela-crise-do-coronavirus-venezuelanos-sofrem-abusos-ao-voltar-a-pais.html+&cd=1&hl=pt-BR&ct=clnk&gl=br. Accessed on 10 Apr. 2021.

[5] More data and information regarding the financial assistance to migrants in Brazil during the pandemic are available here: https://www.sbtnews.com.br/noticia/governo/150705-quase-150-mil-estrangeiros-receberam-auxilio-emergencial. Accessed on 11 Jun. 2021.

[6] For further details on the Operation, see https://www.gov.br/acolhida/. Last accessed on 30 Jan. 2021.

Population Fund (UNFPA): it is organised around three main axes, namely (1) the orderly management of cross-borders movements; (2) providing for shelter, food, and healthcare; and (3) encouraging voluntary interiorisation and providing assistance for socioeconomic inclusion to migrants.

From 2018 until the end of December 2020,[7] the operation has sought to benefit 46,500[8] Venezuelans who voluntarily chose to remain in Brazil and opted into the program of interiorisation to more than 600 cities in Brazil. From the total of Venezuelans benefited by the operation, 19,300 of them correspond to the numbers in the year 2020, which denotes that the effort has been continued all through the year of 2020, despite the COVID-19 pandemic in Brazil.

The Welcome Operation's work resonates with our discussion, as it allowed the application of social work, albeit on an agenda dominated by security and defense dimensions, that is, militarised, towards Venezuelan immigrants and refugees, especially during the pandemic. Logistical operations, such as moving patients to the capital of Roraima, Boa Vista, and other cities in Brazil, were essential to prevent the collapse of the health system and for immigrants not to be left without the proper care.

Not only the work of military physicians and nurses from Welcome Operation is noteworthy, but mainly that of social workers, psychologists, and civil society volunteers. The traumas of forced migration have been duplicated with those of the pandemic. In other words, the challenges for the reception and integration of immigrants in times of pandemic have multiplied, largely because of social distancing, a sanitary measure necessary to contain the circulation of the new coronavirus, however, which represented the seclusion and direct person-to-person reception of Venezuelans.

The social work carried out by the operation also directly impacts Venezuelans' access to essential services in addition to healthcare, such as education, housing, and, especially, feeding. In a context of 19 million people in a situation of hunger in Brazil (Gaglioni, 2021), this welcoming process was necessary so that a generalised humanitarian crisis among migrants would not happen during the pandemic, which was lessened, also to some extent, by the Emergency Aid that we analysed in previous sections.

The main question that remains is the extent to which the militarisation of the migration issue in Brazil impacts social work and the humanisation of the reception and welcoming of migrants and refugees, as the security agenda tends to remain. This question will remain open until the end of the pandemic, at least.

Those facts show a commitment from both state and international organizations, and entities from civil society. However, immigrants are not free from suffering different forms of vicissitudes. As Brigido et al. show (2020), even before the moment when COVID-19 hit Brazil, a diffuse sentiment of xenophobic feelings towards Venezuelans was gaining momentum in Brazil, which has been evidenced by means of the analysis of the Portuguese text corpus extracted computationally from 2404 *tweets* posted by the users of the *Twitter* social network platform within the period starting 1 January 2016 until 29 February 2020. The text corpus extraction attained to query search "out Venezuelans" (in Portuguese, "fora venezuelanos") and only those which applied to this condition entered the analysis. The total corpus of empirical evidence harvested from the social network platform was processed using unsupervised machine learning algorithms, mainly by means of use of the word embedding technique from the "word2vec" library available for Python programming language developed in 2013 (Mikolov et al., 2013).

[7]By January 19, 2021, the International Organization for Migration (IOM) has contributed providing air tickets for 10,000 people who adhered to the program. See: https://brazil.iom.int/news/em-apoio-direto-%C3%A0-opera%C3%A7%C3%A3o-acolhida-oim-chega-10-mil-passagens-fornecidas-para-interioriza%C3%A7%C3%A3o. Accessed on 21 Jan. 2021.

[8]Up until January 15, 2021, more than 600 cities across Brazil had received Venezuelan immigrants. See: https://www.gov.br/acolhida/noticias/acolhida-realizou-a-interiorizacao-de-mais-de-19-mil-venezuelanos-em-2020/. Accessed on 19 Jan. 2021.

Based on the lexicon of words posted by *Twitter* users within their own tweets captured by the authors, it was possible, by using techniques of natural language processing and by visualising word correspondence through corpus lexicon dispersion plotting (Brigido et al., 2020, pp. 13–24), to note an overall noticeable difference exists between, on one hand, those opinions that make explicit reference to words such as "dwelling," "safety," "health," and "employment" (which sheds light on the concerns over material aspects of real people's life), and, on the other hand, those opinions which make explicit reference to words such as "liberty," "security," "disease," and "criminality." It is possible to catch sight of the difference between these two groups of ideas when the mutual correspondence between them has been made explicit: where the textual contexts contained words such as "liberty" and "safety," there were not frequent occurrences of words such as "dwelling," "health," "employment," or others related to concerns with those material aspects of real life and protection of the immigrant. Therefore, a dual typology has been suggested as means of contrasting the contexts of discriminatory and xenophobic discourse against the context of more conciliatory and immigrant-prone discourse (idem). The evidence collected from the text of those *tweets* referring to the discriminatory verve made clear the xenophobic intent, since Venezuelans are taken as "carriers of diseases" that are considered as "been eradicated in Brazil" by the users of the social network platform. Other mentions express the "wish that Venezuelans recover their sense of shame and go claim their rights in their own country." There are many occurrences of such derogatory nature throughout the corpus. Some other manifest opinions depict Venezuelan migrants as scapegoats for the hurdles lived by Brazilian nationals; opinions that seek to justifying the scarcity of resources to nationals by conflating this scarcity with the benefits lawfully granted to immigrants. All the users in the extraction have been anonymised.

These thoughts, captured from the text corpus analysed, evidenced sentiments of xenophobia, manifested through derogatory language, and displayed by either oblique or direct attitudes against immigrants.

14.5 Perspectives

In December 2020, the British government announced[9] what would become the first authorisation for vaccination against COVID-19 in the world. In the same week, the Brazilian government announced its National Immunization Plan for the disease,[10] divided into four priority groups, with four corresponding stages, which began in the second week of January 2021.

Although all the perspectives of epidemiologists and from the WHO signal that the pandemic will end in 2021 or early 2022, its end will be gradual and unequally distributed in the International System; the first countries to vaccinate will be those with more resources, especially in the Global North, such as the United Kingdom, the United States, and Germany, and the last ones will be those in the Global South, such as African, Latin American, and Asian countries (with the exception of China, Taiwan, Japan, and South Korea). In other words, an international division of the vaccine, in which global inequalities and asymmetries once again emerge (Wallerstein, 2004).

From this context, three main questions are raised in the case analysed in this chapter: (a) when Brazil will start immunising its population in general; (b) whether immigrants and foreigners will have the right to be vaccinated in the Brazilian territory through the Unified Health System (SUS); and (c) the extent of the economic, social, political, and health impacts of the pandemic on immigrant life and on the transnational migration flows as well, which allow us to

[9] "Covid-19: Pfizer/BioNTech vaccine judged safe for use in UK from next week." Available at: https://www.bbc.com/news/health-55145696. Accessed on 02 Dec 2020.

[10] "Vacinação contra a Covid vai começar com profissionais de saúde, maiores de 75 anos e indígenas." Available at: https://www1.folha.uol.com.br/equilibrioesaude/2020/12/vacinacao-contra-a-covid-19-vai-comecar-com-profissionais-de-saude-idosos-e-indigenas.shtml. Accessed on 02 Dec 2020.

question if the pandemic will impose more restrictions on the admission of migrants and foreigners in the next months with the current application of vaccines.

These questions allow us to point out some perspectives for the post-pandemic scenario in the migration field and to consider the most relevant aspects of this context at the scale's level (Rückert & Rambo, 2010); as we discussed in the previous sections, both the spread of the new coronavirus and the impacts of the pandemic occurred in a scaled and networked way.

Regarding this scenario, about the beginning of the immunisation of the general population in Brazil, on December 1, 2020, the Ministry of Health released a plan divided into four phases, with their respective priority groups, which include the elderly, health professionals, persons deprived of liberty, teachers, and public security professionals. In this first plan, which should be applied in the first quarter of 2021, the general population was not included, given the availability of vaccines purchased by the Federal Government and subnational entities, such as the Butantan Institute, and the interest in immunising the entire population of 210 million inhabitants.

In this context, immigrants, and foreigners in general, would be supported by SUS and would therefore have the right to be vaccinated against Covid-19, if they were within the priority groups. The question that arises is that the Brazilian Vaccination Plan is silent on this point. Under the Brazilian Federal Constitution and the Inter-American Human Rights System, the right to health must be guaranteed to all, without distinction. In fact, the Brazilian Plan classifies refugees as a vulnerable group, equating them with people living on the streets. However, by explicitly defining the four priority groups, it does not include them. We understand, however, that the objective contemplated in the document is to equate refugees with the population living on the streets and, therefore, would they be included in group 1.

Regarding the other immigrants, if they are regularised and are within the priority groups, we believe that they also will be vaccinated. The most preoccupying issue is with irregular migrants, as they are not supposed to exist for the government. The ideal, therefore, would be the creation of a plan to regularise immigrants, to guarantee not only the right to health, but also emergency aid. In addition, it would also help to control the circulation of the coronavirus. After all, if immigrants do not have their rights guaranteed, they will become a risk to the whole society, as they live in precarious conditions, susceptible to being contaminated and, therefore, to spread the virus.

Despite the daily update of the number of confirmed cases and deaths by COVID-19 in Brazil by the Ministry of Health, this information is not disaggregated by nationality, which makes it difficult to establish a parameter for the number of immigrants who contracted the disease. It would be important to create a confidentiality system for identifying nationalities in hospitals and health posts, to monitor who and how many immigrants are (especially irregular ones). Confidentiality must be mandatory and guarded from any form of abuse so that the focus is on obtaining and keeping track of data and never conceding a way for the State to divert.

One of the only states to report these data is Rio Grande do Sul, whose last update, on April 10, 2021, indicated 16,106 confirmed cases of the disease in immigrants, which corresponded to 1.82% of the total contaminated population, a number slightly less than that of health professionals (3.39%) and higher than that of the population deprived of liberty (0.13%), which leads us to question whether they are also not priority groups for immunisation.[11]

As the universal coverage of SUS without discriminating because of the person's nationality, unlike the health systems of most countries, these populations had free access to exams and treatments against COVID-19, so, observing the normative aspects, there were no restrictions to receive the vaccine in the doses recommended by the Ministry of Health.

[11] According to data compiled daily by the Secretary of Health of the State of Rio Grande do Sul. Available at: https://ti.saude.rs.gov.br/covid19/. Accessed on 10 Apr. 2021.

The third aspect, which points to the most important perspective in the socioeconomic field, refers to the extent of the impacts of the pandemic on the *modus economicus* and on the labor life of immigrants in Brazil, who were the ones who suffered most from the measures of social distance and lockdown, mainly because they work in the economic sectors most impacted and vulnerable to these public norms, mainly decreed by mayors and state governors.

With the non-renewal of the Emergency Aid benefit[12] at sight and with the lack of credible signs that the overall economic indicators, such as unemployment rate, shall resume and recover to pre-pandemic levels, measures to mitigate financial losses of immigrants are one of the most important points to be observed.

The decrease in international remittances and the reiterated interruptions to migration flows since March 2020, with the closure of national borders, accentuated the hardships in this context. In the case of Brazil, future perspectives point to a gradual reopening of land and air borders for foreign residents and nonresidents, as well as to an increase, albeit slow, of remittances to their countries of origin in 2021. Some digital banking tools, such as the instant payment system implemented by the Central Bank of Brazil, called PIX,[13] in service since November 2020, allowed immigrants to circulate money in a more dynamic and less bureaucratic way, also because of fewer requirements for immigrants to open bank accounts.

Despite these issues, we emphasise the maintenance of episodes and the sentiments of xenophobia in the corpus of Brazilian society, with potential to deepen during tumultuous times of the COVID-19 pandemic. This challenge facing the preservation of social rights to migrants, which is certainly not a new phenomenon, nor an exclusive phenomenon relating to the pandemic, ultimately indicates the need for people's engagement in more comprehensive considerations on the dilemmas affecting migrants. Only upon agreeing to a profound reflection may the civil society and state authorities become able to surpass the hurdles to the processes of integration of migrants and come to the realization that it is not enough to be a receiving country, but also a hosting and welcoming country.

14.6 Final Remarks

We conclude the writing of this chapter in January 2021, at a moment when the COVID-19 pandemic in Brazil and all over the world has taken a turn for the worst in terms of the emergence of new strains of the virus, albeit the great efforts being made internationally for widespread vaccination. Whereas countries of the Global North, such as the United Kingdom, the United States, Germany, and Italy started introducing mass immunisation campaigns throughout the society, countries of the Global South, amongst which are Brazil, Mexico, and India, are struggling with challenges to implement vaccination campaigns while also facing peaks of new rises in contamination and deaths as the second wave of contamination sets in.

This duality of perspectives signals to something that deserves our attention, that is, this pandemic comprehends a certain form of discriminatory setting. It is aggravated by elements such as socioeconomic inequalities, access to primary care in health centers and hospitals, to the ultimate access to the vaccine. This paradox also finds resonance in groups of transnational migrants, especially those most vulnerable, such as asylum seekers.

In the case of Brazil, as discussed throughout this chapter, to face the difficulties imposed by vulnerable conditions to groups of transnational migrants—special attention to the case of Venezuelans more recently in Brazil—political,

[12] "Guedes diz que auxílio emergencial não será prorrogado e acaba em dezembro." Available at: https://jovempan.com.br/noticias/economia/guedes-diz-que-auxilio-emergencial-nao-sera-prorrogado-e-acaba-em-dezembro.html. Accessed on 02 Dec. 2020.

[13] "Pix começa a funcionar nesta segunda-feira; entenda quais as funcionalidades disponíveis". Available at: https://www1.folha.uol.com.br/mercado/2020/11/pix-comeca-a-funcionar-nesta-segunda-feira-entenda-quais-as-funcionalidades-disponiveis.shtml. Accessed on 02 Dec. 2020.

economic, and social challenges should be overcome.

Regarding economic aspects, it is possible to identify harsh impacts on migrants means and resources for subsistence (Fernandes & Baeninger, 2020) which certainly includes concerns with abrupt impacts the pandemic produced in the labor market. Further aggravating these difficulties are the provision of access to health and treatment.

Thus, these final remarks include a critical reflection on the role of the Brazilian State and its national and subnational governments in the management of migration flows and, mainly, in mitigating the effects of the pandemic. It was clear that state governments and local governments assumed responsibilities that belonged to the Federal Government in providing social, health, economic, and administrative assistance to immigrants and asylum seekers.

In addition, another aspect to be considered because of the pandemic is the increase in xenophobic tensions and the expression of anti-immigration, anti-globalization, and anti-vaccine sentiments within Brazilian society, also as a reflection of political inaction by the federal authorities.

In summary, it is possible to conclude that the COVID-19 pandemic has given cause to a worsening of vulnerable situations for international migrants in Brazil. Authorities shall remain cautious and wary of the possibilities in deteriorated scenarios that may risk giving cause for xenophobic violence aimed at immigrants and refugees. The outlook for the migration social issue in post-pandemic Brazil presents a surmounting challenge encompassing the political, economic, and social spheres, and will certainly demand the types of care from humanitarian leadership. Only the broadening of this debate may serve to raise further awareness throughout society.

References

Brazil. Presidência da República. *Lei n° 13.445, de 24 de maio de* 2017. http://www.planalto.gov.br/ccivil_03/_ato2015-2018/2017/lei/L13445.htm

Brazil. Presidência da República. *Portaria n° 652, de 25 de janeiro de* 2021. http://www.planalto.gov.br/CCIVIL_03/Portaria/PRT/Portaria-652-21-ccv.htm#:~:text=Portaria%2D652%2D21%2Dccv&text=Disp%C3%B5e%20sobre%20a%20restri%C3%A7%C3%A3o%20excepcional,Nacional%20de%20Vigil%C3%A2ncia%20Sanit%C3%A1ria%20%2D%20Anvisa

Brigido, E. V., Uebel, R. R. G., & Ribeiro, V. E. A. (2020). Evolução da governança migratória no Brasil desafios teóricos, mudanças normativas e ecos sociais de sentimentos xenofóbicos. *Idéias, 11*, 1–30. https://doi.org/10.20396/ideias.v11i0.8658545

Brigido, E. V., & Zibetti, F. W. (2020). Protection of forced migrants with irregular status during the pandemic generated by Covid-19, an analysis of the Inter-American Court of Human Rights on migrants rights. *Novos Estudos Jurídicos, 25*, 757–773. https://doi.org/10.14210/nej.v25n3

Fernandes, D., & Baeninger, R. (Eds.). (2020). *Impactos da pandemia de Covid-19 nas migrações internacionais no Brasil - Resultados de Pesquisa / Duval Fernandes*. Campinas, SP.

Gaglioni, C. (2021). A fome que atinge 19 milhões de brasileiros na pandemia. *Nexo Jornal*. https://www.nexojornal.com.br/expresso/2021/04/06/A-fome-que-atinge-19-milh%C3%B5es-de-brasileiros-na-pandemia

Inter-American Court of Human Rights. (2012). *Case of Nadege Dorzema et al. v. Dominican Republic*. 24 out. 2012. https://www.corteidh.or.cr/docs/casos/articulos/seriec_251_ing.pdf

Inter-American Court of Human Rights. (2020). *Covid-19 and human rights: the problems and challenges must be addressed from a human rights perspective and with respect for international obligations*. 09 abr. 2020. http://www.corteidh.or.cr/docs/comunicados/cp_27_2020_eng.pdf

Mikolov, T., et al. (2013). Distributed representations of words and phrases and their compositionality. In *International Conference on Neural Information Processing Systems, 26, 2013. Sydney. NIPS' 13: Proceedings of the 26th International Conference on Neural Information Processing Systems* (Vol. 2, pp. 3111–3119). Curran Associates Inc.. https://dl.acm.org/doi/10.5555/2999792.2999959

Rückert, A. A., & Rambo, A. G. (2010). Metodologia das escalas geográficas de poder e gestão aplicada à análise de desenvolvimento em quatro territórios rurais no Brasil. *Confins, 8*. https://doi.org/10.4000/confins.6370

Sayad, A. (1998). *A Imigração: Ou os Paradoxos da Alteridade*. Edusp.

Wallerstein, I. (2004). *World-systems analysis: An introduction*. Duke University Press.

15 From the Absence of Public Policies to a State of Emergency: The COVID-19 Pandemic and the Migrant Subject Condition

Giuliana Redin
and Maria do Carmo dos Santos Gonçalves

15.1 Introduction

The 2020 COVID-19 pandemic has exposed social economic structures based on social inequality, as well as the importance of public social security policies. In this context, the social group of migrants and refugees, already vulnerable by their nonnational status, which tends to imply greater difficulty in accessing rights and precarious social and labor conditions, suffers, in an aggravated way, from the consequences of the absence of public policies for migrants in the country. This study presents the empirical research carried out from 13 May to 8 June, 2020,[1] which included, through a structured interview answered by Google form, 42 civil society organizations[2] working to assist the migrant population in the state of Rio Grande do Sul, Brazil. The period corresponds to the 3 months that followed the beginning of the social distance measures resulting from the pandemic in Brazil. The organizations interviewed are linked to the following sectors of civil society: 24 religious, 4 universities, 7 immigrant associations, 6 associations/collectives/volunteers, and 1 nongovernmental organization (Brazilian Red Cross). Of these organizations, of which more than half have operated throughout the state of Rio Grande do Sul, 85.7% develop social assistance actions, 66.7% citizenship and development, 66.7% social inclusion actions, such as Portuguese Language courses, 54.3% inclusion actions in the world of work, and 40.5% provide legal advice.

According to the survey, the Social Assistance Policy[3] is the main gateway for the immigrant and

G. Redin (✉)
Department of Law, Universidade Federal de Santa Maria - UFSM, Santa Maria, Brazil

MIGRAIDH, International Human Mobility and Human Rights, Santa Maria, Brazil
e-mail: giuliana.redin@ufsm.br

M. d. C. d. S. Gonçalves
Centro Scalabriniano de Estudos Migrató, Brasilia, Brasília, Brazil
e-mail: diretora@csem.org.br

[1]This research was an initiative of the Fórum Permanente de Mobilidade Humana do Rio Grande do Sul – FPMH/RS (Permanent Forum of Human Mobility of Rio Grande do Sul) to support demands addressed to the Public Power in the period of the pandemic and actions to face its impacts on the migrant and refugee population. The research was carried out by researchers Doctor Maria do Carmo Gonçalves, from the Centro Scalabriniano de Estudos Migratórios – CSEM/DF (Scalabrinian Center for Migratory Studies), Post-doctor Giuliana Redin, from MIGRAIDH/Sérgio Vieira de Mello Chair at UFSM and Doctor Patrícia Graziottin Nochang, from the Fórum de Mobilidade Humana de Passo Fundo – FMHPF (Passo Fundo Human Mobility Forum).

[2]See Appendix.

[3]The National Social Assistance Policy (PNAS) was approved in 2004 and presents the guidelines for the realization of social assistance as a right of citizenship and places it under the responsibility of the State to provide services to people in situations of vulnerability and social risk. It represents a major advance in the field of social

M. C. S. Gonçalves et al. (eds.), *The Coronavirus Crisis and Challenges to Social Development*,
https://doi.org/10.1007/978-3-030-84678-7_15

refugee population to other policies, such as Education, Health, and Work. Although this is a prerogative of this policy, it is also noted that, regarding care for the migrant and refugee population, the contribution of public resources still remains a major challenge. Within the scope of the *Sistema Único de Assistência Social* (SUAS)[4] (National Unified Social Assistance System), there are a series of recommendations on assistance to migrants and refugees, which are contained in the document prepared in 2016 by the Technical Chamber of Migrants, instituted within the scope of the Tripartite Intergovernmental Commission, but which were regulated at the government level.

In addition, the research pointed out that these organizations carry out their activities predominantly without public resources.[5] Likewise, it shows that the social assistance of the migrant and refugee population has been a great challenge for the State since civil society entities directly occupy the empty space of the State in the absence of a National Migration and Refugee Policy that provides the provision of specific services and programs for this portion of the population.

The humanitarian crisis resulting from the impacts on the daily lives of people already vulnerable by social and economic inequalities has generated a movement to mobilize different subjects and institutional actors. During this period, for example, immigrant associations, such as Haitians and Senegalese, mobilized to provide mutual assistance such as food. These actions were mapped by the research, which outlined priorities in a situation of emergency and action strategies of the institutions and organized groups, allowing us to point out the role of these actors in terms of seeking to expand rights, dialoguing directly with those already established demands for social rights in the field of social work in Brazil.

The current immigration to Brazil, which constitutes that of the population served by the organizations interviewed, is predominantly the result of migration for socioeconomic reasons (95.2%), followed by asylum seekers (47.6%) and refugees (45.2%), whose most present nationalities are Venezuelan, Haitian, and Senegalese. These are mostly populations known to have experienced social exclusion processes in their countries of origin, organizing their migratory project as a strategy to overcome the difficulties of social insertion and access to basic services, such as education, health and safety, and social mobility.

Based on the research, the present study, carried out in the context of the pandemic, analyzes the category of "subject of rights" incorporated in the Migration Law, through the theoretical dialogue on migration and foreignness, inspired by Sayad (1998), Said (2003), and Fanon (2020), its relationship with public policies and, paradoxically, their absence. In this context, the research allows us to understand the agency and the role of civil society in this emergency scenario, enhanced by the absence of public policies, as a space occupied by organizations with different performance profiles, the place they reserve for migrants as agents and its role in the discursive construction of this new subject of rights.

---

work by systematizing and placing under the responsibility of the State actions that were carried out in a fragmented and discontinued manner by governments and civil society. Its principles are the provision of territorialized, decentralized public services, inter-sectorial action with other social policies, social participation, and the right of access to anyone who needs these services due to their condition of vulnerability and social risk.

[4]The Unified Social Assistance System (SUAS) is a management model used in Brazil to operationalize the social assistance actions provided for in the National Social Assistance Policy. The system was regulated by the Organic Law on Social Assistance (federal law No. 8742, of December 7, 1993).

[5]Given the context of the pandemic (COVID-19), what is the risk level for the institution to have suspended resources or private funds (maintainers or companies) or donations linked to assistance? (question 12 of the form) Only 2, in a group of 42 organizations, responded that there was a high risk for the institution to have public resources suspended in the context of the pandemic, that is, the activities carried out by 95.2% of the organizations do not depend on or have public resources for their activities. For 19% the questioning was not applied, as they did not receive any type of public resource, and for 76.1% this risk was pointed out as none, low, or moderate, which means that their activities are not determined by the receipt of public resources.

15.2 The Migrant's "Subject of Rights" Condition

The research, when indicating the limits of articulation of existing public policies to cover the demands of a specific vulnerable population, such as that composed of immigrants and refugees served by civil society associations, takes us back to the process of building the subject as citizen in the Brazilian Constitution, which defines the Democratic Rule of Law. On the basis of the nonrecognition of the right of access of this population to Brazilian public policies is the paradox of the foreigner (Sayad, 1998) who is a subject without rights given his condition as a nonnational. This condition was dramatically strained in the context of the health crisis of COVID-19, including with regard to the way in which social workers welcomed or not these demands in the context of claims for rights for the vulnerable Brazilian population in general, that is, how the State and social organizations acted in the face of emergency security demands. This is an important fact, because social work in Brazil has been incorporated into historical struggles for the recognition of vulnerable populations as subjects of rights, as citizens. In the case of the migrant and refugee population, the new Law on Migration incorporated not only the accumulations of advances in guaranteeing human rights enhanced in the process of democratization in the country put in place with the 1988 Constitution, but also dialogues directly with the struggles for recognition of social rights as the translation of that. Proof of this is that many of the debates on assistance to migrants had as their dispute the access to assistance rights already established for Brazilians in SUAS. In this context, it is relevant to associate the processes triggered by the health crisis of COVID-19 with regard to social work in Brazil, with the new perspectives of reworking the paradigms that support the demands for social rights and public policies. In the debate on decolonial thinking, in which the migratory agenda finds support when integrating the demands of a new subject, that is, the subject of rights whose legitimacy as a subject of rights is no longer strictly based on his national belonging, but simply on his inalienable condition as a human person.

In 2017, the new Migration Law, Law 13.445, came into force in Brazil that completely revoked the Foreigner Statute of 1980, conceived still in the dictatorial period and which guided the State policy for migrations based on security and economic interests. The new legal paradigm, recognized during the struggle of civil society,[6] inverted this logic to insert human rights at the center of State policy for migration,[7] with the recognition of migrants as a subject of rights. An extraordinary advance from a society and its institutions structured in the exclusion of the other: the nonnational, but not only, "that other who does I not want to be", the one that translates all foreignness (Redin, 2020). And it is the foreignness, according to Redin (2020, p. 14), that "is directly linked to the theme of recognition as a subject, because the foreigner is the one who is not represented or representable, what one does not want to be, the one without name, without inscription in order, not recognized, is the lack."

The more the subject demands public security policies from the State, the more foreign he becomes, the more undesirable, more threatening, and less citizen, as it is a cost to the State.

---

[6]In 2014, the Brazilian Federal Government, through the Ministry of Justice, took the initiative to debate with civil society the direction of a new National Policy for Migration and Refuge. This process was triggered by the first National Conference on Migration and Refugee (Comigrar), as the last stage of other preparatory conferences, which had the direct participation of immigrants and refugees in Brazil. There were five axes of dialogue: (a) equal treatment and access to services and rights; (b) social, economic, and productive insertion; (c) cultural citizenship and recognition of diversity; (d) addressing rights violations and means of prevention and protection; (e) social and citizen participation, transparency and data (Brasil, 2014).

[7]The Article 3 of the Migration Law establishes a list of human rights principles and guidelines to govern "The Brazilian immigration policy," followed by Article 4, which establishes the content of fundamental rights for migrants (Brasil, 2017).

Thus, the State and its expression of national identity are associated with the idea of protection, and in that order, little or no space is reserved for foreigners "of this" order. The first excluded from this order is the nonnational who carries the foreignness that we are talking about, which is related to the undesirable subject. At the same time, this order does not exclude the nonnational inserted in a "conditional hospitality", based on reciprocity, advantages, and benefits, translated into certain social origins, which Derrida (2003) speaks of as "lineage," or "name." This recognition, therefore, is determined by class and race, constitutive of national identity (Souza, 2018). Thus, the speeches that speak of immigrants as a threat, who will steal jobs, overburden public services, which should serve nationals before, are aimed at the poor, black, indigenous, non-Western immigrant, speeches updated by the rhetoric of the health crisis. They are the scapegoats made up of that most human fear of helplessness, of lack of assistance. Instead of understanding that it is the unequal economic system that implies helplessness, institutions define, for example, that it is the foreigner. Thus, the social institutions that constitute us as subjects and which determine our understanding of the different, the strange, tend to find mechanisms for this other to be annulled, paralyzed, either by controlling it as a working body, assimilating it, or preventing it from having rights, or reserving a priority place for nationals, for example. An example of this is the government policy[8] that determined the closure of the Brazilian border with Venezuela in the pandemic, an intense influx of Venezuelan refugees, justifying the need to reserve the health system to nationals, with the following argument: "Difficulty for the Brazilian Unified Health System to handle the treatment of foreigners infected with the SARS-CoV-2 coronavirus" (Brasil, 2020, article 3, I).

Sayad (1998), in his classic work that analyzes Algerian immigration in France, brings the dynamics of the exclusion of immigrants from the two contradictory representations of immigration, which:

> imposes on all [immigrants and the host society] the maintenance of the collective illusion of a state that is neither provisional or permanent, or what is the same, of a state that is only admitted now as provisional (in law), with the condition that this 'provisional' can last indefinitely, now as definitive (in fact), with the proviso that this 'definitive' should never be stated as such. (Sayad, 1998, p. 46).

So, the immigrant tends to be a tolerated presence, according to Sayad (1998), based on the advantages offered to the economy, worth its perpetuation exactly as an immigrant, or disadvantages, rated as parasites by the social costs. In the context of the emergency arising from the pandemic, this became even more evident. In addition to the closure of the border for Venezuelan refugees already mentioned, migratory regularization has come to be considered "non-priority" for the government, whose service has been suspended. The difficulty with issuing documents was pointed out by 69% of the institutions, behind the difficulty with the issue of work, mentioned by 81% of them; therefore, a population was inserted in the emergency aid policy, approved by the federal government in the period. The difficulty of access of immigrants and refugees to emergency aid was mentioned by 64.3% of the organizations, a difficulty linked to documentary issues. Therefore, it is a marginalized presence in a society that "denies you all right to a presence recognized as permanent" (Sayad, 1998, p. 46).

Although the New Law on Migration in Brazil has inserted human rights at the center of State policy on migration, which presupposes the recognition of a "subject of rights," her condition of subjects to a "presence recognized as permanent" transits through a political-social field. In other words, her condition as a "subject of rights" for a real and prospective "subject of rights" is not abstract and finished. Therefore, the presence of the immigrant as a subject requires recognition, of a full existence, which is a paradox given the exceptions to formal equality brought by the Migration Law itself (right to access public offices and political rights) and the social or collective imaginary that defines them or can only see them as provisional within the "foreignness" of their presence. In the context of the pandemic,

[8]Interministerial Ordinance 120, of March 17, 2020.

the provisionality of migrants before the law, despite the guarantees and principles of the new legal framework, proved to be constant. What we saw was as a government policy, formulated from the discretionary power of the State on entry and permanence, aimed at closing borders to the most vulnerable in a time of emergency and generalized crisis and the non-prioritization of document regularization, as a use of migration control for the purpose of reducing State costs.

In the emergence of the pandemic, with the need for social distancing and its economic implications and in the productive sectors, immigrants became "costs" and the absence of the State was potentially felt, despite being subject to rights, recognized by the law. That is why, according to Sayad (1998, p. 54), immigration and work or provisional workforce is a pleonasm. The research mentions that one of the greatest difficulties of immigrants in the context of the pandemic is finding work (81% of the organizations pointed out this difficulty), added to the difficulties faced by this population to measures to combat dissemination, such as social exposure by the type of labor insertion (61.9%).

The real and prospective subject, not provisional, but participant, is a recognized one. Recognition is a prerequisite for the subject of rights; it is mutual, intersubjective, and the law is "a necessary and indispensable intermediate instrument in this process" (Douzinas, 2009, p. 279). Even though, says Douzinas (2009, p. 280), rights are an auxiliary in the constitution of the subject "through the recognition of the Other," they do not attribute an atomized and isolated existence, they are "deeply intersubjective" and "deeply political: they presuppose logically and politically build a community" (Douzinas, 2009, p. 280). In a context of emergency or crisis, the foreigner is more easily stripped of the condition of the subject. In the idea of subject recognition, there is the notion that the Other talks about themselves, and that I also recognize myself from that other, from what does not constitute me and what does constitute me. Therefore, the presence of the migrant is spoken by him, either by his agency, or by the demand he brings in the context of his reality. The right based on public policies is the instrument for this Other to be recognized, therefore, considered a subject. Research has shown that in the performance of organizations the Other, the immigrant and the refugee, appears as a subject both for the demands it brings and for its own mobilization as an association for access to rights. The survey was answered by 16.7% of civil society organizations made up of immigrants, that is, 7 of the 42 interviewees. As demands that stood out during the pandemic period, organizations mainly pointed to the issue of documentation (migratory regularization by 27 institutions or 64.3% of the interviewees and issue of documents by 29 of the institutions or 69% of them), family reunion with the impact of the closing of borders (69%), access to information (50%), access to emergency assistance (64.3%) and housing conditions (45.2%).

Relating these demands to the issue of "recognition," we find in Fanon [1925–1961], in his writings that contributed to decolonial thinking, the idea of the Other that speaks of himself, therefore, it is not the Other defined by an order, a society, a State, but it is the Other that defines himself and therefore shows his difference, his existence and presence. For Bhabha (2013, p. 80), when Fanon asks "What does the black man want?", by privileging the psychic dimension, "he not only changes what we understand by political demand but transforms the very means by which we recognize and identify his human agency", that is, he addresses his question "not to a unified notion of history nor to a unitary concept of man," which is forged by order (Bhabha, 2013, p. 80). Although Fanon outlines his thesis on the racial issue, it brings important aspects to reflect on diversity, minorities, excluded social groups and their agency, or the conditions for a subject within a society or a predetermined order, based on relationships of domination. The difficulty of accessing emergency aid in the pandemic period because of the issue of documentation and access to information shows the difficulty that institutions must recognize this Other because they deny the context of their own reality and experience (documentary difficulty, family reunion, access to language); that is, they assimilate a generalized difference, such as the economic need, such as that experienced by nationals, for example. The immigrant here is reduced to a "unitary concept."

The unitary concept is crossed by colonial thinking. Immigration in Brazil is representative of this reality translated by the term "colonized." According to Said, the term has expanded since the independence processes to "include women, the subjugated and oppressed classes, the national minorities [...] Therefore, to be one of the colonized is potentially to be many different but inferior things, in many different places, in many different moments" (Said, 2003, p. 116).

At the heart of this debate is the issue of equality before the State, demonstrated by the fact that it is civil society organizations that make the discursive elaboration of the migratory agenda as relevant to the State. Despite rising to the condition of subjects of law, under the Brazilian constitutional framework, the difficulty lies in being accepted and recognized as subjects under equal conditions and opportunities.

A State policy based on human rights is one that produces conditions for the migrant subject to leave the circle of exclusion. What is noticeable are government policies that establish relations of tolerance based on the advantages of immigration. The answer to the integration processes, which should be given by a State policy, is not a reality. In the context of the pandemic, the response during the emergency on the migration issue was to reinforce the circle of exclusion and not to promote integration. Rather than creating criteria based on the law, on the guaranteed rights, a state of exception was created with suspension of rights, under the argument of emergency. Examples are the situations already mentioned and pointed out, such as the suspension of migratory regularization services, bureaucratization for access to emergency aid, closing the border for vulnerable groups as asylum seekers, who are subject to a protection system.

Therefore, as important as the dispute in the legal field of the definition of the subject of immigrant's rights, whose advances in the Migration Law are important, the protagonism of civil society in which the migrant takes place is the possibility of establishing his presence in the face of multiple situations of exclusion, impositive situations of absence, denial, or "permanent provisionality," according to Sayad (1998). And, in this sense, the way in which the social workers themselves and the principles of social security dialogue with the decolonial perspective that presents us with a re-elaboration, from which the assumption of the subject of rights is based, no longer restricted to the premise of a given national belonging, but as someone imbued with the ability to integrate, to be present. This is a major theoretical and practical challenge that the pandemic has highlighted.

15.3 Conclusion: State of Emergency Resulting from the Pandemic and the Absence of Public Policies for Migrants in Brazil

The data collected by the survey indicate the limits and difficulties of access that immigrants and refugees encounter in Brazil, which were aggravated by the health crisis of COVID-19. Despite having ample legislation regarding social policies, there was considerable difficulty in articulating this right of access to the immigrant and refugee population, much of it as a result of the absence of a national migration and refugee policy that integrates specific demands of this population to other public policies that exist in an intersectoral way.

These demands are located in the social workers' action, whose ordinary work of assisting the migrant and refugee population is predominantly focused on actions of social assistance, citizenship, and development, social inclusion, local integration (linguistic accessibility and inclusion in the world of work), and legal advice, according to the survey. These are demands that mark international human mobility. With the health emergency of the pandemic, the difficulties of migratory regularization, access to documentation, access to information, and the problem of food, jobs, and income insecurity stood out. In this way, 61.9% of these organizations also started to act on the demand related to food safety and to expand their own interaction and mobilization with other organizations (69% of them), as alternatives to manage the demands in the emergency.

The ongoing elaboration of this new subject of rights, who is the international immigrant, on whom the right of access to public policies is articulated, also raises its own agency. The health crisis of COVID-19 broadened the debate and strengthened new actors in the field of social work. Among these actors we find associations of immigrants and refugees who, in the context of the COVID-19 crisis, took on an important role in the tension of Brazilian social policies by placing the right of access and coverage to immigrants under the same conditions offered to nationals on the agenda. Immigrant associations focused on the demands of assistance from their nationals in this context indicated that social policies, in particular health, social assistance, and food and nutrition security policies, are configured as fields of dispute from which these collectives seek to articulate their rights of recognition of citizenship in a concrete and discursive way. Despite the legal establishment of a new migration law, the recognition of migrants and refugees as a subject of rights must still inevitably confront the discursive constructions on the subject of rights in Brazil, many of which have been historically elaborated in theoretical and practical social work.

Appendix

Pastoral do Imigrante de Erechim [Pastoral of the Immigrant of Erechim], *Pastoral do Imigrante de Rio Grande* [Pastoral of the Immigrant of Rio Grande], *Centro Batista de Referência em Ação Social - CEBRAS de Canoas* [Baptist Center of Reference in Social Action - CEBRAS in Canoas], *Migraidh/Cátedra Sérgio Vieira de Mello UFSM* [Migraidh/Sérgio Vieira de Mello Chair UFSM], *Centro de Atendimento ao Migrante (CAM) de Caxias do Sul* [Center for the Migrants of Caxias do Sul], *Projeto Araguaney em Porto Alegre* [Araguaney Project in Porto Alegre], *Fórum de Mobilidade Humana de Passo Fundo* [Human Mobility Forum of Passo Fundo], *ADRA SUL de Porto Alegre, GAIRE da UFRGS, Associação dos Haitianos do Rio Grande do Sul* [Association of Haitians of Rio Grande do Sul], *ELO grupo de Voluntários/GEPEC (Grupo de Estudos de Português, Espanhol e Crioulo) de Porto Alegre* [ELO group of Volunteers/GEPEC - Portuguese, Spanish and Creole Study Group], *A Igreja de Jesus Cristo dos Santos dos Últimos Dias de Santa Maria, A Igreja de Jesus Cristo dos Santos dos Últimos Dias de Charqueadas* [The Church of Jesus Christ of Latter-day Saints in Charqueadas], *A Igreja de Jesus Cristo dos Santos dos Últimos Dias de Viamão* [The Church of Jesus Christ of Latter-day Saints in Viamão], *Igreja de Jesus Cristo - Estaca Moinhos de Vento* [Church of Jesus Christ - Moinhos de Vento Stake], *Núcleo dos LMS São Rafael de Casca* [LMS Center São Rafael de Casca], *A Igreja de Jesus Cristo dos Santos dos Últimos Dias de Bagé* [The Church of Jesus Christ of Latter-day Saints in Bagé], *A Igreja de Jesus Cristo dos Santos dos Últimos Dias de Porto Alegre* [The Church of Jesus Christ of Latter-day Saints in Porto Alegre], *Associação Antônio Vieira - Serviço Jesuíta a Migrantes e Refugiados de Porto Alegre* [Antônio Vieira Association – Jesuit Service for Migrants and Refugees in Porto Alegre], *Cruz Vermelha Brasileira* [Brazilian Red Cross] *Estaca Partenon IJCSUD* [Estaca Partenon IJCSUD], *COMIG - Serviço de Acolhida e Orientação ao Migrante de Porto Alegre* [COMIG - Reception and Migration Service for Porto Alegre Migrants], *Cáritas Brasileira - Regional do Rio Grande do Sul, Comitê Municipal de Atenção ao Migrante de Porto Alegre* [Municipal Committee for Attention to Migrants of Porto Alegre], *SAJUR Migrações da UPF* [SAJUR Migrations of the UPF], *Cooperativa Migrantes do Sul de Porto Alegre* [Migrant Cooperative in the South of Porto Alegre], *Movimento Leigo Scalabriniano de Encantado* [Encantado Scalabrinian Lay Movement], *Associação do Voluntariado e da Solidariedade de Porto Alegre* [Porto Alegre Volunteer and Solidarity Association],

Associação dos Senegaleses de Porto Alegre [Porto Alegre Senegalese Association], *Associação Senegalesa de Passo Fundo* [Senegalese Association of Passo Fundo],*Instituto Anglicano Unidade Caxias do Sul* [Anglican Institute Caxias do Sul Unit], *Arquidiocese de Passo Fundo* [Archdiocese of Passo Fundo], *Testemunhas de Jeová de Pelotas* [Jehovah's Witnesses of Pelotas], *Cáritas Arquidiocesana de Pelotas* [Caritas Archdiocesan of Pelotas], *Mães Gestantes de Piratini* [Pregnant Mothers of Piratini], *Gemigra/UCPEL, Associação Senegalês de Pelotas* [Senegalese Association of Pelotas], *Cáritas Diocesana de Santo Ângelo* [Caritas Diocesan of Santo Ângelo], *Projeto Haiti da Associação de Imigrantes Haitianos de Santo Ângelo (Projeto de Extensão Interação Linguística Português Francês)* [Haiti Project of the Association of Haitian Immigrants of Santo Ângelo - Portuguese French Linguistic Interaction Extension Project] and *Cáritas Diocesana de Cruz Alta* [Diocesan Caritas of Cruz Alta].

References

Bhabha, H. K. (2013). *O local da cultura* (2nd ed., pp. 77–116). UFMG, Interrogando a identidade.

Brasil. (2014). Ministério da Justiça. *1ª Conferência Nacional sobre Migrações e Refugiados.* https://reporterbrasil.org.br/documentos/comigrar.pdf

Brasil. (2017). Lei de Migração n. 13.445, de 24 de maio de 2017. http://www.planalto.gov.br/ccivil_03/_ato2015-2018/2017/lei/l13445.htm#:~:text=Institui%20a%20Lei%20de%20Migra%C3%A7%C3%A3o.&text=Art.,pol%C3%ADticas%20p%C3%BAblicas%20para%20o%20emigrante

Brasil. (2020). *Portaria Interministerial n. 120, de 17 de março de 2020.* https://www.in.gov.br/en/web/dou/-/portaria-n-120-de-17-de-marco-de-2020-248564454

Derrida, J. (2003). *Anne Defourmantelle convida Jacques Derrida para Falar da Hospitalidade.* Escuta.

Douzinas, C. (2009). *O Fim dos Direitos Humanos.* Unisinos.

Fanon, F. (2020). *Pele Negra.* Máscaras Brancas.

Redin, G. (2020). *Psicologia Social da Vulnerabilidade do Migrante Internacional.* Postdoctoral thesis, Social Psychology Institute, USP, São Paulo, SP, Brazil.

Said, E. (2003). *Reflexões sobre o Exílio e outros Ensaios.* Companhia das Letras.

Sayad, A. (1998). *Imigração ou os paradoxos da alteridade.* EdUSP.

Souza, J. (2018). *Subcidadania Brasileira: Para entender o país além do jeitinho brasileiro.* LeYa.

16 Social Justice in the Time of COVID-19: Transcend Borders—From the Micro to the Macro, from Patagonia Argentina to the World

Marina Anahí Curzio

16.1 Introduction

The coronavirus pandemic (COVID-19) has changed the lives of people around the world, and the world will not be the same again. As a society we must accept the threat that this virus represents and the consequences it has generated, such as social distancing, the use of masks, and hand sanitizing. However, the coronavirus has also revealed the great underlying problem that the world is facing: inequality.

In this chapter I analyze and reflect on how the concept of social justice plays in the light of the pandemic that COVID-19 has generated in Argentina, starting with the reality that the province of Chubut is enduring.

The Argentine Patagonia is made up of six provinces, one of which is Chubut with an approximate population of 556,300 inhabitants spread over 224,700 km². There is a deep political-economic crisis in which sectors of the State, many of them linked to direct assistance to the population (health, education), are in constant tension because of assets owed as well as the lack of inputs. This crisis makes it difficult for the health service to address and adequately care for possible cases of contagion, generating in turn a deterioration of working conditions and institutional infrastructure. Health begins to be seen as a public expense and not as a human right.

I propose a series of questions that lead us to focus on the issue of social justice. Questions such as: What happens to the mental health of the general population that is in a process of permanent change? What happens when some of the towns of the province suddenly recede into this almost unsustainable but necessary isolation or social distancing? How does social justice have a role in the framework of equalities/inequalities when the phases of isolation/distancing might allow us to leave home to work, visit family and friends, bond with others, have a coffee, perform recreational activities and/or entertainment, get the children out of confinement? How is social justice visualized if we think about the relationships of equalities/inequalities in terms of availability and accessibility at the time of virtual education for infants, young people, and adolescents from different social strata?

The social transformations in terms of links, ways and forms of relating between human

M. A. Curzio (✉)
Graduate in Social Work, National, Faculty of Humanities and Social Sciencies, University of Patagonia San Juan Bosco (UNPSJB), Comodoro Rivadavia, Chubut, Argentina

Research Group: Action and Territory Research Group (GIGAT-Patagonia Geographical Research Institute-UNPSJB), Cultural Heritage Research Group (LUPAT Civil Association "Activate from Knowledge" – UNPSJB) – Comprehensive Learning and Development Center (CADI-Inclusion Support Program), Comodoro Rivadavia, Chubut, Argentina
e-mail: marycurzio@live.com.ar

M. C. S. Gonçalves et al. (eds.), *The Coronavirus Crisis and Challenges to Social Development*,
https://doi.org/10.1007/978-3-030-84678-7_16

beings, as well as the policies implemented by the States to face this new reality, share some basic preventive premises, although they also contain profound differences according to the particularities of each context. A whole system of beliefs, practices, habits, and cultural customs is put under strain and is impossible to sustain, such as customs rooted in the heart of the Argentine community such as sharing, meeting every weekend, celebrating birthdays, greeting each other with kisses, hugs, caresses, and shaking hands.

At the same time, empathy toward others comes into play, toward the well-being of others; relationships of social equality/inequality are highlighted with a deepening of the gap for access to technologies as a means of communication, information, and training (Stolkiner, 2020). In an interview with Carolina Brandariz,[1] published in August 2020, the phenomenon of the growing inequality gap in Argentina is visualized; for instance, 6 of 10 boys will be poor by the end of 2020. The data, put on the table these days by UNICEF, not only expose the structural poverty of Argentina, but also challenges and forces us to accelerate the times of discussion about what type of country will be built once the COVID-19 pandemic ends. Brandariz states that the Emergency Family Income has made this point clear, estimating that "*four million people would apply, but twelve signed up and finally nine million received it. The Renater is a tool that allows you to build a clear diagnosis. Thirty or forty percent of the population does not receive a salary in relation to dependency (…).*" (Mandy, 2020; author translation.)

16.2 The Pandemic Challenges Us to Think of the Other as a Brother

The transformations that the COVID-19 pandemic has generated in people's daily lives, in the practice of professionals—especially social workers and health personnel—and in the form of social relationships typical of the community, feel like a profound social transformation around the world. Therefore, international borders are forced to constantly be configured and reconfigured, showing the capacity of solidarity of states.

The National Decree of Necessity and Urgency 297/2020 of Argentina marked the beginning of a social, preventive, and compulsory isolation for a certain period, which lasted approximately 7 months. Later, periods of social distancing began with certain restrictions, measures at the national level. At the local level, the provinces and municipalities were controlling the measures according to the development of the pandemic, taking into account the number of infections.

The isolation measures of people in their usual residences, or in the place where they were, and refraining from going to their places of work, had different phases. The phases and dates set out as follows belong to the official website Argentina.gob.ar and to the national Decrees: 260/2020 (03/12/2020), 274/202003/16/2020 (), 297/2020 (03/20/2020), 310/2020 (03/24/2020), 311/2020 (03/25/2020), 313/2020 (27/03/2020), 320/2020 (03/29/2020), 325/2020 (03/31/2020), 332/2020 (04/01/2020), 355/2020 (04/11/2020), 408/2020 (04/26/2020), 459/2020 (05/11/2020), 493/2020 (05/25/2020), 520/2020 (06/8/2020), 576/2020 (06/29/2020), 605/2020 (07/18/2020), 641/2020 (08/02/2020).

The first phase, from 21 March to 30 March, consisted of strict isolation prohibiting all citizens from leaving their homes with the exception of going out to buy food or medicine. From that moment on, no one could move away from their residence. In the second phase from 1 April to 10 May, the quarantine was extended again, only for agglomerates with more than 500,000 people. The measure was also made more flexible to allow recreational outings of 1 h per day and within a radius of 500 m from the residences, children having to be accompanied by their parents or adolescents.

In the third phase, from 11 May to 7 June, President Alberto Fernández ordered the end of the quarantine for the entire territory of Argentina, moving to phase 4 (distancing), with the excep-

[1] Carolina Brandariz is a sociologist, teacher, and researcher. She is currently the Director of Comprehensive Care of the Ministry of Social Development of the Nation and a member of the National Board of the Evita Movement.

tion of the Metropolitan Area of Buenos Aires, which remained in phase 3. On 23 May, President Fernández extended the quarantine in the AMBA and three other urban areas until 7 June.

From 8 June to 17 July, eight provinces ended the quarantine over their entire territory and went into a "distancing" regime with hygiene protocols. Only four urban areas remained isolated: the Buenos Aires Metropolitan Area (AMBA), the San Fernando Department of the Chaco Province, the Rawson Department of the Province of Chubut, and the Córdoba Metropolitan Area. A few days later, two more were added, the departments of Bariloche and General Roca of the Province of Río Negro. In the distancing stage, social gatherings and sports that require 10 people or less were allowed, so long as health and distance precautions were maintained.

From 18 July to 2 August, calls on the population to become aware of the seriousness of the situation and the need to respect sanitary regulations were emphasized in the AMBA, Chaco, Jujuy, and Río Negro. Some activities were reopened, such as recreational outings for boys (days of outings were extended) 500 m from the residence address, with social distancing and use of face masks for people over 6 years of age and maximum duration of 60 min per day; opening of squares and parks without use of playground or aerobic posts; and nearby shops and neighborhood galleries joined the neighborhood clothing and footwear shops according to the completion of DNI for customers; churches were opened for administrative tasks, online celebrations, and individual prayer within limit (maximum of 10 people at the same time in the same room); opening of carwash locations, authorized dog walkers, authorization for the toy industry; removals enabled only on weekends, lawyers authorized to work in their offices; opening of art galleries, hairdressers, hair removal, manicure, and pedicure salons; psychologists, educational psychologists, occupational therapists, and kinesiologists who work with neurodevelopmental disorders and the elderly; speech therapists who work with autism spectrum disorder (ASD). From 20 July factories were open, with their own transportation system. From 27 July other legal, notarial, accounting, and auditing services were also authorized. In addition, health professionals and others who offer "home maintenance services" (such as gardeners and pool keepers) were allowed to work.

From 3 to 16 August, the pandemic was on the rise again in Argentina, attacking areas of the territory that had remained free of contagion and worsening in most of the other affected areas. The most serious situation continued to be in the AMBA and Jujuy regions. On 31 July, the heads of the national government, the City of Buenos Aires, and the Province of Buenos Aires reported in a press conference that the quarantine would be kept in the AMBA for another 14 days, until 16 August.

On 2 August, DNU No. 641/2020 was published, extending the mandatory distancing status (DISPO) throughout the country, with the exception of five areas, which had to continue in quarantine (ASOP): the AMBA (City of Buenos Aires and 35 parties of the Province of Buenos Aires), all 54 departments of the Province of Jujuy; the departments of Atreucó, Catriló, Capital, and Toay of the Province of La Pampa; the department of Güer Aike of the Province of Santa Cruz; and the department of Río Grande of the Province of Tierra del Fuego, Antarctica, and the South Atlantic Islands.

In the midst of social distancing, on 12 August 2020 it was announced that Argentina had signed an international agreement that would allow it to be part of the vaccine production chain and access it in 6–12 months. The agreement was signed between the University of Oxford, the Swedish-English company AstraZeneca, and the Slim Foundation, with the participation of the governments of Argentina and Mexico, to produce between 150 and 250 million vaccines destined for all of Latin America with the exception of Brazil, which was not part of the agreement. Argentina was selected to produce an active part of the vaccine in a laboratory inaugurated in February 2020 in the town of Garín (Province of Buenos Aires), belonging to the company mAbxience, part of the Insud group. The general director of mAbxience Argentina, Esteban Corley, explained that the decision was motivated by the high quality of Argentine pharmacological research and industry: the country has a flourishing relationship between a powerful, modern, and competitive pharmaceutical industry, and, on the other hand, highly trained human resources. The agreement allowed the production of the vaccine to begin on 14 August, before the verification phases were completed, to save time in the event that the drug is finally effective so that vaccinations can begin in the first half of 2021.

From 17 to 30 August, the pandemic continued to increase in Argentina, attacking new areas of the territory that had remained free of contagion and worsening in most of the other affected areas. The most serious situations continued to be in the AMBA and Jujuy region, with considerable peaks in the cities of Mendoza, Córdoba and Rosario. Decree No. 677/2020 was published on August 16, extending the mandatory distancing status (DISPO) throughout the country, with the exception of seven areas (two more than in the previous decree), which had to continue in quarantine (ASOP): the AMBA (City of Buenos Aires and 35 parties of the Province of Buenos Aires); the departments of Manuel Belgrano, Ledesma, El Carmen, and San Pedro of the Province of Jujuy; the department of Güer Aike of the Province of Santa Cruz; the department of Río Grande of the Province of Tierra del Fuego, Antarctica, and the South Atlantic Islands; the departments of Capital and Chamical, of the Province of La Rioja; the department of General José de San Martín of the Province of Salta; and the departments of Capital and Band of the Province of Santiago del Estero.

From 31 August to 20 September, social distancing continued with the respective measures mentioned in the previous paragraph.

From 21 September to 11 October, social, preventive, and compulsory isolation (ASPO) continued to be applied in the Metropolitan Area of Buenos Aires (AMBA) and in the Buenos Aires towns of Mar del Plata, Bahía Blanca, and Tandil. It was also applied in the Jujuy departments of Manuel Belgrano, Ledesma, El Carmen, Palpalá, Susques, Yavi, Rinconada, and San Pedro, and in the Capital department of the province of La Rioja, all cities with a very high level of coronavirus infections. Other localities where it was applied were located in the agglomerates of the cities of Bariloche and Dina Huapi and the department of General Roca, in the province of Río Negro; in the departments of General José de San Martín, Cerrillos, Rosario de Lerma, General Güemes, La Caldera, Orán, and Capital of the province of Salta; in the agglomeration of the city of Río Gallegos, Santa Cruz; in the departments of Capital and Banda, in Santiago del Estero, and in the department of Río Grande, in Tierra del Fuego.

The remaining districts of the country continued under the measures of distancing, social, preventive, and mandatory (DISPO), with the same conditions as until now (February 2020, the time of writing). The DISPO applies in those jurisdictions in which the health system has "sufficient and adequate capacity to respond to the health demand," the doubling time of confirmed COVID-19 cases is not less than 15 days, and they are not defined "by the national health authority as those with sustained 'community transmission' of the SARS-CoV-2 virus."[2] The provincial governments continued to maintain the power to, in case of detecting situations of risk of spread of the virus, order preventive isolation from people who enter the provinces from other jurisdictions for a maximum period of 14 days. For its part, in the province of Santa Fe, despite being in DISPO, commercial activities of shopping malls and pedestrians were restricted, neither did they open gastronomic establishments nor wholesale and retail stores of more than 100 m^2. It did not allow the exercise of freelance professionals, the services of domestic staff, and religious activities. Neither did they allow sports practices nor private work.

From 12 to 25 October, Decree 792/2020 detailed how the restrictions and flexibilities would continue in the different provinces, according to their particular epidemiological situation,

[2] Decree DNU 641/2020 of the NATIONAL EXECUTIVE POWER OF ARGENTINA (P.E.N.) published on August 02, 2020. Retrieved from http://servicios.infoleg.gob.ar/infolegInternet/anexos/340000-344999/340612/norma.htm

during the next two weeks. The Government mentioned that "at this stage in the evolution of the pandemic, epidemiological indicators, the weight of cultural, social and behavioral factors, must be evaluated when taking measures for the future" to contemplate the extension of the quarantine. The percentage of bed occupancy was 63.3%: in the Autonomous City of Buenos Aires, it was 69% and in the metropolitan region of the Province of Buenos Aires it was 60.1%." "In Mendoza it is 81%, reaching 92% in Greater Mendoza."[3] The City and Province of Buenos Aires and the 35 municipalities that make up the Metropolitan Area would continue in the ASPO phase. The Government of the City of Buenos Aires authorized social gatherings of up to ten people in public outdoor spaces. In addition, the following continued in the ASPO phase: the departments of San Fernando, Comandante Fernández, Mayor Luis Jorge Fontana, and Chacabuco of the province of Chaco; the departments of Biedma and Escalante in Chubut; the departments of Capital, Santa María, Punilla, Colón, Tercero Arriba, and General San Martín in Córdoba; the departments of Manuel Belgrano, Ledesma, El Carmen, Palpalá, Susques, Yavi, Rinconada and San Pedro de Jujuy; the departments of Capital and Chilecito of La Rioja; the departments of Capital, Luján de Cuyo, Las Heras, Maipú, Guaymallén, Godoy Cruz, Tunuyán, and Tupungato de Mendoza; the agglomerations of the cities of Neuquén, Plottier, Centenario, Senillosa, Cutral Có, Plaza Huincul, and Zapala, in Neuquén; the agglomerates of the cities of Bariloche and Dina Huapi and the department of General Roca de Río Negro; the departments of Cerrillos, Rosario de Lerma, General Güemes, La Caldera, and Capital of Salta; the Rawson and Capital department in San Juan; the department of General Pedernera in San Luis; the agglomerates of the City of Río Gallegos, El Calafate, and Caleta Olivia de Santa Cruz; the departments of Rosario, La Capital, General López, Caseros, Constitución, San Lorenzo, Las Colonias and Castellanos, in Santa Fe; the Capital and Banda departments of Santiago del Estero; the department of Río Grande de Tierra del Fuego; the Capital department in Tucumán.

Public transport continued to be available for essential workers, so that in the activities, employers had to continue to guarantee the transport of workers and the safety and hygiene conditions to prevent contagion. Social or family gatherings in private homes, cinemas, theaters, cultural centers, libraries, museums, clubs, and any public or private space that involve the attendance of people continued to be prohibited; as well as tourism. Also, circulation is restricted in 18 provinces in the interior of the country: Chaco, Chubut, Buenos Aires, Río Negro, Neuquén, Jujuy, Salta, Tucumán, Córdoba, La Rioja, Mendoza, Santa Cruz, Tierra del Fuego, Santiago del Estero, Santa Fe, San Juan and San Luis, and the city of Buenos Aires. Corrientes, Misiones, La Pampa, Entre Ríos, Formosa, and Catamarca are excluded.

From 26 October to 8 November, the social, preventive, and compulsory isolation (ASPO) continued for eight provinces (Santa Fe, Chubut, Córdoba, San Luis, Mendoza, Neuquén, Río Negro, and Tucumán) and the Metropolitan Area of Buenos Aires (AMBA) under the same conditions; 55% of infections were concentrated in these places. The provinces of Misiones, Corrientes, Formosa, Entre Ríos, Catamarca, Jujuy, La Pampa, and San Juan will be under the modality of preventive and compulsory social distancing (DISPO). Some departments and cities of 16 provinces will be under the ASPO modality: AMBA, Buenos Aires, Chaco, Chubut, Córdoba, La Rioja, Mendoza, Neuquén, Río Negro, Salta, San Luis, Santa Cruz, Santa Fe, Santiago del Estero, Tierra del Fuego, and Tucumán.

Toward the end of 2020, from 9 November to 31 December, the Preventive and Mandatory Social Isolation (quarantine) was extended until 29 November in some departments of 10 provinces. For the first time since March 20, the Metropolitan Area of Buenos Aires (AMBA) was

[3] Decree DNU 792/2020 of the NATIONAL EXECUTIVE POWER OF ARGENTINA (P.E.N.) published on October 12, 2020. Recovered in https://www.argentina.gob.ar/normativa/nacional/decreto-792-2020-343033

excluded from the situation of isolation (quarantine) and became a situation of distancing (DISPO). Public transport would continue exclusively to serve those who were authorized because they perform essential activities. Any activity that involved an agglomeration of people in closed places will continue to be prohibited, for example, theaters, cinemas, and recitals in closed places. Bars or restaurants can only function in conditions set by the local authorities.

In the Province of Buenos Aires, five measures were announced to go from flattening the curve of cases to crushing it: sustain and deepen the active search, strengthen care guidelines, pursue a policy of intelligent distancing, apply active surveillance of the close contacts (for this to be asymptomatic or not, a test is also going to be done), and finally, isolation and targeted quarantine were allowed: Schools went back to classes (in 26 municipalities considered low risk, face-to-face classes were being resumed, for certain groups and under certain conditions, and in 82 risk-free municipalities it has been possible to implement relinking activities in buildings, but outdoors). Other activities that had to stay closed were auxiliary staff of private homes (multi-domicile); restaurants and bars in the interior with capacity; gyms as well as collective sports activities for up to ten people in closed spaces; and expansion of private construction.

Meanwhile, the City of Buenos Aires authorized the following for education: school activities of all levels, including the garden rooms of 2, 3, and 4 years and adults who continue with their primary or secondary studies in shifts and on a noncompulsory basis. Nursery schools (children from 45 days to 2 years): they would be put into operation as early stimulation encounters of a baby with a teacher plus a companion; 3- and 4-year-old rooms: sports, recreational, and artistic activities would be set up in the open air in bubble groups of up to 8 students: the activity would last 2 h. The second to sixth grade of primary school, and second to fourth year, plus fifth year of technical schools in secondary schools: sports, recreational, and artistic activities will be opened in the open air in bubble groups of up to ten people, with a duration of 2 h.

Since December 24, the borders would remain closed to tourism: then, only Argentines and residents can enter the country, or foreigners for exceptional reasons duly accredited or with a work permit. Tourism was focused on circulation within each province mainly, with the use of the CARE Application, processing a summer certificate, wearing a mask, and Obra Social or COVID-19 Insurance. To travel between provinces or from another country, a negative PCR swab test was necessary; if you enter from another country, it was a requirement to perform a mandatory 10-day isolation from the PCR test required upon arrival in the country. Some of the reasons given for the measures were (a) the declaration by the World Health Organization (WHO) of the outbreak of the new coronavirus as a pandemic; (b) the WHO report dated 19 March 2020, which confirms the spread of cases of the coronavirus COVID-19 worldwide, reaching a total of 213,254 infected people, 8843 deaths, and affecting more than 158 countries on different continents, having reached our region and our country. Country a few days ago; and (c) we are facing a potential unprecedented health and social crisis, and for this it is necessary to take timely, transparent, and consensual measures based on the available evidence to mitigate its spread and its impact on the health system (Candusso & Pereyra, 2020).

For this reason, the exemptions have been officially limited to activities and services declared essential in the emergency, fixed by a list of activities. This stage gave way to a process of virtualization or rather digitization of activities that are not declared essential. Teachers and students plead to use platforms such as Zoom, Meeting, Jitsi. At the same time, countless conferences, talks, webinars, workshops, training cycles, cultural activities, and other offers were given online. Suddenly platforms and social networks, that is, virtuality entered homes and monopolized spaces that were considered "family."

This variance gives people the opportunity to celebrate birthdays, or organize family and friend gatherings. Here are possibilities to connect with others who are far from home, perhaps in another city, province, or outside the country. The range of talks and webinar allows us to generate exchanges with different professionals from different countries of the world, to generate or strengthen ties, networks that allow working on issues and/or problems that affect humanity. The house becomes the space where work, education, bonds, and social relationships meet and are formed. But everyone who works and studies from home must do so with their own means: tables, computers, Internet, etc. Employers do not recognize the obligation to pay the expenses generated by working at home. Internet connection begins to be considered an essential service because it is essential for daily life: it allows you to study, work, connect with family, friends, acquaintances, and professionals who work in solving social problems, make purchases, pay for different services, and a range of activities that are channeled virtually.

However, it became a problem that access to Internet service is not so simple for those who do not have the necessary financial resources. In his article "*Internet access: vital in times of pandemic but unequal in terms of access to study at a distance*" (author translation), Francisco Argerich mentions that that approximately 19.5% of students at primary level do not have access to the Internet, and at the secondary level 15.9%, according to a report by the Observatorio Argentinos por la Educación. These percentages are even higher in villages and settlements, and also in the provinces with the highest poverty rates. The installation of antennas such as those used in public spaces is one of the possible solutions. Water, electricity, and gas are services that were always considered essential. But today there is a service that reflects inequality more than ever: Internet access. Inequality obviously also varies by region. In the north of the country, accessing the Internet is even worse. In provinces such as Santiago del Estero, up to 40% of the homes of primary students do not have an Internet connection. CABA has the lowest rate in the country with 7.2% (Argerich, 2020).

This availability is where the gap between those with less and those with more becomes even more pronounced. In addition, a number of workers who only have jobs occasionally are affected, people who work in the informal sector or day laborers, called "Workers of the Popular, Social or Solidarity Economy" in Argentina. Even more, there are several problems that drag down the most disadvantaged neighborhoods or villages such as access to water, unemployment, overcrowding, lack of sewage, and gender violence. In particular, in the province of Chubut there is a problem that reveals a strong and deep crisis that the provincial State has not been able to resolve, namely the wages owed to state workers, who occupy approximately 80% of the province's workforce. A newspaper article from a Chubut digital newspaper stipulated that the plant of State agents totals 61,570 agents, according to the payroll of salaries consigned for the month of August. In 2019, in which the number of agents was established for each of the salary ranges, the payment of salaries was problematic, which creates a serious conflict. This problem includes active workers and also those in the passive sector, both retired and pensioned. In rank 1, a total of 26,424 agents were included in that month, in rank 2, 17,724, and in rank 3, 17,422, reaching a global salary mass of 3400 million pesos, without incorporating the salary increases planned since June onward. A separate discussion can be based on the growth of this mass of agents in recent years, but the official numbers reflect a situation far from what the national media shows. The total population is also higher: 481,500 inhabitants, if one considers the sad fact that Chubut's debt per capita amounts to 1900 dollars for each inhabitant, of a stock recorded at 915 million dollars until September 3, as officially recognized by the provincial government (Alonso, 2019).

However, Infobae reveals that of a total of 580,000 inhabitants of Chubut, about 46,000 are state employees; which represents about 80% as a wage group; among them are health, educational, judicial, and banking personnel. This situation has caused a tension that is increasing between the governor of the province and state workers. At the end of the year at least 3 months of salaries are owed, plus the July bonuses. Despite the debt that the State maintains with the workers, they have continued to face the vicissitudes that this pandemic has generated.

Since February 2018, the governor of the province Escribano Mariano Arcioni had to appeal the staggered payment to meet the salaries, which lasted until November. Half a year later he had to resort to that modality again. According to data provided by the provincial executive to the newspaper Infobae in a note made on 13 August 2019 (Diario Infobae). On the other hand, the digital newspaper *El Chubut* reveals on 8 November 2020 that they will continue with the staggered payment of said wage bill in response to the ongoing financial and economic crisis in the province (Daily Note, El Chubut, 2020).

16.3 Spearhead Social Justice

> *Inequality is a key obstacle to mental health globally. Many risk factors for poor mental health are closely associated with inequalities in the conditions of daily life. Many risk factors are also linked to the corrosive impact of seeing life as something unfair.* —Dr. Dainius Pūras, UN Special Rapporteur on the right of everyone to the enjoyment of the highest attainable standard of physical and mental health (United Nations, 2019).

In the context of deep social inequalities and injustices that do not only involve social classes, but also transcend other dimensions of social life, it is necessary to be clear that social justice is the axis of all social intervention, even more so if we talk about social work. But in a context where the daily struggle involves not being excluded from the system (not only from the health system), it is vital to rethink the concept of social justice from a restorative, redistributive, and recognition point of view (Cifuentes & Vallejos, 2018). A notion of social justice closely linked to human rights is proposed here, emphasizing economic redistribution as a problem of social justice. Prioritizing equal positions, social cohesion, and the consolidation of the social structure to create a system of rights and obligations, is a reformism of the State that, with certain social and civil measures, tries to return to the concept of the welfare state (Dubet, 2011).

A key point of Dubet (2011) suggests the prioritization of the equitable position model, that is, in fact, equality of opportunities that rests on a narrow conception of the Rawlsian principle of difference. By virtue of this principle, it is required that inequalities produced by meritocratic competition are not unfavorable for the most vulnerable. He maintains that the equal opportunities model says nothing about unacceptable social inequalities; from the moment people are born into equal competition, they consider it fair. Equality of opportunity assumes that all individuals should be proportionally distributed at all levels of the social structure regardless of their origin. This conception does not seek to affect the hierarchies of positions, but to guarantee that they are accessible to all, marking an equal starting point for all.

Dubet adds that social relations are tense, often aggressive; people have little confidence in themselves and in others, they always have a lot to lose or a lot to gain; people become distressed and develop illnesses related to that stress. At this point, he takes up a study by who shows that inequalities pervert the social capital of individuals, reducing their trust in the circle of their peers and accentuating mistrust between communities. Inequalities increase hostility between groups and individuals. Your peers are the same as you in terms of personal tastes, same economic level, you only help those closest to you, that is, friends, family, acquaintances, neighbors. Free to choose or forced to live together, individuals protect themselves by placing the greatest possible distance between themselves and others, always perceived more or less as dangerous strangers. That is, the emphasis is always placed on the "individual" as a single being, who helps those closest to him, with freedom to choose. But the pandemic shows us that the context always conditions that freedom to choose, because individuals become people when they begin to think and act that their actions have consequences for others, although they are not part of their closest bond. That is, all the people who know each other and those who do not know each other need the community. In this sense, social organizations have had a fundamental role because they see all people in the same way, and therefore they provide services such as food packages, providing internet access, providing school help, offering bags of clothes and materials for the construction of adequate housing for the families of unknown people, who have nothing to do with those who are members of these social organizations.

Continuing with the analysis proposed by Dubet, inequalities also degrade the collective life of affluent societies. The richest are grouped in closed communities or closed neighborhoods, and the poor are grouped in quasi-ghettos, popular neighborhoods, or villas. Public space is divided between rich and protected areas and poor and dangerous areas.

If we refer to the societies in which we live, as the so-called democratic ones, Dubet presents an interesting analysis because it is in them where inequalities increase the frustrations of those who cannot reach the ways of life and consumption of others:

> *The richest are so rich who no longer feel tied to the societies in which they live, while the poorest feel rejected by that same society that 'blames the victims; and accuses them of being responsible for their misery'.* (Dubet, 2011, p. 96).

In June 2019, Argentina was already talking about the richest and the poorest. The article "Rich getting richer and poor getting poorer" provides data established by INDEC (National Institute of Statistics and Censuses): the poorest population in Argentina received 1.2% of the income while the richest sector of the population obtained 31.2%; which means that the richest earn 26 times more than the poorest. Almost 70% of the population received an average individual income of up to 22,404 pesos, below the cost of the basic food basket in March, which was 28,750 pesos. The richest 10% of the population has an income 30 times higher than that of the poorest sector, widening the gap that had reached a 20-fold mark in December 2018 (El Patagónico, 2019).

Peronism as a social movement had promoted the reduction of social inequalities in Argentina. It is clear that the more inequalities are reduced, the more opportunities increase. It is easier to move on the social scale when the distances between different positions are relatively narrow. In other words, social mobility is one of the objective indicators of equal opportunities. In that case, the "social elevator" does not go up or down very much, but many more people can use it. For instance, if the City of Buenos Aires were made up of relatively wealthy neighborhoods, others a little less rich, and others a little less rich, people who live in neighborhoods a little less wealthy could move to those that are a little richer and then, perhaps, to the richest. Also, people who live in the richest neighborhoods would not be haunted by the fear of living in slightly fewer wealthy neighborhoods. But if you have inequalities as in Argentina today, those who are below will never rise and those who are above will never descend. In a certain way, there is something mechanical that one sees clearly in school: if one regulates inequalities of positions, it mechanically increases equality of opportunity. On the contrary, if one increases equality of opportunity, one does not increase equality of positions. It can even increase inequality.

Argentina is a country where Peronism or Justicialism still persists as a national and popular movement that flies five flags, one of them fully dedicated to social justice. General Juan Domingo Perón, creator and ideologist of this movement, put into practice the idea that justicialism promotes social justice, which gives each person their right to a social role, as one of the 20 basic truths of the movement.

Perón argues that the world is divided between capitalists and communists, and justicialism is neither one thing nor the other. In this framework, the person is the only beneficiary of social justice that, applied rationally, is the only way. The "political economy" is therefore exchanged for the "social economy." In other words, capital is at the service of the economy and capital is at the service of social welfare. People are capitalized and each person has the possibility of realizing his destiny, according to his qualities, within a community that is realized by the action of all. Social law is basically about putting into practice the solidarity of the community and justice on their part, and it is that everyone has the same opportunities and the same rights. Social justice lives in love for the other; therefore, the community has a central role:

> *The community is like the mother: it is loved for its self-denial, its sacrifice and its solidarity; not for its mother. A just and supportive community, in which we are all equal and equally helped by her, will instinctively defend itself out of solidarity and convenience without need for speeches or nonsense like that.* (Gómez, 1999: 149).

Social justice is manifested through health, education, the economy, freedom of worship, culture, sports, and various aspects of life that make the development of the social welfare of the community. In this sense, the Peronist government that took office on 10 December 2019, with Alberto Fernández, and that has faced not only the coronavirus pandemic, but also the economic restructuring of a country devastated by the economic policy of the previous government of Cambiemos led by Eng. Mauricio Macri, had to implement a package of economic measures to deal with this situation, to mention a few: the IFE (Ren Economic Family Fee of 10,000 pesos), the Emergency Assistance Program for Work and Production (ATP), extraordinary bonuses, benefits for companies, tax payers and self-employed, credits for research of companies, cooperatives, and institutions, and temporary suspension of services such as electricity and gas.

Inequalities are not new, but they have been exacerbated by the pandemic and have become even more radical, putting stress on the relationship between capital accumulation and redistribution. It is fundamental from where we analyze these inequalities to give meaning and orientation to our profession, to the social sciences, to the construction of citizenship, to the construction of the collective. It seeks that the State is efficient and professionalized to build more egalitarian public policies. The objective is to achieve a more egalitarian society, with an emphasis on favoring the less fortunate and those who are beginning to be excluded from the system.

At the same time, it makes it clear that when speaking of poverty, it is done from a reality very different from that shown by the media. Families live in one room; there is no Internet. There is much demand for public space because of overcrowding. For this reason, at one point in the pandemic, the president stopped talking about social isolation and started talking about community isolation, because the conditions that the Villas go through are different from those of the neighborhoods.

The word "Villa" is a term with various uses linked to different types of populations and to certain particular styles of housing. In its classical sense, a town is a population that has some privileges that differentiate it from villages or towns, but that is not considered as a city. In Argentina, the notion of town is used to refer to the neighborhood of precarious and crowded houses with one another and with infrastructure deficiencies. The original concept spoke of a shantytown (coined by Bernardo Verbitsky in one of his books), although in everyday language it is simply referred to as a "Villa". The villages are usually located in or around the big cities and are formed from migrations (with people who come from different towns or countries in search of work).

Lucia Dominga González Duarte (2015) defines the villages as unorganized occupations of one or several families, to which others are added, in a more or less long time, until some of more than 50,000 inhabitants live there. Population density is very high. They produce very irregular urban patterns, with intricate corridors, where generally no vehicles can pass. The houses are built with waste materials and with time some inhabitants build their masonry houses. The inhabitants considered them in their origins a transitory habitat towards a 'possible' and longed for social ascent, an expectation that failed to materialize for the majority of its inhabitants.

"Staying at home" becomes "staying with the neighbor, that is, entire neighborhood communities isolate themselves in a kind of bubble isolated from the rest of society". They add that "The neighborhood program takes care of the neighborhood" seeks to strengthen community isolation, giving an account of the reality in which, we live. It works to promote the necessary care measures, although it starts from the idea that those who live in this type of neighborhood are already trying to take care of themselves in unequal conditions, totally different living conditions from the rest of society.

The writer Cristian Carillo relates that the Secretariat for Economic Policy reveals that, according to data from the IMF Fiscal Monitor (April), with regard to fiscal policies, the Argentine response is sixth, with packages similar to those of Germany and the United Kingdom. It is above Brazil, China, Korea, Italy, Spain, and France. Social protection assistance against the pandemic reaches 1.7 trillion pesos. After the social, preventive, and compulsory isolation was decreed, economic and productive measures were outlined to serve the most vulnerable population and the affected sectors of activity. To mention some, fiscal measures were applied, such as the IFE (10,000 pesos), and the ATP (payment of salaries) or extraordinary bonuses, which until now have had a monthly frequency. On the other hand, a loan package linked to the financing of productive loans aimed at companies and sectors affected by the emergency was outlined. These lines are financed with contributions from the Treasury to subsidize interest rates or offer guarantee programs.[4]

16.4 Social Work: Post-challenges

In this pandemic, people undergo a transformation in the networks of connection, and social relationships are changing their commonly practiced forms. It still remains to be seen whether the population complies with the necessary restrictions for healthcare, complying with the policies applied by the national government in pursuit of the mental healthcare of the people. The actions of those who govern the province of Chubut put people's health at risk because the limited control over the circulation of the population causes the coronavirus to spread rapidly. This control affects people especially when family events are approaching, and they long to meet family, friends, and they long to be able to return to normality.

The Doctor in Psychiatry of the Regional Hospital of Comodoro Rivadavia and Mental Health Coordinator Marta Rodríguez tells us about a "psychosocial crisis," and emphasizes the need to "*maintain personal and virtual ties in the face of uncertainty, because they allow us to move forward and we do not know how long it will happen until this is over.*" At the same time, it provides very important information regarding the appearance of mental illnesses such as insomnia, anxiety disorders, and symptoms related to affective problems such as anxiety, crying, and irritation, as expressed in an interview with a local newspaper *Daily Note* (2020, author translation).[5]

Two issues are crucial in this psychosocial crisis that affects people's mental health. On the one hand, people begin to have difficulties in satisfying their basic material (house, food, clothing) and immaterial (social relationships) needs. On the other, the ability to physically establish socio-affective relationships is difficult. It is key to become aware of our social problems. The condition of social isolation caused an absolute alteration of daily life as we know it (Stolkiner, 2020), and the fact of having infections or not gives us no hope of returning to that long-awaited daily life, of being able to return to the "normal" work, to hug each other, to take up future projects, and to be able to bring daily bread to the family table. The wear and tear that is generated by not being able to make sense of this new reality has its origin in people, generating fears, anxieties, and uncertainty for not knowing when to leave: from home, from the city, from the region, from the countryside; and to be able to know the "other." That is to say, the pandemic:

> *As a process, it impacts differently depending on the place, the space where it appears, the nutri-*

[4]Daily Note Page 12. Cristian Carillo. Argentina on the social protection podium., Buenos Aires. Published 29/04/2020. Recovered in https://www.pagina12.com.ar/262678-argentina-en-el-podio-de-la-proteccion-social?fbclid=IwAR0j9XJGAdEvCt_ieNeqCW0VIkOe-JOH11SpdkTTfmB6dpZ7FV12xcT52yAg.

[5]Daily Note: The Southern End of Patagonia. Sanchez, Lola. COVID in Commodus: "We start to be afraid of each other and it seems that the virus is getting closer and closer every day." Published on 07/09/2020. Recovered in https://www.elextremosur.com/nota/26216-covid-en-comodoro-emperamos-a-tener-le-miedo-al-otro-y-parece-que-el-virus-se-acerca-cada-dia- más/.

> *tional and housing characteristics, previous illnesses, the construction conditions of daily life and especially the possibility of perception of feeling ill, healthy or exposed to it in relation to the subjectivity of each one and the social and economic conditions that inevitably dialogue with these issues.* (Carballeda, 2020a, b, c).

Empathy toward others needs to be put into practice toward the well-being of others. The relationships of equality or social inequality stand out more than ever now with a deepening of the gap caused by access to technologies as means of communication, information, and training (Stolkiner, 2020).

The struggle for human rights, the struggle for integrating others, is a struggle that is collective, because subjectivity is constituted from the other, becomes stronger and more intense. Mental construction is the construction of subjectivities with new parameters. Talking about the reconstruction of a present state as an articulator of social life gains strength in this collective character (Rozas Pagazza, 2020). This new social relationship that has been generated is a unique process, traversed by suffering and mental wear-and-tear that causes anguish and desolation, not only from isolation/ social distancing, but also from the anguish of not making ends meet, or not to be able to collect some "remunerative benefit" from the State to combat this harsh situation. A situation of total uncertainty that requires a bond of involvement with the Other, with the problem that is suffering, with attentive listening, and with a word that accompanies and keeps alive the call of hope.

Undoubtedly, we as social work professionals are challenged by the coronavirus pandemic. Not only because it is a social problem that concerns us when our intervention is interrupted, but also because social justice represents a priority objective for the profession. It is necessary to reflect how the pandemic challenges us and affects intervention scenarios in complex ways. We must understand the disease as a collective phenomenon both for development and for solution (Carballeda, 2020a, b, c).

Social work is the profession whose concern is linked to the design, elaboration, and implementation of public policies; in general and in particular, we are State makers. The Federal Law of Social Work No. 27072 of Argentina understands the profession of Social Work based on practice and an academic discipline that promotes change and social development, social cohesion, and the strengthening and liberation of people. The principles of social justice, human rights, collective responsibility, and respect for diversity are fundamental to social work. For this reason, our professional practice is linked to the promotion of people's rights, with a specific contribution regarding the needs that differentiate us from other professions. We are the ones who intervene in the complexity of the daily life situations of the subjects where rights are not guaranteed, and with that specific role and knowledge.

I agree with Alonso (2019) that inequality is a key obstacle to mental health globally. Poor or rich, mental health depends largely on inequalities in the conditions of daily life. In turn, many of the risk factors are linked to the aggressive impact of looking at and perceiving life as unfair.

The question is how do we improve this situation? What can we do as professionals? We certainly need to improve education, health and social development systems to reduce inequality and social exclusion.

Some key guidelines in this challenge are linked to the generation of global networks, a concept such as solidarity and exchanges that cross borders, in a kind of collective confrontation to which we are forced by circumstances. At the same time, we must maintain the local networks that we have been able to build and continue to strengthen them, but the momentum and exchange with other disciplines and with colleagues from all over the world prevail.

Another important point is the demand and the implementation of collective actions that include nontraditional forms of promotion and defense of human rights. Social movements and organizations such as nongovernmental organizations have become a collective force that raises the flag in defense of human rights. Consolidate nontraditional strategies such as people who sit on the sidewalks of public organizations with banners and songs, dance during marches, show naked and drawn bodies, disguise themselves as trees, are some examples. Movements are rational adaptive responses to conflict situations, when members participate to achieve a collective good that is considered possible. Social movements are made up of available resources, organization, selective incentives, and opportunities for collective action. Social movements become a political actor that defends human rights and fights for the eradication of inequalities. Examples of collective strength in Latin America include the Landless Movement of Brazil, Not One Less in Argentina, Self-convened by the No to La Mina in Chubut.

The great problem of inequality historically haunts us because humanity involves us all, notably states and professionals. Aiming for social justice should be the ultimate goal. We need to develop intervention strategies that guarantee accessibility to essential resources and services and to the objective conditions of existence, particularly for the most vulnerable population groups.

It is necessary to create meeting spaces, to meet face-to-face and virtually, to debate, discuss, and question current issues. It is important to share experiences, generate joint action plans, and draw up intervention guidelines that adapt to different scenarios. As the pandemic has made it clear to us, it is that being connected is the collective key to facing social problems and finding all possible solutions, that working locally is recommended but not enough.

16.5 Conclusion

The challenge that awaits us professionally is to think about how we handle the post-pandemic, how we work with this inequality gap, and what is the meaning we give to our practice. The situation of uncertainty, malaise, and social insecurity challenges our professional practices. However, in the search for transformation of social reality based on the principles related to human rights and social justice, Carballeda (2020a, b, c) proposes that the intention of our practice is linked to the right to accessibility from the essential to the most important: accessibility to water and food, to vaccines, to the health system, to work, to the management of closed spaces with the necessary healthcare, to how to achieve the opening of those closed spaces. Aim to recover the human condition of getting involved with the other, of being in solidarity, recovering that ability to sensitize ourselves to the difficulties and conditions that the other person is experiencing. To recover the concern for the other from the sensation, the perception and the slogan are taking care of ourselves and of the Other Therefore, it is necessary to think about a mobile, dynamic, changing, and articulated border. A frontier where the design of public policies is reflected in a comprehensive, inclusive, and strategic way that aims to reduce these relationships of social equality/inequality. Think of the Other as an equal, a couple, a conscious subject with rights and dignity as a human being. Think of the Other as a brother.

Social justice as a concept, definition, and implementation is put into play not only in micro realities but also in macros. The global pandemic of COVID-19 does not recognize static and immobile borders, nor does it make distinctions by skin color and creeds: much less does it distinguish social status, class, or if you are rich or poor. The coronavirus is present in all places, in all spaces, in all regions, in all countries; it has become a global phenomenon that generates an unprecedented impact on the general population and on health systems.

The implementation of solidarity and exchange at the local, provincial, regional, national and international levels is key. In other words, it is essential to understand that the only alternative to be able to combat this pandemic, and what it has made visible, is to restructure global network schemes, strengthen international ties, and design joint strategies to combat the great social problems that have afflicted humanity for decades.

The measures taken in each country to face the economic consequences of the pandemic are also measured on a global scale. For this reason, borders are key for the post-pandemic, recognizing that COVID-19 is a common problem as are its consequences, in terms of health, education, economy, politics, and all human concerns. Grimson (2005) affirms that borders are diverse interstate relationships, links between border societies and national states, networks where the sociocultural peculiarities of both countries come into contact. The nation, territory, and population links are put into play.

A clear example of transnational links represents being able to employ a vaccine that, thanks to the technological characteristics of our country, is necessary to import from states that have the necessary means to produce it, such as the United States or Russia. In this sense, it is important to note than in early 2021 about 300,000 doses of "Sputnik V" vaccines from Russia have arrived in Argentina, which is setting the course for foreign policy and international ties that go beyond the border. The consolidation of networks, that is, a network of relationships between states around the world, is important to face the great problem that COVID-19 creates: inequality.

References

Alonso, M. F. (2019). Social justice is more important to mental health than therapy and medication, declared the UN spokesman. *Psyciencia Magazine*. https://www.psyciencia.com/la-justicia-social-es-mas-importante-para-la-salud-mental-que-la-terapia-y-la-medicacion-declaro-el-vocero- de-la-onu /? fbclid = IwAR0j9XJGAdEvCt_ieNeqCW0VIkOeJOH11SpdkTTfmB6dpZ7FV12xcT52yAg

Argerich, F. (2020). *Acceso a internet: vital en tiempos de pandemia pero desigual en cuanto a su acceso para estudiar a distancia*. https://www.redaccion.com.ar/acceso-a-internet-vital-en-tiempos-de-pandemia-pero-desigual-en-cuanto-a-su-acceso-para-estudiar-a-distancia/

Candusso, P., & Pereyra, P. B. (2020). *Reflexiones sobre nuestro papel en el territorio durante la pandemia. Colegio de Profesionales en Servicio Social de la Provincia de Córdoba*. http://cpsscba.org/confluenciasvirtual/?p=7488&fbclid=IwAR0j9XJGAdEvCt_ieNeqCW0VIkOeJOH11SpdkTTfmB6dpZ7FV12xcT52yAg

Carballeda, A. (2020a). *Notes for the intervention of social work in times of the Covid-19 Pandemic*. La Plata, Faculty of Social Work. https://www.margen.org/pandemia/index.html

Carballeda, A. (2020b). *Social work in times of pandemic* [Audio podcast]. https://www.margen.org/pandemia/carba_charla.html

Carballeda, A. (2020c). Social theme, contexts and intervention. Comodoro Rivadavia, Secretary of Extension of the Faculty of Humanities and Social Sciences of the National University of Patagonia San Juan Bosco. In *Virtual Conference Held on 04/17/2020*.

Cifuentes, M. R., & Vallejo, S. Y. (2018). Social work and social justice in times of transition. *Eleuthera Magazine, 18*, 150–165. https://doi.org/10.17151/eleu.2018.18.9

Decree DNU 641/2020 of the NATIONAL EXECUTIVE POWER OF ARGENTINA (P.E.N.). (2020). http://servicios.infoleg.gob.ar/infolegInternet/anexos/340000-344999/340612/norma.htm

Decree DNU 792/2020 of the NATIONAL EXECUTIVE POWER OF ARGENTINA (P.E.N.). (2020). https://www.argentina.gob.ar/normativa/nacional/decreto-792-2020-343033

Dubet, F. (2011). *Rethinking social justice. Contra el mito de la igualdad de oportunidades*. siglo XXI..

El Patagónico, D. (2019, June 27). *Rich getting richer and poor getting poorer*. https://www.elpatagonico.com/ricos-cada-vez-mas-ricos-y-pobres-cada-vez-mas-pobres-n5039571?fbclid=IwAR3KJMdCo8e8EK60EYS98-Knc0nYVLyOJRv8ytkggapzE7gEmanti

Gómez de Mier, E. (1999). *Obras completas Juan Domingo Perón*. Editorial Docencia SA, Tomo XX.

González Duarte, L. D. (2015). *Villas miseria: la construcción del estigma en discursos y representaciones (1956-1957)* (1st ed.). Universidad Nacional de Quilmes.

Grimson, A. (2005). Fronteras, Estados e identificaciones en el Cono Sur. In D. Mato (Ed.), *Cultura, política y sociedad. Perspectivas latinoamericanas* (pp. 127–142). CLACSO.

Mandy, M. F. (2020). *Niños de barrios vulnerables y derecho a la conectividad: el impacto pospandémico*. https://www.bigbangnews.com/politica/los-chicos-y-los-barrios-post-pandemia-como-estan-toy-los-sectores-mas-vulnerables-y-el-proyecto-de-base- popular-202082212410? fbclid = IwAR0j9XJGAdEvCt_ieNeqCW0VIkOeJOH11SpdkTTfmB6dpZ7FV12xcT52yAg.

Nota de Diario El Chubut. (2020). *Antes del 10 de diciembre el Gobierno pagaría otra masa salarial*. https://www.elchubut.com.ar/nota/2020-11-7-23-4-0-antes-del-10-de-diciembre-el-gobierno-pagaria-otra-masa-salarial

Rozas Pagazza, M; y otros. (2020). *Ciclo de diálogos: Neoliberalismo, pandemia y desigualdad: reflexiones desde Trabajo Social*. Facultad de Trabajo Social de la Universidad de La Plata. https://www.youtube.com/watch?v=R_6Anx2OcHs

Stolkiner, A. (2020). *Conversación sobre pandemia, derechos humanos y salud mental.* Buenos Aires, Secretaria de Derechos Humanos de la Nación Argentina. https://www.youtube.com/watch?v=rsm9ulp4fR4.

United Nations. (2019). 41st Session of the Human Rights Council (24 June–12 July 2019). Report A/HRC/41/34. Right of everyone to the enjoyment of the highest attainable standard of physical and mental health. Report of the Special Rapporteur on the right of everyone to the enjoyment of the highest attainable standard of physical and mental health. https://www.ohchr.org/EN/HRBodies/HRC/RegularSessions/Session41/Pages/ListReports.aspx

17 Colombian Women Between the Pandemic and Armed Conflict and Poverty

Maria Mauersberger

17.1 Introduction

A few days ago, I experienced a drastic situation in front of a little food store in a place called Gran Via (Big Street), near the municipality Tena in the Department of Cundinamarca. I was not allowed to enter, but the owner served the people outside. In front of me stood a woman, maybe 45 years old. She looked like she was from the countryside. She was wearing a mask, as were almost all the people, and rubber boots. I saw two packages of milk, some rice, and some meat at the counter. When counting her money, she gave back the milk and rice. There was not enough money to pay for all of it. I know that is an everyday situation for many of the Colombian people. I thought about the impact of the pandemic on poor people. This woman is just an example of many. It is a very worrying situation that must be resolved quickly because, among other reasons, children's well-being often depends on their mother. And women's well-being depends often on their partner or other family members. According to the Organization of American States:

> In the framework of the pandemic, (…) that the loss of income and reduction of economic activity is an additional factor to the rise of the inequality and poverty levels, especially affecting women, particularly women heads of households. The Commission highlights the need for a specific approach towards the 126 million female workers in the informal economy, as well as domestic workers, rural women and sex workers, and other groups disproportionately affected by the pandemic, such as migrant women, homeless women and trans women.[1]

This chapter shows the position of women in societies marked by inequality, poverty, and lack of human rights, and how women try to manage their lives in the pandemic. It is meant to draw attention on the difficult situation faced by millions of women worldwide, but especially in the Global South. Human rights for women are established in law, but the reality is different. Colombian women daily face violation of their rights to live a life of dignity, free from violence, stigmatization, and marginalization. This chapter is divided into three sections. Section 17.2 reviews the incidence of poverty and illegal armed groups in relation to the pandemic and how it affects women. Section 17.3 describes the domestic violence and patriarchal structures related to a historically strong gender discrimination against women. And finally, Sect. 17.4 presents the challenges for social workers in the time

M. Mauersberger (✉)
Fundación Mujeres en Paz Colombia (Women Peace Foundation), Barrio Recreo, Cundinamarca, Colombia
e-mail: mmauersberger@unal.edu.co

[1] http://www.oas.org/en/iachr/media_center/PReleases/2020/074.asp.

M. C. S. Gonçalves et al. (eds.), *The Coronavirus Crisis and Challenges to Social Development*,
https://doi.org/10.1007/978-3-030-84678-7_17

of a pandemic and the importance to contribute to the public politics, create social support networks and special care routes and protocols to prevent violence.

Since the beginning of the pandemic, people in the District of Cundinamarca (Bogotá and neighboring zones), are allowed to go to the market only once per week: this day depends on the last number of the identification card and the gender. However, literally no one can save money to buy food and other products for the next 7 days. Those who fail to comply with the lockdown are punished with fines. The Government does not provide the minimum conditions as financial support to those unable to work because of the pandemic. Therefore, there is a permanent situation of hunger in the country, with permanent conditions of vulnerability to poverty, which is further aggravated by food insecurity.[2]

Vulnerable groups, such as indigenous people, children, and women experience a high risk to starve or catch the virus:

> Indigenous Peoples in Colombia are on high alert. The government is implementing preventive measures for COVID-19 in the country without adequately guaranteeing their fundamental rights. Historically they have not had access to health, water or food and in the context of this pandemic, this situation is much more serious because they do not have the sanitary and social conditions to deal adequately with COVID-19 (…).[3]

For children living in countries where conflict and violence are already present, the impact of this crisis further increases the risk of instability and of families falling into poverty. Children in Colombia are still starving because of the lack of drinking water and food and the inadequate public health system. In 2015, 10.8% of children under 5 years had chronic malnutrition.[4] In indigenous groups, the risk is even higher, with 1 of every 3 children living with malnutrition. During the period from 2005 to 2017, there were 4956 deaths caused by malnutrition in children under 5 years, an average of 381 dead per year. Similarly, 80% of mortality from malnutrition in children under 5 years of age is concentrated in 50% of the vulnerable population.[5]

Whereas some people in the industrialized countries are worried about where to spend their vacation in the full pandemic, Colombian people must cope with lockdowns, the armed conflict, displacement, hunger, and the insufficient healthcare system. It is a sign of a growing crisis in Colombia that almost 50%[6] of its population work in the informal sector and are running out of food and money under lockdown. Despite the equality and non-discrimination clauses that protect women in the Colombian Constitution from 1991, Article 43, they are still negatively affected in getting employment by a series of societal and biological reasons such as pregnancy, childbirth, or even just the possibility to get a child (Ramirez et al., 2015, p. 2). The International Labour Organisation (ILO) protects pregnant workers from being dismissed during pregnancy and with 14 weeks[7] of paid maternity leave (ibid., pp. 2–3). Among other reasons, that seems to make it more attractive to employ men than women. According to a study of Bank of the Republic, the increase in duration of the maternity license can be attributed to a lower probability of reenlisting in other jobs and a higher probability of quitting permanently the formal labor market for women (Romero, 2018, p. 28).

[2]"In its Judgment C-644/12, the Constitutional Court defines food security as the degree of guarantee that the entire population must have, to be able to have timely and permanent access to food that meets their nutritional requirements, trying to reduce the external dependence and taking into account the conservation and balance of the ecosystem for the benefit of future generations." (https://www.corteconstitucional.gov.co/relatoria/2012/C-644-12.htm).

[3]https://www.amnesty.org/en/latest/news/2020/04/colombia-pueblos-indigenas-covid19-hambre/, access 8 of June 2020.

[4]Análisis de Situación de Salud (ASIS). (2018). *Dirección de Epidemiologia y demografía* (p. 117). Ministerio de Salud y Protección Social, Bogotá.

[5]Ibíd.: p. 255.

[6]According to the Colombian National Administrative Department of Statistics (DANE), between December 2019 and February 2020 the informal occupation for men was 45.2% and for women 48.6% (https://www.dane.gov.co/index.php/estadisticas-por-tema/mercado-laboral/empleo-informal-y-seguridad-social).

[7]Law 1468 of July 2011.

Colombian women have a 70% higher unemployment probability than men,[8] which makes them very vulnerable to poverty and marginalization.

17.2 Poverty and Illegal Armed Groups

> Women and girls in Colombia are seen as rewards and trophies of war, and as a mean to punish the enemies.[9]

It is assumed that today, 5 years after the signing of the peace agreement in Colombia, the population affected by the armed conflict is in a process of transition to the disarmament phase and post-conflict. Some people believe that they live in peace now. But there are still many challenges. One is the ongoing war, and restitution of land, especially for women.

> One of the most sensitive areas of 'delivering justice' to the displaced population is the restitution of land and housing as part of a reparations programme. However, displaced women face more obstacles than men when they claim their right to land and property restitution. The reason is that their land rights had not often been formally registered before being moved (Meertens, 2011, p. 41).

Girls and young women in Colombia, and particular those living in areas of the armed conflict and without school education, are the most exposed to different forms of violence, such as sexist, ethnic, and class violence (Ramirez & Gómez, 2007, p. 99). Historically women and children were the most vulnerable population in times of war, seen as trophies to punish the enemies. And still, they are. "(…) Violence against women is used as a war strategy by the actors of the armed conflict, in their struggle to control territories and the communities they inhabit."[10] According to the Single Victims Registry (RUV) during 2019, 52.08% of women were affected by victimizing acts in the context of the armed conflict. At the same time, every 16.5 h, at least 1 woman was sexually assaulted in the context of the Colombian armed conflict (Sisma Mujer, 2020, p. 12).

And besides the cruel violence, with nowhere to go, victims and displaced women cannot expand their life project any further or build a new one. Another problem is the instability of the labor market and discrimination against women. Therefore, many Colombians, especially women, not only have to fight for their land, from which they were displaced, but also for their daily survival. Most of the people are poor; they can hardly get the essentials to survive. There is only a small middle class and a few rich people. The vulnerable middle-class and lower-income households are more affected by the current crisis caused by the COVID-19 pandemic and its future consequences. These effects will be reflected in both poverty, and inequality (Nota Macroeconómica, 2020, 20:2). The current paralysis of activities and the possible future destruction of jobs and productive activities will return the country to at least a decade ago (ibid., p. 2). In consequence, the most vulnerable population such as women, children, and poor people carry the burden of the ongoing crisis on their shoulders. It is recommended to act quickly to prevent an even worse situation for thousands of women.

> (…) the faster policy makers and business leaders act to push for greater gender equality, even as the COVID-19 crisis continues, the bigger the benefits not just for gender equality but also for economic growth. Conversely, there is a real risk of losing even more economic output—and the economic security it could mean for millions of women—than COVID-19 would normally affect all workers. Women stand to lose both in terms of parity and in terms of economic benefits if nothing is done and the stagnating record of the past five years settles in as the norm—on top of the gender-regressive shock we are seeing because of COVID-19.[11]

---

[8] https://colombiareports.com/unemployment-among-colombias-women-70-higher-than-among-men/, access 23 of February 2021.

[9] Susan Lee, Americas Director at Amnesty International.

[10] https://www.cidh.oas.org/countryrep/ColombiaMujeres06sp/III.htm, access 28 of May 2021.

[11] McKinsey Global Institute. (2020). *COVID-19 and gender equality: Countering the regressive effects*. https://www.mckinsey.com/featured-insights/future-of-work/covid-19-and-gender-equality-countering-the-regressive-effects#.

According to World Bank, the GINI Index, which measures the economic differences in a population's income, was 50.4%[12] in Colombia in 2018.[13] People live in absolute poverty if they cannot satisfy or cover their basic needs such as housing, nutrition, healthcare, and drinking water. Quantitatively speaking, their income is less than $1.25 a day.[14] The number of people in Colombia living in absolute poverty is, at 2.2 million, alarmingly high.[15] The National Statistical Office in Colombia determined in 2018 that people who earn more than 257.433 pesos (approximately 70 dollars!) a month are not considered poor.[16]

In 2020, Colombia's total population was 50,883,000 people. In 2018, the overall poverty rate was 29.9%, 26% in cities and 43.4% in the countryside. In the same year, the percentage of people without income was 27% for women and 10.9% for men.[17] Women are particularly vulnerable economically. Usually they earn less than men; they experience various disadvantages in getting a full-time job because they are the primary caretakers of children and elderly people.[18] According to the Organisation for Economic Co-operation and Development (OECD), there is a large gender gap in terms of employment and unemployment.[19] The day laborers are the most affected because of the fragility of their sources of income in periods of economic shocks (Nota Macroeconómica 20:1). Rarely are they part of the health system and social insurance. They can survive only if they are able to work every day.

In addition, many Colombian villages and cities are still affected by the armed conflict. Although the peace treaty between the government and the Colombian Revolutionary Forces (FARC) was signed in 2016, civil society, especially well-known social leaders, such as human rights defenders, indigenous and Afro-Colombian leaders, and reporters, are still subject to violence. The number of killed social leaders[20] and incidents of violence against women since the pandemic are increasing. According to the Institute for Peace and Development Studies (INDEPAZ), up to 18 May 2020, 105 social leaders were killed, 24 of them during the lockdown in the pandemic time, and 8 family members of social leaders.[21] The Non-Government Organization "Somos Defensores" in 2020 confirmed 969 attacks against social leaders and 199 murders, which means an increase of 60.4% relative to 2019, the highest figure documented in 11 years.[22] Female activists and leaders face every day high risks of violent attacks. The militarized masculinity of the armed groups does not

[12]A GINI coefficient of 50 represents 50% concentration in a country's income distribution; that could mean, that half the people share all the income, while the other half get nothing, or only a small part. See: http://iresearch.worldbank.org/PovcalNet/methodology.aspx: "To measure poverty in the developing world as a whole, the World Bank's "$1 a day" measures apply a common standard, anchored to what "poverty" means in the world's poorest economies. The original "$1-a-day" line was based on a compilation of national lines for only 22 developing economies, mostly from academic studies in the 1980s (Ravallion et al., 1991). (…). Since October 2015, the World Bank uses a poverty line of $1.90 a day at 2011 PPP to estimate global poverty. This new poverty line (referred to as the International Poverty Line) is the average of the same 15 national poverty lines that yielded the $1.25 line at 2005 PPPs (Ferreira et al., 2016).

[13]https://datos.bancomundial.org/indicador/SI.POV.GINI, access 8 of June 2020.

[14]https://www.goethe.de/ins/co/de/kul/sup/fot/20876633.html

[15]https://www.eltiempo.com/economia/sectores/informe-mundial-de-pobreza-extrema-deja-a-colombia-en-puesto-70-282948

[16]https://www.dinero.com/pais/articulo/crecen-los-niveles-de-pobreza-en-colombia/270504.

[17]https://estadisticas.cepal.org/cepalstat/Perfil_Nacional_Social.html?pais=COL&idioma=spanish

[18]See about the disadvantage and barriers facing women: https://www.project-syndicate.org/commentary/women-progress-and-hurdles-advanced-economies-by-laura-tyson-and-anu-madgavkar-2020-04, access 12 of June 2020.

[19]http://unperiodico.unal.edu.co/pages/detail/muerte-por-desnutricion-en-colombia-otro-virus-cronico-sin-aparente-solucion/, access 22 June 2020.

[20]In Colombia social leader means "líder social" and that is a person who fights for the human rights, for justice and equality. The "Lideres Sociales" try to build a bridge between their community and the government.

[21]http://www.indepaz.org.co/paz-al-liderazgo-social/, access 25 May 2020.

[22]https://somosdefensores.org/2021/05/20/la-mala-hora/, access 26 May 2021.

approve of women who transgress traditional gender roles and that empower local communities. Often their families and lives are threatened.[23]

This threat exists because some of the guerrillas of the Colombian Revolutionary Forces did not participate in the peace pact and did not surrender their weapons. Others surrendered their weapons, but then joined other armed groups, partly in response to the government's deficit reintegration programs and lack of alternatives.

In May 2017, the Colombian Revolutionary Forces dissidents included more than 2300 members.[24] Armed groups remain highly active, particularly in Arauca on the border with Venezuela. People continued to be murdered or abused, minors recruited, forced to work, and others kidnapped all the way to Venezuela. The National Liberation Army (ELN) is still active and committed violent crimes against the civilian population, such as displacement from their land and murders.[25] In the District of Magdalena (Caribbean), the Gaitanis Self-Défense Forces of Colombia (the government calls them the Gulf Clan) are disputing with other illegal groups about the drug trafficking routes, because in the Caribbean territory "they profit from the entire chain: planting, processing, transportation, marketing (distribution and export) and money laundering" (author translation).[26] According to sources from the Prosecutor's Office, today this Clan controls the ports of Barranquilla, Cartagena, and Santa Marta, and a part of the natural ports of the Guajira peninsula, in alliance with Guajirá's criminal organizations.

A recent article from the daily paper "El Espectador" mentioned how poverty and the COVID-19 pandemic affects children in Colombia. Most families who live in the countryside cannot afford a computer in their homes. Therefore, the children cannot take the virtual classes and have no real access to school education. Armed groups take advantage of this miserable situation. They recruit the minors telling them to get some quick money smuggling guns and drugs. For lack of alternatives and because the children must economically help their families, "they consent." Actually they have no choice to make, because if they refuse, armed groups will force them by killing or threatening their families; thus, the numbers of recruited boys, girls, and teenagers in Colombia increased to 113% from January to May 2020. According to the Colombian ombudsman, between March and September 2020, 83 minors between 8 and 18 years of age were recruited, more than 80% of them at the countryside.[27]

To prevent and mitigate these phenomena in the full pandemic of COVID-19, Colombian society needs policies and strong public politics that focus on strengthening victims and marginalized people with constant economic support in crisis to protect and secure their nutrition, shelter, healthcare, and education as well as micro business. At that point, social workers should start to move and demand enforcement of the rights of vulnerable people. "(…) social sciences and social work research contribute not only to the academic debates but also by researching on how to prevent, minimize, and respond to inequalities and cover the social urgent needs of vulnerable groups particularly affected by COVID-19" (Redondo-Sama et al., 2020, p. 2).

So, the gender focus should not only seek to restore the right to property, protection, food security, access to education, and political participation but also transform discriminatory practices and strengthen the effective enjoyment of these rights and other human rights for women over the long term. Protecting women and ending war need durable solutions with impact in communities, municipalities, and departments. State workers should be aware and sensitized on gender issues.

[23] https://carnegieendowment.org/2020/05/07/in-colombia-pandemic-heightens-risks-for-women-social-leaders-pub-81736, access 26 of May 2021.

[24] https://www.hrw.org/es/world-report/2020/country-chapters/337323.

[25] Ibid.

[26] https://www.elespectador.com/colombia2020/territorio/el-rebrote-del-conflicto-armado-en-el-caribe/, accessed on 10 June 2020.

[27] https://www.semana.com/nacion/articulo/por-la-pandemia-aumento-riesgo-del-reclutamiento-forzado-de-menores-de-edad/202106/, access 26 May 2021.

Colombian women need empowerment and independence through economic and politic stability. All of them, but especially victims, need formal and material access to justice; it must be accessible for them. On the other hand, a piece of land and economic stability would be the first step in achieving the path to independence and dignity for women. And it could be a prevention mechanism for femicide because of the liberation from dependence of unhealthy relationships between women and men. The following section shows the consequences of this kind of relationship.

17.3 Domestic Violence and Patriarchal Structures

Many women continue to be discriminated against through cultural laws or patterns, which limit their rights within the family, through discriminatory attitudes by police, judicial staff, health personnel, and many other sectors. Combating and eliminating gender-based violence remains a global challenge: "Despite the tremendous progress made in national, regional and international legal frameworks, millions of women around the world claim to have experienced some form of violence in their lives, usually at the hands of their partner" (UN, Women, 2011–2012, p. 8).[28] Women's rights are less protected: we see this in the private sphere, where many women are exposed to abuse and violence. They cannot make decisions about their sexuality, marriage, divorce, and reproductive health (UN, 2011–2012, p. 13). We know, for example, that in peacetime the most unsafe place for 65% of women is their own home. This situation is not limited to one region of the world or any precise time (Serret, 2006, p. 8).

In the first quarter of 2020, more than 15,000 cases of domestic violence were reported in Colombia. According to the forensic institute report, of the 15,440 registered cases, 11,840 (76.7%) were against women, whereas 3600 cases (23.3%) had men as victims.[29] Between January and September 2019, The Nacional Institute of Legal Medicine registered 14,501 cases of sexual violence against girls and teenagers and 17,068 against women.[30] Comparing data of domestic violence against women, there was an increase of 228% during the period from March to May 2020.[31] During 2020, a woman was sexually assaulted approximately every 35 min (Sisma Mujer, 2020, p. 10).

COVID-19 disproportionately affects women and girls in several ways, including "adverse effects on their education, food security and nutrition, health, livelihood, and protection".[32] Lockdowns bring women closer to violent situations with their partners, who can take advantage of the situation. Often there is no way to escape because the financial situation does not allow separation. Victims sometimes not even can make a phone call to report violence, which is why the number of abuses and violence against women increases in the Global South.[33]

The UN mentions four fundamental issues analyzing how gender operates as a primary cause of violence against women in the family. The first is the harmful masculine-based beliefs in male privilege, control, and dominance; the second is the submission and subordination expected of women; the third is the lack of long-term economic autonomy and security for

[28] See about the Colombian case in the UN Report WOMEN AND MEN: GENDER GAPS IN COLOMBIA. EXECUTIVE SUMMARY, and DANE (2020), p. 17 and up.

[29] https://www.elespectador.com/noticias/nacional/mas-de-15000-casos-violencia-intrafamiliar-en-primer-trimestre-en-colombia-articulo-912254/, access 12 June 2020.

[30] https://www.sismamujer.org/wp-content/uploads/2020/01/7-01-2020-Boletín-25-de-Noviembre-de-2019_SISMA-MUJER-VF-1.pdf, access 27 May 2021.

[31] http://www.senado.gov.co/index.php/prensa/lista-de-noticias/1333-las-mujeres-asumen-el-impacto-mas-alto-de-la-pandemia-el-de-las-violencias-y-el--socioeconomico, access 25 of May 2021.

[32] Gender Implications of COVID-19 Outbreaks in Development and Humanitarian Settings. CARE.

[33] Apoyo a la respuesta nacional en VBG en el contexto de la pandemia de COVID-19. (2020, 1). Fondo de Población de las Naciones Unidas (UNFPA), UNU Mujeres.

women; and the fourth, the ideal of family harmony, which emphasizes the family as a private space (UN, 2018–2019, p.185).

Even though the Colombian Government has taken measures against violence, this is not covering the existing demand,[34] especially because of the gap between the law and its correct application and interpretation by the judges. An example of the strength of cultural patterns in interpreting specific cases is the revictimization of the female victim by public officials. Thousands of women who report domestic violence by their (ex)-partner or other man are assigned stereotypes by public intuitions, by putting them in a more vulnerable and disbelief situation with stereotypical questions: "What have you done to get him to hit you?" "Did you provoke him?" This example shows that prejudices about women are in the unconscious, in culture, permeating societies. The great danger, besides denying justice to victim, is that violence against women becomes normal and is seen as a private matter, accepted by society.

Thus, legal issues are extremely important. Women's rights are vulnerable in all areas and at any time, referring especially to their right to live in dignity without violence, labor protection, pregnancy protection, equality between men and women, political participation, land access, and food security. The law is supposed to protect women from violence and simplify the access to justice, to a fair process. Even the Colombian Constitution from 1991 in Article 42 refers to family protection and equality: "Family relationships are based on equal rights and duties of the couple and in reciprocal respect among all its members."[35] But the reality is different.

According to Obando, "The law may become an instrument for social change or an obstacle to the empowerment of half the world's population" (1999, p. 166). It all depends on whether there is awareness, that "there is never a single correct, definitive and valid interpretation for all cases and at any time" (ibid., p. 166).

It is assumed that the concept of interpretation as hermeneutics, or Theory of Comprehension, considers all the confluent elements in the interpretive act, the subject, object, social reality, culture, tradition, among others, and therefore fits more to the three-dimensional conception of law (ibid., p. 181). This dimension of law considers that the norm, the social fact, and the legal value influence are related to each other, and must be considered when interpreting a case (ibid., p. 166). Therefore, to make fair decisions, we would need high consciousness and gender focus in public institutions. For an argument that eliminates discrimination against women and men from marginalized groups, the six-step model for the analysis of any case, text, or law should be considered. The first step is to become aware and understand in depth discrimination against women and their subordination. Next one is to deepen understanding and identify forms of sexism in texts or contexts. The third step is to identify which woman is unvisitable in the text or context. The fourth step is the identification and recognition of stereotypes. The fifth step is to analyze the text or context, considering the legal phenomenon beyond the norm. And as a last and sixth step, collective awareness must be deepened, to achieve a strict elimination of prejudices, stereotypes, and preconceptions still present regarding the value of the feminine and the masculine.[36]

A fundamental concept is the legal-feminist one that starts from an integral vision of the law, contemplating the contradictions between the written norm, its application in practice, and its interpretation (Obando, 1999, p. 186). This concept includes formal equality (before the law) to achieve gender equality. Therefore, it is not enough to create law, it only makes sense when people who interpret law are aware of the gender issues, disadvantages, and stereotypes that women must experience in their daily life. The

[34] https://colombia.unfpa.org/sites/default/files/pub-pdf/Comunicado%20UNFPA-ONU%20MUJERES.pdf, p.2, access 29 May 2021.

[35] https://www.constitucioncolombia.com/titulo-2/capitulo-2/articulo-42.

[36] Recovered from the Regional Programme for the Formation of the Diploma in Gender and Justice (PRIGEPP http://prigepp.org).

gender focus on women and other vulnerable people or groups is essential for protecting their human rights.

As indicated by Onofre de Alencar:

> Stereotypes become a much more serious problem when they are assumed by institutions. Their widespread use in different spheres can naturalize them, especially when they influence the development of legal norms and are reflected in attitudes and practices of state agents. Its use hinders the exercise of rights and generates a climate of discrimination and defenselessness, justifying, in some cases, acts of violence, which maintains the status quo of subordination of women (Onofre de Alencar, 2015–2016, p. 26).

What partly explains the high level of violence against the female population is pointed out by Onofre de Alencar, clarifying that the legal norms reflect the acceptance of gender stereotypes. Often, they are included in the justification and content of a legal text. It is a way of perpetuating stereotypes by naturalizing them and legitimizing acts of discrimination. This practice shows the establishment of distinctions between men and women, especially in the family, placing women in a situation of subordination with respect to their husbands, which does not allow them to exercise control over relevant aspects of their lives (2015–2016, p. 36).

The stereotypes that permeate public institutions and state agents reflect the objectification and subordination of women related to their way of dressing, their work occupation, and their sexual experience and behavior. In addition, they do not allow an in-depth analysis of the facts of the case and the evidence,[37] because they focus more on the relationship with the aggressor, the reaction to the violence, and the veracity of the account of his aggression, especially when there are no witnesses or visible marks of violence (Onofre de Alencar, 2015–2016, p. 39). The IACHR has indicated that stereotypes have a negative impact on access to justice for women victims of violence. They affect the objectivity of State officials charged with investigating complaints, influencing their perception to determine whether an act of violence, in its assessment of the credibility of witnesses and of the victim herself, and in the evaluation of the evidence.[38]

Even though the facts speak for themselves, women are obligated to prove that there was violence and that it was not their fault. This handling of violence is extremely dangerous because it provides the perpetrator with an easy way out, which in part explains the high rate of femicides. According to the Colombian Femicide Observatory, in 2020 there were 630 femicides, and between January and Abril in 2021 there were 208 femicides.[39] Another problem is the extremely high demand of violence, but in effect only a few cases are attended in court. According to the Inter-American Commission on Human Rights (IACHR), it is especially important to investigate the facts and bring offenders to trial quickly, convict those responsible, and protect the victim and their family. Procedures should be based on a gender focus for the protection of the victim.[40]

Social workers can contribute realizing sensibilization workshops with public and private institutions that attend victims and decide about sentences referring to violence. Knowledge of social workers about special cases and challenges for women to get a fair trial, and the intensive contact with victims, can bring their difficult situation closer to the institutions. Demonstrating the numbers of femicides and explaining what is prevention work could save women's lives. Often women who are victims of violence ask for help,

[37]Wrongful gender stereotyping is a frequent cause of discrimination against women. It is a contributing factor in violations of a vast array of rights such as the right to health, adequate standard of living, education, marriage and family relations, work, freedom of expression, freedom of movement, political participation and representation, effective remedy, and freedom from gender-based violence. https://www.ohchr.org/en/issues/women/wrgs/pages/genderstereotypes.aspx. Accessed on 29 of May 2021.

[38]http://www.oas.org/es/cidh/informes/pdfs/violencia-discriminacion-mujeres-Anexo1-es.pdf, p.17, accessed on 28 May 2021.

[39]https://www.observatoriofeminicidioscolombia.org, accessed on 29 of May 2021.

[40]http://www.oas.org/en/iachr/media_center/PReleases/2020/074.asp, accessed on 12 of June 2020.

try to report violence, but state agents such as an attorney or the police do not believe them and thus they would not offer any help or solutions. And every woman not attended is a potential case of femicide. Nobody should take the risk to be responsible for another dead woman because of negligence. Consequently, social workers could help to prevent nonintegral decisions or sentences, showing typical stereotypes against women. Further, they can accompany and empower women to fight for their rights and not accept unequal treatments. They can as well strengthen families, including men, with sensibilization work, showing what domestic violence, women rights, equality, and so on mean. Unquestionably, it would be useful to organize social movements with women to influence in public politics to achieve gender-focused public policies that protect them from violence. To achieve social transformation, we must start in the family, in communities, in schools, in universities, and in public institutions. Women must understand themselves as subjects of law. Gender equality means that women, regardless of their stratum,[41] their race, their sexual and political orientation, can access the legal system the same as men.

The gender perspective must be included in the dominant or main culture of each institution to transform the patriarchal paradigm. Jaramillo says that "(…) by introducing gender as a social structure, men of flesh and blood ceased to be the main targets of attack, as well as women of flesh and blood ceased to be always the victims" (2009, p. 106).

17.4 Challenges for Social Work in Pandemic Times

Social work promotes, among the various collectives and social groups, the use of legislative and legal instruments that enable them to exercise citizenship as a mechanism for political participation, which leads to social inclusion through the exercise of power making qualified and informed decisions (Ramirez & Gómez, 2007, p. 101). For some reason, the prevailing approaches to care for violence against women have focused on individualized care and treatment, not prevention (ibid., p. 98). The idea of prevention work is to identify populations at risk, to identify risk factors and protection factors that avoid harmful effects. This intervention is based on values of democracy and human rights as ethical foundation, because professional action is oriented toward respecting the social and human rights of individuals and groups that experience degrading and discriminatory treatment (ibid., p. 99).

Social workers as human rights defenders are at the front door in direct contact with a vulnerable population. Normally they identify households exposed to more violence, because of the contact with victims. Thus, a social worker could act as a first alarm system, knowing the needs of this kind of people, and prevent violent situations. In a pandemic, it is fundamental to identify vulnerable population groups and offer them quick consultation.

In a pandemic, social workers can strengthen, support, and motivate victims to stand up for their lives, to report violence, search for shelter if necessary, and accompany them constantly

To begin preventive work, first, we must ensure that there are reliable statistics of the homes with previous violence, which will serve as the basis for monitoring in times of pandemic. Certainly, data collection and the privacy of victims could be a challenge in pandemic times. The essential point is the safety and privacy of victims, because if the violent offender notices the file charge, violence can lessen.[42] So perhaps a strategy of protection could be analyzing the first data recollected before the pandemic: probably the victims still need help and counseling.

The Convention on the Elimination of All Forms of Discrimination against Women

[41] In Colombia we have six Estratos (stratums), Estrato 1 belongs to the poorest and vulnerable people, Estrato 6 the richest.

[42] Violencia contra las mujeres y las niñas: La recopilación de datos en el contexto de COVID-19 (2020, 3). ONU Mujeres, Organización Mundial de Salud.

(CEDAW), as an international treaty adopted by the United Nations General Assembly, has the purpose of protecting and promoting respect for the rights of women. This convention is based on the concept of substantive equality, that focuses on the results and material impacts of gender laws and policies, as well as a support network, which provides direct and dynamic support and advice.

The social support received in the most difficult moments of a life can certainly change our world. Social support networks are a basic communication tool for women as victims of violence. In critical situations they become important resources that strengthen human resources and the mobilization of alternatives. Contact with the outside world is fundamental, and even more so in times of a pandemic, when most of the time they are locked up with the perpetrator. The creation of support networks for women in general, and specifically for victims of violence, is an important tool for their strengthening, and to create an alarm system and to prevent violence. These groups will work on issues related to stereotypes against women, emergency care, legal advice, gender equality, access to justice for women, shelters, regulations, restraining orders, and accompaniment to report violence, among others.

At a political level it is fundamental to design prevention and protecting programs for women and children, based on empirical bases that minimize risk in the pandemic and after, as well as:

> to design health emergency programs for pandemic that also are useful after. As well as the actualization/update of care routes to gender-based violence to reflect changes in access to services, support continuity of response comprehensive to sexual violence, and the spread of information on the rights and resources of GBV[43] survivors (2020, p. 4).[44]

Returning to the four UN issues, mentioned in Sect. 17.3, first, the network supports the awareness of society on the issue of gender equality: that means we must see women as a subject of rights, and ensure that these rights become material. This gender focus work should begin in schools, families, universities, and public entities, on radio, television, and other social networks. Second, the empowerment of women is required to prevent violence and combat sexism in societies such as the Colombian. Empowered and confident women will probably and hopefully end unequal and harmful relationships. For this, third, the security of having a paid job and long-term security, kindergartens, participation equal to the barons in political issues and positions, design of public policy—especially on issues regarding to gender—as well as knowledge and easy access to report violence, are needed. And finally, if women actively participate in public life, they automatically leave the private sphere of the family and will get attention having voice and a vote.

The pandemic shows clearly how unequal social structures disadvantage marginalized and vulnerable people even more. Social workers should participate actively in public policies because they are aware of the needs of marginalized populations. If social workers, with support of the government and civil society, could offer holistic attention that prevents hunger, marginalization, suffering, recruiting of minors, homelessness, and violence generally, the situation would change.

17.5 Conclusions and Recommendations

In relationship to the social context of Colombia, the ongoing armed conflict, social structures, and violence permeating the Colombian culture, institutions, and families for a long period, it will require some time to prevent and combat this structure. And it is not just about combating gender-based violence, but eradicating it, which means that we must identify causes of violence against women and search for protection mechanisms. To achieve real equality and prevent poverty, we need a transformation of society with equal access to resources. That ideal begins with

[43] Gender-based violence.

[44] Apoyo a la respuesta nacional en VBG en el contexto de la pandemia de COVID-19 (2020).

a basic income, protection and access to the healthcare system, social security at workplaces, education and study opportunities, political participation, and access to the labor market for all people.

In a pandemic, more than ever, women need low-threshold offers, "niedrigschwellige Angebote." To prevent, address, and punish violence against women and girls in the pandemic, the Colombian Government should strengthen their institutionality and capacity to quickly respond. Procedures for victims of violence should be more flexible and efficient. These women need psychological care, shelters for themselves and their children, consultation, kindergartens, and money. Civil society and women's organizations can participate in public policy decisions with a gender focus and human rights perspective. The implementation of agreed measures should reach all sectors of population and all areas of the country. When States fail and cannot offer protection for victims of violence, NGOs can support victims through medical and psychological assistance and advice. Even in the presence of the State, victims may feel more comfortable and more trusting with the civil society. Local protection networks in the community help to prepare and strengthen victims for trial.

A particularly influential point in women's access to justice, highlighted by CEDAW, is the concept of substantive equality, which focuses on the material outcomes and impacts of gender laws and policies. "(...) laws mean little unless they are implemented. It is essential to draft laws that enable their effective implementation, with clear mandates and procedures for those providing the services, as well as integrated accountability and adequate financing mechanisms" (UN Women, 2011–2012, p. 45). Therefore, the State has the responsibility and duty to create substantive equality through (1) the elimination of historically determined male paradigms (Art. 5), (2) to accelerate the attainment of equality through temporary special measures (Art. 4.1), and (3) to create an environment in which women can live free from violence.

The best recipe to prevent violence against women is through campaigns and a specific public policy, creating access to justice in an uncomplicated way and constant accompaniment. That plan implicates agents in communities, villages, and municipalities who help victims taking their cases to the municipality's institutions. Women should actively participate in the definition and application of justice, to combat discrimination and demand substantive results. In the same way, the cases should be followed up, ensuring that the perpetrators cannot continue to exercise their power over women.

Solidarity in community and neighborhood care as a social help network can mitigate the traumatic effects of the pandemic as well.

References

Jaramillo, I. (2009). La crítica feminista al derecho. In *Género y derecho*, Santiago de Chile, American University/ILANUD; Ediciones La Morada.

Meertens, D. (2011). *La dimensión de género en el desplazamiento interno: respuestas institucionales en el caso colombiano. Yearbook on Humanitarian Action and Human Rights* (pp. 41–52). Universidad de Deusto. ISSN: 1885-298X.

Mujer, S. (2020). *La pandemia antes del Covid-19. Violencias hacia las Mujeres y Niñas en Colombia durante 2019 y 2020* (Boletín No. 22). Corporación Sisma Mujer, Colombia.

Nota Macroeconómica. (2020). *Efectos en pobreza y desigualdad del Covid-19 en Colombia: un retroceso de dos décadas*. Facultad de Economía, Universidad de los Andes.

Obando, A. E. (1999). Las interpretaciones del derecho. In *Género y derecho*, Santiago de Chile, American University/ILANUD; Ediciones La Morada.

Onofre de Alencar, E. (2015). Mujeres y estereotipos de género en la jurisprudencia de la Corte Interamericana de Derechos Humanos. Eunomía. *Revista en Cultura de la Legalidad, 9*, 26–48.

ONU Mujeres. (2011) 2011-2012. *El progreso de las mujeres en el mundo*. En busca de la justicia. Naciones Unidas.

ONU Mujeres. (2019). *El progreso de las mujeres en el mundo 2019-2020* . Familias en un mundo cambiante. Naciones Unidas.

ONU Mujeres, Entidad de las Naciones Unidas para la Igualdad de Género y el Empoderamiento de las Mujeres, Departamento Administrativo Nacional de Estadísticas (DANE), & Consejería Presidencial para la Equidad de la Mujer (CPEM). (2020). *Brechas de Género en Colombia*. Resumen ejecutivo.

Ramirez, M. H., & Gómez, J. C. (2007). *La intervención del trabajo social en la prevención de la violencia contra las mujeres*. Revista del Departamento de Trabajo Social, Facultad de Ciencias Humanas, Universidad Nacional de Colombia.

Ramirez, N., Tribin, A. M., & Vargas, C. (2015). *Maternity and labor markets: Impact of legislation in Colombia*. Inter-American Development Bank. Andean Group. IV. Title. V. Series. IDB-WP-583. Colombia.

Ravallion, M., Datt, G., & van de Walle, D. (1991). *Quantifying absolute poverty in the developing world*. Wiley Online Library. https://doi.org/10.1111/j.1475-4991.1991.tb00378.x.

Redondo-Sama, G., Matulic, V., Munté-Pascual, A., & de Vicente, I. (2020). Social work during the COVID-19 crisis: Responding to urgent social needs. *Sustainability, 12*, 8595. https://doi.org/10.3390/su12208595. https://www.mdpi.com/2071-1050/12/20/8595

Romero Prieto, J. (2018). *La maternidad y el empleo formal en Colombia. Documentos de trabajo sobre economía regional y urbana*. Banco de la República, Centro de Estudios Económicos Regionales (CEER). Núm. 268. Cartagena.

Serret, E. (2006). *Discriminación de género. Las inconsecuencias de la democracia. Cuadernos de Igualdad No. 6*. Consejo Nacional para prevenir la discriminación, México.

Part II

Strategies and Responses in Social Work: Globally and Locally

18 Ecuador's and Iran's Response to Protect Refugees and Migrants in Vulnerable Situations During the COVID-19 Pandemic

Cesar Castilla and Samaneh Kachouie

18.1 Introduction

At the end of December 2020, 83 million people worldwide had been infected with COVID-19, and more than 1.8 million had died of the virus (Corona Virus Resource Centre – JHU, 2020). The COVID-19 pandemic had dire consequences for the world economy. The International Monetary Fund's forecasting issued in October 2020 envisioned a −4.4% drop in global gross domestic product (GDP) because of confinement and a new normal imposed in different regions, including both Latin America and the Middle East, with an expected −8.1% and −4.1% fall, respectively, for this year (IMF, 2020). Given these figures, the outlook does not look very encouraging, especially for migrants in vulnerable situations.

At the beginning of the pandemic, several countries, including those that have applied an open-door migration policy, had to close their air and land borders. Besides, states implemented a curfew, which caused the Venezuelan and Afghan diaspora to consider the idea of returning to their countries. Both Venezuelans living in Ecuador and the Afghan in Iran became seriously affected by the measures adopted to face the pandemic. Especially when the migrant's mobility in different cities became dramatically restricted, and most of these migrants need to work daily on the streets for surviving

Given this situation, Ecuador and Iran have adopted some actions in response to the crisis unleashed by COVID-19, all aiming at easing the suffering of these migrants.

This chapter seeks to answer the following research question: What was the response of the Ecuadorian and Iranian states to protect Venezuelan and Afghan migrants, respectively, during the COVID-19 crisis?

18.2 Part I: A Look at the Situation of Migrants and Refugees in Ecuador and Iran Before and During the Pandemic

Ecuador and Iran are developing countries and share something in common. Both nations enjoy great geostrategic importance, innumerable natural resources, oil-dependent economies, and open their borders for those who escaped from conflicts. Ecuadorian State has experience dealing with the Colombian refugees and migrants and currently with the Venezuelan diaspora. The Islamic Republic of Iran, since its foundation in

C. Castilla (✉)
CLACSO's Research Group in the Middle East and North of Africa, Buenos Aires, Argentina
e-mail: ccpublications99@gmail.com

S. Kachouie
Kish - International Campus, University of Tehran (UT-KIC), Kish, Iran
e-mail: kachouie.samaneh@ut.ac.ir

M. C. S. Gonçalves et al. (eds.), *The Coronavirus Crisis and Challenges to Social Development*,
https://doi.org/10.1007/978-3-030-84678-7_18

April 1979, has welcomed Iraqi and Afghan citizens for more than four decades.

These two countries have stood out for their solidarity, especially with migrants and refugees fleeing conflict. Ecuador has become the first country in Latin America with the largest refugee population at the beginning of the twenty-first century. This country has mainly welcomed Colombian citizens escaping the internal conflict (UNHCR, Fact Sheet Ecuador, 2020c). Ecuador is home to nearly 70,000 recognised refugees, and 97% are from Colombia (Pugh et al., 2020). From 2015 to the present, this Andean country has welcomed more than 400,000 Venezuelans, including refugees, migrants, and an estimate of people who have entered through informal steps (IOM-UNHCR, 2020). The Islamic Republic of Iran is home to one of the largest urban refugee populations in the world and has been hosting refugees for four decades. In Iran, there are about 980,000 documented refugees, mostly Afghans (97%) and Iraqis (3%), supported by the UN Refugee Agency (UNHCR, Fact Sheet Iran, 2020d). However, more than 2.5 million undocumented Afghans are living in the Persian country (UNHCR, 2020a, b, c, d, e, f, g).

Since the adoption of a new political constitution in October 2008, Ecuador applied a novel approach to human mobility during the Rafael Correa administration. As a result, Ecuador has become one of the most important references in the field of Human Mobility at a regional level. Notwithstanding, the administration of President Lenin Moreno required a visa for Venezuelan citizens entering Ecuadorian territory. Regulations came into force on 26 August 2019. For this reason, Venezuelan citizens must apply for a tourist, humanitarian, or other visa shown within the Organic Law of Human Mobility of Ecuador (Ministry of Government of Ecuador, 2019). At the beginning of 2020, more than five million people would have left Venezuela (EEAS, 2020), and most of them had settled in countries such as Colombia, Peru, Chile, Argentina, and Ecuador (IOM-UNHCR, 2020).

At the beginning of the COVID-19 pandemic, the concern of Venezuelan migrants living in Ecuador began on the night of Monday, 16 March 2020; when President Lenin Moreno declared a State of Exception to the Ecuadorian territory because of the pandemic: "If we do not nip the problem in the bud, we can have over 800,000 infected people." Besides, he added that "No one infected will enter our borders" (Ministry of Government of Ecuador, 2020). Later, he added he would extend the curfew from 14:00 p.m. until 5:00 a.m. from Wednesday, 25 March (General Secretariat of the Presidency of Ecuador, 2020), which lasted until 3 June, when it changed from 18:00 p.m. to 5:00 a.m. This order affected the migrant labour aspect as their status as regular or irregular required them to work daily on the streets.

Against this background, the economic situation of Venezuelan migrants, which was already critical before the beginning of the pandemic, became drastically affected. About 80% of Venezuelan refugees and asylum seekers interviewed at the regional level by UNHCR in 2019 stated that they were working with no contractual agreement. Most of these migrants depended on the informal economy to survive (UNHCR, 2020a, b, c, d, e, f, g). In Ecuador, 65% of the 161,761 Venezuelan citizens that make up the Biometric Registry do not have any job (Ministry of Foreign Affairs and Human Mobility of Ecuador, 2020).

Because of the problems affecting the Venezuelan diaspora throughout the region, the budget of the RMRP 2020 (Regional Refugee and Migrant Response Plan) has increased from 1.35 to 1.41 billion dollars. The third part of this budget is for specific COVID-19 activities to help refugees and migrants in precarious situations, especially those in urgent need of food, shelter, and health services (EEAS, 2020).

The Islamic Republic of Iran has become one of the most relevant homes for refugees in the past four decades. Since the occupation of Afghanistan by the Soviet Red Army in late 1979, Iran has hosted millions of Afghan refugees. According to published statistics, about 4% of Iran's population are Afghan immigrants, and the number of legal and illegal immigrants in the country reaches three million people. In this way, Iran has provided various sanitary, medical, and educational facilities. Immigrants mostly live in Kerman, Khorasan Razavi, Yazd, Tehran, Isfahan, Bushehr, Fars, Sistan, and Baluchistan (IRNA, 2020).

Including during the Iran-Iraq war (1980–1988) and subsequent problems such as the US sanctions against the Persian country, Iran tried to provide services to Afghans, including education and health. Regarding education issues, according to an order issued by Iran's Supreme Leader Ayatollah Syed Ali Khamenei in 2015, Iranian schools should enrol all migrant Afghan children living in Iran, including those undocumented (Mashregh News, 2015).

Concerning health issues, the ongoing dialogue between UNHCR and Iran's government counterparts has been productive. Both sides have agreed to expand universal health coverage. The Government of the Islamic Republic of Iran has covered the health of refugees from Afghanistan and Iraq. The decision came into force in May 2015 with the signing of a memorandum of understanding between the Ministers of the Interior, Health and Welfare (Ministry of Health and Medical Education of the Islamic Republic of Iran, 2018). As do Iranians, Afghan migrants have also faced economic problems because of restrictions imposed on some jobs under the Government measures to prevent the spread of the pandemic.

18.3 Part II: Common Actions Adopted by Ecuador and Iran to Protect the Migrant and Refugee Population in the Framework of the COVID-19 Pandemic

To identify the common actions taken by Ecuador and Iran to protect the migrants in vulnerable situations during the COVID-19 pandemic, we have classified these in terms of migration, welfare, and international cooperation.

18.3.1 In the Migration Field

The Ecuadorian State showed flexibility concerning the regularisation of Venezuelan migrants. For this reason, the government implemented a Biometric Registry allowed by the Supreme Decree No. 826 of July 25, 2019. To accomplish this goal, the Ecuadorian State adopted an executive decree and two ministerial agreements during the first months of the health emergency. The Ministerial Agreement No. 035 of March 19, 2020, which in its second article provides: "Extend, since March 19 2020, and for the duration of the health emergency, the terms that are running or those that have expired as of that date, so that foreigners can stay in Ecuador…" (Chancellery of Ecuador, 2020a, b).

Ecuadorian State also adopted Executive Decree No. 1020 of 23 March 2020 to extend the amnesty and regularisation on humanitarian grounds for Venezuelans who entered Ecuador illegally (Chancellery of Ecuador, 2020a, b). The government finally adopted Ministerial Agreement No. 006, of 13 April 2020. It established the "Procedure for the regularisation of foreigners, parents of Ecuadorian children and adolescents, who have not registered their entry through the official immigration control points." This initiative aims to help migrants, mainly Venezuelan citizens living in Ecuador, but in an irregular migratory status (Chancellery of Ecuador, 2020a, b).

According to the Coordination Platform for Refugees and Migrants from Venezuela (R4V), until August 19, 2020, Ecuador had granted 178,246 residence permits. This platform also shows that, as of 16 September 2020, 417,199 Venezuelans were in Ecuadorian territory. This figure includes Venezuelan refugees and migrants, plus an estimate of people who would have entered through informal steps (IOM-UNHCR, 2020).

Because of these actions, the Ecuadorian State achieved the creation of the Biometric Registry. It meant access data of 161,761 Venezuelan citizens, of whom 38,243 can get the Exception Visas for Humanitarian Reasons (VERHU)

(Ministry of Foreign Affairs and Human Mobility of Ecuador, 2020).

Simultaneously, during the Nowruz holidays and the beginning of the pandemic, the repatriation of Afghan refugees in Iran increased between March and April 2020. Both the Iranian ministry of internal and foreign affairs refused to issue visas to those suspected of being infected with COVID-19. As a result, Iran prohibited the re-entry of expelled citizens into the country. Iran announced the closure of borders by the Afghan government and, in addition, decided the prohibition of the repatriation of Afghans in the first days of the expansion of the coronavirus. Then Iran contacted the Afghan side to accept the return of its citizens to their homeland (Poursohein, 2020).

18.3.2 In the Welfare Field

In the same way, Ecuador and Iran have worked on welfare to protect Venezuelan and Afghan migrants, respectively. Ecuador has not adopted an exclusive policy focused on Venezuelan migrants. Notwithstanding, they benefited when the Ministry of Economic and Social Inclusion (MIES) enabled 33 temporary emerging shelters to serve people in vulnerable situations (CMV, 2020). Besides the social bonus granted by the Ecuadorian state to people in vulnerable situations, another implemented welfare mechanism has been the delivery of food kits. In this manner, Ecuador has benefited those Venezuelan migrants that appear in the social registry, without regard to nationality (EFE, 2020).

Iran intended to establish public health insurance for the benefit of all refugees. It should cover about 100,000 vulnerable groups, especially patients, using the free medical services brochure with the financial support of the UNHCR and the Islamic Republic of Iran. This country has also tried to prevent the spread of the coronavirus among refugees by actively detecting the disease and making available free treatment for those infected by COVID-19, among the measures carried out by Iran's interior ministry (Mehr News, 2020).

The spokesperson of the Iranian government, Ali Rabiei, stated we established seven health centres in Tehran during the current context of the coronavirus outbreak, where Afghan and Iraqi immigrants live. Iran does not discriminate between Iranians and immigrants in terms of treatment. Similarly, officials of the Ministry of Health and Medical Education said around one million Afghan immigrants, and between 2.5 and three million undocumented Afghan immigrants, have received the same medical care as the Iranian population (IRNA, 2020).

In addition, the Iranian government carried out the plan to detect those migrants infected by the coronavirus in the areas inhabited by Afghans, such as the Shahr-e Rey district (southern Tehran). In this zone live more than 150,000 Afghans registered by the Ministry of Health system (IRNA, 2020).

18.3.3 In the Field of International Cooperation

The Ecuadorian Foreign Ministry negotiated with national public institutions and the delegation of the European Union in Ecuador to get financial support through Team Europe for an amount of US$37 million (Chancellery of Ecuador, 2020a, b). Among the initiatives framed in this project, the Northern Border project stands out, which indirectly benefits Venezuelan refugees or migrants. However, a second phase of the Europe-Ecuador Package is expected, with new resources to work on water and sanitation, risk management, migration, and economic recovery (Delegation of the European Union to Ecuador, 2020).

The Ecuadorian Foreign Ministry has also attempted to boost multilateral cooperation by relying on international organisations to protect migrants in vulnerable situations, such as the International Organization for Migration (IOM). It provided accommodation kits, medical and hygiene supplies. In the same way, UNHCR provided 2000 food kits, triage tents, adaptation of shelters, and donation of cleaning supplies. It also provides technical assistance through 15 experts to care for migrants in vulnerable conditions (Chancellery of Ecuador, 2020a, b).

The Ecuadorian State has coordinated with foreign embassies and consulates the organisation of humanitarian flights for the return of their nationals. Concerning Venezuelan citizens, until May 2020, there were more than 17,000 registered in their Consulate in Quito for repatriation (EFE, 2020). However, the repatriation flights continued even in November 2020. The Ecuadorian Foreign Ministry coordinated with the Venezuelan consulates in Guayaquil and Quito. As a result, they agreed to six flights for transferring Venezuelan citizens living in vulnerable situations. Both sides agreed to cover the cost of the free PCR test (Velez, 2020).

The economic conditions resulting from the sanctions against Iran have left their impact on the migrant community. It has also influenced their desire to return to Afghanistan or emigrate to other countries. However, UNHCR has also acknowledged that the Iranian government has generously included refugees in its national programs to fight against COVID-19, including free testing, treatment, and hospitalisation. Notwithstanding, there is still an urgent need for more support from the international community. Thus, UNHCR can provide more to the Iranian government and host society in supporting refugees. It happens while the Iranian government and UNHCR are looking for more ways to assist the growing number of refugees struggling to meet their needs. Until October 2020, UNHCR has received only 36% of the US$99.9 million that is needed for supporting refugees and host communities (UNHCR, 2020a, b, c, d, e, f, g).

18.4 Part III: Analysis of the Measures of the Ecuadorian and Iranian States Implemented for Protecting Venezuelan and Afghan Migrants During the COVID-19 Pandemic

During this crisis, many governments have adopted an approach conceiving the pandemic generated by COVID-19 as a matter of national security. Stefan Elbe states, "The epidemics have exotic names and enigmatic acronyms, and they are fast becoming too many to list—like HIV/AIDS, SARS, H5N1, H1N1, Middle East respiratory syndrome (MERS), Ebola, and Zika. Together they have made the question of how to better protect populations against lethal infectious disease outbreaks politically much more urgent. Governments now take such outbreaks so seriously that they even consider them as threats to national and international security" (Elbe, 2018). For this reason, some states have closed their borders, believing that this would stop the contagion.

However, most decision makers never have considered that this measure could seriously damage migrants in vulnerable situations. Given that, there was no immediate response from the States to ease their economic, social, or health problems. Notwithstanding, Ecuador and Iran closed their borders. But their humanitarian approach and engagement with people in human mobility have immediately reacted to protect refugees and migrants in their territories.

The humanitarian approach of Ecuador has its origin in the Quechua word "Sumaq Kawsay" (good living), which is the principal focus of its 2008 Constitution. It is a worldview and legacy of the original Andean peoples. Concerning the Islamic Republic of Iran, this derives mainly from the basis of Islam established on its Constitution of 1979 that underlines the principles of freedom and human dignity.

Regarding the response of the Ecuadorian state at the migration level, this relies on the Ministerial Agreement No. 035 adopted on March 19, 2020, the Executive Decree N°1020 issued on March 2?, 2020, and Ministerial Agreement No. 006 adopted on 13 April 2020. It allowed granting 178,246 residence permits and regular stay for Venezuelan citizens during the pandemic. It has also helped to build a biometric registry with Venezuelan citizen data.

At the welfare level, the Ecuadorian administration did not adopt any measure toward Venezuelans directly. However, the installation of 33 shelters by the Ministry of Economic and

Social Inclusion (MIES) attended to people in vulnerable situations, among them Venezuelans. In addition, The State granted subsidies through the Human Development Bonus, supplemented by the delivery of food kits.

This humanitarian measure indirectly benefited Venezuelan migrants, because many of them are in a particular state of need, and they must resort to begging in the worst case. According to MIES figures, until December 2019, the 29.77% of people in a state of begging were foreigners in human mobility (Machado, 2020). At the international cooperation level, the Ecuadorian government just got donations from UNHCR and IOM for people in human mobility.

Regarding Iran, despite the economic problems, because of the US policy of maximum pressure imposed by the Trump administration, which aims to strangle the Iranian economy, this country has also adopted measures to protect refugees and migrants in vulnerable situations during the COVID-19 pandemic. Notwithstanding, there is a pleasant disposition from the Iranian authorities to protect Afghan refugees and migrants. It includes the Iranian support for voluntary repatriation coordinated with the Afghan authorities during the COVID-19 crisis.

However, it is worth mentioning that the public health insurance for the refugees will cover 100,000 vulnerable groups. It would help prevent the spread of the coronavirus among refugees by detecting the disease in time and allowing them to access treatment in case of being infected. In addition, another action took place with the opening of seven health centres in Tehran for those who need to benefit from this service. Regarding international cooperation, there was a joint effort between UNHCR and the Bureau for Aliens and Foreign Immigrants Affairs under the Ministry of Interior (BAFIA) to get funds to protect refugees and migrants.

In contrast, some countries in the Northern Hemisphere, such as the United States, did not care about protecting refugees and migrants in vulnerable situations. The conditions of illegal migrants worsened during the administration of President Trump. Since the beginning of the pandemic, this became much more complicated. "Tens of thousands of people remain in immigration detention despite the high risk of COVID-19 transmission in crowded jails, prisons, and detention centres that US Immigration and Customs Enforcement (ICE) uses to hold noncitizens. The pandemic led to the suspension of many immigration court hearings and limited the functioning of the few courts which remain open or reopened. Meanwhile, Congress left millions of immigrants and their families out of legislative relief, leaving many people struggling to stay afloat in a time of economic uncertainty" (Loweree et al., 2020a, b).

Concerning the European countries, the situation for migrants became complicated. Another example is France, where there was less support of the migrant population in vulnerable situations. In this sense, the head of the migration service of the "Catholic Committee against Hunger and Development"—CCFD Terre Solidaire, Nina Marx, stated, "Currently, this is true that vulnerable populations, especially migrants, become the Forgotten of this health crisis that invades France. We can see this in the shelters for migrant workers, where people live in overcrowded situations, which makes confinement impossible and that privileges the condition of the virus" (Marx, 2020).

If we wanted to compare the situation with some countries in the Northern Hemisphere, we would immediately know that the actions undertaken by Ecuador and Iran allowed protecting refugees and migrants. Despite the economic and financial problems in recent years, those nations from the Global South have allocated domestic and international funds to protect migrants in the middle of this global pandemic. After analysing the response of Ecuador and Iran to protect people in human mobility, we can affirm that the most efficient way has been the welfare actions. In case of a recent wave of COVID-19 or any other health emergency, both nations should reinforce their welfare actions by focusing on social work.

18.5 Discussion

An efficient approach to social work helps people finding positive ways forward in the challenges to face in their lives. In addition, it paves the way to build environments in which they want to live. Therefore, it promotes social change through social cohesion and targeting the liberation of the people (International Federation of Social Worker, 2014). Malcolm Payne points out three views of social work objectives: Empowerment, Problem Solving, and Social Change. Perhaps this latter becomes the most important because it seeks a synergy based on social cohesion. "These see social work as seeking cooperation and mutual support in society so that the most oppressed and disadvantaged people can gain power over their own lives. Social work facilitates this by enabling people to take part in a process of learning and cooperation that creates institutions which everyone can own and take part in" (Payne, 2014). And to achieve this, it is mandatory to get the cohesion between the key actors such as the state, NGOs, Institutions (private and public), civil society, and migrants. In this way, people in situations of human mobility not only well be eligible for aid but empowered to achieve true emancipation.

After the pandemic COVID-19, governments must strengthen their approach to political and critical social work. Political-social work paves the way to set up a mechanism where the decision-making process aims to optimal social change. For this reason, states must build public policies that promote the good practice of social work, which plays a transcendental role as a facilitator between the state and society. In this sense, specialist in public policy Professor John Forester argues, "to make new things happen, and to discover what can be done effectively in politically uncertain environments, you have to learn and to learn it is necessary to ask questions and listen carefully, where we become "planners" and policy analysts in the broadest sense" (Forester, 2006). It is a muss to elaborate efficiently public policies with and an optimal level of institutionalisation. It can privilege political-social work to improve the quality of life of those migrants in vulnerable conditions. Also, we should implement a mechanism of control to evaluate the outcomes of those practices. "Assessment is at the heart of all good social work practice. It covers a spectrum of activities, from observation and judgments made within the context of an initial encounter through to more formal and complex frameworks of assessment" (Watson & West, 2006).

Apart from the agenda of governments, it is necessary to strengthen the practices of social work carried out by the universities through social cohesion. The research projects related to social work at university departments are precious because of the student collaboration. They can understand better the needs of marginalised groups, especially refugees or migrants in vulnerable situations.

Critical social work comprises empowering the "forgotten people" and makes visible those hidden in social structures. In this manner, the Iranian journalist Faranak Bakhtiari considers important the role of social work in this health crisis. Given that people have faced situations of fear and anxiety because of the isolation during this pandemic, the importance of social work is increasing. It is worth mentioning that the role of social workers has been essential to support people in vulnerable situations. In this sense, they have promoted social solidarity (Bakhtiari, 2020).

To conclude, the challenges of political and critical social work are the lack of financial aid. The countries in the Global South do not have the resources to invest in an optimal social change. Most of the time, this latter is a victim of populism. It is clear, the nonexistence of a mechanism for evaluation of outcomes to measure the progress of the social work practices becomes a major barrier. Another challenge is the bureaucracy of public institutions because this does not allow approaching people in need: and the absence of social cohesion, given that some nondemocratic governments cannot work with private institutions and other social actors.

18.6 Conclusions

At the end of 2020, we have witnessed that this pandemic has reconfigured the way of life. Losing loved ones and a fragile world economy has been the ultimate result. Most of the migrants lost their jobs or could not go out to work on the streets because of restrictive measures such as the curfew, caused by many trying to return to their countries, crossing closed borders through illegal passages or even losing their lives in the attempt.

To answer the research question and subsequently analyse the response of Ecuador and Iran during the COVID-19 crises, we classified actions in terms of migration, welfare, and international cooperation. Among them, the most relevant activities are welfare actions. It is the fastest way to ease the suffering of migrants.

This pandemic brought out the humanitarian aspect of some states and the indifference of others towards those migrants in situations of need. In contrast, the rich countries based in the Northern Hemisphere did little or nothing to protect migrants and refugees during this global pandemic. Both Ecuador and Iran enjoy an excellent reputation for tradition and experience in human mobility at the international level. In this sense, the actions undertaken by those nations are something to be highlighted, despite economic and social crises affecting them in recent years.

However, those countries should empower their approach to political and critical social work. First, both countries must increase the budget destined for their social work programmes. Their social work approach must be more pragmatic, aiming for an optimal social change through social cohesion. This change will create new social work practices aiming to promote greater inclusion, especially for those migrants who are in vulnerable situations. Both States must consider that social work emancipates people from the moment that empowers them and addresses inclusion within society.

References

Bakhtiari, F. (2020). Social work's vital role in fight against pandemic. *Tehran Times* 1–7, December 8.

Chancellery of Ecuador. (2020a). *Press Release*. https://www.cancilleria.gob.ec/2020/06/18/ayuda-humanitaria-y-cooperacion-internacional-frente-a-la-covid-19/

Chancellery of Ecuador. (2020b). *Press Release*. Quito, Pichincha, Ecuador. https://www.cancilleria.gob.ec/2020/06/18/extranjeros-migrantes-y-refugiados-tambien-fueron-preocupacion-de-la-cancilleria-durante-la-emergencia-sanitaria-de-la-covid-19

CMV. (2020). They give help to those who live in a situation of begging. *El Mercurio*. https://ww2.elmercurio.com.ec/2020/04/01/dan-ayuda-a-quienes-viven-en-situacion-de-mendicidadessed

Corona Virus Resource Centre (JHU). (2020). Corona Virus Resource Centre, JHU. https://coronavirus.jhu.edu/map.html.

Delegation of the European Union to Ecuador. (2020). Delegation of the European Union to Ecuador. *Press Release*. https://eeas.europa.eu/delegations/ecuador/80663/

EEAS. (2020). *EEAS*. https://eeas.europa.eu/headquarters/headquarters-homepage/79328/donors-conference-solidarity-venezuelan-refugees-and-migrants-countries-region-amid-covid-19_en.

EFE. (2020). Ecuador acknowledges concern about the transit of those who return to Venezuela. *El Nacional*. https://www.elnacional.com/mundo/ecuador-reconoce-inquietud-sobre-transito-de-los-que-regresan-a-venezuela/

Elbe, S. (2018). *Pandemics, pills and politics: Governing global health and security*. JHU Press.

Forester, J. (2006). Policy analysis as critical listening. In M. Moran, M. Rein, & R. Goodin (Eds.), *The Oxford handbook of public policy*. Oxford University Press.

General Secretariat of the Presidency of Ecuador. (2020). *From Wednesday, March 25, the curfew in the country runs between 2:00 p.m. and 5:00 a.m.* Quito, Pichincha, Ecuador. https://www.comunicacion.gob.ec/desde-el-miercoles-25-de-marzo-el-toque-de-queda-en-el-pais-se-extiende-entre-1400-y-0500/#:~:text=%E2%80%93%20Desde%20el%20d%C3%ADa%20mi%C3%A9rcoles%2025,de%20la%20Rep%C3%BAblica%2C%20Len%C3%ADn%20Moreno

IMF. (2020). *World Economic Outlook*, October 2020, New York. https://www.imf.org/en/Publications/WEO/Issues/2020/09/30/world-economic-outlook-october-2020

International Federation of Social Workers. (2014). *Global definition of social work*. https://www.ifsw.org/global-definition-of-social-work

IOM-UNHCR. (2020). *R4V*. https://r4v.info/en/situations/platform.

IRNA. (2020). IRNA. *Astanha va khdmata keh beh penahjwaan afghan araah mi shawad (Provinces and services provided to Afghan asylum seekers)*. https://www.irna.ir/news/83835255

Loweree, J., Reichlin-Melnick, A., & Ewing, W. (2020a). American Immigration Council. Obtenido de tens of thousands of people remain in immigration detention despite the high risk of COVID-19 transmission in crowded jails, prisons, and detention centers that U.S. Immigration and Customs Enforcement (ICE) uses to hold noncitizens.

Loweree, J., Reichlin-Melnick, A., & Ewing, W. (2020b). *American Immigration Council*. https://www.americanimmigrationcouncil.org/research/impact-covid-19-us-immigration-system.

Machado, J. (2020). *Primicias*. https://www.primicias.ec/noticias/sociedad/mendicidad-pobreza-secuela-coronavirus-pandemia

Marx, N. (2020). *Coronavirus and migrants, what is France doing?* Paris, France. CCFD-Terre Solidaire: https://ccfd-terresolidaire.org/actualites/covid-19/coronavirus-et-migrants-6584

Mashregh News. (2015). *Mashregh News*. News (2020) Mashregh News, Tehran.

Mehr News. (2020). https://www.mehrnews.com/news/5042059

Ministry of Foreign Affairs and Human Mobility of Ecuador. (2020). *Results of the immigration registration process and the issuance of VERHU Visas*. Quito, Pichincha, Ecuador: MREMH. https://www.youtube.com/watch?v=x6i5VSjTdWY

Ministry of Government of Ecuador. (2019). *The visa for Venezuelan citizens entered into force*. Quito, Pichincha, Ecuador. Ministry of Foreign Affairs and Human Mobility: https://www.ministeriodegobierno.gob.ec/entro-en-vigencia-el-visado-para-ciudadanos-venezolanos/

Ministry of Government of Ecuador. (2020). *President Lenín Moreno decrees a State of Exception to prevent the spread of COVID-19*. Quito, Pichincha, Ecuador. https://www.comunicacion.gob.ec/el-presidente-lenin-moreno-decreta-estado-de-excepcion-para-evitar-la-propagacion-del-covid-19/

Ministry of Health and Medical Education of the Islamic Republic of Iran. (2018). *Press Release*. Tehran, Iran. https://behdasht.gov.ir/%EF%BA%8E%EF%BA%A8%EF%BA%91%EF%BA%8D%EF%BA%AD-%EF%BA%8E%EF%BA%A3%EF%BA%98%EF%BA%BB%EF%BA%8E%EF%BA%BB%DB%8C/%D8%B4%DE%8C%D9%88%D9%87-%D8%AB%D8%A8%D8%AA-%D9%86%D8%A7%D9%85-%D9%88-%D8%B5%D8%AF%D9%88%D8%B1-%D8%AF%D9%81%D8%AA%D8%B1%DA%8

Payne, M. (2014). *Modern social work theory* (5th ed.). Palgrave Macmillan.

Poursohein, R. (2020). *Borna News*. https://www.borna.news/%D8%A8%D8%AE%D8%B4-%D8%A7%D8%AC%D8%AA%D9%85%D8%A7%D8%B9%DB%8C-4/997395-%D8%A8%D8%A7%D8%B2%DA%AF%D8%B4%D8%AA-%D9%85%D9%87%D8%A7%D8%AC%D8%B1%D8%A7%D9%86-%D8%A7%D9%81%D8%BA%D8%A7%D9%86-%D8%A8%D9%87-%DA%A9%D8%B4%D9%88%D8%B1-%D9%BE%D8%B3

Pugh, J. D., Jimenez, L. F., & Latuff, B. (2020). *Welcome wears thin for Colombians in Ecuador as Venezuelans become more visible*. MPI: https://www.migrationpolicy.org/article/welcome-wears-thin-for-colombians-ecuador

UNHCR. (2020a). *UNHCR*. https://www.unhcr.org/news/briefing/2020/5/5eabdc134/displaced-people-urgently-need-aid-access-social-safety-nets-coronavirus.html

UNHCR. (2020b). https://www.unhcr.org/ir/fa/refugees-in-iran/

UNHCR. (2020c). *Fact Sheet Ecuador*. New York. https://reporting.unhcr.org

UNHCR. (2020d). *Fact Sheet Iran*. New York. https://www.unhcr.org/ir/wp-content/uploads/sites/77/2020/05/UNHCR-Monthly-Factsheet-IRAN_Jan-Mar-2020-Eng.pdf

UNHCR. (2020e). *Refugees in Iran*. UNHCR. https://www.unhcr.org: https://www.unhcr.org/ir/wp-content/uploads/sites/77/2020/05/UNHCR-Monthly-Factsheet-IRAN_Jan-Mar-2020-Eng.pdf

UNHCR. (2020f). *UNHCR*. UNHCR: https://www.unhcr.org/ir/fa/refugees-in-iran

UNHCR. (2020g). *UNHCR*. https://www.unhcr.org/ir/fa/2020/10/13/unhcr-covid19-gift-cards

Velez, R. (2020). *El Comercio*. https://www.elcomercio.com/actualidad/ecuador-venezuela-vuelos-humanitarios-pandemia.html

Watson, D., & West, J. (2006). *Social work process and practice: Approaches, knowledge and skills*. Macmillan Education.

"Am I an Essential Worker?" COVID-19 and (Re)shaping of the Social Work Profession in Uganda

19

Laban Kashaija Musinguzi, Janestic Twikirize, Agnes Kyamulabi, and Denis Muhangi

19.1 Introduction

Following the declaration of COVID-19 as a global pandemic on 11 March 2020 (WHO, 2020; Cucinotta & Vanelli, 2020),[1] several countries instituted varying degrees of prevention and control measures. Uganda, as did other countries, introduced a national lockdown, closed education institutions and places of worship, and restricted nonessential travel (Nakkazi, 2020). Besides the universally adopted behavior change measures of social distancing, hand-washing, use of hand sanitisers, and wearing of face masks (MoH, 2020), the government embarked on a mass awareness campaign about COVID-19 including messages on signs and symptoms, prevention measures, management of the symptoms, and guidelines on self-isolation, among others (MoH, 2020).[2] These measures were justified on the premise that they would contain the spread of the virus, save people's lives, and prevent overwhelming an already fragile and ill-equipped healthcare system. By 30 January 2021, Uganda had a recorded cumulative total of 39,188 cases and 318 confirmed deaths (MoH, 2021).

One of the critical COVID-19 control and prevention measures announced by Uganda's President Yoweri Museveni was a restriction of movements except for what was termed 'essential services.' The services designated as essential included "the medical, agriculture and veterinary, telecommunication, door-to-door delivery of goods, financial institutions, all media, private security companies, cleaning services, garbage collection, fire-brigade, fuel stations, water departments, funeral services, and some staff of Kampala Capital City Authority (KCCA)[3]" (Museveni, 2020, p. 6). All other providers of what was considered nonessential services were expected to work from home. As soon as the classification of essential and nonessential workers was announced, some professional bodies and individuals came out to claim that the services they offer were very important, especially in times of an epidemic, and that ought to have been included among the essential workers. Lawyers

[1] See also, WHO Director General remarks during press briefing on March 11, 2020; https://www.who.int/director-general/speeches/detail/who-director-general-s-opening-remarks-at-the-media-briefing-on-covid-19%2D%2D-11-march-2020.

[2] See https://www.health.go.ug/covid/category/iec-materials//.

[3] Kampala Capital City Authority (KCCA) is a management and governance structure of Uganda's capital Kampala, responsible for everyday running and management of city affairs.

L. K. Musinguzi (✉) · J. Twikirize · A. Kyamulabi · D. Muhangi
Department of Social Work and Social Administration, Makerere University, Kampala, Uganda
e-mail: musinguzilaban16@gmail.com; janestic@gmail.com; aggieiss2012@gmail.com; denmuhangi@gmail.com

M. C. S. Gonçalves et al. (eds.), *The Coronavirus Crisis and Challenges to Social Development*,
https://doi.org/10.1007/978-3-030-84678-7_19

argued that the President had not understood the importance of judicial services in society and questioned the legitimacy of the directive (Okiror, 2020), and in some cases also petitioned courts to compel governments to include them with those designated as essential workers (see *Daily Monitor*, 23 April 2020). Social workers were equally not pleased that they had not been included among the essential workers category.

The classification of essential and nonessential services greatly affected the services of frontline social workers, including government social workers in ministries and local governments. In particular, social service agencies argued that the exclusion of social workers from the COVID-19 response left glaring gaps in addressing some of the social concerns arising from COVID-19 and the associated lockdown measures such as the increasing cases of domestic violence and the mental and psychosocial effects. Reports suggested that the COVID-19 control measures led to escalation of gender-based violence, loss of livelihoods, and mental distress (Twinomugisha, 2020; Sali, 2020; Waiswa, 2020; Musisi, 2020) and other non-COVID-19 concerns such as child abuse, child labor, and increased teenage pregnancies. The closure during the initial days of the lockdown of the national child helpline (known as Sauti 116), used for reporting cases of violence against children,[4] affected response to violence against children amidst these increasing incidents of violence. In addition, it was reported that more than 2372 girls became pregnant during the lockdown and 128 girls were married off in the Ugandan districts of Kitgum, Ngora, Kyegegwa, Kasese, and Lyantonde in the first few months of the lockdown (*Daily Monitor*, 2020). Many of the ongoing abuses against children and women were being reported in both the mainstream media and social media, often with frightening graphic images and video clips. The escalation of social ills emanating from the lockdown generated a debate around the role of social workers. Could stronger social work involvement in COVID-19 response have reduced the scale of the magnitude of the problems that emerged?

It is fair to say that Uganda's response to COVID-19 was largely biomedical, top down, and militaristic. True to its biomedical nature, the response focused on contact tracing, isolation and quarantining of contacts, testing of travelers (mainly truck drivers from across borders), and hospitalization and treatment of those who tested positive, many of whom were asymptomatic. To a large extent the biomedical approach seemed to be justified on the premise that the coronavirus and COVID-19 were medical phenomena. Nevertheless, the biomedical response excluded other fields such as social work and the social sciences in general. The Ministry of Gender, Labour and Social Development (MGLSD), the ministry that regulates social work services in Uganda, had a limited role in the initial response to COVID-19, including relief such as food distribution in Kampala. However, the dominance of biomedical approaches is not new to management of epidemics in Uganda. Biomedical interventions have previously been applied during control and management of Ebola in Uganda (De Vries et al., 2016; Lamunu et al., 2004; Hewlett & Amola, 2003).

Similarly, enforcement of adherence to COVID-19 control measures was largely militaristic, characterised by heavy involvement of security personnel. The militarization of relief aid such as food distribution in Kampala, for example, created several challenges. The food was delayed in reaching the beneficiaries, no clear eligibility criterion was issued, some of those in critical need never received the food rations, although those who never needed the food were given rations, and the quality of the food itself became an issue of contention (Macdonald & Owor, 2020). Social workers who are well trained in needs and vulnerability assessment could have been better placed to direct such relief interventions, especially in setting the eligibility criteria and ensuring that the most vulnerable and most deserving would be reached.

The exclusion of social work only changed after concerted advocacy involving social development actors and academics. Some nongovern-

[4] See: https://www.usaid.gov/uganda/news/prioritizing-child-protection-during-covid-19-response.

ment organisations and other development partners led by USAID, the U.S. President's Emergency Plan for AIDS Relief (PEPFAR), and UNICEF lobbied for opening of the Child Help Line and recognition of the importance of Probation and Social Welfare Officers (PSWO) as frontline workers (see Footnote 4). Social workers from Makerere University working closely with the National Association of Social Workers of Uganda (NASWU) wrote position papers and technical guidance notes on addressing the social side of the epidemic and strengthening community response. Their initial write-ups directed to the Ministry of Health and the National Task Force initially seemed to fall on deaf ears. It was not until June 2020 that some space begun to be opened for the MGLSD to participate in the National Task Force and the social workers at district level to be part of the district response to COVID-19.

Could the situation have been different had social workers been involved early enough? Did COVID-19 present an opportunity for social workers to reflect on the years of marginalization and therefore rethink the strategies of claiming the space? This chapter seeks to contribute to the debate on the role of social workers and challenges the profession to rethink their position in society in addressing social ills. This is particularly critical because marginalization of the social work profession is not only historical but also reverberates in several other countries. Acceptance of decades of neglect and historically endured marginalization by social workers (Guerrero et al., 2020) does not position the profession well to fulfill its critical roles. Yet even when they are pushed almost to the point of invisibility, social workers undoubtedly remain the backbone of social service delivery and healthcare systems (Lipe, 2020). In this chapter, we attempt to situate the discussion of the role of social work in these debates and show how the COVID-19 has shaped and reshaped social work as a profession that fosters social solidarity and resilience during pandemics. We attempt to show how COVID-19 has created the urgency for social work to rethink not just its position but also its image and how to respond when faced with such crises. We also draw from experiences of a few social workers who had key roles in Uganda during COVID-19. To put this discussion into context, we present a brief overview of the situation of professional social work in Uganda.

19.2 Social Work in Uganda: A Brief Overview

In Uganda, social work was introduced during the British colonial administration to handle a wide range of social problems (Twikirize, 2014). Since 1969, the country has been training social work professionals at university level, and currently an estimated 1000 students graduate every year from social work programmes offered in at least 18 universities in the country. As the government lacks a strong social welfare system, more than 70% of social workers are employed in the nongovernmental organisations (NGOs) (Twikirize, 2017), which are key actors in implementing programmes for vulnerable groups, particularly children, persons with disabilities, older persons, and in general the poor and marginalised. According to available data, the key sectors in which social workers are currently engaged are community development (37%), health (27%), and education (14%), with almost a third (32.1%) of the agencies that employ social workers providing services to children (Twikirize et al., 2013). Government social workers mostly work at the district and lower local government levels as Probation and Social Welfare Officers, Community Development Officers, and rehabilitation and gender officers. Others work in medical and psychiatric hospitals, in refugee and other humanitarian programmes, while at the macro level they are engaged in policy, programming, advocacy, research, and education, albeit in a very limited capacity (Twikirize et al., 2013).

Social workers contributed enormously to stemming the HIV and AIDS pandemic in Uganda through aggressively educating and mobilizing communities to respond appropriately to the epidemic and to adopt protective behaviours and practices (Ankrah, 1992), a challenge that could not be simply resolved through biomedical interventions. Social work professionals continue to play critical roles in responding to the various epidemics and emergencies that have hit the country almost perpetually, including the Ebola epidemic and the nodding disease syndrome that affected much of conflict-ridden Northern Uganda in the aftermath of the 20-year armed conflict.

Despite its undeniable contribution to welfare and socioeconomic development, the social work profession in Uganda has suffered from low recognition and validation by the government and low visibility and community sanction. The current government leadership has openly classified it among the 'useless courses' that do not deserve government funding (Tusasiirwe, 2020). It should be noted here that the government of Uganda pursues a neoliberal development agenda, with private sector-led development seen as the panacea for the attainment of a middle-income status. It is in this context that when the COVID-19 crisis struck, social work professionals, whether in government or elsewhere were not recognised as essential, with government instead, choosing to pursue an almost exclusively medical model to respond to the crisis. Social workers faced insurmountable challenges to position themselves as essential, recognizing that total lockdown of services to the most vulnerable populations served by social work agencies could only exacerbate their situation.

19.3 Methods and Sources of Data

Content for this chapter drew from three main sources, namely (a) existing local (Ugandan) and international literature on debates around the role of social work, as well as that on the response of social workers during epidemics; (b) the authors' experiential knowledge, drawing from their many years of experience as social work academics, researchers, and practitioners; and (c) key informant interviews with selected social work practitioners and managers. With regard to the latter, a total of six key informants were contacted, consisting of two social work practitioners working at the frontline (one in a district local government and another in a national mental referral hospital), and four working in different roles as managers or coordinators of social care, advocacy, and support programmes in NGOs and development partner organisations. One key informant worked with the National Association of Social Workers of Uganda and another with the child protection working group, which coordinates more than 50 organisations in the child protection sector. Interview data were transcribed and analysed manually using thematic analysis. Key themes in the analysis included (a) experiences and perceptions on the exclusion of social work from essential services during the COVID-19 lockdown, (b) the effect of COVID-19 lockdown on provision of social work services, (c) the historical marginalization of social work, (d) the actual role held by social workers during the COVID-19 response, and (e) repositioning social work for future emergencies.

19.4 Social Workers' Experience of Being Excluded from the "Essential Services"

Following the President's pronouncement about essential and nonessential services, heads of various organizations wrote to their staff specifying who could stay at work and who should go home. District staff retained to work during the lockdown often consisted of heads of departments, the health staff, and the sub-county chiefs at the lower local government level. Social work practitioners across the country accordingly went home and their services came to a halt: these providers included all categories of social workers ranging from medical social workers in hospitals, those working with childcare agencies and even those working with statutory services such as the Child and Family Protection Unit of the Police. Social workers interviewed for this paper reported on this situation:

> *The lockdown affected the social work services in our Hospital because the department was closed. Let me say it was closed because we could not access the office or the hospital to support our patients. Most, if not all of us the social workers stay far from the hospital, no one has a house in the staff quarters, so we were all cut off. Remember at*

first there were no even taxis moving. Then for private cars, one had to have a sticker and we were not given any sticker and so the department was closed (Interview, Medical Social Worker, Mental Referral Hospital).

Besides specifying the services that were considered essential and listed to continue operating, and excluding social work services, the lockdown also imposed practical and logistical challenges that made it impossible for social work services to continue functioning. The first was public transport was not operational and nonessential workers were not given passes for private means of transport. The second was that at district level, for instance, all government vehicles were put under the command of the District Health Officer (DHO) and were to be deployed for only COVID-19-related work. The social workers who continued to work, or who resumed work early, managed to do this mainly through informal contacts and networks, not because it was allowed by government policy at the time. Social workers from dwelling places (a local NGO working with children on the streets), for instance, managed to do a bit of work during lockdown because they were collaborating with Kampala Capital City Authority to affect resettlement of children on the streets.

An important question that arises is whether the social workers themselves think that their services are essential and should have been treated as such. Equally important to ask are the criteria used to categorise services as essential or nonessential. Some informants believed that whether social work services were essential depends on the setting. One respondent for instance argued that for social workers based in hospitals, their services were essential because they, among other matters, needed to handle COVID-19 patients, while for those working in community settings, their services were probably less essential.

19.5 Why Social Work Was Not Considered Essential

The criteria that government used to categorise some services as essential during the COVID-19 lockdown and others as not was not clear. The social workers interviewed for this chapter did not know what criteria were used. It all seemed that what was categorised as essential had to be medical- and security related (Museveni, 2020). Government clearly saw the virus as a medical problem, and the measures to curb its spread as ones to be achieved through medical and security measures. At that point, no one seemed to think about the likely impacts of the measures being implemented.

I think in the context of COVID-19 being a disease emergency, the focus was more on prevention and cure of the disease, so in the mind of the leaders, they were only looking at disease control. But we in the social services know that even while the doctors and nurses are providing curative services, the psychosocial aspects are very essential in ensuring recovery and even prevention, so that was, I could say, an error from the leadership (Key Informant, UN Agency Official).

Others believed that it is typical that in a health emergency the priority areas of focus are usually health and food (Lamunu et al., 2004; De Vries et al., 2016). Some of the problems that emerged from the lockdown, such as increasing cases of domestic violence, were not anticipated. It was only later, when other needs of a social nature arose, that they were recognised.

On the other hand, some of the social workers interviewed believed that social work was not considered essential because the government of Uganda has never understood or recognised the critical role and contribution of social work in such a crisis or even in other settings (Twikirize et al., 2013). Thus, the exclusion of social work services from the essential services list could arguably also be linked to the long-standing broader discourse that has sought to undermine social work (and humanities and social sciences in general) in Uganda. This discourse has particularly been propagated by President Museveni, who has several times questioned why universities continue to offer 'useless" courses such as social work that produce unemployable graduates (Tusasiirwe, 2020). Even during his several presidential addresses on COVID-19, the President often hailed the importance of scientists and played down the role of arts and humanities. At one time he said the problems in the country (including COVID-19) were being handled by scientists and not the 'Shakespeares' of this world (referring to the famous poet Shakespeare). Many social workers in Uganda therefore believe that this bashing and negative narrative coming from the head of state himself fuels the marginalisation and lack of recognition of social work.[5] Social workers have sometimes protested this, such as through letters and newspaper articles by NASWU and others (Tusasiirwe, 2020). The narrative by the President is not well received amongst social workers and other professionals, and many commentators recognise that a country cannot develop only through science to the exclusion of the social and arts disciplines. The government's lack of prioritization for social work-related services is also reflected in the long-standing underfinancing of the MGLSD, the ministry responsible for social development issues and social work services. This underfunding has existed through many years, even before the advent of COVID-19.

Other respondents linked the exclusion and marginalisation of social work to the deep-rooted culture of not seeking professional help for issues such as child abuse, domestic- and gender-based violence, or even mental health. They pointed to a tendency to plan and cost other services, while hoping that social services will naturally be provided through traditional structures facilitated by volunteers and communities. This approach seems to have persisted and affects the planning, budgeting, branding, and publicity of social work, which in turn affects the recognition received by social workers.

The question of effectiveness of social workers and the impact of the social services they provide was also argued. Categories of social workers such as probation and social welfare officers work in a context where they interact with police, with judicial officers, and other professions. Do they make a mark when they work with others? Do other professionals feel or see the value that these social workers are adding to the collaborative work? There is a sentiment that if social workers were able to make a valuable contribution wherever they are, they would be recognised and their services would always be demanded. And yet at the same time, it is impossible to be effective without adequate resourcing and tooling of the social services sector. Hence, it becomes a vicious cycle and blame game between government and the social service sector stakeholders, coupled with the difficulties faced in measuring or quantifying the output from services provided by social workers, including, for example, psychosocial support.

19.6 Effect of the COVID-19 Lockdown on Social Work Services Functionality

The COVID-19 lockdown in Uganda affected the provision of social work services. Normal service procedures could not take place during the time of the lockdown. Many social workers could only work remotely, and tasks requiring physical contact with other service providers or clients suffered. Those tasks that required movement to the field were curtailed. One informant explained:

> *Most of the work that social workers do involves physical interaction; for example, if it is taking children on remand to court for case hearing, you have to physically transport the children ... Sometimes there are things that require multidisciplinary intervention and you could not have access to the other experts to work with* (Interview, Government Ministry Official).

Thus, one of the clear effects of the lockdown was that the clients of social work services missed the services during the lockdown, sometimes with potential adverse effects. Their challenges and needs continued to prevail, and probably got worse. Some of the planned events such as meetings, trainings, and conferences had to be cancelled or turned into a virtual format. The child helpline, which is a critical service in responding to cases of child abuse, was shut down. The lockdown resulted into a slow response to cases which were identified at the

[5] Through the directive of the President, government in paying scientists (including university science staff) better/more than it pays arts/humanities staff at the same rank/level.

community level because such cases could not be reported through the helpline. Even when the child helpline was eventually reopened, there were few staff available to attend to the cases being reported.

Even after the social service workforce was allowed back to work, provision of services and response to cases was slow. Some informants reported that upon reporting back for work, they found a huge backlog of work. In line with MoH SOPs, offices had to retain a few people and people returning to the office had to work in shifts. A social worker in one of the district local governments tells her story:

> *When we returned to work in May [2020], … work was too- too much. Imagine just two months of being under lockdown, we found a lot of work that we are still grappling with up to today. I found very many juveniles in the cells that did not have any legal representation. So I had to interview all those juveniles, and conduct social inquires under very difficult conditions because transport was still restricted.* (Interview, District Official).

Other agencies reported that the lockdown and cutting back of staff, as well as changing the work modalities, slowed down their pace of planned implementation.

A social worker at a National Mental Referral Hospital reported that her patients were affected because they were no longer receiving the counselling services from Social Workers. But the patients also overstayed on the ward because they were not being taken back to their communities, which led to some of them relapsing. The challenge also led to overcrowding because new patients were being brought in, while those ready for discharge were not being discharged.

Social work agencies reported that the lockdown affected their field activities, and even after the relaxation of the lockdown, they kept field-based activities at low key, only going into the field when it was essential. Many resorted to doing their field monitoring through telephone calls. Others reported that they now relied more on their field-based implementing partners and use the reports they receive from them, but with minimal opportunity of physically going to verify such reports.

> *When we get a case, we are supposed to interface with the client in question, assess him/her, and go out for a social inquiry before we intervene. So all that was put to a standstill;… Even when we later came on board, transport was still restricted. The vehicles were basically committed to doing surveillance for COVID-19 cases so everything was committed to issues of coronavirus forgetting the other effects that the virus was causing* (Interview, District Official).

> *We had to call back all the staff that were in the field. We had some staff in Karamoja and we had to call them back. They were dealing with a lot more in livelihood support and prevention of children coming to the streets and then we also had ones who were going to the streets and into the slums working from there, we had to also cut back their work. We were telling social workers to make phone calls and use other forms of communication to follow up children* (Interview, NGO Official).

Social workers reported that working remotely or via the phone was not as effective as their usual community visits. Community visits would benefit from the rapport they have built over time and people would recognise their faces. A voice at the other end of the phone line does not generate as much effect on the client. Take an example of a child who is probably at risk of sexual abuse or has already been sexually abused and when they call the helpline, a social worker picks up the call but he/she do not have the power and the means to travel to reach the child. Some counselling may be offered by the social worker on the phone, but he/she cannot be entirely sure that this will provide the safety that the child needs.

There were also other practical challenges to social work agencies that affected their operations in the COVID-19 context. Most of the social work agencies, like most other organizations, were affected financially as some of their grants were suspended or deferred. As a result, some had to lay off workers; thus, after the lockdown, such organizations could not work at full capacity.

Social work agencies reported how they had made adjustments to their work modalities and procedures to cope with the lockdown. The adjustments included working from home, through telephone calls, and working virtually. Later, when the lockdown was eased, they cut back the number of staff at offices and many started coming to office in turns. Such adjustments have not been as effective in delivering social work services as the previous, mostly community oriented social work approaches.

> *Social work is not effectively delivered via a phone call arrangement. Working on phone should be really the last option. It's more of a physical agenda; you have to have conversations because with a phone, you cannot look at someone. Remember that social work is not only about what you hear but also what you see. So you go to the home and you hear them saying I am fine but when you are looking, you see medicine around and then you know there was some one sick here. You look and say do they have a mosquito net because that also shows you a sign if they are prone to malaria which is one of the killer diseases. So, it's not about what is in the phone call but also what is in the environment.* (Interview, NGO Official.)

Some of the agencies recognised the limitations and indeed the dangers of remodeling their approaches and went an extra mile to mitigate these risks and quality improvements and checks into their new models. MGLSD reported that when child protection actors moved from face-to-face to telephone child counselling, the Child Protection Working Group was concerned about the quality and effectiveness of this mode of service delivery. They had to call in experts to train workers in effectively delivering child counselling via the phone.

In an effort to respond to emerging needs, some social work agencies innovatively tried to restructure their budgets to cater to the new needs that emerged in their clientele as a result of the lockdown. Some were, for instance, working with families that previously did not need food support or shelter because there was an income earner in the family. But now, with businesses and workplaces locked up, some families were at risk of hunger and destitution. Some of the agencies therefore had to craft a welfare budget line within their development work to be able to meet these emerging needs. Paying house rent was found to have been a major emerging need among vulnerable groups in urban areas.

There were positive experiences as well. Organizations like NASWU which had planned face-to-face capacity-building activities in social work agencies had to repackage them and offer them as virtual webinars. The association quickly realised the virtual option was actually a useful way to deliver these services, which they could continue to use in the post-COVID period.

The various adjustments adopted by social work agencies in response to the lockdown restrictions raise various lessons and implications. First, successful adjustments point to the limitless opportunities for social work innovation and adaptation in the face of challenging circumstances. Social work therefore does not have to remain stagnant or to resist change. The capability for social work to adapt implies that the profession can maintain its relevance even in times of difficulty, as one informant aptly puts it:

> *One of the implications for me is that it has helped social workers to remain relevant to their clients and it has also opened a new challenge for us as social workers not to think that we shall always do things the way we are used to. It points to the fact that we have to change based on changed circumstances and context but how fast we can adapt and change is another one.* (Interview, Government Ministry Official).

Others reported how beyond turning their monitoring and coordination mechanisms from physical to virtual, they had to do a lot more to ensure that these processes were still meaningful and effective.

19.7 Positive Contributions of Social Workers to the COVID-19 Response

Despite the initial lockdown of social work services, the social work contribution both during and after the lockdown turned out to be indispensable. Some agencies conducted media campaigns on COVID-19, featuring issues of child protection. Others provided ongoing support to community volunteers, providing technical guidance through phone calls, while some continued to pay allowances to facilitate the volunteers' work. Some of the agencies worked with the District Task Forces in their respective districts of operation, equipping the response teams, working alongside the medical teams and providing psychosocial support. Many in child protection such as Child's i Foundation, Plan International, World Vision and Save the Children worked closely with district Task Forces to ensure that child protection issues were integrated in the COVID-19 response.

Medical social workers were deployed to work with COVID-19 patients in multidisciplinary teams at various treatment centres across the country, especially at national and regional referral hospitals. Social Workers were engaged in community sensitization and preparing communities and families on how to support COVID-19 patients being discharged from treatment centres. They addressed issues of stigma which was threatening to affect the prevention and response to COVID-19 within the communities. A pool of trained social workers, mobilised through the national association of social workers, supported the MoH to offer psychosocial support to people under quarantine.

Many social work agencies including those operating in refugee settings distributed masks, hand-washing facilities, soap, and relief food items. Social work agencies that do coordination work adjusted quickly with much effort given to coordination roles virtually and through other innovative means. They were able to bring their partners together in virtual space to continue sharing their updates and lessons. Some used this opportunity to expand the scope of their participants to include international ones. In this way, there has been ongoing improvements in the delivery of social work services as organisations adapt to the COVID-19 context.

19.8 Missed Opportunities and Missing Links as a Result of Excluding Social Workers

It can be argued that if social workers had been involved from the start of the COVID-19 response, probably the spread of the virus and subsequent deaths would have been different. This scenario is probable because the initial government response was top down and lacked any community involvement strategies. A strong community engagement process from the start would have strengthened the acceptance of prevention efforts. The levels of stigma would probably have been nipped in the bud if social workers had been involved from the start. Social workers would have helped to prepare communities to accept suspected COVID-19 cases being released from quarantine and recovering patients who were discharged from hospital. Social workers are also well placed to prepare families for home isolation and home-based care. A few weeks after the start, it was clear that institutional quarantine of suspects would not be sustained for long, and home-based isolation would be the option. It was equally evident that the few Ugandan hospitals that were offering care to COVID-19 patients would very soon be overwhelmed, and home-based care would be eminent. However, the government response lacked the element of preparing communities and families for this obvious occurrence, a gap that could have been possibly filled by social work services.

Social workers would have filled key roles in the whole spectrum of COVID-19 response including prevention, care and support, and mitigation. They would have played critical roles in awareness raising about COVID-19, psychosocial support, supporting relief food distribution and distribution of masks, preparing families for home isolation and home-based care, addressing stigma, and supporting bereaved families.

Even the health workers themselves would have made use of the social workers' support for their own self-care. Several health workers were stressed by the overwhelming work, lack of PPE, and the sheer risk of contracting the infection. Moreover, health workers handling COVID-19 patients were not being allowed to return home and had to be resident at the hospitals for the duration of the lockdown. Their accommodation facilities at the hospitals were just improvised. Media reports indicated that their allowances had been delayed. Some eventually contracted the virus in the line of duty and a few died. The health workers therefore certainly needed psychosocial support to handle this challenging work situation.

Overall, the country missed recognizing that this was a crisis which required a multi-sectoral response from the start, in which social workers would be useful, working alongside medical, security and other response teams, and making the response holistic.

19.9 Positive Outcomes and Opportunities: More Recognition for Social Work?

Some organizations such as NASWU and the Department of Social Work at Makerere University proactively sought to assert the social work profession's relevancy and to increase its visibility during the COVID-19 response. These organizations initiated innovative work around COVID-19 including writing guidance notes, research proposals and conducting research, advocating community engagement, and harnessing the use of information and communication technology for networking and linkages across the country.

Besides, COVID-19 re-shaped the social work approaches from the conventional face-to-face to more innovative and technology-based approaches such as online meetings and trainings, telephone counselling, and the use of social media. NASWU reported that the jump into these approaches opened their doors to extend their reach and involve a wide range of participants in their trainings and webinars. With the use of these new technologies, the limitations of physical distance and logistical travels are overcome.

The advocacy for social work that was conducted in the wake of COVID-19 increased the acknowledgement of the role of social work not only during COVID-19 response, but in all emergency response situations as well as in development work. It indeed sparked off more advocacy for strengthening of the social service workforce to be able to respond to diverse needs. Key informants reported that as a result, other sectors such as Health, Justice, Law and Order sector (JLOS) and Ministry of Local Government are beginning to demand for the involvement of social service professionals in their programs.

> *It is now very common for you to hear the other sectors – I want to give examples of health and justice – asking if social work aspects are incorporated in their guidance notes even in their implementation. For example, when there was a training for local councils recently organised by the Ministry of Local government, there was this outcry about the linkages between justice and social services. People argued that during COVID-19, we need to apply child-friendly procedures which encourage mediation and amicable resolution of cases, rather than taking people to detention centers where they would face the risk of exposure to the Coronavirus.* (Interview, UN Agency Official).

In the wake of the COVID-19 crisis, for instance, the Ministries of Health and that of Gender, Labor and Social Development have developed several guidance notes related to service provision in the context of COVID-19. Most of these guidance notes now incorporate the social work services such as child protection and child-friendly services as well as addressing the needs of the poor and the most vulnerable, which has been largely attributed to the advocacy for social work services that happened in the wake of COVID-19. Other informants reported that they are beginning to see the multisectoral and integration of services that includes social work services that they had been 'singing' about for long but attracting no attention. The realities of COVID-19 demonstrated to other sectors, especially the health sector, that emergencies such as COVID-19 and their ramifications would not be addressed through medical responses alone.

The COVID-19 crisis certainly opened new areas and opportunities for research. Social workers in universities, NGOs, and other agencies are undertaking a diversity of interesting and pioneer research on social issues in relation to COVID-19. Much of such research is focusing on vulnerable groups: refugees, children, slum dwellers, informal sector workers, women, people with disabilities, and so on, hence expanding the breadth and width of locally generated research and evidence for social work practice and training in the country.

19.10 Conclusions and Implications

This chapter has outlined the struggles, challenges, successes, and resilience of social workers and the social work profession in a developing country context during epidemics. We have shown that social work's current marginalised role in COVID-19 response in Uganda stems from an entrenched marginalisation of the profession by the current regime and generally reflects the neglect the profession has endured for many years. We have also shown how resilient the profession has been and the potential to overcome adversity to continue to fulfil their professional mandates and commitments to the vulnerable populations.

Whereas the government response to COVID-19 as a disease was to the exclusion of social work, the ramifications of the government responses ignited the search for the social work function to fill the emerging gaps in the broader response. As indicated, it is no doubt that the "crisis was an opportunity not just for social work to reinvent itself, but for societies to reinvent themselves too" (Truell, 2020, p. 548). The changing stance of government towards social work was triggered by strong advocacy by the MGLSD and its partners. This advocacy was not just for the involvement of social workers in the COVID-19 response, but also for multisectoral and integrated action on all matters whose scope cuts across sectors, including the social development sector. However, this also means that social workers must be ready to occupy the most critical spaces where they will become more effective.

The marginalisation of social work in COVID-19 response is also a wake-up call that unless we amplify professional action and voice, then "the profession may continue to be accorded a second-fiddle status, or brusquely have its relevance called to question" (Amadasun, 2020, p. 755). We agree with Dauti et al. (2020) that the exclusion from initial COVID-19 challenges social work to engage in political spaces and decisions that affect programing for social policies. Social workers must engage in political spaces and decisions that affect programing for social policies (Dauti et al., 2020). Their argument is that if social workers fail to engage in political spaces that largely centralise decision-making that affect the marginalised, then the voices of those that social workers serve will remain unheard. This was the case in Uganda. Therefore, as social workers, it is time to actively be involved in political spaces where decisions about social policies and programs are made. Lipe (2020) challenges social workers to become strong advocates of their positions and role in society.

Social workers in Uganda and the world over must work towards a more recognised, robust profession whose role becomes appreciated in the future. In this sense, repositioning the role of social workers requires that social workers become more forceful in advocacy.

References

Amadasun, S. (2020). Social work and COVID-19 pandemic: An action call. *International Social Work, 63*(6), 753–756.

Ankrah, E. M. (1992). Aids in Uganda: Initial social work responses. *Journal of Social Development in Africa, 7*(2), 53–61.

Cucinotta, D., & Vanelli, M. (2020). WHO declares COVID-19 a pandemic. *Acta Biomedica Atenei Parmensis, 91*(1), 157.

Daily Monitor. (2020). *Man petitions court to list lawyers as essential staff.* https://www.monitor.co.ug/uganda/news/national/man-petitions-court-to-list-lawyers-as-essential-staff-1886608

Dauti, M., Dhëmbo, E., Beqko, E., & Allmuça, M. (2020). Rethinking the transformative role of the social work profession in Albania: Some lessons learned from the response to COVID-19. *International Social Work, 63*(5), 640–645.

De Vries, D. H., Rwemisisi, J. T., Musinguzi, L. K., Benoni, T. E., Muhangi, D., De Groot, M., Kaawa-Mafigiri, D., & Pool, R. (2016). The first mile: Community experience of outbreak control during an Ebola outbreak in Luwero District, Uganda. *BMC Public Health, 16*(1), 1–12.

Guerrero, L. R., Avgar, A. C., Phillips, E., & Sterling, M. R. (2020). They are essential workers now, and should continue to be: Social workers and home health care workers during COVID-19 and beyond. *Journal of Gerontological Social Work, 63*(6–7), 574–576.

Hewlett, B. S., & Amola, R. P. (2003). Cultural contexts of Ebola in northern Uganda. *Emerging Infectious Diseases, 9*(10), 1242.

Lamunu, M., Lutwama, J. J., Kamugisha, J., Opio, A., Nambooze, J., Ndayimirije, N., & Okware, S. (2004). Containing a haemorrhagic fever epidemic: The Ebola experience in Uganda (October 2000–January 2001). *International Journal of Infectious Diseases, 8*(1), 27–37.

Lipe, L. (2020). Social workers are essential workers. *The New Social Worker*. https://www.socialworker.com/feature-articles/practice/social-workers-essential-workers

Macdonald, A., & Owor, A. (2020). *Food distribution and corona-politics in Uganda: The view from Kampala*. https://blogs.lse.ac.uk/africaatlse/2020/06/15/food-distribution-coronapolitics-uganda-lockdown-elections-kampala/

MoH (2020). IEC Materials for COVID-19. Accessed from https://www.health.go.ug/covid/category/iec-materials/

MoH. (2021). *Coronavirus (pandemic), COVID-19*. https://www.health.go.ug/covid/

Museveni, Y. K. (2020). *Address to the nation: Latest updates on matters regarding corona virus (COVID 19) on 4 May, 2020*. Nakasero.

Musisi, S. (2020). *COVID-9 and mental health in Uganda: How COVID-19 and the response of the Uganda Government may affect mental health*. https://www.jasprogramme.ug/publication/covid-19-and-mental-health-in-uganda-how-covid-19-and-the-response-of-the-uganda-government-may-affect-mental-health

Nakkazi, E. (2020). Obstacles to COVID-19 control in east Africa. *The Lancet Infectious Diseases, 20*(6), 660.

Okiror, S. (2020). *Access to justice: Lawyers fight to be recognized as 'essential' workers in COVID-hit East Africa*. https://www.ibanet.org/Article/NewDetail.aspx?ArticleUid=46ea57e0-6a2b-43a1-8194-1c0868b8aef0

Sali, S. (2020). *Covid 19 and gender: Examining the gender dynamics of Uganda's national response*. https://www.jasprogramme.ug/publication/covid-19-and-gender-examining-the-gender-dynamics-of-uganda-s-national-response

Truell, R. (2020). News from our societies–IFSW: COVID-19: The struggle, success and expansion of social work—Reflections on the profession's global response, 5 months on. *International Social Work, 63*(4), 545–548.

Tusasiirwe, S. (2020). *Remarks that social work is 'useless' raises questions*. https://www.monitor.co.ug/uganda/oped/commentary/remarks-that-social-work-is-useless-raises-questions-1877572

Twikirize, J. M. (2014). Social work education and practice in Uganda: A historical perspective. In H. Spitzer, J. M. Twikirize, & G. G. Wairire (Eds.), *Profession social work in East Africa. Towards social development, poverty reduction and gender equality* (pp. 136–148). Fountain Publishers.

Twikirize, J. M. (2017). Social work practice in the NGO sector in Uganda and Kenya. Opportunities and challenges. In M. Gray (Ed.), *The handbook of social work and social development in Africa* (pp. 367–381). Routledge.

Twikirize, J. M., Asingwire, N., Omona, J., Lubanga, R., & Kafuko, A. (2013). *The role of social work in poverty reduction and the realization of millennium development goals in Uganda*. Fountain Publishers.

Twinomugisha, B. (2020). *Covid 19 and the right to health in Uganda: Analysis of the national response and its implications for the realization of the right to health*. https://www.jasprogramme.ug/publication/covid-19-and-the-right-to-health-in-uganda-analysis-of-the-national-response-and-its-implications-for-the-realization-of-the-the-right-to-health

Waiswa, P. (2020). *Sexual reproductive health and Covid-19 in Uganda: Avoiding the pitfalls of unintended consequences for maternal newborn, child, adolescent and nutritional health in the national response*. https://www.jasprogramme.ug/publication/sexual-reproductive-health-and-covid-19-in-uganda-avoiding-the-pitfalls-of-unintended-consequences

WHO. (2020). WHO Director General remarks during press briefing on March 11, 2020. https://www.who.int/director-general/speeches/detail/who-director-general-s-opening-remarks-at-the-media-briefing-on-covid-19%2D%2D-11-march-2020

20 Responses of Social Work Students and Teachers to COVID-19: Experiences from Crisis Relief in Urban Slum and Rural Communities of Maharashtra, India

Sanaya Singh, Prabha Tirmare, and Apurva Shinde

20.1 Introduction

This chapter presents the experiences of social workers from a field action project that was initiated in urban slum and rural communities in Maharashtra (India) as a response to COVID-19 and the Indian states responses to the pandemic. The initiative was undertaken by a group of social work students and academicians as an immediate crisis relief intervention outreach. Their actions reflect situational leadership approaches characterised by youth engagement, community participation, and local-level advocacy. In a locked-down and confused state in the face of a crisis, these young social workers were involved in everything from fundraising to providing essential material for survival to counselling and educating the marginalised masses about the new reality. In this chapter, we shed light on the vulnerable groups and social problems that were accentuated by the pandemic, document the work of the field action project and the voices of grassroots-level social workers, and discuss developmental responses recognised in the process. The chapter is based on the firsthand experiences of social workers who worked in the field when COVID-19 was at its peak, to reflect the grassroots realities at large both during but also pre- and post-COVID.

Methodology: The data for this chapter were collected by interviewing five social workers from the Project Jeevan Pravaah team, three of whom were at the threshold of graduating with the Master's degree in social work and two who are academicians, all of whom became connected to each other during the COVID-19 peak in India. Purposive sampling was used as all these social workers were active on the project and connected via it in their efforts to respond to the pandemic. In addition, short interviews were conducted with another four social workers with long-term experience of activism with marginalised groups and academic work in India to gain expert views on directions for policy post COVID-19. The commonality that connects these participants was their own initiative and prompt response to rising social problems around them accentuated by the pandemic. All the authors of this chapter are

S. Singh (✉)
Department of Social Work and Psychology, University of Gävle, Gävle, Sweden
e-mail: Sanaya.Singh@hig.se

P. Tirmare
Nirmala Niketan College of Social Work, Mumbai, India

A. Shinde
ICMR Indo-Swedish Ageing Care Project; Non-profit Organization Consultant on Environment, Health, and Educational Issues, Mumbai, India

M. C. S. Gonçalves et al. (eds.), *The Coronavirus Crisis and Challenges to Social Development*,
https://doi.org/10.1007/978-3-030-84678-7_20

members of project Jeevan Pravaah and were involved in interventions on the field during the lockdown in India, and we draw hugely on our own reflections from the actions we felt imperative to take during this time. The authors had several focus group discussions which, along with the interviews we conducted with other social workers, led to generation of themes that are broad on the areas expanded further in this chapter.

20.2 Corona Crisis: Background

The year 2020 began with unprecedented alterations across the globe as transmission of the novel coronavirus COVID-19 began and spread quickly across a globalised world. The onset of a fast-spreading virus brought about humongous uncertainties as borders began closing down, a pandemic was declared, confinements and lockdowns of militaristic nature were implemented, death reports of an unpredictable disease were rising, and widespread panic among civilians grew. Nearly three million deaths owing to the virus are reported even as this chapter is written in March 2021 (Worldometer, 2021). Vaccinations have started rolling out, but the global situation remains uncertain and highly imbalanced.

In the early phases, COVID-19 was considered a nondiscriminatory virus and everyone was at risk, making this global pandemic an equaliser of sorts. "We are all in this together" became a common slogan to call for cooperation and compliance of restrictions for combating the virus, and global solidarity was infused to 'flatten the curve' and support clogged-up healthcare systems. However, evidence soon showed that some groups were more vulnerable than others. The elderly, especially people older than 80 years, were at a fivefold higher risk of dying; a higher mortality rate was reported for people with underlying medical conditions (Verity et al., 2020). As time progressed, the social discriminatory tendencies of the virus showed how its effects were neither uniformly nor universally felt. The pandemic disproportionately affected the Global South (Soutphommasane, 2021) as well as the psychological and social well-being of society's undervalued and underserved populations (Amadasun, 2020). Studies ranging from Asia (Pawar, 2020) to Europe (Rambaree & Nässén, 2020) to Africa (Dafuleya, 2020; Amadasun, 2020) showed how the most socially marginalised groups in these countries, which include indigenous groups, ethnic minorities, immigrants, and prisoners, were the worst affected in terms of both high case ratios and the shadow effects of the crisis.

In India, one of the most affected areas was Dharavi, the biggest slum of Asia. Dharavi has a population density of 800,000 people living in every 2.5 km^2. Up to 10 people are living in small hutments of 10 × 10 ft (Bhalerao, 2021). Maintaining physical and social distance to break the mode of transference of the virus was not possible for the millions of slum dwellers there, axiomatically making them more vulnerable than those afforded by the basic human right of a decent shelter. As Lingam and Suresh Sapkal (2020) have shown analysing India's readiness for the pandemic, poorer households in India were unequally endowed for observing physical distancing, which led to increased case fatality and incidence ratios among the poor.

State action in most countries globally directed their resources into the health sector, given COVID-19 was a public health concern. Accordingly, nations began producing and buying medication and masks, personal protective equipment, and pumping up hospitals and training staff to prepare for the oncoming crisis. Owing to media reports and data released throughout the world, the healthcare sector became attributed to front-line work done in terms of the pandemic and flattening the curve. However, at the same time, problems of socioeconomic nature were arising as a 'shadow' of the pandemic. Deteriorating mental health, increasing domestic violence and the sex trade, and destitution of migrants were issues brought to the forefront by social justice actors (UN, 2020a, b). However, there was a clear lack of focus on governmental agendas on the socioeconomic impact of the pandemic on deepening marginalisation of already excluded people and communities. Social workers have an important role here responding to hunger, destitution, displacement, mental health problems, and protecting lives from gross violation of human rights. Despite COVID-19 being a new virus, social workers are proficient in managing disasters, and so they became front-line workers in tackling the growing marginalisation and injustice during the crisis. The data for this chapter are collected by interviewing five social workers who worked actively in local communities during the first COVID-19 wave in India between March and September 2020. Through this chapter, we intend to inform the readers about local actions taken by a group of social workers in Maharashtra, India during this public health crisis, without any formal support. Their work at the grassroots involved a broad spectrum of interventions. But not all problems they needed to tackle arose from the pandemic alone; most of the problems were multi-layered, building on long-standing societal inequalities and injustices and negligence of the same by the state and social policy.

20.3 The Indian Context

India has a population of 1.3 billion, and cities like Mumbai have a population density of 199,430 people per square kilometer; 1.8 million people are homeless (Thelwell & Alexander, 2021). Although having an economy of $2.9 trillion, the country faces extreme income inequality: that is, nearly 176 million people struggle to survive on $1.90 a day or less (World Poverty Clock, 2021). The 93% of India's workforce that has helped to build India's economy works in the informal or unorganized sector (Government of India Union Budget and Economic Survey, 2008), which is tinged by the absence of social security measures such as healthcare and pensions, fair welfare legislations, negation of social standards and worker rights, and a denial of minimum wages. So these populations live hand to mouth, inhabiting urban slums in poor social conditions or rural destitution. In Mumbai alone more than 55% of its 22 million population lives in slums (World Population Review, 2021). These slums are characterised by poverty, deteriorated housing and buildings, and unhygienic and poor living conditions. Slums are defined as informal settlements that lack access to clean water, toilets, and nondurable overcrowded houses (UN-Habitat, 2018). Additionally, Mumbai, as a metropolis mega-city, sees a big influx of migrants from rural India and neighbouring countries. High real estate prices with high unemployment rates leads to most of the migrants settling down in the slums and undertaking unskilled daily wage labor. Even most populations of rural areas depend on seasonal farming and seasonal employment. Living conditions within villages see a huge disparity, and the caste system creates a divide in terms of how villages are planned and how access to resources is provided. In these circumstances, it is evident how these communities are extremely vulnerable to transference of the virus. Thus, even before the global pandemic, extreme inequalities and social injustices have existed in the Indian society. The pandemic reinforced these.

Following the outbreak of COVID-19, the government of India proclaimed a national 'lockdown' to stop the transmission of the virus and help prepare the health-care sector for the upcoming demands. The declaration of the lockdown was made at short notice, less than 24 h, and in periods of 2 weeks at a time, and a long-term plan was never rolled out, causing increased confusion and panic. The lockdown lasted from 24 March to mid-June 2020 with unlocking in phases afterwards. The sudden lockdown encapsulated the 'stay-in' measure to maintain social and physical distancing, effectively shutting off all public movement and activities, schools, businesses, workplaces, factories, and transportation to prevent transmission of infection. No one was to be outside except for the purchase of bare necessities. Police monitoring and punitive actions by state authorities were put in place to maintain the lockdown, pushing the general public into further fear and confusion. Lingam and Suresh Sapkal (2020) analysed India's preparedness for a lockdown using the readiness index of Jones et al. (2020). The study showed that the majority of the Indian states were least prepared for the pandemic, not having all the necessary physical infrastructure in place that was needed to enable people to stay indoors to maintain physical distance. This picture was reflected in what actually happened in the country.

The lockdown led to the millions of daily wage laborers working as landless agricultural laborers, construction workers, workers in brick kilns and stone quarries, bonded laborers, migrant workers, rag-pickers (waste management) and scavengers, carriers of head loads, drivers of animal-driven vehicles and other such unorganized sectors, suddenly losing their livelihood and employment (Vikaspedia Domains, 2021). The sudden cease of employment and income meant the loss of sudden inflation and the shortage of food supply meant hunger, starvation; the halt of country-wide public transport led to thousands being stranded in big cities far away from home and emotional support, police actions to punish those violating orders reportedly resulted in abuses against people in need, lack of hygiene and essential supplies meant more disease, resorting to violence, and a deeper fall into poverty for the marginalised. This situation was reported throughout the country. A number of media articles and sources (Sengupta & Jha, 2020) reported in detail the plight of some 40 million migrants from different parts of the country stranded, starving, and suffering, some even dying of exhaustion trying to walk thousands of kilometers back to their villages, as a consequence of the lockdown measure. Those who were able to make it home found, in some instances, villages refusing entry because of fears of transmission, leading to destitution and further poverty. All of this rendered the marginalised groups bearing the brunt of the worst to come out of the pandemic (Sengupta & Jha, 2020). These people were brought down to essentially choosing starvation or infection (Chen, 2020).

Parallel to the lockdown as a strategy to contain the spread of COVID-19, there were no social security plans or measures provided by the state for protecting the health, well-being, and basic human rights such as food, water, and shelter guarantee of these highly vulnerable groups (Human Rights Watch, 2021). Public welfare measures such as housing, safe drinking water, sanitation facilities, waste management, and sewerage systems—all pre-conditions required to handle a public health crisis—were already highly dysfunctional (Lingam & Suresh Sapkal, 2020). In addition to this backdrop, the country has a long history of neoliberal policies, half-hearted social protection measures, and underfunding of healthcare services (Sengupta & Jha, 2020). So, when cash transfer and food subsidy measures were announced by the state, they were meagre in proportion, amounting to only 0.2% of India's GDP (IMF Policy Tracker, 2020), and were not easily accessible at grassroots. All this has meant widened socioeconomic and health inequalities following the pandemic.

20.4 Project Jeevan Pravaah

Even as the world grappled to understand this strange new reality, and the healthcare sector toiled to cope with the surmounting pressures of a global pandemic, social work's principal endeavor to strive for social justice made it imperative for social workers globally to leap to support and assist these most vulnerable in any way possible. Amidst the lockdown and state of confusion and lack of knowledge, in Mumbai a small group of social workers began organizing themselves as relief workers under the project name 'Jeevan Pravaah.' Jeevan Pravaah essentially means the 'stream of life.' The name signifies that the efforts undertaken by the social workers during the pandemic are not enough and cannot be isolated, and that sustainable empowerment of communities and individuals for an improved, safe, and dignified livelihood are the end goals of social work. A call for sustainable empowerment of especially the vulnerable communities comes out as an even more urgent need in the light of the pandemic.

Jeevan Pravaah was developed based on academic research conducted by young social work students from the same community in which the interventions take place. At its core it follows a people-centered participatory and community-based model for sustainability and inclusive development of urban and rural marginalised poor. The project was developed on the idea of consolidating the potential, skills, and local wisdom of the community in ecology with their environment to strengthen the abilities and empower individuals and the community as a whole.

The project involves a group of social work graduates and teaching staff, who got together originally to work for sustainable life enhancement of rag-picker women, children, and elderly in the slums of Mumbai with a vision to spread their work ahead to adjacent towns. However, as COVID-19 struck, Jeevan Pravaah and its members redirected their efforts into crisis intervention, assistance, and aid to groups such as ragpickers, slum dwellers, displaced daily wage labourers, and the rural poor. At this stage the efforts of Jeevan Pravaah were not formally registered and there was no funding. But the initial stages of project planning were underway, and the areas for intervention were mapped and recognised.

The main interventions took place in two geographic areas: the first, the Bhim Nagar slum area in Thane, Mumbai, and the other in the small villages of Marathwada in Maharashtra. Bhim Nagar is characterised by slum communities constituting deprived migrants, mostly from the drought-prone rural areas of Marathwada. These migrants largely resource their livelihood from garbage disposal grounds as rag-pickers, who make for one of the most vulnerable communities in urban settings. Their livelihood depends on daily labour as garbage sorters; they work in unhygienic and risky areas without protection. In the context of India, it is critical to consider that along with class, and religious or gender marginality, 'caste' as an intersection has a big role in excluding groups. This group we put the spotlight upon in Bhim Nagar mainly consists of the socially excluded lower-caste Dalits, Muslims, and Nomadic tribes. Working in some form of unorganised sector on a daily wage basis as rag-pickers means they had generally no monetary savings or other social security benefits when the pandemic hit.

20.5 Community Mapping

Before beginning our work in the field, we conducted a community mapping of pilot areas in both urban slums and rural communities in Maharashtra (Thane in Mumbai and Beed in Maharashtra). What we found was that the women, youth, and children of the communities where we planned to work are more vulnerable and economically further resourceless in these regions. Alcohol and drug addiction is rampant in the community, and many women are widowed or left on their own because of the alcoholism of their husbands, hence without any earnings for livelihood. Prevailing gender disparity leads to exploitation of girls and women. Child marriage practices, sexual abuse, lack of education, superstitious beliefs, taboos about female menstruation being impure, and wife and child beating are regular occurrences in the community, which violate human rights. This is not an unusual scenario for most of the slum-dwelling population in urban cities in India. The spread of the pandemic, and the ensuing draconian steps undertaken by the state, meant that socioeconomically backward slum communities and the especially marginalised such as the women and children became even more vulnerable to hunger, starvation, impoverishment, gender discrimination, and violence.

20.5.1 Initial Lack of Appropriate Information and Relief Work

As mentioned earlier, the first line of action taken in India to curb the transmission of the virus was initiating a lockdown, but with a warning of a mere 24 h. Up until this time, the infection was relatively unknown, with sporadic news reported, which is not accessible to all in the context of India. Here, *Dr. Prabha Tirmare, an Associate Professor at Nirmala Niketan College of Social Work, Mumbai and the co-founder of Jeevan Pravaah,* reflects:

> This sudden news was rather strange, scary and hard to understand. Even for educated people, it took a long time to realize what the COVID-19

> pandemic was, how to deal in a lockdown, how to maintain social and physical distancing were all new. Then we began seeing problems related to livelihood faced by excluded communities in rural and urban India. Initially it was challenging to connect the crisis with the role of the social work educator or practitioner or researcher; there were no clear directives to intervene. However, gradually by reading more newspapers, WHO reports, watching local-global news, talking with family and friends, we developed an understanding about COVID pandemic and the crisis. She further adds as a social work professional I was personally involved in many crisis relief situations before. This led me to developing a strong feeling to reach out and help, especially the marginalized poor migrants. My continuous thought process became a push factor for an action plan. But the big question was, how and where and when to start? The pandemic seemed huge, there was no clarity, everyone feared catching the infection, and they were scared for their loved ones. But something needed to be done for the ones suffering the most!

Whilst Prabha reflects the emotions felt by several regarding the initial lack of guidance but the nagging values of the social work profession demanding responses, *Datta, a graduate of Master of Social Work from Nirmala Niketan College of Social Work, Mumbai and an active member of Jeevan Pravaah,* had to relocate back to his village as the pandemic spread. After a few days of staying indoors feeling helpless and restless, he began to try and make sense of the situation around him on his own, as no help or assistance was being provided otherwise. He describes the situation around him:

> During the Corona period, complete closure was observed in the villages. No one was going to anyone's house, farm work, offices were closed, and farm produce was not available, only darkness was visible everywhere. I was in the village at my home quietly, scared like everyone else for a while but after a while I thought we should do a little survey of the village, me being a social worker, to understand the condition of my village. I saw widows in the village, the landless families and farmers, daily wagers, and the poor people who had been living in poverty for more than 18 years, thinking that it was all over now, everything was going to end. And this pandemic will finish everyone now. In some houses, they didn't even have grains for their hunger. All were starving for food.

To this Sanaya, who is a lecturer in social work at a university in Sweden but was visiting her hometown Mumbai and became a part of Jeevan Pravaah, adds:

> We had been working with a small but zesty group of social workers to get a project running for the rag-picker women in Mumbai slums. However, all that suddenly came to a halt when the lockdown was announced. On the one hand, my friends with privileged socioeconomic backgrounds were posting social media messages about how this lockdown was a wonderful opportunity to rest and unwind, almost like a vacation. On the other hand, one saw stories of pain and suffering and hunger, starvation, and tragic deaths of poor migrants. That there is this inherent disparity and lopsided injustice in our society was never more obvious than at that time. I could not sit without acting. There was no clarity of the situation for anyone, but I began writing to all my friends and colleagues in Sweden for help and support, and we diverted the project to crisis relief with whatever little we had.

In this rather confused and limited knowledge phase with a lot of worries attached to it, the Jeevan Pravaah team began discussing the issue of loss of livelihoods of the marginalised urban and rural groups and decided to take matters into their own hands. As this was a project only initiated but not completely developed in this stage, they did not have to limit themselves to certain target groups, but instead took cognisance of those most affected all around them and conducted semi-systematic reviews to understand their situation first. As Prabha observes:

> As an entry point and an experiment, an attempt was made to contact my postgraduate and alumni students from urban and rural communities. Upon discussing my concerns, they began assessing the situation of their native geographical regions and showing a willingness to be part of interventions. Here we had to stand in solidarity and know that something had to be done. Seeing the young social workers' willingness to help their own communities we began to think of mobilising contacts for fundraising and material help to ease immediate relief. I reached out to numerous students, and from them the ones who responded back we connected to assess the local situation as a first step.

20.5.2 Challenges in Raising Funds, Providing Relief, and Advocacy

Given that the project was only in its initial planning days, there were no inherent funds at disposal of the Jeevan Pravaah team. Add to that the lockdown, and extreme punitive actions of the police, meant people, including social workers well-meaning to help, were unable to move around for fund and resource mobilisation. However, results from the initial survey of various localities and media reports evidently showed how people were lacking basic essentials because of the overnight loss of employment and lockdown. And so began the process of fundraising. As one of the members of the team notes:

> As a social worker, the first instinct was to mitigate the suffering of the people. However, not knowing where to turn to, we began writing appeals to family, friends, colleagues, social media contacts. But the challenge was, since we were asking for funds informally, where could the funds be collected? Who could be accountable? Since there was still so much uncertainty to the pandemic, we also had to cope up with feelings of uncertainty and maintaining transparency was key. The funds that began getting collected, based on the surveys conducted, were then redirected to our students and social workers in their native districts (Rural-Beed, Aurngabad, Baramati, Jalana, and urban Thane). There locally along with local volunteers the funds were used to purchase and distribute food like rice, lentils, oil, salt, sugar, and sanitation material. This process was time consuming, risky and made social workers face ample challenges.

While we acknowledge that is it problematic to focus social work efforts of provision of services vis-a-vis engaging with a rights-based approach for sustained social justice, and while relief work has the potential to reducing communities to mere receivers rather than taking ownership of the problems, it was assessed on the field that basic provision of essentials was a dire need. The elderly, children, and communities were starving, and crisis relief was an important first step and one that went on throughout the lockdown.

As Datta stresses further:

> When I, as a social worker, started visiting the village with some young friends from the village, I realized that the situation was very serious. Many people were looking at me with hope, everyone was worried, scared thinking that their survival is difficult without food. Baba, Corona will finish us soon. I even saw empty vessels in the house with no food grains left. Watching such miserable conditions of people, I decided to mobilize food grains for them and play my role of being a social worker in my village.

Once assistance was provided to a group or community, we would be bombarded with phone calls of more people who had heard of the material support we had provided. These were generally migrants from other states but stuck in Mumbai by the lockdown, or families from slum areas who had exhausted their small savings. Once they got in touch with us, we would have to begin finding logistics and ways in how to reach them with the material—this was a real challenge. Local networking and finding connections were of utmost importance then. It was not easy for us to reach the people in need because of the police checks and controls, refusal of transportation, and basic widespread fear, so networking with residents, communities, and engaging youth from the locality became a strategy we soon realized worked.

However, as mentioned earlier, efforts of the state came across as opposing the actions of social workers here. Punitive and custodial action by police and local politicians meant it was extremely difficult to find vehicles to transport the material purchased to its end locations. Students and social workers purchasing essentials in bulk were suspected of hoarding and were restricted from access to purchase. On the other hand, ration shopkeepers (the state public distribution system of subsidized goods) were not selling and providing food grains to local women. There were cases of cheating and inflation. Several of our Jeevan Pravaah members had to intervene and sort out such matters. Several letters were to be written, signed, and stamped by professors and the principal of the College of Social Work or approved by local municipal heads for the essentials to be transported and supplied. Here, situations leadership and the quick thinking of young social workers helped to get positive actions.

As Datta further mentions:

> With all these things in mind, I first wrote a letter to the police station, tehsil (local governance) office, and shared negative practices like above with him. This led to immediate action of police on the essentials of life. I can now reflect over how I worked at advocacy level, albeit at the grassroots.

Following that, many of the Jeevan Pravaahmembers, especially in the rural areas, saw the plight of migrants who had started walking back to their villages, trying to cover thousands of kilometers walking because there was no public transport. Here Datta, whose actions were exemplary, says:

> Those migrants and daily wagers who were walking down the street to reach their home, we arranged houses for them to stay in one place for two three days, following all the corona guidelines of the government. Since these groups of people had been walking for days without any proper places to stay, we conducted medical tests with all of them. After that, I went to tehsil (local governance), the regional collectors office, presented them with a request letter and took official government permission for arranging a tempo truck for all these migrants. Finally in three days they all were sent home safely by a tempo.

This was a widespread case of migrants who began walking back on foot to their villages. Many died in the process and many suffered excruciating health challenges. So, team Jeevan Pravaah's intervention in helping these migrants by arranging camps for overnight sleep, working with local communities to arrange food and water, and working with local authorities to arrange transportation was a much-required assistance where state measures were absent.

20.5.3 Arranging Livelihood Documents

Other important problems that came to the forefront in the face of displacement and loss of livelihoods of the migrants and daily wage laborer was how many of them lacked official identification cards or papers of any kind and what a big gap this is in statutory provision of basic verification essentials. Vishal, one of the other members interviewed in this study, came across and worked on this area during the pandemic:

> As the prevalence of Corona increased, work in many areas gradually ceased/reduced. All of these factors had a greater impact on daily laborers. One such group of people had set out on foot from Panvel to go home. It included children, women, men, and the elderly. A total of 80 to 85 people set out on foot to reach their village. But his village was at least 500 to 600 km away from Panvel. All these people were caught by the police mid-way while walking in their village and were put in camps. But in these camps, they had to face many difficulties. Proper provision of place to stay, food and water was not made. So, local communities united to help provide this. In addition, most of these migrants lacked any sort of identification documents that were needed for travel, a so-called e-pass. There were e-pass agents who were available, but they were charging extraordinarily high sums of money from these poor people. So in this situation, I started making e-pass appeals and applications for these people. These applications would get rejected more often than not. So I needed to assess on the spot what was going wrong and what needed to be done differently.

This goes to show how already, pre-Corona, the poor migrants were living without essential documents, but with the sudden situation in the pandemic, they became further vulnerable to being mismanaged by the state.

20.5.4 Women's and Children's Situation

In April 2020, UN Women reported that violence against women and girls had intensified the world over because of the pandemic and referred to it as 'the shadow pandemic' (United Nations statement by Mlambo-Ngcuka, 2020b). Increase in instances of violence against girls and women during the pandemic became apparent. Along with evidence of violence, which already reflected at the community mapping stage, at Jeevan Pravaah we had a rather eye-opening experience regarding this. In India, menstruation is still largely considered taboo with many myths attached to the topic, such as menstruation being an unclean time for the woman who should be banished and shamed from common spaces during these days. As Santosh, another one of the social workers, brings to notice:

> For women living in slum communities, it became a burden purchasing sanitary pads during lockdown. They would be subject to embarrassment and eve-teasing while walking back from the shops with sanitary pads or face humongous embarrassment purchasing these from male salespersons at the shop. So for many women lockdown meant not being able to purchase menstrual products, and asking a male in the family to purchase this was out of question due to the taboo subject. So many girls and women started suffering from increased infections and reproductive problems, as they had nowhere to turn to for support.

This was an urgent appeal from Santosh's community, which he recognised, and Jeevan Pravaah then networked with NGOs working specifically in this area. Myna Mahila Foundation, one such NGO, provided us with required supplies of sanitary pads, which were transported to the community and redistributed by the community youth. This is another such area that needs sustained action from the state for ending these myths and misconceptions and making women's reproductive and sexual health a priority and safety.

There are 472 million children in India under the age of 18 years, representing 39% of the country's total population. Lockdown also meant that schools were shut down and these children were out of school, those engaged in labor work were out of work, and those belonging to poor families were highly at risk of being trafficked or married off. As basic needs of the vulnerable groups began to taken care of and relief measures from the state began coming through, Jeevan Pravaah began undertaking more work for the psychological and physical well-being of children in the urban slums. Community libraries were set up by Santosh and others, computer labs were arranged, workshops in physical training such as dance were made regular, small-level competitions in arts and crafts and engagements in local festivals for mental and physical stimulation of the children were conducted. This activity was recognised as a dire need as parents were not able to focus on this need because of their own worries, and state intervention in this front was not seen.

20.5.5 Mental Health

The widespread social and economic disruption of the pandemic has produced a psychosocial impact unheard of in modern times. Mental health issues following the COVID-19 pandemic stemmed from normal people being exposed to 'extraordinary situations.' The presentations are myriad, and included emotional difficulties such as anxiety, depression, biological effects such as sleep and appetite disturbances, as well as severe mental illness and substance misuse. All these effects have been further fueled by information overload of new generation media platforms that have relentlessly spread a mix of accurate as well as inaccurate information and even conspiracy theories. Apurva, a social work graduate who worked with mental health during the pandemic, observes:

> In India, the first and foremost responses to the pandemic has led to fear and a sense of clear and imminent danger. Fears have ranged from those based on facts to unfounded fears based on information/misinformation circulating in the media, particularly social media. The social distancing and lockdown have also led to several changes in day-to-day activities, redistribution of home chores, extensive working from home and greater time spent with those living together in small spaces. Uncertainty and a sense of loss of control are undoubtedly the pathogenic agents for anxiety, panic, and depression. For families separated from patients admitted with COVID-19 complications, the separation was excruciatingly painful from a psychological viewpoint leading to worry, helplessness and frank depression. There were situations when people faced the unexpected instance of the death of a family member and prepared for negative outcomes. Children have lost access to spaces like schools, no opportunity for outdoor play and socialisation, they become increasingly engrossed in social media which makes them even more socially isolated when they emerge out of this situation.

So as interventions, parents were educated about means of keeping the children engaged, providing an opportunity to learn new skills at home, as well as encourage children to participate in activities, get them engaged in "edutainment" and hone their extra-curricular skills as well. Young people going through anxiety were given spaces to talk and express while receiving counselling. Similarly, the impoverished poor who had given up trying to survive needed a lot of mental support by the social workers on the field to be able to move past the most critical phases of the pandemic.

20.6 Directions for the Future

This chapter presented a selection of the interventions undertaken by a handful of social workers during a public health crisis in specific areas in Maharashtra, India. The extent of the work conducted by all of us jointly is vast, and it will take more time to reflect on what we did, and why and how things were done to provide help and assistance to the suffering that arose from COVID-19 and the lockdown in India. There are many more unnamed supporting actors such as the College of Social Work faculty and students, local leaders and authorities, other NGOs and funders, and friends and family, who helped us in our work.

But the work done by the Jeevan Pravaah team and the 92,000 other nongovernmental actors (NITI Aayog, 2020) has been emergency crisis relief and disaster management work. Thus, the work undertaken, and even the relief provided by the state during the pandemic, is short term—it assists the affected groups only momentarily. The evidence of this is seen, as this chapter is written 1 year after the COVID-19 pandemic began, and yet the most affected communities, which emerge as the already impoverished and marginalised groups, are still scattered, unorganized, in search of daily wages, unemployed, homeless, and without basic needs being fulfilled (Chen, 2020). As this chapter is written, parts of India are moving towards a second major lockdown due to the second and more harsh wave of COVID-19, but once again domestic workers, construction workers, and sanitary workers find themselves in a similar state.

20.6.1 Support for the Most Vulnerable: Women

As the pandemic has shown globally, women are one of the most vulnerable groups affected by COVID-19 and the shadow pandemic. In this context, the suggested directions for social work and policy are as follows.

Helplines of the government of persons calling to report gender-based violence should be connected to existing service providers, Family Counselling Centres, and protection officers to provide professional help. All local protection officers need to be issued a directive to attend to domestic violence cases in districts to reduce these increased incidences. An increase in the number of allowed days in shelter homes for women in distress, which is currently a maximum of only 4 days. Supply of sanitary pads, maternal health care, neonatal and child health, immunisation, and the nutritional needs of pregnant and lactating women need to be declared and provided as essential services. Additionally, an increased budget for nutrition in pre-primary school centers needs to be mandated to ensure food security. Vitamins should be made an integral part of the nutrition of children and pregnant and lactating mothers as the basic immunity of the population needs to be bettered. Schemes for market-oriented and sustainable employment of women in the sex trade, a highly marginalised and hidden group and seeking rehabilitation, are needed. And to conclude, special efforts need to be taken to identify single women, women-headed households, transgender people, elderly, beggars, and the homeless for making direct cash transfers to them as these are some of the most affected groups.

20.6.2 Strengthen Local Self-Governance

Community strengthening and local regional leadership need to be harnessed and supported by the state. Communities and locally elected leaders were actors who were closely connected to the people, helping those in need of basic rights like food, water, shelter, and sanitation, and made available resources that were lacking and not provided by the state. Thus, all local self-governments need complete autonomy with proper intime monitoring, guidelines and resource support, and sustained incentives for best efforts. In addition, the elected local representatives need to check the demand–supply chain and to communicate gaps with the local self-governments. Also, a labour helpline in Hindi and regional languages need to be instituted for the entire country, particularly given the high rate of intrastate migration within the state borders. Locally the expansion of free Internet access for online educational platforms and material in both urban and rural settings is a requirement. Additionally, authentic Information-Education-Communication platforms for the public with online consultation boards to get in-home treatment and medical attention need to be created and made accessible to all corners of the country. Indigenous voices and communities need to be considered formally, as with their support and knowledge, social workers were able to seek assistance from communities and local leaders to help out the most affected groups.

20.6.3 Social Security Provision

The situation of the unorganized labor market, urban slum communities, seasonal migrants, and daily wage laborers is evidence of livelihood uncertainties and disparity. Although social workers and local leaders provide support, national policy needs to take on sustained social justice measures to regulate safety nets and welfare support for these groups. For example, to maintain public health of all, decent housing, private toilets, and water and other basic needs need to become a priority for the state. When cash transfer and compensation has been announced by the state, the lack of clear guidelines on how to obtain these, lack of basic identification documents to attain any benefits, and mid-level corruption has often led to the most needful not obtaining the benefits. This impediment needs to be rectified, not only in the context of a global pandemic but even in general, as this situation was only highlighted in the lockdown but exists in general. The unorganised sector, which constitutes more than 90% of India's workforce, needs to become formalised in the sense of attaining basic welfare and safety benefits attributed to the labour they contribute in the long term. Contractual employment, health insurance, parental leave, and unemployment benefits are some measures to be considered to be enforced by the state on employers for long-term development. Apart from this, in the situation of a crisis, ration supplies and financial assistance per person needs to be mandated and provided as a right to daily wagers and slum dwellers who have lost their source of income from the lockdowns and curfews enforced by the state. Nongovernmental organisations and community-based organisations need to be actively included with the cooperation of the government to conduct rapid needs assessment, especially in slum pockets and rural areas. These actors can then be supported to undertake ration provision, monetary assistance, and various kinds of support in these areas.

20.6.4 Advocacy

COVID-19 came at a time when the country was already in crises from other social stressors. The past few years have seen a surge in right-wing extremism, characterised by hate crimes and mob lynching towards Muslims and other socially backwards castes and communities (Kaul 2017). Hindu nationalism or Hindutva, the political ideology that advocates Hindu supremacy, specifically over Muslims who comprise about 14% of modern India's population, is being promoted openly in the country This environment in the country and among the people who are starving for food and water has meant the media, politicians, and state bureaucrats are able to dilute issues of public health, collective resources, and social justice and instead divert masses into religious sentiments and segregation. Ordinary people are hypnotised and are made to forget their basic needs and human rights, which is the state responsibility. There is fear among people, and they are pressurised and controlled into not raising their voices for their basic rights. In this situation, it is the responsibility of academicians, teachers, students, researchers, field practitioners of all interdisciplinary faculties, and the social work fraternity to intervene and advocate by framing welfare policies based on relevant research studies and field experiences.

The most vulnerable groups that have come to the forefront during COVID-19 are, in fact, the ones most vulnerable in society even outside the public health pandemic. So long-term action plans to support victims of the COVID-19 pandemic are required and at the same time policy and its implementation to prevent any victims of social discrimination and future disasters becomes the challenge for the state and social work in India.

Acknowledgments The authors thank Dr. Geeta Balakrishnan for giving her expert advice from her extensive experience of work with women and children and social work in India. We also thank Bhim Raskar for his expert advice on local self-governance from his extensive experience of work in this area in India.

References

Amadasun, S. (2020). COVID-19 pandemic in Africa: What lessons for social work education and practice? *International Social Work, 64*(2), 246–250. https://doi.org/10.1177/0020872820949620

Bhalerao, S. (2021, April 19). Mumbai: With rise in Covid cases in Dharavi, BMC returns to last year's strategy. *The Indian Express*. https://indianexpress.com/article/cities/mumbai/mumbai-with-rise-in-covid-cases-in-dharavi-bmc-returns-to-last-years-strategy-7280518/

Chen, M. (2020, April 10). *To die from hunger or the virus*. UNU-WIDER. https://www.wider.unu.edu/publication/die-hunger-or-virus

Dafuleya, G. (2020). Social and emergency assistance ex-ante and during COVID-19 in the SADC Region. *The International Journal of Community and Social Development, 2*(2), 251–268. https://doi.org/10.1177/2516602620936028

Government of India Union Budget and Economic Survey (http://indiabudget.nic.in). (2008). *Indian Budget*. https://www.indiabudget.gov.in/budget_archive/ub2007-08/ubmain.htm

Human Rights Watch. (2021, April 22). *India falters amid growing Covid-19 crisis*. https://www.hrw.org/news/2021/04/22/india-falters-amid-growing-covid-19-crisis

International Monetary Fund (IMF). (2020). *Policy responses to COVID-19 policy tracker*. https://www.imf.org/en/Topics/imf-and-covid19/Policy-Responses-to-COVID-19. Google Scholar.

Jones, N. R., Qureshi, Z. U., Temple, R. J., Larwood, J. P. J., Greenhalgh, T., & Bourouiba, L. (2020). *Two metres or one: What is the evidence for physical distancing in Covid-19?* BMJ Publishing Group. https://doi.org/10.1136/bmj.m3223

Kaul, N. (2017). Rise of the political right in India: Hindutva-development mix, modi myth, and dualities. *Journal of Labor and Society, 20*(4), 523–548. https://doi.org/10.1111/wusa.12318

Lingam, L., & Suresh Sapkal, R. (2020). COVID-19, physical distancing and social inequalities: Are we all really in this together? *The International Journal of Community and Social Development, 2*(2), 173–190. https://doi.org/10.1177/2516602620937932

NITI Aayog. (2020, November). *Mitigation and management of Covid-19 practices from India's states and union territories*. National Institution for Transforming India (NITI) Aayog. https://doi.org/10.7910/DVN/7MHJEM

Pawar, M. (2020). *COVID-19 pandemic: Impact on and implications for community and social development* (1st ed.). SAGE.

Rambaree, K., & Nässén, N. (2020). 'The Swedish Strategy' to COVID-19 pandemic: Impact on vulnerable and marginalised communities. *The International Journal of Community and Social Development, 2*(2), 234–250. https://doi.org/10.1177/2516602620936048

Sengupta, S., & Jha, M. K. (2020). Social policy, COVID-19 and impoverished migrants: Challenges and prospects in locked down India. *The International Journal of Community and Social Development, 2*(2), 152–172. https://doi.org/10.1177/2516602620933715

Soutphommasane, T. (2021, May 4). Criminalising citizens returning from India signals some are more Australian than others. *The Guardian*. https://www.theguardian.com/commentisfree/2021/may/04/criminalising-citizen-returns-from-india-signals-some-are-more-australian-than-others

Thelwell, K., & Alexander, L. (2021). Homelessness in India | *The Borgen Project*. https://borgenproject.org/tag/homelessness-in-india/

UN-Habitat. (2018). SDG Indicator 11.1.1 Training Module: Adequate housing and slum upgrading. United Nations Human Settlement Programme (UN-Habitat), Nairobi.

United Nations. (2020a). The Shadow Pandemic: Violence against women during COVID-19. *UN Women*. https://www.unwomen.org/en/news/in-focus/in-focus-gender-equality-in-covid-19-response/violence-against-women-during-covid-19

United Nations. (2020b). Statement by Phumzile Mlambo-Ngcuka, UN Women Executive Director, on the International Day for the Elimination of Violence against Women. *UN Women*. https://www.unwomen.org/en/news/stories/2020/11/statement-ed-phumzile-international-day-for-the-elimination-of-violence-against-women

Verity, R., Okell, L. C., Dorigatti, I., Winskill, P., Whittaker, C., Imai, N., Cuomo-Dannenburg, G., Thompson, H., Walker, P. G. T., Fu, H., Dighe, A., Griffin, J. T., Baguelin, M., Bhatia, S., Boonyasiri, A., Cori, A., Cucunubá, Z., FitzJohn, R., Gaythorpe, K., … Ferguson, N. M. (2020). Estimates of the severity of coronavirus disease 2019: A model-based analysis. *The Lancet Infectious Diseases, 20*(6), 669–677. https://doi.org/10.1016/s1473-3099(20)30243-7

Vikaspedia Domains. (2021). https://vikaspedia.in/social-welfare/unorganised-sector-1/categories-of-unorganised-labour-force

World Population Review. (2021). *Mumbai Population 2021*. https://worldpopulationreview.com/world-cities/mumbai-population

World Poverty Clock. (2021). *World Poverty Clock*. https://worldpoverty.io/map

Worldometer. (2021). *COVID-19 coronavirus pandemic*. https://www.worldometers.info/coronavirus/

21 COVID-19, Hyper Vulnerabilities, Silenced Traumas, and Colonial Scars: Social Work Scholars Engaging in Critical Dialogue with Racialized Communities

Sophie Hamisultane, Edward Ou Jin Lee and Roxane Caron

21.1 Introduction

Within the context of the COVID-19 pandemic, many countries have further restricted and secured their national borders, which has also shaped the contours of symbolic borders on individual liberties, human rights, and collective struggles. During the periods of confinement that have followed, communities which were already disproportionately impacted by socioeconomic and racial inequalities were further rendered vulnerable (Diversité Canadienne, 2020; Cleveland et al., 2020). A succession of tragic and traumatic events triggered deeper levels of collective anger and rage, particularly within racialized communities, including those experiencing multiple and intersectional forms of oppression. As social work educators and scholars situated in Tiohtià:ke on the unceded Mohawk et Kanien'kehá:ka territories, otherwise known as Montréal, Québec, Canada, the following events were highly mediatized in our area, in ways that resonated with each of us and resulted in collective expressions of grief.

- May 25, 2020: The murder of George Floyd at the hands of police resulted in spontaneous uprisings across the United States and generated a worldwide reaction against police violence and anti-Black racism, reminding everyone of the potent power of the virus of racism (Laferrière, 2020).
- August 4, 2020: Multiple explosions at the main port in Beirut, Lebanon, caused hundreds of deaths and thousands of injured, further exacerbated by a failing political system and a heavily privatized health system already over capacity from COVID-19 (Le Monde, 2020a). After the explosions, people came out to provide food and medical support while also cleaning the streets.
- September 28, 2020: Joyce Echaquan, an Indigenous woman from the Atikamekw First Nation in Quebec, shared a live Facebook video of healthcare workers making derogatory, racist, and anti-Indigenous comments toward her, only hours before her death on a hospital bed (Riopel, 2020). Public condemnation of the incident included collective protests against a colonial healthcare system that continues to perpetuate systemic racism (Radio Canada, October 3, 2020a).
- March 16, 2021: The massacre of eight people at Asian massage parlors of mostly Asian women, by a 21-year-old white man. This

S. Hamisultane (✉) · E. O. J. Lee · R. Caron
School of Social Work, Université de Montréal, Montreal, QC, Canada
e-mail: sophie.hamisultane@umontreal.ca; edward.lee@umontreal.ca; roxane.caron.2@umontreal.ca

M. C. S. Gonçalves et al. (eds.), *The Coronavirus Crisis and Challenges to Social Development*,
https://doi.org/10.1007/978-3-030-84678-7_21

mass shooting occurred in the shadow of a longer history of anti-Asian racism and Asian people in Canada, the United States (U.S.), and Europe being more recently targeted and serving as scapegoats in the COVID-19 era, in what was labeled by former U.S. president Donald Trump as the "China" virus.

We aim to engage in critical self-reflection and dialogue about these realities as individuals with differing positionalities in relationship to COVID-19 and the various events shared earlier. In this chapter, we examine our fields of research and community involvements, as well as our educational institution, to critically re-assess how we, as social subjects, became vulnerabilized. Indeed, many scholars and educators, especially those who hold marginalized identities, are not solely "insider" or "outsider" to what is being studied or taught (Naples, 1996), but instead navigate "insider/outsider dynamics, understanding these dynamics as fluid, on-going and ever-changing" (Caron et al., 2020, p. 12).

Thus, we asked ourselves these questions: In what ways do I engage in insider/outsider dynamics with respect to these situations? How am I affected by socioeconomic and racial inequalities? What informs my commitment to social change and transformation in light of the colonial and racial violence that is occurring in this global pandemic context? These questions are meant to elicit our critical self-reflections about our individual experiences and perspectives, which we subsequently put into dialogue with each other.

In the following sections, the key theoretical frameworks that inform our analyses will be presented as well as the methodological approach that was used to scaffold this chapter. Each author subsequently shares their 'testimonies' in relationship to events related to racial and migrant injustices, as overlapping with the inequalities entrenched by COVID-19. The chapter concludes with strategies to engage in actions committed to social justice.

21.2 Vulnerability, Colonial Scars, and the Resurfacing of Historic and Silenced Traumas

To anchor our perspective, we draw from the interdisciplinary concept of vulnerability by articulating it within a reflection that integrates two dimensions (Spini et al., 2017): the internal (subjective and psychic construction) and the external (life pathways, historical contexts, social events). Vulnerability is expressed in different forms depending on the subject's experience. For people affected by racism and intersectional forms of oppressions, vulnerability is shaped by people's perceptions of them, which is consistent with current understandings of vulnerability as an individual, affective, and physical experience (Garrau, 2018). The vulnerability of people experiencing oppression and post-colonial domination must be understood in relationship to questions of power, inequality, and the ability or inability to act (Naepels, 2019).

The feeling of vulnerability is also associated with the feeling of 'risk:' the risk of encountering a cumulative number of threatening events, the risk that these events will actually materialize, and the risk of lacking protections to confront or avoid these threats (Sirven, 2007). The different forms of racism that have emerged since the arrival of COVID-19 brought to the surface overlapping sociohistorical processes of domination and oppression within Quebec/Canadian history, such as the Indian Act and its genocidal impacts on Indigenous Peoples (Monture-Agnes, 1995),[1] immigration laws that explicitly surveilled and excluded Asian people (Thobani, 2007),[2] and the

[1] See The National Inquiry into Missing and Murdered Indigenous Women and Girls (2019), https://www.mmiwg-ffada.ca/final-report/ and the Truth and Reconciliation Commission Report (2015), http://www.trc.ca.

[2] The Chinese immigration law of 1923, the internment in camps of the Japanese in 1942, the exclusion of South

history of slavery, state surveillance, and racial segregation of Black people (Gay, 2004). The intensification of acts of racism and intersecting oppressions have 'fragilized' racialized people who struggle against this persistent risk of recurrence as a form of violence onto itself and also as a historical return to the suffering of their ancestors (Hamisultane, 2020). This risk of recurrence operates as a colonial scar, carried as an intergenerational heritage of oppression reactivated by the events that we raise to the surface here. They can result in a commitment to the preservation of the self, when one is directly impacted, but also to other oppressed peoples (Fanon, 1952).

Post/decolonial theories reveal how colonial heritages have shaped current inequalities experienced by racialized people. Indeed, the foundations of capitalism, European empire building, and white settler colonies emerged from the gendered racialization of labor, as demonstrated by conquest, the slave trade, and indentured labor (Lowe, 2015; Vergès, 2019; Wynter, 2003). Moreover, analyzing the coloniality of power (Mignolo, 2007; Quijano, 2000) and the colonial/modern gender system (Lugones, 2008) reveals how dominant narratives declaring the progress of 'Western civilization' as a market-based democracy and the defenders of the human rights of oppressed women and queer and trans people can obscure complex historical colonial legacies (Caron & Lee, 2020). The colonial management of labor and intimacy (Lowe, 2015) shapes the origins of social work in Canada (Caron & Lee, 2020) through the promotion of 'moral and social reform and hygiene' (Lee & Ferrer, 2014). Even as contemporary social work promotes social justice, the framing of social workers as benevolent (Heron, 2007) obscures how "this 'helping' is so often invested in managing the morality of those being 'helped', thus reinforcing a set of racialized, gender, and sexualized norms" (Caron & Lee, 2020, p. 74).

From a clinical sociological perspective, these colonial heritages reveal the ways in which "the individual is the product of a story of which he seeks to become the subject" (de Gaulejac, 2009, p. 186; author translation). Whether it is regarding one's family history or a broader social history, this formulation makes it possible to understand how history operates within oneself (de Gaulejac, 2009), even if it is not told but is transmitted by what is unspoken or what is denied (Hamisultane, 2017a). Indeed, the denial of the colonial past is characterized by the refusal to integrate and recognize the colonial past in the understanding of contemporary social phenomena (Bancel et al., 2006).

These historical erasures can operate in the present as colonial scars that were never fully healed and suddenly break open. When these colonial histories are denied and unspoken, its colonial scars can surface in collective forms of trauma. For example, as a result of colonial and genocidal practices such as forced relocation, the reservation system, and the separation of children from their families and communities through residential schools, Indigenous Peoples in Canada/Quebec have endured collective forms of historic and intergenerational trauma that when "ignored…there is no support for dealing with it, the trauma will be passed from one generation to the next" (Wesley-Esquimaux & Smolewski, 2004, p. 2). Thus, intergenerational trauma can be viewed as the breaking open of colonial scars, haunting the lives of historically colonized peoples. Intergenerational and silenced traumas are "like the shadowy thing that lives in empty spaces… (and) reveals how the past is in the present" (Cho, 2008, p. 29).

Thus, we suggest that the hypervulnerabilities experienced by racialized communities during this pandemic are shaped by colonial heritages within Quebec and globally, resulting in colonial scars and the resurfacing of historic and silenced traumas. These colonial scars, and the ways they become infected and break open, inform the current reactions against the racial and colonial injustices that COVID-19 has amplified. In the following section, we share our individual testimonies of how we situated ourselves within this reality.

Asianss in 1908, etc. (Thobani, 2007).

21.3 Methodological Approach

To answer these questions, we engaged in multiple discussions to collectively reflect upon these different levels of vulnerability. This chapter is the result of these exchanges. We recognize that our differing social locations places us within complex and shifting dominant versus oppressed groups. Our social locations shape the nature of our engagements and how we navigate tensions between our experiences and professional engagement. How might one feel legitimate about their responses to colonial and racial injustice when one has been afforded 'white privilege?' How might one critique and analyze racism when one is racialized? How might one recognize the ways in which multiple intersecting forms of oppression shape these dynamics?

As a discipline anchored by the 'helping relationship,' anti-oppressive and decolonial feminist social work approaches pushes us to lean into these discomforts. According to Cifafi (2019), "we are there with our history and our affects" (p. 62; author translation). It is the intentional and reflexive process of distancing from our own history and affects that allows the social work scholar and practitioner to not project their own history onto others and thus be able "to carry out this work of lucidity" that sometimes discovers what "has pushed us to" (Cifafi, 2019, p. 62; author translation). When a public health emergency was declared in Quebec in mid-March 2020, we were literally and figuratively immobilized, as the government raced to impose shutdown measures to contain COVID-19. This sudden inability to 'take action' compelled each of us to turn inward and reexamine our social locations and histories. This reflexive process ultimately pushed us to re-engage in our collective desire for social change toward a more just and equitable society, as we were reminded that "a margin of freedom is essential to our humanity" (Cifafi, 2019, p. 62; author translation). As Cifafi (2019) argues, feeling powerless is "most of the time a construction, a representation of the possible scope of our actions: often therefore a mode of defense which justifies our inaction" (p. 264; author translation).

In the following section, we share our individual testimonies of how we situated ourselves within this reality. Sophie begins with sharing the ways in which her social location of mixed Asian origins informs the ways in which she engages in research related to racist micro-aggressions and racial justice. Roxane then shares how the constant tension between her long-term engagement with refugee women in Lebanon versus her social location as a white settler woman has animated her research and teaching. Finally, Edward describes how being part of the queer and trans Black, Indigenous, and other People of Color (QTBIPOC) community in Montreal/Tiohtià:ke is intrinsic to the challenges of being part of and outside of this community. Each of us shares our initial responses to the arrival of COVID-19 and reflects deeply about how the COVID-19 public health measures impacted ourselves and the communities of which we are a part, are connected to, and with which we have a profound relationship.

21.4 Our Testimonies

21.4.1 Sophie Hamisultane: Tensions of Being Directly Impacted Versus Fostering a Reflexive Process

My research interests focus on the issues of interculturality and, particularly, on the complexity of the identity of descendants of migrants. On a personal level, I am of Vietnamese and French origins, therefore within this broad category of Asian people. Before the arrival of COVID-19, my sensitivity to issues of racism and my personal experiences brought me closer to communities who were victims of racism and discrimination. Social work, as well as the humanities and social sciences in general, allow me to question these social relationships and the historical contexts that anchor them. This questioning includes interrogating the needs of racialized people that do not feel recognized as equal citizens in comparison to white people. However, although discrimination and racism are experienced as injustices, sometimes their damages are described solely from a legal lens, when in fact, these damages are lived in silence. I have worked on the question of this silence (Hamisultane, 2021), resulting in invisible racial microaggressions that are considered as nonexistent not only within the workplaces where they take place and also sometimes within the victim's close family and friends.

The context of the pandemic, yet again, entrenched people into their community, through the creation of groups on social networks to denounce the injustices that targeted them. In particular, for example, the Groupe d'entraide contre le racisme envers les Asiatiques du Québec (GECREAQ) was created during the pandemic. Indeed, Asian people were the targets of racism (Braun, 2020) because COVID-19 originated in China. So I myself was sucked into the phenomenon of stigmatization and of community belonging. I became a member of the GECREAQ Facebook group. I noticed the alarming number of testimonies of racial micro-aggressions. I became invested in these testimonies because of both my understanding of this Asian community and my role as a researcher on issues of interculturality. Therefore, I applied for a grant, which I obtained,[3] to work toward building a reflection on the context that our society was living, precisely from the point of view of descendants of Asian migrants.

My approach to this issue questions the researcher's involvement in the objectification of her data (Giust-Desprairies, 2004). My vulnerability propelled my desire to do research and my desire to act. This vulnerability, which was both internal (as subjective and psychic) and social (from experiencing racism as an Asian person) pushed me toward action. Through a reflexive process, I gained a sense of what I describe as 'resonance'—the ways in which our historical heritage informs what we experience in the present and within the current social context (Hamisultane, 2018). This resonance, which cannot be strategic nor premeditated, serves as a tool for my work. It is the strained bond between me and the other, between me who is also the other, or as Ricoeur (1990) suggests, *oneself as another*.

21.4.2 The Recurrence of Vulnerability

This vulnerability is again materialized in a new event amplifying the previous ones (the pandemic and its consequences and racism): the death of George Floyd. This event affected me as a racialized person because I experienced racism and harassment when I was young, living in the French countryside where virtually no Asian people lived. This kind of injustice made no sense to me, as with the death of George Floyd, which had a resonance with my own heritage. In the context of a pandemic, exacerbating the social inequalities particularly affecting Black people in the United States (U.S.) (CDC, 2020; Eichengreen, 2020), the death of George Floyd created a general anger that had worldwide repercussions (Radio Canada, June 6, 2020b). Protests in the U.S. following the death of a Black person as a result of a police altercation are recurrent (Tellier, 2020). However, as Black people are disproportionately more vulnerable to negative health consequences caused by COVID-19, as this overlaps with other social inequalities, Black Lives Matter protests continued to surface and caught international attention. This anger is significant in a temporal process of oppression experienced by Black people and other racialized people. For example, the history of Black people in Quebec has largely been made invisible (Gay, 2004). During these collective demonstrations, many statues of historical colonial figures in several white settler/Western countries who were involved in colonization and the slave trade have been overthrown (Ducourtieux, 2020; Le Monde, 2020a, b).

I experience these societal phenomena as a reality of what the postcolonial theories strive to show and that I try to transmit in my teachings, namely, the colonial legacy of the domination and oppression dynamics that shape current social inequalities.

[3]Descendantes de migrants faisant l'objet de racisme dans un contexte de pandémie. Subvention institutionnelle CRSH-2020–2022.

21.4.2.1 Roxane Caron: Vulnerabilities and Trouble in the Insider/Outsider Positionality

What I recall from the earliest weeks of living in this "COVID-19 time" was, first, denial: "it will not last." I was rapidly confronted, as everyone else, at the long-lasting scope and scale of this new reality. If media outlets focused their attention on the situation "here"—the local realities in Quebec and Canada—my attention was dedicated to "over there." In light of what Al-Ali (2020) highlights: "While much of the focus so far has been on the original epicenters of the outbreak (…) we know that many people in the Global South will bear the long-term effects (of the pandemic) in even more horrific ways" (p. 334). For me, this "over there" is the Bourj el Barajneh refugee camp in Lebanon. For more than 15 years now, my research in Lebanon has given rise to questions that have led me to question my capacity as a scholar to write and communicate "through cultures." I have previously written what had led me to work with refugees and to continue my commitment to this community (Caron et al., 2020).[4] Although I (re)plunge into identity questions that I (re)visit regularly (see Caron, 2012; Richard & Caron, 2020; Caron & Lee, 2020; Caron et al., 2020), this is not "just-another-reflexive-exercise" as it reveals what I call a "disturbance in my insider/outsider positionality."

21.4.2.2 COVID-19: Deepening Conditions Lived, Imposed, and Attributed

As with many governments around the world, the "stay home slogan" during the present pandemic is widely used in Lebanon, regardless of the fact that it makes no sense given the situation of many refugees in the country and highlights huge disparities (Al-Ali, 2020). A widely quoted tweet by a South Asian doctor illustrates this idea: "Social distancing is a privilege: you need running water, space in your house, and the means to afford not going out to earn money" (Horn, 2020). Indeed, it is very difficult to practice social distancing given many refugees often live in overcrowded conditions lacking adequate hygiene and sanitation. However, if Horn evokes the notion of privilege, it is the notion of condition that refugees I work with put forward; conditions that are imposed and attributed. I recall the powerful testimony of someone who affirmed her conditions of confinement and encampment as a protracted Palestinian refugee, and her description of the refugee camp as a 'kind of blockage or siege' and an 'open prison.' These words have haunted me for a long time, and they were the first to emerge from my memory as COVID-19 took hold of my life and of the refugees with whom I have worked with for many years. Measures, in particular social distancing and confinement, are not only "non-sense" as Horn (2020) points out; they exacerbate protracted colonial scars and the protracted condition of refugees; scars and conditions revealing ongoing overlapping systems of oppression: orientalism and neo/colonialism.

Over the years doing research with Palestinian and Syrian refugees in Lebanon, many refugee women have reminded me of their neo/colonial[5] experience; colonial relationships that resurface and respond to each other in situations such as the global pandemic. The individual experiences of refugees in this COVID time are certainly essential to grasp, but the testimony that I recalled, like so many others, put forward the historical forces, which attribute or even impose

[4] I cannot continue this exercise without revealing my positionality and saying "from where I speak" by identifying certain identities that have often emerged in my work with refugee women. Therefore, I am a western woman, citizen (Canadian), researcher, and teacher… I am not Palestinian or Syrian and I never experienced refuge or forced migration myself.

[5] The end of the First World War marked the dismantling of the Ottoman Empire. As a result, geopolitical changes took place through colonial mandates: France administers Lebanon and Syria while Britain is mandated over Palestine, Transjordania, and Iraq. The institutionalization of communitarianism in Lebanon took place under the French mandate (Corm, 2007), the same system contested in the streets of many Lebanese cities in the fall of 2019 and then again, after the explosion at the port of Beirut. The Lebanese population was indignant about long-standing and ongoing political corruption as well as exacerbated economic devastation shaped by COVID-19.

conditions, of the refugee and of encampment. I have discussed elsewhere the limits of human rights discourse and international law (Caron et al., 2020) in advancing social justice. Most of the refugees in Lebanon do not benefit from international protection frameworks and, as a result, regularly face high risks of arrest, detention, abuse from security forces, exploitation by landlords and employers, coercive practices, and illegal expulsions (Save the Children, 2020).

21.4.2.3 "I Am a White-Settler-Woman"

March 2020. We're in a worldwide pandemic. Shock. Denial. I begin to learn about COVID-19 and its impacts. Quickly, I turn my attention to the Global South. May 2020. I have a Skype call with Lina Abou Habib (2020a, b), a Lebanese feminist activist whom I had met in a previous research-stay in Lebanon. Lina and I discussed potential research collaborations, an idea that strengthened in the context of the world pandemic as this situation consolidates the relevance of a collaboration given the exacerbation of the precarious situations experienced by many vulnerable groups in both Canada and Lebanon. May 25, 2020. The tragic death of George Floyd in the hands of a white police officer marks my mind. I'm reminded of my white-settler-woman condition. August 4, 2020. The explosion at the Port of Beirut. This event hits me—full force. This catastrophe is a third wave that throws me to the ground. It's not images that reach me first but the cries and distress of "my loved ones" in refugee camps.

Through the present exercise, I (re)visit my positionality, meaning "where I speak from" and "where I (re)act from… or don't." If I was well aware of my white-settler-woman condition, the process of writing and more specifically of hearing and reading my colleagues' testimonies highlighted this condition, disorganizing my insider/outsider positionality. Being this outsider person—namely not being a refugee, not being racialized—shook me once again. Should I step back? Should I react? But more importantly, can I understand and feel their experiences? Audre Lorde (1981) reaffirms my response so far. She reiterates that turning my back on these emotions expressed such as anger of various minority groups "with the excuse or pretext of being intimidated does not give anyone any strength—it is just another way to preserve racial blinders, the power of established, untouchable, untouched privileges. Guilt is just another way of treating ourselves as an object" (p. 10). Decolonization cannot be placed solely on minorities alone. As a white-settler-woman I recognize that "decolonization demands that we uproot long-standing structures of our world, that we must struggle against our own self-interests and our identities, for we have come to recognize ourselves in the institutions of settler-colonialism and in the prospects of settler futurity" (Shaw, 2019).

21.4.3 Edward Ou Jin Lee: Crisis Upon Crisis, Silenced Traumas, and the Insistence of Collective Survival

As part of queer and trans Black, Indigenous and other People of Color (QTBIPOC) community building and organizing over the past two decades, I was aware of the urgent needs of QTBIPOC people, especially those who were street involved, migrants with precarious status, living with HIV, etc. The material deprivation and social isolation experienced by various QTBIPOC communities were caused by multiple, intersecting forms of structural violence, and informed by intergenerational colonial and imperial histories (Lee, 2018). When COVID-19 first hit, time seemed to simultaneously slow to a crawl, while also accelerating at an unimaginable pace. Time slowed down as I spent hours watching COVID-19-related news, trying to absorb as many details as possible. At the same time, time accelerated, as I began to realize how destructive COVID-19 was going to be on oppressed communities, including and perhaps especially QTBIPOC communities.

In a different way, timeframes in my mind also seemed to warp as intense thoughts and emotions triggered at times past childhood experiences and at other times pointed to apocalyptic futures. I imagined what it would have been like if I had lived in this new COVID-19 reality, as a suicidal queer and gender-creative Asian child and then youth whose main forms of survival included escaping into queer and trans social spaces as well as traveling outside of the city. I honestly do not know if I would have survived if I lived through COVID-19 as a youth. The colonial scars that I had worked so hard to heal broke open as the silenced and intergenerational traumas embedded within my family and the broader Korean diaspora resurfaced. By tracing the historical legacies of Japanese colonialism and U.S. imperialism, Cho (2008) argues that the silenced traumas from this heritage surfaces in the artistic expressions of diasporic Koreans in the U.S. and elsewhere. As such, the production of haunting (Gordon, 1997) reveals how oppressed and colonized peoples make sense of themselves, their suffering, and their collective will to survive, as "unspeakable trauma does not die out with the person who first experienced it. Rather, it takes on a life of its own, emerging from the spaces where secrets are concealed" (Cho, 2008, p. 6). This realization brought me back to the present and the urgent future of QTBIPOC people in Montreal/Tiohtià:ke—particularly those who are Black and Indigenous, Arab, Muslim, migrants with precarious status, trans, street involved, etc. How were we going to survive?

In response, I leaned into these multiple crises and took action in the ways that I could. I spent time supporting QTBIPOC community workers in the transition to develop digital outreach strategies and co-facilitated space for community workers to address the various crises: mental health distress (i.e., suicide), addictions, financial and housing precarity, extreme social isolation, etc. Some queer and trans migrants, for example, who had recently arrived in Montreal/Tiohtià:ke did not know French or English and had difficulties meeting their basic needs. Each crisis situation that arose revealed the ways in which the multiple and intersecting forms of structural violence faced by QTBIPOC people and migrants rendered many vulnerable to a particular set of living conditions that deepened people's exposure to premature death. These crises have broken open colonial scars left by the colonial management of intimacies and current forms of hetero-cis-normative and patriarchal violence that haunt QTBIPOC and migrant communities (Lee, 2018). What is at stake, for many QTBIPOC people and migrants, is not simply a lesser quality of life, but literally accelerated pathways to profound social isolation, material deprivation, and death.

This urgency led me to accelerate the pace of building research and intervention projects, especially those that diverted resources to initiatives which included peer outreach programs. This diversion allowed more QTBIPOC people to be paid and trained to address the multiple crises in our communities. Somehow, the time warp during this COVID-19 reality, and my position as professor, created pathways to mobilize research funds to create innovative practices that could respond adequately to the devastation caused by COVID-19. At the same time, my position as a non-Black and Indigenous university professor pushed me away from my community, as I was perceived by some community members as outside of the crises that were unfolding. As I navigated these tensions, I strove to center QTBIPOC people survival and resistance and humbly contribute to opening and holding new spaces and futures that honor QTBIPOC lives and life-worlds.

21.4.4 Mobilizing for Change Within Social Work Programs: How to Give Voice, How to Be Heard?

As government-imposed public health measures to contain COVID-19 became the new reality, our university and school of social work entered into crisis mode. University classes were abruptly forced to transition into online delivery and field placements were cancelled. Faculty, instructors, staff, and students alike had difficulty in adapting and entered into differing levels of crisis. This step was especially difficult for racialized students, including those who were international, queer, and trans students. This difficulty forced us to reorganize how we taught and supervised to make space for emergent student needs and to realign how we navigated classrooms, meetings, and projects.

The subsequent events related to continued anti-Asian attacks, the deaths of George Floyd and Joyce Echaquan, as well as the explosion in Beirut further disorganized all of our lives. In some ways, it was like everyone in Quebec was bearing witness to the historical, social, and political conditions that led to the continued suffering and premature death of racialized communities. The colonial scars were breaking open with silenced collective traumas resurfacing from a plurality of voices and experiences haunted by historical colonial legacies. These "vulnerabilities" expose the ways in which underlying historical, geopolitical, social, and political conditions of racialized communities are intimately tied to colonial logics, anti-Black racism, white supremacy, and orientalism. However, many racialized communities refuse to be reduced to being "vulnerable"—as they come together, with allies, to protest, to resist, to provide mutual support, and to collectively mourn and demand for human dignity and equitable living conditions.

These multiples crises, overlapping with the crisis of COVID-19, compelled us into action within our school of social work. We organized on-line mutual support spaces for Black students and instructors impacted by the murder of George Floyd and ongoing anti-Black racism in Quebec as well as for those impacted by the explosion in Beirut, especially those who belonged to the Lebanese and Armenian diasporic communities. These initiatives were created to make space for people who wanted to be heard and from which we could learn collectively. As a response to multiple crises, these spaces challenged the presumptions of how learning occurs within the university, as textbooks were put aside and peoples' voices and emotions were prioritized. Bearing witness to people's pain and suffering, as well as engaging in critical dialogue allowed for, to some degree, the transforming of feelings of powerlessness, to collective mobilizing for future actions.

However, fostering these spaces were not without its challenges. COVID-19 had forced everyone in our school of social work to be in "crisis mode" about every aspect of the program. Within this context, it was difficult to find space and energy to respond to the multiple events that we referenced above that particularly impacted racialized communities in Quebec and migrant communities in the Global South. In the days following the murder of George Floyd, many people wanted to make a declaration about the school's commitment to racial justice and equity Upon recognition of the underrepresentation of Black people within the faculty, this led to the online support spaces that were created with Black members of the school and subsequently with Arab members of the school and those who were impacted by the explosion in Beirut. These discussions have led to the creation of committees focused on anti-racism and solidarity in the face of natural disasters that will perhaps permit racialized people to give an account of oneself, to make space for what is silent to be spoken and where an emotional incomprehension is explained. To give the possibility that an "I" may express itself. Within oppressive environments for racialized people, how can we give an account of oneself (Butler, 2007)? In other words, how does one foster critical consciousness about not only oneself but also the social context within which one lives?

Moreover, as non-Black professors within a school of social work with a significant number of Black students, how do we engage in a reflexive practice that will allow us to take an ongoing stance of humility for the ways in which we may unintentionally perpetuate anti-Black racism? As Asian professors, Sophie and Edward are not only 'insiders' to racialized communities and exposed to anti-Asian racism, but, like Roxane, they are also 'outsiders' to Black and Indigenous communities that are disproportionately exposed to COVID-19 and vulnerabilized by the intertwined historical colonial legacies of genocide and slavery, and the ways these legacies haunt contemporary social institutions, including child welfare and health and social services, leading to hypersurveillance and premature death, as was the case with Joyce Echaquan. As non-Black, Indigenous, and Arab professors with a degree of institutional power, how might all three of us navigate the ways in which we are implicated within systems of domination?

Part of how we respond to these questions has been shared in this chapter, through our individual testimonies and our collective analysis of how we responded to societal racial injustices that were heightened during this COVID-19 era, especially through our involvement within our school of social work to engage in solidarity alongside communities. This is, of course, only a partial way to respond to these questions. We encourage readers to develop similar questions for themselves, so that they can used in an ongoing and reflexive manner, so that they can be asked and answered every time racial injustice occurred within and outside of social work educational settings.

21.5 Discussion–Conclusion

In this section, we conclude by providing a brief synthesis of how we "collectivized" our individual testimonies related to how COVID-19 shaped our initial reactions and subsequent responses to racial injustice experienced by communities in which we were in deep connection and relationship. We critically reflect upon how the critical dialogue we share in this chapter is informed by the ways in which our vulnerabilities are differently shaped by colonial logics. In naming these colonial scars, we explore how a decolonial feminist approach in social work may lead us to more liberatory and anti-normative futures.

21.5.1 Reflecting on the Question of Belonging, Borders, and Coloniality

The starting point of our chapter was the arrival of COVID-19 in our lives and how this pandemic shaped local and global events related to racial violence informed by colonial legacies. Each of us engaged in critical self-reflection to explore how these events were shaped by the hypervulnerabilities that we witnessed within directly impacted communities and by the vulnerability that we felt during this time period, based on our respective social locations and experiences. Subsequently, we critically reflected upon how we responded to our feelings of powerlessness to take action within the communities that we are part of, rooted within, and committed to—both through our research and community mobilization efforts as well as within our school of social work. The result of this collective exercise exceeds individual testimonials as it reveals to what extent 'the act of speech,' of speaking, of saying, and of speaking to oneself, is crucial to gaining deep insight into the historical, political, and social contexts that shape the ways in which racialized communities have become vulnerabilized by COVID-19. This echoes what Gayatri Spivak (1988) has evoked as the problem of 'voice'—who gets to speak and who is listened to?

Our testimonies highlight the ways in which our experiences intimately shaped our belonging to and rejection from various groups by overlapping lines of domination from race, gender, sexuality, citizenship status, etc. As Nassira Hedjerassi (2017) suggests, critical dialogue can serve as a tool for liberation in ways that build cohabitation despite colonial logics shaped by practices of domination. Critical dialogue counters "colonial arrogance" (Dor, 2017) and the imposition of the prevailing racist, classist, sexist, hetero-cis-sexist, capitalist, and imperialist social and epistemic order. Thus, our critical dialogue defied a binary understanding of the world, such as foreigner–national, Indigenous–migrant, here–there, etc. Instead, our dialogue helped to gain insight into each other's thoughts and perspectives, in ways that allowed us to decrypt mechanisms of domination and oppression that govern our lives and put into words how different people and communities feel (Perrochaud et al., 2018).

COVID-19 led to a closing of borders, forcing us to rethink our own personal boundaries. These boundaries are also informed by our experiences of belonging and rejection. Within this context, this requires a certain type of translating of how one feels a sense of belonging within a community because one's proximity to others' vulnerability and how to navigate feeling rejected by dominant communities, because of the reactivation of racial violence and discrimination. These dynamics signals to the ways in which we often sit on the borders of a group, between inclusion and exclusion (Hamisultane, 2017b). This insider/outsider tension needs continued attention, especially within social work. We have attempted to keep in mind this question in our engagement of this chapter: How do we negotiate these borders?

Scholars have described the close association between vulnerability (Goldstein, 2017), the need (or disregard) for recognition and empowerment. Racism, colonialism, and discrimination are experienced as a denial of the right to be treated as any other citizen and calls for the need to resist. As such, social work views care as the recognition of one's humanity (Marzano, 2017). Moreover, it is imperative to take into account how centuries of colonial mechanisms shape 'vulnerabilities' within the Global South and Global North. Such realities require a long-term and deep work of deconstructing our patterns of thought and actions. Our collective reflections in this chapter reveal how colonial mechanisms—and their consequences—are still present, notably through the internalization of social asymmetries.

The reproduction of injustices suggests that fostering a decolonial process is difficult and profound (Perrochaud et al., 2018). Our commitment to dialogue and recognizing the perspectives that are outside of ourselves help to shake up the dominant social order and hegemonic Western-Eurocentric epistemology, as previously silenced voices are intentionally brought forward alongside "other intertwining and entanglement of words and imposing of other knowledges" (Perrochaud et al., 2018, p. 293; author translation). As such, we aim to engage in practices of decoloniality to highlight the conditions under which our current debates take place: minoritization, forgetting or erasure of knowledges, voices, worldviews, and perspectives from a plurality of experiences (Quijano, 2000). Furthermore, a decolonial feminist approach to social work may point to ways for social work scholars and practitioners to decolonize epistemologies and frameworks, and work toward a liberatory and anti-normative politics to build egalitarian life-worlds, especially for racialized (cis and trans) women and queer and trans people (Caron & Lee, 2020).

Finally, these events permit us to reexamine the place of social work in research and practice: in what ways do events impact us and render us vulnerable, based on our social location and our varied degrees of belonging to directly impacted communities? In what ways do we need to foster an ongoing and iterative reflexive practice to go through a process of distancing ourselves from our experiences and engage in critical thinking and analysis about the broader colonial logics and social relations that shape our everyday experiences? To answer these questions, we must take a closer look at the subject's discourse to understand the suffering that was felt: deep listening without being too directive, without waiting for a 'right answer' and by allowing for time to unfold, taking into account that a testimony can only be shared within a trusting and safe space and resonance, that is, a space for talking where experiences of oppression can be heard and affirmed, not solely in one's own story, but as a way of giving an account of oneself. In other words, a space where we recognize that "there is a causal relationship between the self and the suffering of others" (Butler, 2007, p. 12; author translation) to act for the collective. To listen, one must be aware that intercultural relationships are anchored in colonial legacies of relationships of domination and oppression. Thus, decolonizing social work knowledge requires taking into consideration the multiple challenges that we have outlined in this book chapter, which includes reconsidering not only the structural but also the relational aspects of training.

References

Abou Habib, L. (2020a). Unequal gender relations and the subordination women in the MENA region: What the Covid-19 pandemic has taught us. IEMed Mediterranean Yearbook 2020 (pp. 160–164).

Abou Habib, L. (2020b). *Feminist perspectives on care work in the MENA Region.* https://www.fes-mena.org/

fileadmin/user_upload/pdf-files/publications/FES-Care_Work.pdf

Al-Ali, N. (2020). Covid-19 and feminism in the Global South: Challenges, initiatives and dilemmas. *European Journal of Women's Studies, 27*(4), 333–347. https://doi.org/10.1177/1350506820943617

Bancel, N., Blanchard, P., & Lemaire, S. (2006). *La fracture Coloniale*. La Découverte.

Braun, D. (2020) *Des actes racistes commis envers des Asiatiques à Montréal*. Radio Canada. https://ici.radio-canada.ca/nouvelle/1710914/racisme-anti-asiatiques-discrimination-montreal-motion

Butler, J. (2007). *Le récit de soi*. Presses Universitaires de France.

Caron, R. (2012). *Entre refuge et exil: l'expérience de femmes palestiniennes du camp de Bourj El Barajneh (Doctorat)*. Université de Montréal. https://papyrus.bib.umontreal.ca/xmlui/handle/1866/9112

Caron, R., & Lee, E. O. (2020). Towards a decolonial feminist approach to social work education and practice. In T. Kleibl, R. Lutz, N. Noyoo, B. Bunk, A. Dittman, & B. Seepamore (Eds.), *Postcolonial social work and indigenous development perspectives from the South* (Routledge international handbook) (pp. 71–88). Routledge.

Caron, R., Lee, E. O., & Pullen Sansfaçon, A. (2020). Power, locations and tensions: Social work professions building anti-oppressive ethical frameworks for research, teaching, practice and activism. *Ethics and Social Welfare Journal, 14*(3), 298–214.

Cho, G. M. (2008). *Haunting the Korean diaspora: Shame, secrecy and the Forgotten War*. University of Minnesota Press.

Cifafi, M. (2019). *Préserver un lien. Éthique des métiers de la relation*. Presses Universitaires de France.

Cleveland, J., Hanley, J., Jaimes, A., & Wolofski, T. (2020). *Impacts de la crise de la COVID-19 sur les «communautés culturelles Montréalaise.» Rapport de Recherche*. Institut Universitaire Sherpa.

Corm, G. (2007). *Histoire du Moyen-Orient. De l'Antiquité à nos jours*. La Découverte.

de Gaulejac, V. (2009). Colloque «Famille, couple: transmission et transformation»: Conférences: Le sujet face à la transmission. *Dialogue, 186*(4), 117–129.

Diversité Canadienne. (2020). Covid 19. *Immigration en temps de pandémie, 17*(3).

Dor, T. (2017). Rencontres radicales: un positionnement trans/formateur. In M. Dans, T. D. Altamimi, & N. Guénif-Souilamas (Eds.), *Rencontres radicales. Pour des dialogues féministes décoloniaux?* (pp. 231–260). Éditions Cambourakis.

Ducourtieux, C. (2020). Des manifestants s'en prennent aux statues, symboles du passé colonial et esclavagiste du Royaume-Uni. Le Monde, 10 juin 2020. https://www.lemonde.fr/international/article/2020/06/10/au-royaume-uni-les-manifestants-s-en-prennent-aux-statues-symboles-du-passe-colonial-et-esclavagiste_6042317_3210.html

Eichengreen, B. (2020). Aux Etats-Unis, la révolte anti-raciste est aussi un effet de la pandémie due au coronavirus. Le Monde 24 juin 2020. https://www.lemonde.fr/idees/article/2020/06/24/aux-etats-unis-la-revolte-anti-raciste-est-aussi-un-effet-de-la-pandemie_6044024_3232.html

Enquête nationale sur les femmes et les filles autochtones disparues et assassinées. (2019). https://www.mmiwg-ffada.ca/fr/final-report/

Fanon, F. (1952). *Peau noire, masques blancs*. Éditions du Seuil.

Garrau, M. (2018). *Vulnérables et libres. Entretien par Philippe Worms, Matière à penser, France Culture*. https://www.franceculture.fr/emissions/matieres-a-penser-avec-frederic-worms/vulnerables-et-libres

Gay, D. (2004). *Les Noirs du Québec, 1629–1900*. Septentrion.

Giust-Desprairies, F. (2004). *Le désir de penser. Construction d'un savoir clinique*. Tteraèdre.

Goldstein, P. (2017). Vulnérabilité et théorie des capacités. In D. Jousset, J.-M. Boles, & J. Jouquan (Eds.), Penser l'humain vulnérable: de la philosophie au soin (pp. 47–56).

Hamisultane, S. (2017a). *Trouble dans l'Interculturalité*. L'Harmattan.

Hamisultane, S. (2017b). *Interculturalité et trajectoires socio-professionnelles. Intervenants descendants de migrants et enjeux dans la relation avec leur public: la reconduction de formes d'inclusion et d'exclusion*. Rapport de recherche postdoctoral FRQSC. Collection METISS.

Hamisultane, S. (2018). La résonance interpersonnelle: une attention épistémologique à la clinique en sociologie. In I. Fortier, S. Hamisultane, I. Ruelland, J. Rhéaume, & S. Beghadadi (Eds.), *Clinique en sciences sociales: sens et pratiques alternatives*. Presses Universitaires du Québec. Collection Problèmes sociaux et interventions sociales.

Hamisultane, S. (2020). *Vulnérabilité et engagement: enjeux identitaires des jeunes personnes descendantes de migrants faisant l'objet de racisme dans un contexte de pandémie. Recherche-Subvention exploration*. CRSH.

Hamisultane, S. (2021). Personnes descendantes de migrants racisées face aux micro-agressions: silence, résistance et communauté imaginaire d'appartenance. *Nouvelles Pratiques Sociales, 31*, 2.

Hedjerassi, N. (2017). Postface. In M. Altamimi, D. Dor, & N. Guénif-Souilamas (Eds.), *Rencontres radicales. Pour des dialogues féministes décoloniaux?* (pp. 287–299). Éditions Cambourakis.

Heron, B. 2007. Desire for development. Whiteness, gender and the helping imperative. Waterloo: Wilfrid Laurier University Press.

Horn, J. (2020, April 9). *Surviving Covid-19: Why we need to listen to African women's organisations*. African Women's Development Fund. https://awdf.org/surviving-covid19-why-we-need-to-listen-african-womens-organisation/

Laferrière, D. (2020). Le racisme est un virus. Le Devoir 10 juin 2020. https://www.ledevoir.com/opinion/libre-opinion/580494/opinion-le-racisme-est-un-virus

Le Monde. (2020a). *Face à des hôpitaux débordés, le Liban se reconfine pour deux semaines*. https://www.lemonde.fr/international/article/2020/08/21/face-a-des-hopitaux-debordes-le-liban-se-reconfine-pour-deux-semaines_6049528_3210.html

Le Monde. (2020b). *Des Américains s'en prennent aux statues de Christophe Colomb, dénoncé au même titre que les esclavagistes*. https://www.lemonde.fr/international/article/2020/06/10/des-americains-s-en-prennent-aux-statues-de-christophe-colomb-denonce-au-meme-titre-que-les-esclavagistes_6042433_3210.html

Lee, E. (2018). Tracing the coloniality of queer and trans migrations: Resituating hetero-cis normative violence in the Global South and encounters with migrant visa ineligibility to Canada. *Refuge: Canada's Journal on Refugees, 34*(1), 60–74.

Lee, E. O., & Ferrer, I. (2014). Examining social work as a Canadian settler colonial project: Colonial continuities of circles of reform, civilization and in/visibility. *Journal of Critical Anti-Oppressive Social Inquiry, 1*(1), 1–20.

Lorde, A. (1981). The uses of anger: Women responding to racism. In *Speech-opening pronounced in June 1981 at the Conference of National Association Studies Women*, Storrs, Connecticut.

Marzano, M. (2017). Préambule. Penser et vivre. La vulnérabilité. In D. Jousset, J.-M. Boles, & J. Jouquan (Eds.), *Enser l'humain vulnérable: de la philosophie au soin* (pp. 17–24). Presses Universitaires de Rennes.

Monture-Agnes, P. (1995). *Thunder in my soul: A Mohawk woman speaks*. Fernwood Publishing.

Naepels, M. (2019). *Dans la détresse: une anthropologie de la vulnérabilité*. Éditions de l'École des hautes études en sciences sociales.

Naples, N. (1996). A feminist revisiting of the insider/outsider debate: The "outsider phenomenon" in rural Iowa. *Qualitative Sociology, 19*(1), 83–106.

Perrochaud, A., Hébert, P., & Wélépa, P. (2018). Vers un dialogue décolonial au pays du non-dit. In M. Altamimi, T. Dor, & N. Guénif-Souilamas (Eds.), *Rencontres radicales. Pour des dialogues féministes décoloniaux?* (pp. 261–284). Éditions Cambourakis.

Quijano, A. 2000. "Coloniality of Power, Eurocentrism, and Latin America." *Nepantla: Views from South 1*(3): 533–580.

Radio Canada. (2020a). *Mort de Joyce Echaquan: Enquête publique sur fond de manifestations*. https://ici.radio-canada.ca/espaces-autochtones/1738492/joyce-echaquan-manifestation-montreal-racisme-justice-nakuset

Radio Canada. (2020b). *Un mouvement de colère mondial aux ramifications locales*. https://ici.radio-canada.ca/nouvelle/1709742/george-floyd-racisme-discrimination-colere-monde

Richard, M., & Caron, R. (2020). Réalités (in)visibles et vulnérabilités ambivalentes: dialogue autoethnographique autour d'un terrain de recherche auprès de femmes réfugiées au Liban. *Nouvelles Perspectives en Sciences Sociales, 16*(1), 145–179.

Ricoeur, P. (1990). *Soi-même comme un autre*. Seuil.

Riopel, A. (2020). Les dernières heures de Joyce Echaquan. Le Devoir, octobre 2020. https://www.ledevoir.com/societe/587114/les-dernieres-heures.

Save the Children. (2020). *Economic crisis combined with COVID-19 is pushing Lebanon towards a hunger crisis*. https://www.savethechildren.org/us/charity-stories/lebanon-economic-hunger-crisis

Shaw, D. Z. (2019). *We settlers face a choice: Decolonization or white supremacy*. https://anthrodendum.org/2019/02/28/we-settlers-face-a-choice-decolonization-or-white-supremacy/

Sirven, N. (2007). De la pauvreté a la vulnérabilité: évolutions conceptuelles et méthodologiques. *Mondes en Développement, 140*, 9–24.

Spini, D., Hanappi, D., & Jousset, D. (2017). La vulnérabilité : un concept au carrefour des disciplines. In D. Jousset, J.-M. Boles, & J. Jouquan (Eds.), *Penser l'humain vulnérable: de la philosophie au soin* (pp. 69–76). Presses Universitaires de Rennes.

Spivak, G. C. (1988). Can the subaltern speak? In L. Grossberg & C. Nelson (Eds.), *Marxism and the interpretation of culture* (pp. 271–313). University of Illinois Press.

Tellier, M. (2020). États-Unis: les violences policières contre les Noirs en quelques grandes dates. France Culture 1 juin 2020. https://www.franceculture.fr/societe/etats-unis-les-violences-policieres-contre-les-noirs-en-quelques-grandes-dates

Thobani, S. (2007). *Exhalted subjects: Studies in the making of race and nation in Canada*. University of Toronto Press.

Vergès, F. (2019). *Un féminisme décolonial*. La Fabrique.

Wesley-Esquimaux, C. C., & Smolewski, M. (2004). *Historic trauma and Aboriginal healing*. Aboriginal Healing Foundation.

22 The Kerala, India Experience of Facing the COVID-19 Pandemic

Anu George

22.1 Introduction

The COVID-19 pandemic has significantly changed the world. It has caused devastating effects on not only people's health but also on economic and social situations. The global economy has sunk into the deepest recession in decades (The World Bank, 2020). The social crisis caused by the pandemic has deepened inequality and exclusion (UN, 2020). This unprecedented crisis has affected every nation on earth and is refusing to back down. The first of the COVID-19 cases in India were imported from outside the country among persons who returned to the country. Social distancing had become necessary for containing the spread of the virus as in a matter of a few days the number of infected cases rose among the returnees from abroad and gradually spread to others. As a result, India went into a nationwide lockdown on 24 March 2020, but with just four hours notice. The impact of such a sudden and unplanned lockdown was huge and brought a string of other problems. It caused the largest departure of people en masse from cities to villages and from one state to the other since the partition of India (Ellis-Petersen & Manoj, 2020). There are 450 million informal workers in India who suddenly lost their work and were left without food or money for survival (GoI, 2020). There were depressing scenes of men, women, and children walking many kilometers to reach their distant villages. The already cash-starved informal sector, because of the ill effects of demonetization was most affected, pushing millions of people into deeper poverty, starvation, and death (Shekar & Kashif, 2020). The implementation of lockdown measures was rested upon the federal states although the lockdown was ordered by the central government. In spite of the grave pandemic situation in India, the state of Kerala drew the world's attention for the arrangements it made to face the pandemic in stark contrast to the realities of the rest of India.

This chapter analyzes the COVID-19 crisis management by the government of Kerala. The duration focused in this study is from March 2020, when India went into a lockdown to contain the spread of the virus, to March 2021. It is divided into three parts. The first part summarizes the measures accomplished by the government of Kerala as the COVID-19 crisis hit the state. The state's COVID-19 strategies worked out as per the plan because of Kerala's robust public system and the public trust in the government's decisions (Heller, 2020). The second part considers how, over the years, Kerala managed to build a strong healthcare system along with other achievements, such as in education and social reforms. The third part focuses on Kerala's decentralization of powers to local governments. Decentralization

A. George (✉)
Christ (Deemed to be) University, Bangalore, India
e-mail: anushacj@gmail.com

M. C. S. Gonçalves et al. (eds.), *The Coronavirus Crisis and Challenges to Social Development*,
https://doi.org/10.1007/978-3-030-84678-7_22

encouraged people's participation, especially that of women, in governance. Having a robust healthcare system along with the common public that joined forces with the government stood in good stead for Kerala while facing the COVID-19 pandemic. This chapter examines the relatedness of Kerala's social development to the successful management of the COVID-19 crisis. The purpose is to assess some components in the politics of Kerala that have contributed to Kerala's laudable performance. The information used in this chapter is derived from books, studied articles, journal publications, and news stories on Kerala. The empirical information on the situation was collected from the news stories from some of the leading Indian and foreign media. Some of the favorable arguments on the Kerala model of development are reproduced here to highlight that Kerala was in a better position to manage the pandemic because of the social development it had achieved and sustained.

22.2 The Model State and Its Response to the COVID-19 Pandemic

A few decades ago, the Kerala model of development rose to be a curious example of study globally (Jeffrey, 1992; Franke & Chasin, 1994; Heller, 1995). The state achieved remarkable advances in social development, especially in domains of female literacy, life expectancy, and child mortality through extensive politicization of the Kerala society much before the other states of India (Jeffrey, 1992). The collective public involvement brought about successful reforms in society, which led to land reforms, poverty reduction, education and healthcare access, and child welfare (Franke & Chasin, 1994; Dreze & Sen, 2002; Jeffrey, 1992; Parayil, 1996; Tharamangalam, 2006). These changes contributed to shaping a new public environment, which eventually affected the quality of people's lives in Kerala (Parayil, 1996; Sen, 1999). When the COVID-19 crisis hit the state the advantages of Kerala's social development began to show. Here we will look at the immediate response of the state, which made Kerala stand out from the rest of the country as the pandemic was catching on.

Kerala reported the first COVID-19 case in India. On January 30, 2020, the first COVID-19 virus infection was confirmed in a Wuhan returnee in Kerala's Thrissur district. At the time when other countries reported cases of COVID-19, Kerala was already drafting measures for the containment of the virus (Shailaja, 2020). The state already has a record of successfully containing the NIPHA virus in 2018 and 2019. COVID-19 has high risk factors, as it is highly transmissible and poses a higher danger to the elderly population and people with underlying health conditions (CDC, 2021). These factors caused greater worry for Kerala, because of the density of population (860 persons per square kilometer), a high proportion of the elderly population (13.1% of the population more than 60 years of age against the national average of 8.3%, Pandey, 2020), and the international mobility of its citizens. The preparation was intensified when the first case was reported. Headed by the Health Minister, K.K. Shailaja, the health ministry drafted measures for the COVID-19 containment. A 24-member State response team was formed including experts from various branches of medicine with K.K. Shailaja as its chairperson (Nileena, 2020). They meticulously planned every stage. The clinical guidelines and advisory were provided by the Directorate of Health Services, which included details of the precautionary measures and treatment of the COVID-19 patients. These measures were followed strictly by everyone who had to interact with a person suspecting COVID-19 or who had already contacted it. Hospitals were equipped to meet the needs of emergencies with special COVID wards.

The health ministry also had an action plan for strengthening and managing human resources. A three-tier system was put into place to avoid burnout among doctors. The doctors were divided into three groups and when two groups were on duty one was on standby. After a week of COVID-19 duty, every group had 2 weeks off (Rajiv, 2020). A medical College block was converted into a COVID-19 treatment center in 4 days, and a COVID hospital with a 553-bed facility was built in record time in the Kasargod district of Kerala. Under K.K. Shilaja's supervision, the health ministry closely followed the guidelines of the WHO and tested, contact traced, and isolated for containing the virus. The immediate manner in which Kerala acted when the COVID-19 cases were reported resulted in containing the virus in the first phase when in the other parts of the country cases continued to rise. By the end of April 2020, there were very few cases and on May 1 there were no cases reported, flattening the curve. However, when the interstate movement was restored and people were repatriated from abroad, the cases started to rise again. The number kept spiking with a large number of people returning to the state after the lockdown period, but unlike other states with many cases, the death rates remained very low. Kerala's COVID-19 death rate showed 0.37% when other major COVID states, such as Maharashtra, had 2.6%, Karnataka 1.3%, Delhi 1.6%, and Tamil Nadu 1.5% (Newsclick, 2020). Kerala's health system could accommodate everyone even when the numbers surged.

The immediate action by the Kerala government to tackle the virus gained national and international attention. The British magazine, *Prospect*, announced the Health Minister, K.K. Shailaja, as the winner of the world's top thinkers for the COVID-19 age (Prospect Team, 2020). The Guardian published two articles on K.K. Shailaja: it described her as the "corona slayer" and "rockstar Health Minister" (Spinney, 2020a) and praised her and her "COVID brigade" for their efforts to keep the COVID-19 deaths lower than anywhere else in India (Spinney, 2020b). The *Financial Times* chose her among the list of the most influential women in 2020 (Financial Times, 2020), and Vogue India featured her on its cover as the "woman of the year" (Rajan, 2020). This international recognition brought attention once again to the Kerala model of development, which is the basis of the discussion here.

COVID-19 brought also a humanitarian crisis along with the health crisis. Kerala declared COVID-19 as a state disaster when the third COVID-19 case was reported. With the Disaster Act in place, the Chief Minister took over the coordination work among various ministries (police, revenue, electricity, water, and public works), which was needed to assist the health ministry in implementing plans effectively (Nileena, 2020). The Chief Minister of Kerala held a daily press meet at 6 p.m. for 1 h to communicate to the public the decisions and plans of the government. The citizens had first-hand information and daily updates from the Chief Minister himself. Some of the major decisions made by the government were aimed toward alleviating economic hardships caused by the pandemic. Kerala is the first and the only state to announce a financial package (200 million rupees) to mitigate the economic crisis caused by COVID-19 and the successive lockdown. This financial package was utilized in various ways. Two months of welfare pension was given in advance, and 1000 rupees in cash was given to the poor not eligible for pension to steady their purchasing power. Every ration cardholder received food kits from the public distribution system, irrespective of the type of the card. A subsidized meal program was made available, in addition to the interest-free loans availed through the women's community network known as *Kudumbashree*. A special health package was used for creating isolation facilities to treat the COVID-19 patients. The financial package also earmarked cash for reviving the rural economy through employment guarantee schemes. The water and electricity bill payment was extended, and entertainment taxes were waived. Financial assistance was provided to the artists and performers who were left without work in the lockdown.

The urban laborers' crisis was the most immediate and visible crisis that resulted from the lockdown. Kerala has a considerable number of migrant workers. Kerala's demand for low-skilled workers for jobs, such as agriculture and construction, has brought 2.5 million workers from other states of India to the state (Jalan & Sen, 2020). When the lockdown created a humanitarian crisis with the migrants walking en masse back home to other parts of the country, Kerala took measures to prevent such tragedies. The government ran 15,541 shelter camps for them to be housed during the lockdown; 65% of such shelters in the entire country were in Kerala (The Hindu, 2020).

One of the major factors of Kerala's good performance in COVID-19 management was the coordination between government, bureaucracy, and the public. The citizens united behind the Chief Minister as he communicated with the public daily to evade the fears, clear doubts, and give the right information on the situation. The district collectors were in charge of executing the plans. It was evident that "across all levels, the actions of bureaucracy have embodied a spirit of self-sacrifice for the collective welfare of the state" (Singh, 2020). Prerna Singh (2016) attributes this to the historically shared solidarity among the people of Kerala, which goes beyond the religious and caste groups. This deep interconnection between the people as one single Malayalee society or the social capital of Kerala has worked as the influencing factor for its pandemic management success (Babu, 2020). This unifying factor about the Kerala society was manifest previously also during the 2 years when Kerala was hit by severe floods (Babu, 2020). People spontaneously formed networks to provide help and support, especially taking care of and protecting the vulnerable. Jalan and Sen (2020) comment that during COVID lockdown the state and the public worked in such accord that state actions were transformed into public action and the trust people have in the government made spontaneous. The biggest network of organized social capital is an all-women's self-help group known as *Kudumbashree*, a government-sponsored civil society initiative. The details of the role *Kudumbashree* played during the COVID-19 crisis are described in the later section. The rise of Kerala as a welfare state did not happen all at once but developed over the years of planning and efforts. Heller (2020) says that it is the social democracy that has been built and fostered in Kerala, which proved to be beneficial during the crisis.

22.3 The Kerala Story of Development

Kerala's development experience is hailed as a model in global academic circles (Franke & Chasin, 1994; Jeffrey, 1992; Parayil, 1996; Heller, 2005). Several factors have contributed to building current Kerala other than its historical, cultural, or geographic exceptionalism (Heller, 2020). The factors that are fundamental to Kerala development are related to political and social processes that have taken place since the formation of Kerala State in 1956. Kerala's story of development evolved through many social mobilization practices that took place under the first elected communist government at the beginning of the State's existence and then continued by the successive governments (Heller, 1995). The strengthening of democratic institutions by people's active participation in the decision-making process has been at the base of Kerala's development story (Dreze & Sen, 1995). This democratization beyond the electoral participation happened by strengthening the social democracy in Kerala (Heller, 2005; Sen, 2009). Here, as Sen (2009) says, the social policies were politicized and the "need for universal education, basic health care, elementary gender equity and land reforms has received effective political backing" (p. 350). The early public investment in education and health improved the social inclusion of various sections of the people (Jeffrey, 1992; Dreze & Sen, 2002). The government was guided by public reasoning (Sen, 2009) and enhanced by the decentralization of powers at the local level, which served the interest of the people (Heller et al., 2007). This action also furthered women's participation in political matters, which had already been strengthened by educational opportunities (Jeffrey, 1992).

Kerala became a state in the Indian union in 1956. It did not start off as a promising state but as a problem state. The rise of communism in Kerala was viewed suspiciously, and there was a lingering notion about Kerala as the Yan'an of India (Yan'an being the center of the Chinese communist revolution) (Jeffrey, 1992). Contrary to such judgment, Kerala began to change in different ways. The state carried out social and economic reforms, focusing on the poor majority population and their needs (Jeffrey, 1992). It made distinguishable advances in healthcare and education, making them accessible to all without class/caste or male/female discrimination. These advances brought many changes to Kerala's social fabric. The people lived longer; fewer children were born and more of those who were born survived; there were more women than men (1084 women for 1000 men); and people could read and write (Franke & Chasin, 1994; Dreze & Sen, 2002; Jeffrey, 1992; Parayil, 2000). Kerala distinguishes itself from the other Indian States in matters of female/male ratio and development in areas of education (literacy rate, 93.91%) and health. The state ranks first among the states of India in Human Development Index ranking, with the advances in areas of sanitation, health, education, and poverty reduction (Suryanarayana et al., 2011). These changes improved the living conditions of people, without industrializing the state or without a political revolution, but by institution building (Jeffrey, 1992). The changes included the Minimum Wage Legislation (1958).

The political mobilization of the Kerala society was at the core of its development. As Heller points out, there were many people's movements in Kerala's history, such as the temple entry movement (1930s), peasant and workers' movement (1950s and 1960s), literacy movement (1980s), people's campaign for the decentralized government (1990s), and recent gender and environmental movements that were significant to change (Heller, 2020). These movements advanced the "politics of social citizenship," and here the style of association among the people was more "horizontal, cutting across primary identities of caste and communities" (Heller, 2005, p. 84). Therefore, it boosted democratic rights along with social rights (Heller, 2005). The politically active citizens placed high demands on the state government, and the demands of the poor majority became the priority of the state (Jeffrey, 1992). This closeness of the state with the working class and poor developed a social pact that is linked with the political will to provide social security to people (Heller, 2005, 2020). This was the pattern set in Kerala politics, and all governments in Kerala, regardless of the party, are forced to work toward expanding the social security of people or else be voted out of power.

Dreze and Sen (2002) link Kerala's social achievements to its promotion of "social opportunities based on public action" (p. 15). Public action involves "policy and governance, on the one side, and cooperation, disagreement and public protest, on the other" (Dreze & Sen, 2002, p. 7). The state initiatives and social movements brought about successful outcomes that include land reforms, equal rights for all sections of society for education and healthcare, and access to various public services. The public action has influenced the Kerala society. As Dreze and Sen (1995) find, it has affected the public discussion and has created awareness against gender bias, which in turn increased the freedom of women and a gradual decrease in the birthrate. The empowerment of women led to their political assertiveness and social involvement (Jeffrey, 1992, Dreze and Sen, 1999). Education in Kerala, especially of girls, is seen as the backbone of Kerala's development and the basis for the advancement of human and social development (Dreze & Sen, 1995, 2002; Jeffrey, 1992). Education influenced the political culture of Kerala, and people who could read and write laid the foundation for the public discussion practices in the state.

Another, equally important, factor is universal primary healthcare. Like education, healthcare was demanded by the people from the government (Sen, 2009). During the first half of the twentieth century, people of Kerala suffered from outbreaks of illnesses, such as cholera, smallpox, and other communicable diseases. People found the solution to this by socially mobilizing and creating awareness. There was an anti-cholera campaign by the communists in the 1950s, and volunteers (Red guards as they called them) went from house to house to inform people about the illness and to instruct them on cleanliness and prevention (Jeffrey, 1992). The people's awareness made them seek medical treatment, and the government was committed to providing them medical care because healthcare, like education, was also politicized (Sen, 2009). The health unit of the government, which was established in 1930, provided the public with health education through various campaigns educating the public on hygiene and preventable diseases, creating health consciousness among the public (Panikar, 1975). These measures worked, and people sought treatment for their illnesses, and as a result there was a gradual but sharp decline in mortality rate by the 1970s, and the life expectancy of 48 years in the 1960s grew to 60 years in the 1970s (Panikar, 1975; Jeffrey, 1992). More and more hospitals and dispensaries were opened to meet the health needs of the population. It also opened salaried job opportunities to women in Kerala as the political awareness of health needs expanded and governments could not give in to neglect anymore (Jeffrey, 1992; Sen, 2009). One of the direct effects of public health awareness was the decreased birthrate. People chose smaller families for bringing up healthier children. The infant mortality rate dropped because people made use of prenatal and postnatal healthcare. Institutional childbirth and control of infectious diseases brought the infant mortality rate down (Kannan, 1991). Vaccination in children increased their immunization, and vaccines were freely available to all classes, thereby making both rich and poor immune to diseases (Soman et al., 1990; Kannan, 1991).

Kerala's health service has developed into a robust system that is the best in the country (NITI Aaayog, 2019). The healthcare system has been one of the top priorities of all governments in Kerala. It has a rich legacy of fighting various outbreaks of diseases with the support of public participation. In recent years, the health ministry successfully contained the outbreak of the NIPHA virus and stopped the potential health crisis after the massive floods in 2018 and 2019 by taking maximum precautions. The state has well-equipped primary health centers, which function as immediate contact to the people. Kerala's doctor–patient ratio in Kerala (1:5) is higher than in most of the states (Nagarajan, 2018). Although Kerala always had a well-functioning health system in place, the decentralization of health services has "created conditions for a more effective and efficient extension of needed public health facilities" (Elamon et al., 2004, p. 705). It not only improved the accountability of the public healthcare system but also equipment and facilities at primary and secondary healthcare institutions, thereby benefiting the economically poor and women the most (Elamon et al., 2004; Thomas & Rajesh, 2011).

The Kerala government initiated a healthcare scheme known as *Aardram* with the intention to provide "people friendly outpatient services; reengineer primary health centers to family health centers"; provide "access to comprehensive health services for the marginalized/vulnerable population," and "standardize services from primary care settings to tertiary settings" (National Health Mission, 2017). Transforming primary health centers to family health centers also required administrative and infrastructural change. This scheme in healthcare is one of the four innovative undertakings in *Nava* Kerala Mission (New Kerala), initiated in 2016 by the Left Democratic Front-led government of Kerala, for the benefit of the economically backward and common people of the state. The other schemes include undertakings related to agriculture, education, and housing. The *Aardram* mission was started in Kerala in 2017, aiming to improve the public health sector in keeping with the SDG goals of 2030. Under this mission so far, 461 family health centers have been created, which provide quality medical service to people at the nearest location. Family health centers conducted daily testing of people for COVID-19 and functioned as first-line treatment centers.

22.4 Decentralized Governance and People's Participation

The advantages of decentralization were not only in the health sector but also in bureaucracy. In 1996 the Left Democratic Front government started the People's Planning Campaign for decentralized planning. This move was followed by the 73rd and 74th amendments to the Indian Constitution to encourage more local democratic participation for development. With this plan, 35–40% of the State's development budgeting power was transferred to local self-governments. Assuming this new power (administration, fiscal, and political), the local self-governments were also mandated to make maximum involvement of citizens in planning. Heller et al. (2007) say that in scope and design this was the most ambitious state-led effort undertaken in the subcontinent to bring participatory governance to local institutions. The purpose as well as the outcome of this move was to deepen democracy, and improve the quality of governance and accountability, thereby going beyond electoral participation to direct participation in decision making (Dreze & Sen, 1995; Heller et al., 2007). The result of decentralization was experienced in the following years. It solved the fund shortage of local bodies (Chathukulam & John, 2002). Planning and development was no longer the exclusive right of politicians and officials, as decentralization incorporated civil society into planning; the elected representatives' responsiveness to local needs and opinions increased, participation of women became greater and also had a hopeful impact on social inclusion, and above all the people's campaign created a structure of participatory governance without the help of a model (Heller et al., 2007).

The effects of decentralization were largely visible during the COVID-19 crisis. People's participation under the empowered local government had a larger effect without having to wait for every decision to come from the center. The most visible and powerful effect of decentralization was visible through the undertakings of *Kudumbashree*, a women-only organization that has been acknowledged for its success and contribution to women's participation in Kerala (Oommen, 2008; Willams et al., 2011). The tremendous social capital of *Kudumbashree* has had a significant role in the earlier crises, such as the floods, and so also during the COVID-19 crisis. A number of the State's COVID strategies were executed through *Kudumbashree*, be it implementing the Break the Chain Campaign initiated by the state government for creating awareness or taking care of the elderly and quarantined groups. The *Kudubashree* created social networking groups to control the spread of fake news and quell fears. As COVID-19 was making its way into Kerala, the *Kudumbashree* volunteers started making reusable cloth masks and producing hand-sanitizers on a large scale to avoid the shortage of them. During the lockdown, there were 1300 community kitchens run by *Kudumbashree* to provide food for the COVID centers and the quarantined, the stranded, and the poor people. It also started floating supermarkets to bring essential commodities to the doorsteps of people during the lockdown.

It was a collaborative effort of the *Kudumbashree* and the local self-governments to coordinate the contact tracing, transporting patients, scrutinizing home isolation, and also distributing food to families and migrant workers. The *Kudumabashree* continued to manufacture the food supplement known as Nutrimix, for the *Anganwadi* (child care center) children under 3 years during the lockdown and delivered it to their homes. They brought food and medicine to homebound or bedridden sick and elderly people; they formed a group of community counselors to assist and help the people who were stressed out during the lockdown. The government of Kerala created a volunteer portal to coordinate activities during the lockdown, and more than 50,000 *Kudumbshree* members volunteered as its members. They also worked alongside local self-governments, the police, and health workers.

22.5 Kudumbashree as the Subsystem of Local Governments

Kudumbashree is the outcome of the Women Component Plan that was set up during the decentralized planning process. It became the poverty eradication program of the Kerala government in 1998 through women's mobilization and was named *Kudumbashree*, which means prosperity of the family. *Kudumbashree* has a three-tier structure: the primary level Neighborhood Groups (NHGs), ward level Area Development Societies (ADS), and Community Development Societies (CDS) on the top level. From its establishment, *Kudumbashree* became the subsystem of the local governments for poverty reduction through its micro-finance program (Oommen, 2008).

Kudumbashree is a community network of women. Unlike the Self-Help Groups elsewhere in the country, *Kudumbashree* is an integral part of the government and focuses on the benefits of women and their financial independence (Willams et al., 2011). Although the dynamics of politics weighs on *Kudumbashree*'s functioning (Willams et al., 2011), its neighborhood groups function autonomously by creating credit that contributes to their joined development through active thrift; it provides them income-generating opportunities with micro enterprise undertakings, and they have active participation in the matters of the local government. *Kudumbashree*'s purpose and work have established a connection between participatory politics and poverty alleviation, especially in challenging the gender norms. Over the years, it has expanded to include a broader development vision alongside poverty eradication. Although it is oriented on the development of society through women empowerment, *Kudumbashree* has designed programs for the tribal population, children with disabilities, and transgender people, while continuing the poverty alleviation projects for poverty reduction. This network, 4.4 million members strong, has been successful, as Willams et al. (2011) conclude, in "linking group participation and state resources" (p. 16) for empowering women, strengthening them with access to credit and operation at the local government, while they have served the state through their voluntary labor. *Kudumbashree* has shown that a well-organized group of women can be successful not only in creative and profit-making activities but also in offering selfless service to society. It is also an example of civil society engagement in governance.

22.6 Conclusion

This chapter argues that Kerala successfully managed the crisis caused by COVID-19 because of the long-standing attention the government has paid to expanding, improving, and sustaining universal healthcare and the social safety net in Kerala. What makes Kerala's COVID-19 crisis management story humane is that it also cared about the other needs of people. Kerala has a long story of people-oriented policy making and has cultivated a society that is not only politically conscious but also socially active. During the COVID-19 crisis, Kerala's solid foundation on social democracy, public action, and accountable governance became visible. The state action and public action became unified. People voluntarily trusted their government and extended their unhesitating collaboration and support. This trust in government was crucial for the government to function and execute plans, especially regarding the rules of lockdown. Kerala government showed a humanitarian and compassionate side and extended protection to its citizens when their normal lives were affected. The attitude of the government was not arrogant but empathetic, and it sought public cooperation. During the crisis, the government's actions were guided and influenced by the needs and problems of the common people. This affiliation of the government of Kerala to the common people is historically present.

Kerala society also has its share of hurdles created by highly competitive and adversarial party politics, lousy media reporting, violent protests, police atrocities, and similar disruptions. However, in the face of disaster, the Kerala society displays an amazing sense of solidarity and oneness as they had shown during the severe floods in recent years and now during the COVID-19 crisis. The wide network of social capital served the people and the government. People's participation, especially women's participation in governance through decentralized planning, has brought the government close to people and their needs.

After a year into the pandemic, a second and more deadly wave of the virus is ravaging across India, exposing a broken healthcare system. The hospitals in many cities of the country have run out of beds and oxygen, increasing the number of deaths. The government at the center is guilty of not taking enough measures to prevent the tragedy into which the country has plunged (Ellis-Petersen, 2021) and for the callous attitude of the political leaders that led to this disaster (The Guardian, 23 April 2021). Kerala's distinctiveness becomes notable again by being the only state with surplus oxygen. The state increased the oxygen production after the first wave of the pandemic, and so during the second wave when many states are running short of oxygen supply, Kerala is supplying oxygen to other states (Jacob, 2021). The COVID-19 pandemic has not ended, and the effect of this crisis on societies and peoples is yet to be revealed fully. The people of Kerala can at least be proud that their government fared well through the democratic challenges the pandemic had openly raised.

References

Babu, S. (2020, November 4). How social capital can help deal with the pandemic better. *The Hindu Business Line*. https://www.thehindubusinessline.com/opinion/how-social-capital-can-help-deal-with-the-pandemic-better/article33021238.ece

Centers for Disease Control and Prevention (2021). *Underlying medical conditions associated with high risk for severe COVID-19: Information for healthcare providers*. Author. https://www.cdc.gov/coronavirus/2019-ncov/hcp/clinical-care/underlying-conditions.html

Chathukulam, J., & John, M. S. (2002). Five years of participatory planning in Kerala: Rhetoric and reality. *Economic and Political Weekly, 37*(49), 4917–4926. https://www.epw.in/journal/2002/49/special-articles/five-years-participatory-planning-kerala.html

Dreze, J., & Sen, A. (1995). *India. Economic development and social opportunity*. Clarendon Press.

Dreze, J., & Sen, A. (2002). *India: Development and participation* (2nd ed.). Oxford University Press.

Elamon, J. F., Richard, W., & Ekbal, B. (2004). Decentralization of health services: The Kerala people's campaign. *International Journal of Health Services, 34*(4), 681–708. https://doi.org/10.2190/4L9M-8K7N-G6AC-WHEN

Ellis-Petersen, H. (2021, April 21). The system has collapsed: India's descent into Covid hell. *The Guardian*. https://www.theguardian.com/world/2021/apr/21/system-has-collapsed-india-descent-into-covid-hell

Ellis-Petersen, H., & Manoj, C. (2020, March 30). India racked by greatest exodus since partition due to coronavirus. *The Guardian* https://www.theguardian.com/world/2020/mar/30/india-wracked-by-greatest-exodus-since-partition-due-to-coronavirus

Financial Times. (2020, December 4). Who have been the most influential women of 2020? *Financial Times*. https://www.ft.com/content/469df412-7ed8-4_6e-99c3-2fabf0995ad6

Franke, R., & Chasin, B. (1994). *Kerala: Radical reform as development in Indian State*. The Institute for Food and Development Policy.

Goli, S. (2020, April 20). *COVID-19: The Indian COVID-19 episode: Unprepared lockdown and its impact*. https://www.news.uwa.edu.au/archive/2020042012003/uwa-public-policy-institute/covid-19-indian-covid-19-episode-unprepared-lockdown-and-i/

Heller, P. (1995). From class struggle to class compromise. Redistribution and growth in south Indian state. *The Journal of Development Studies, 31*(5), 645–672. https://doi.org/10.1080/00220389508422384

Heller, P. (2005). Reinventing public power in the age of globalization: Decentralization and the transformation of movement in politics in Kerala. In R. Raka & M. Fainsod Katzenstein (Eds.), *Social movements in India: Poverty, power and politics* (pp. 79–107). Rowman & Littlefield.

Heller, P. (2020, April 18) A virus, social democracy and dividends for Kerala. *The Hindu*. https://www.thehindu.com/opinion/lead/a-virus-social-democracy-and-dividends-for-kerala/article31370554.ece

Heller, P., Harilal, K. N. & Chaudhuri, S. (2007). Building local democracy: Evaluating the impact of decentralization in Kerala, India. *World Development, 35*(4), 624–648. https://doi.org/10.1016/j.worlddev.2006.07.001

Jacob, S. (2021). *Kerala model: How India's only oxygen surplus state is managing the crisis*. Money Control. https://www.moneycontrol.com/news/business/economy/kerala-model-how indias-only-oxygen-surplus-state-is-managing-the-crisis-6805021.html

Jalan, J., & Sen, A. (2020) Containing a pandemic with public action and public trust: The Kerala story. *Indian Economic Review, 55*(1), 105–124. https://doi.org/10.1007/s41775-020-00087-1

Jeffrey, R. (1992). *Politics, women and well-being: How Kerala became 'a model'*. Palgrave.

Kannan, K. P. (1991). *Health and development in rural Kerala: A study of the linkages between socio-economic status and health status*. Integrated Rural Technology Centre of the Kerala Sastra Sahitya Parishad.

Minimum Wage Legislation. (1958) etc.. In the brackets are the years these borads were established.

Nagarajan, R. (2018, September 2). 6 states have more doctors than WHO's 1:1000 guideline. *The Times of India*. https://timesofindia.indiatimes.com/india/6-states-have-more-doctors-than-whos-11000-guideline/articleshow/65640694.cms

National Health Mission. (2017). Government of Kerala. https://arogyakeralam.gov.in/2020/04/01/aardram/

Newsclick Report. (2020). *Kerala has lowest death rate among major COVID states*. Newsclick. https://www.newsclick.in/Kerala-Has-Lowest-Death-Rate-Major-COVID-States

Nileena. (2020, March 28). How Kerala government is shaping and implementing its COVID-19 response. *The Caravan*. https://caravanmagazine.in/health/covid-19-coronavirus-kerala-vijayan-shailaja-healthcare-system

NITI Aaayog. (2019). *Health Index*. Ministry of Health and Family Welfare. http://social.niti.gov.in/uploads/sample/health_index_report.pdf

Oommen, M. A. (2008). *Micro-finance and poverty alleviation: The case of Kerala's Kudumbashree*. Center for Socio-economic & Environmental Studies (CSES). https://kudumbashree.org/storage/files/fqvd6_micro%20finance%20and%20poverty%20alleviation.pdf

Pandey, S. (2020). *Kerala's elderly population on the rise: Finds economic review*. Newsbytes. https://www.newsbytesapp.com/news/india/kerala-s-elderly-population-exceeds-national-average-economic-review/story

Panikar, P. G. K. (1975). Fall in mortality rate in Kerala. An explanatory hypothesis. *Economic & Political Weekly, 10*(47), 1811–1818. https://www.jstor.org/stable/40738370

Parayil, G. (1996). The Kerala model of development: Development and sustainability in the third world. *Third World Quarterly, 17*(5), 941–957. https://library.fes.de/libalt/journals/swetsfulltext/11220652.pdf

Parayil, G. (2000). Is Kerala's development experince a "Model". In G. Parayil (Ed.), *Kerala: The develpment experience* (pp.1–16). Zed Books.

Prospect Team. (2020, September 2–October). The world's top 50 thinkers 2020: The winner. *Prospect*. https://www.prospectmagazine.co.uk/magazine/the-worlds-top-50-thinkers-2020-the-winner

Rajan, M. S. (2020, November 9). K K Shailaja on being the thick of things during COVID-19: "More than fear, I feel an enthusiasm to get involved". *Vogue*. https://www.vogue.in/culture-and-living/content/kk-shailaja-kerala-minister-interview-vogue-india-november-2020-cover-story

Rajiv, G. (2020, June 11). Kerala: Now focus on health staff and hospital beds. *The Times of India*. https://timesofindia.indiatimes.com/city/thiruvananthapuram/kerala-now-focus-on-health-staff-and-hospital-beds/articleshow/76313361.cms

Sen, A. (1999). *Development as freedom*. Alfred A. Knopf.

Sen, A. (2009). *The idea of justice*. The Belknap Press of Harvard University Press.

Shailaja, K. K. (2020, March 23). How to handle a pandemic. *The Hindu*. https://www.thehindu.com/opinion/op-ed/how-to-handle-a-pandemic/article31136612.ece

Shekar, C., & Kashif, M. (2020). *COVID-19. Lockdown impact on informal sector in India*. University Practice Connect Azim Premji University. https://practiceconnect.azimpremjiuniversity.edu.in/covid-19-lockdown-impact-on-informal-sector-in-india/

Singh, P. (2016). *How solidarity works for welfare: Sub-nationalism and social development in India*. Cambridge University Press.

Singh, P. (2020). *How solidarity is controlling contagion in Kerala*. Center for Advanced Study of India. https://casi.sas.upenn.edu/iit/prernasingh

Soman, C. R., Malati, D., Rajasree, S., Ramankutty, V., & Vijayakumar, K. (1990). High morbidity and low mortality: The experience of urban pre-school children in Kerala. *Journal of Tropical Paediatrics, 37*, 17–141.

Spinney, L. (2020a, March 14). The coronavirus slayer. How Kerala's rock star health minister helped save it from covid-19. *The Guardian*. https://www.theguardian.com/world/2020/may/14/the-coronavirus-slayer-how-keralas-rock-star-health-minister-helped-save-it-from-covid-19

Spinney, L. (2020b, December 22). How K.K. Shailaja and her 'covid brigade' won a victory against the virus. *The Guardian*. https://www.theguardian.com/lifeandstyle/2020/dec/22/how-kk-shailaja-and-her-covid-brigade-won-a-victory-against-the-virus

Suryanarayana, M. H., Agarwal, A., & Seeta Prabhu, K. (2011). *Inequality adjusted Human Development Index for India's States*. United Nations Development Program, UNDP.

Tharamangalam, J. (2006). Understanding Kerala's paradoxes: The problematic of the Kerala model of development. In J. Tharamangalam (Ed.), *Kerala: The paradoxes of public action and development* (pp. 1–37). Orient Longman.

The Guardian. (2021, April 23). The Guardian's view on Modi's mistakes: A pandemic that is out of control. *The Guardian*. https://amp.theguardian.com/world/commentisfree/2021/apr/23/the-guardian-view-on-modis-mistakes-a-pandemic-that-is-out-of-control?__twitter_impression=true&s=04&fbclid=IwAR1WWC1_W90q-Ol7CH5vowalC0Nvx6lNFyDL71bv3bsSbrLHUsDuY1I1nB0

The Hindu. (2020, April 7). Coronavirus: Centre files report on migrant workers. The Hindu. https://www.thehindu.com/news/national/coronavirus-centre-files-report-on-migrant-workers/article31283896.ece

The World Bank. (2020). *Covid-19 to plunge global economy into worst recession since World War II.*

Author. https://www.worldbank.org/en/news/press-release/2020/06/08/covid-19-to-plunge-global-economy-into-worst-recession-since-world-war-ii

Thomas, B., & Rajesh, K. (2011). *Decentralization and intervention in health sector: A critical inquiry into the experience of local self governments in Kerala*. The Institute for Social and Economic Change. http://www.isec.ac.in/WP%20271%20-%20Benson%20Thomas%20and%20Rajesh.pdf

UN. (2020). *Everyone included. Social impact of COVID-19*. Author. https://www.un.org/development/desa/dspd/everyone-included-covid-19.html

Willams, G., Thampi, V., Binitha, N. D., Nandigama, S., & Bhattacharya, D. (2011). Performing participatory citizenship: Politics and power in Kerala's Kudumabashree program. *The Journal of Development Studies*, *47*(8), 1261–1280. https://doi.org/10.1080/00220388.2010.527949

23 Responding to COVID-19 and Beyond: Key Recommendations for the Effective Public and Mental Health Response to Support the Well-Being of Aboriginal and Torres Strait Islander Peoples in Australia

Pat Dudgeon, Joanna Alexi, Kate Derry, Emma Carlin, and Rob McPhee

23.1 Preface

The Australian response to COVID-19 demonstrates how Aboriginal and Torres Strait Islander leadership, partnership, and self-determination are critical in ensuring public health measures and pandemic response planning is effective for Aboriginal and Torres Strait Islander peoples.[1] This chapter outlines the key evidence-based recommendations and actions developed by three national Aboriginal and Torres Strait Islander-led groups, in meaningful partnership with government, during the COVID-19 pandemic. The Aboriginal and Torres Strait Islander response to COVID-19, led by Aboriginal and Torres Strait Islander organisations and communities, has been renowned across the world. This chapter highlights the importance of Aboriginal and Torres Strait Islander governance and leadership in leading the pandemic response for Aboriginal and Torres Strait Islander peoples and further illustrates the strengths of the Aboriginal and Torres Strait Islander response to COVID-19 when priority reforms are heard and implemented by government.

Throughout this chapter, mental health and well-being responses related to COVID-19 are particularly emphasised. Mental health experts predict that the mental health and well-being issues exacerbated by the pandemic will persist for many years (Savage, 2020). The mental health and well-being impacts of COVID-19 are of particular significance to Aboriginal and Torres Strait Islander peoples, who experience significant well-being disparities associated with the historical, political, and social determinants of health, arising from colonisation (Dudgeon et al.,

[1]Note on wording: The term Indigenous respectfully refers to Indigenous peoples in a global or international context.

P. Dudgeon (✉) · J. Alexi · K. Derry
School of Indigenous Studies, University of Western Australia, Crawley, WA, Australia
e-mail: pat.dudgeon@uwa.edu.au

E. Carlin
Rural Clinical School Western Australia, University of Western Australia, Broome, WA, Australia

Kimberley Aboriginal Medical Services, Broome, WA, Australia

R. McPhee
Kimberley Aboriginal Medical Services, Broome, WA, Australia

M. C. S. Gonçalves et al. (eds.), *The Coronavirus Crisis and Challenges to Social Development*, https://doi.org/10.1007/978-3-030-84678-7_23

2014). Together, the recommendations outlined here provide an effective base to plan for long-term recovery of the mental health and well-being of Aboriginal and Torres Strait Islander peoples from COVID-19 and ensure the preparedness of Aboriginal and Torres Strait Islander communities for future pandemics.

23.2 Introduction: The Role of Colonisation and Historical, Political, and Social Determinants of Health During Pandemics

Before colonisation, Aboriginal and Torres Strait Islander peoples were a hunter-gatherer and semi-nomadic people, with each group comprising their own language, culture, history, responsibilities, and obligations (Dudgeon et al., 2014). Aboriginal and Torres Strait Islander peoples consider themselves spiritually and culturally interlinked with the land on which they reside, and a strong emphasis was, and continues, to be placed on connection to body, mind, family, kinship, community, spirituality, and Country (Dudgeon et al., 2014; Gee et al., 2014). For Aboriginal and Torres Strait Islander peoples, a harmonious balance and connection to these components are essential in promoting healthy social and emotional well-being (SEWB) and mental health (Gee et al., 2014).

The European settlement of Australia from the 1780s saw a severe disruption to the livelihoods of Aboriginal and Torres Strait Islander peoples, communities, and culture (Dudgeon et al., 2014). War over land and diseases introduced by European settlement, such as measles, smallpox, and influenza, had a profound effect on Aboriginal and Torres Strait Islander peoples, and even led to the death of entire tribes who had not been exposed to such diseases previously (Dudgeon et al., 2014). Subsequent oppressive and racist government legislation throughout the nineteenth and twentieth centuries sought to denigrate and displace Aboriginal and Torres Strait Islander peoples and culture and to assimilate them with European people (Dudgeon et al., 2014). This political and historical mistreatment and oppression of Aboriginal and Torres Strait Islander peoples through colonisation had immensely negative consequences, including intergenerational and transgenerational trauma, displacement of families, and attempted denigration of identity, culture, and SEWB (Dudgeon et al., 2014).

Through the resilience and strength of Aboriginal and Torres Strait Islander peoples, communities have begun to rebuild their health and SEWB. Still, Aboriginal and Torres Strait Islander peoples today experience higher rates of poverty, homelessness, and physical and mental health difficulties, particularly depression and suicide (Australian Government Australian Institute of Health and Welfare, 2019; Commonwealth of Australia Department of Prime Minister and Cabinet, 2020; Dudgeon et al., 2016). Historical and social determinants of health including colonisation, poverty, socioeconomic status, unemployment, overcrowded housing, and continuing systemic and institutionalised racism impact the health and well-being outcomes of Aboriginal and Torres Strait Islander peoples (Commonwealth of Australia Department of Prime Minister and Cabinet, 2020).

Critically, social determinants of health are also known to increase health risks from pandemics (Ahmed et al., 2020; Singu et al., 2020). Social determinants of health contribute to the higher prevalence of health conditions such as cardiovascular disease, hypertension, and diabetes, which can then compromise the ability of one's immune system to fight viruses (Singu et al., 2020). Further, restrictions on the protective factors related to social determinants of health, such as cultural and community activities, and the cultural foundations of Aboriginal and Torres Strait Islander peoples of being together and sharing, can also impact well-being (Zubrick et al., 2014). Pandemic-related restrictions limited these protective factors and exacerbated risk factors. Historically, viral pandemics and transmittable diseases have disproportionately impacted Aboriginal and Torres Strait Islander peoples, primarily from the effects of colonisation and resultant inequalities between Aboriginal and Torres Strait Islander peoples and non-Aboriginal and Torres Strait Islander peoples. The 2009 H1N1 pandemic demonstrates a recent example of the disparate effect of pandemics on Aboriginal and Torres Strait Islander peoples. In Australia, the 2009 H1N1 pandemic resulted in hospitalisations of Aboriginal and Torres Strait Islander peoples as much as 12-fold the rate of non-Aboriginal and Torres Strait Islander peoples (Flint et al., 2010). Although historical, political, and social determinants of health perpetuate inequalities for Aboriginal and Torres Strait Islander peoples during pandemics, a lack of government engagement with Aboriginal and Torres Strait Islander organisations to lead recovery responses is also considered a contributor to this health inequality (Crooks et al., 2020).

For many years, Aboriginal and Torres Strait Islander community leaders and health organisations have called for effective partnerships with the government to work together to improve long-standing health issues for Aboriginal and Torres Strait Islander peoples (i.e., Commonwealth of Australia Department of Prime Minister and Cabinet, 2017a; Social Health Reference Group, 2004). This call was recently reaffirmed in the *National Agreement on Closing the Gap* and the 2020 *Close the Gap* report, with the Australian Government now recognising the importance of meaningful engagement and partnerships with Aboriginal and Torres Strait Islander peoples, communities, and organisations (Australian Government, 2020; Commonwealth of Australia Department of Prime Minister and Cabinet, 2020). In particular, the National Agreement made commitments to four priority reforms: (1) "formal partnerships and shared decision making..." with Aboriginal and Torres Strait Islander peoples, (2) "building Aboriginal and Torres Strait Islander community-controlled sectors to deliver services to support Closing the Gap," (3) "transformation of mainstream government organisations to improve accountability..." and to better meet the needs of Aboriginal and Torres Strait Islander peoples, and (4) "shared access to data and information at a regional level" (Australian Government, 2020). In the *2020 Close the Gap* report, it was acknowledged that this is a shift in the manner in which governments previously worked. However, the report and National Agreement acknowledged that effective partnership with Aboriginal and Torres Strait Islander peoples is the way forward in closing the health gap.

Aboriginal and Torres Strait Islander Population

As of 2016, the Aboriginal and Torres Strait Islander population in Australia is 3.3%, or 798,400 people (Australian Bureau of Statistics, 2018). A large proportion of the Aboriginal and Torres Strait Islander population identified as being Aboriginal (91%, 727,500 people), whereas 5% (or 38,700 people) identified as being Torres Strait Islander and 4% (or 32,200 people) identified as being both Aboriginal and Torres Strait Islander. Approximately 37.4% of the Aboriginal and Torres Strait Islander population reside in major cities (compared to 72.7% of the non-Aboriginal and Torres Strait Islander population), with almost 50% of Aboriginal and Torres Strait Islander peoples residing in inner and outer regional areas (23.7% and 20.3%, respectively), and to a lesser extent in remote (6.7%) and very remote (11.9%) areas (Australian Bureau of Statistics, 2018). In Australia, Aboriginal Community Controlled Health Organisations (ACCHOs) played a vital role in the COVID-19 response, as they represent self-determination and are the appropriate providers of culturally safe and responsive care for Aboriginal and Torres Strait Islander peoples. There are 143 ACCHOs located across Australia, as depicted in Fig. 23.1, which are represented by the National Aboriginal Community Controlled Health Organisation (NACCHO) (NACCHO, 2021).

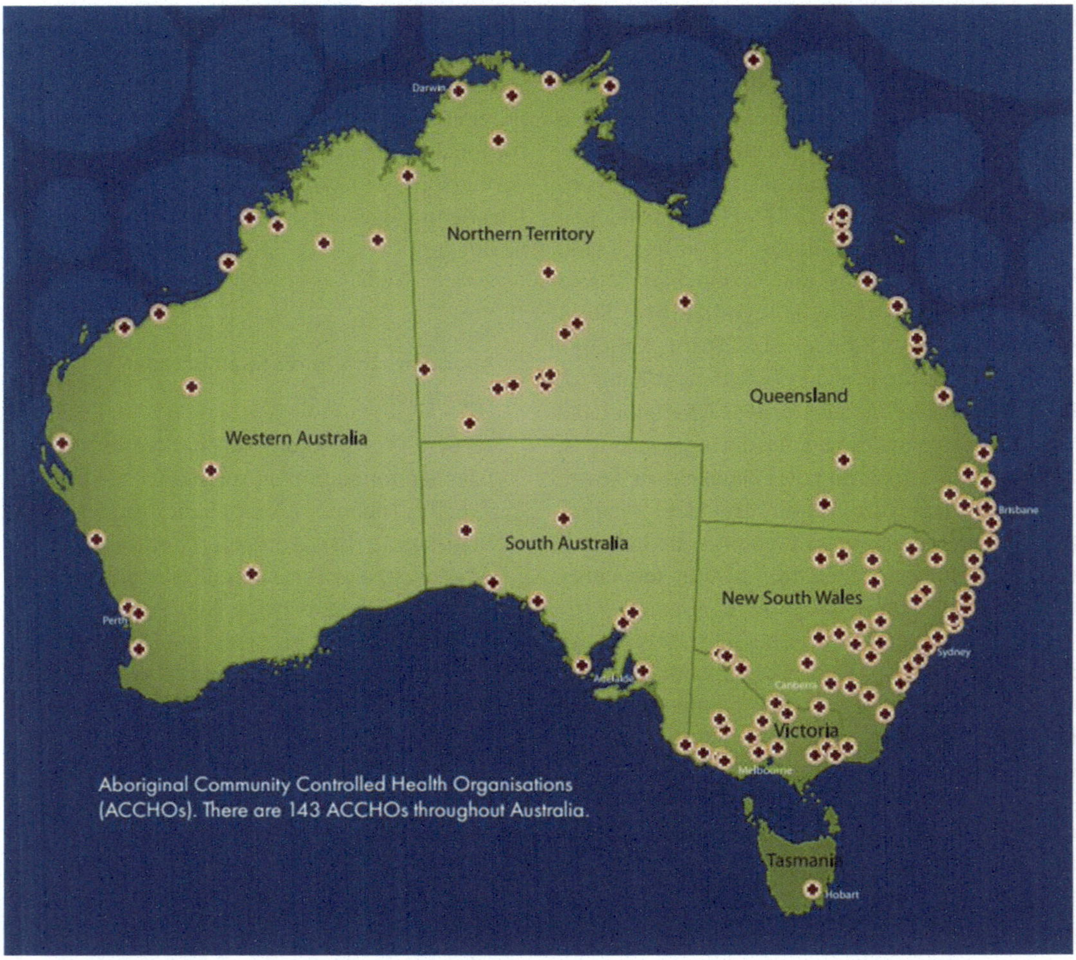

Fig. 23.1 Map of the Aboriginal Community Controlled Health Organisations (ACCHOs) across Australia. (This image has been reproduced with permission from NACCHO, 2020c)

Effective partnerships can facilitate self-determination that enables Indigenous governance principles and community control and incorporates shared decision making (Commonwealth of Australia Department of Prime Minister and Cabinet, 2020). The emergence of COVID-19 provided a further opportunity for the Australian government to establish effective partnerships with Aboriginal and Torres Strait Islander peoples and communities, to lead effectual COVID-19 planning for communities. The Aboriginal and Torres Strait Islander response to, and experience of, COVID-19 in 2020 is a remarkable example of the efficacy of partnership, self-determination, and community empowerment. The responses clearly demonstrate the way forward for the health and healing of Aboriginal and Torres Strait Islander peoples.

23.3 COVID-19 and the Need to Mobilise

COVID-19 is a respiratory illness and a novel form of coronavirus (Australian Government Department of Health, 2020d). The first report of a 'viral pneumonia' in Wuhan, China, was identified by the World Health Organization (WHO) on 31 December 2019 (World Health Organization,

2020). On 30 January 2020, the World Health Organization declared the outbreak a 'Public Health Emergency of International Concern' as it began to spread rapidly across the world (World Health Organization, 2020). The virus was named SARS-CoV-2 and the disease it caused was named COVID-19 in February. COVID-19 presents a grave risk of severe illness or death for individuals who are 70 years and older, have pre-existing medical conditions, or across populations of people where health disparities are already prominent (Australian Government Department of Health, 2020d; Li et al., 2020). WHO officially declared COVID-19 a pandemic on 11 March 2020 (World Health Organization, 2020). In response to the pandemic, Australia declared a human biosecurity emergency on 18 March, with national borders closing just 1 day later (Prime Minister of Australia, 2020). On 23 March, an emergency response plan was published for the health sector, and widespread lockdown restrictions began to be progressively implemented, with a forecast of 6 months, to further curb the spread of the virus (Australian Government Department of Health, 2020b). These measures included travel restrictions, temporary closure of nonessential businesses and places of social gathering, and stay-at-home orders from schools and work and a reprioritisation of healthcare services (Parliament of Australia, 2020).

Learning from recent history of the effect of pandemics on Aboriginal and Torres Strait Islander peoples, Aboriginal and Torres Strait Islander leaders, organisations, and communities were among the first to mobilise and respond to COVID-19 in Australia. For example, before the first Australian COVID-19 case, the community-controlled sector had already initiated effective COVID-19 public health responses, as described next (see NACCHO, 2020b, for further information on the ongoing leadership and contribution by the National Aboriginal Community Controlled Health Organisation to the COVID-19 response). On 6 March 2020, an Aboriginal and Torres Strait Islander COVID-19 Advisory Group (ATSIAG) was convened by the Australian Government Department of Health in partnership with the National Aboriginal Community Controlled Health Organisation (NACCHO). ATSIAG was tasked to lead the development of, and to advise on, the implementation of a national pandemic management plan for Aboriginal and Torres Strait Islander peoples and communities (Crooks et al., 2020; NACCHO, 2020a). In addition, the ATSIAG identified and escalated emerging matters, reviewed and informed key COVID-19 guidelines, documents, and communication materials, and assisted to inform the flow of information within the Aboriginal and Torres Strait Islander health sector.

In April 2020, a taskforce of leading Aboriginal and Torres Strait Islander academics and allies were convened by the university sector to work with the Group of Eight (Go8) Universities to advise the Government on the public health and care of Aboriginal and Torres Strait Islander peoples during the pandemic (Group of Eight Australia, 2020). These recommendations were then outlined in Chap. 9 of the report, which focused on the "care of Indigenous Australians."

In May 2020, a specific Aboriginal and Torres Strait Islander mental health and well-being working party was then convened to ascertain the longer-term consequences of the pandemic. The working party was formed by Professor Pat Dudgeon and the University of Western Australia's Poche Centre for Indigenous Health to provide recommendations to address the mental health and SEWB needs of Aboriginal and Torres Strait Islander peoples during COVID-19 and beyond (Dudgeon et al., 2020).

The relatively low numbers of COVID-19 infection (0.5% of all confirmed cases) and no deaths among Aboriginal and Torres Strait Islander peoples in Australia, at the time of writing, as compared to non-Aboriginal and Torres Strait Islander peoples (99.5% of all cases and 909 deaths; Australian Government Department of Health, 2020c; Government of Western Australia Department of Health, 2021) are, in part, a result of the actions taken by ATSIAG and ACCHOs. The low rates of infection are in contrast to other Indigenous peoples across the globe. In the United States (U.S.), COVID-19 rates in the first half of 2020 were 3.5 times higher compared to non-Indigenous persons and had caused 2689 deaths (Arrazola et al., 2020). Notwithstanding these low rates in Australia, we must remain vigilant in protecting Aboriginal and Torres Strait Islander peoples from the impacts of COVID-19, which must also include working to reduce the societal inequity that creates disproportional risk between Aboriginal and Torres Strait Islander peoples and non-Aboriginal and Torres Strait Islander peoples in Australia. Some of the recommendations developed by and for Aboriginal and Torres Strait Islander peoples during COVID-19 to support long-term and sustainable recovery are outlined next.

23.4 Public Health Responses to COVID-19

23.4.1 Aboriginal and Torres Strait Islander Advisory Group (ATSIAG) on COVID-19

The ATSIAG advisory group is constituted of representatives and members of regional, state, and national Aboriginal and Torres Strait Islander health organisations and ACCHOs (Australian Government Department of Health, 2020a). This group was co-chaired by NACCHO, in partnership with the Department of Health (Moodie et al., 2020). Together, this group reported directly to the Australian Chief Medical Officer and the Australian Health Protection Principal Committee, which provides input to the National Cabinet (Moodie et al., 2020). Critically, NACCHO had an important role in convening key Aboriginal and Torres Strait Islander health organisations and partners to the advisory group, to ensure that COVID-19 response plans were culturally appropriate and beneficial to communities.

A key output from this group was the development of a national Management Plan. This Management Plan detailed clinical guidelines and initiatives to ensure the preparedness of Aboriginal and Torres Strait Islander communities. For example, the Management Plan identified four phases of action. The first phase centred on preparing for potential COVID-19 outbreaks, with actions for preparing the workforce and medical equipment, establishing and targeting health communications accordingly, and preparing Aboriginal and Torres Strait Islander communities. The second phase detailed actions for suspected or initial cases of COVID-19 in the Aboriginal and Torres Strait Islander population, including early identification of the virus, laboratory testing, and supported isolation. The third phase outlined actions for potential outbreaks in communities, emphasising increased support and resources, and safeguarding at-risk groups. The final stage of the plan detailed longer-term measures following COVID-19, particularly monitoring for subsequent waves of the pandemic, and thorough evaluation of data relating to COVID-19 through a cultural lens (Australian Government Department of Health, 2020b). These guidelines were developed to ensure that the needs of Aboriginal and Torres Strait Islander peoples are prioritised in the pandemic response, and to address logistical matters in remote communities, such as COVID-19 screening and infectious disease training for staff (Crooks et al., 2020).

Crooks et al. (2020) note that strong leadership and input by the ATSIAG contributed to important legislative changes; these included recommending biosecurity measures and travel restrictions of nonessential travel to remote communities as well as access restrictions to communities for new visitors (Crooks et al., 2020). Further, Crooks et al. (2020) reported on the efforts of the ATSIAG to: ensure public health messages were culturally relevant and locally delivered, develop a sustainable workforce plan to increase local health staff, and develop rapid testing in remote/regional communities, to reduce the need for isolation and evacuation if results were negative (Crooks et al., 2020).

Because of the efforts by the ATSIAG, including relevant stakeholders and the ACCHOs, who formed part of this group and worked directly with communities, COVID-19 risk mitigation strategies were rapidly developed. In turn, this enabled strong preparedness among communities (Crooks et al., 2020). The rates of COVID-19 among Aboriginal and Torres Strait Islander peoples in Australia are exemplary of the importance of establishing effective partnerships with government and facilitating self-determination, community empowerment, and Indigenous governance in the fight against COVID-19.

23.4.2 The Go8 'Roadmap to Recovery' Report and the Care of Aboriginal and Torres Strait Islander Peoples

To ensure the Australian Government received the best advice to inform evidence-based policy, a coalition of the top eight research universities in Australia (i.e., the 'Group of Eight') established an academic taskforce to develop a COVID-19 *Roadmap to Recovery* report (Group of Eight Australia, 2020). The taskforce comprised more than a hundred research leaders from a range of backgrounds, including public health, mental health, Aboriginal and Torres Strait Islander health, epidemiology, mathematics, economics, and philosophy, who developed the report during an intensive 3-week period in April 2020. The taskforce primarily utilised an online platform to support collaboration through document sharing and drafting (Group of Eight Australia, 2020; Moodie et al., 2020). The published report describes key evidence-based recommendations and options to manage the immediate threat of COVID-19 and facilitate the short-term recovery from the pandemic. Further, the report included a chapter on the care of Aboriginal and Torres Strait Islander peoples, described here (Group of Eight Australia, 2020). The report was presented to the Australian Government on 27 April 2020.

23.4.2.1 Core Recommendations of the 'Roadmap to Recovery' Report

Support the Right to Self-Determination

The first recommendation made by the taskforce was for governments to support Aboriginal and Torres Strait Islander peoples' right to self-determination. The United Nations Declaration on the Right of Indigenous Peoples (UNDRIP; United Nations, 2007) established minimum standards for the dignity, survival, and well-being of Indigenous peoples globally, which have important implications during a pandemic (Department of Economic and Social Affairs, 2020). An abundance of research has affirmed that self-determination is positively related to health and economic outcomes for Indigenous peoples (e.g., Cornell & Kalt, 2010; Dudgeon & Bray, 2018). Because of the continued impacts of colonisation on Indigenous peoples, enabling self-determination is vital to improving health outcomes, particularly during pandemics when health disparities become further exacerbated. Primarily, self-determination during a pandemic means that Indigenous peoples need to have control over their own communities and must be involved in emergency and health responses to the pandemic.

The taskforce advised the continual support from the Government, both financially and logistically, for Aboriginal and Torres Strait Islander COVID-19 planning groups and taskforces for the entirety of the pandemic (Group of Eight Australia, 2020). As outlined earlier, the initial Aboriginal and Torres Strait Islander responses to the pandemic have been highly successful, with Aboriginal and Torres Strait Islander COVID-19 cases representing 0.7% of all Australian cases at the time of the report (Group of Eight Australia, 2020). Importantly, these responses and rates of infection were maintained throughout the pandemic.

Increase Housing Supply and Access

To curb the spread of COVID-19, the Australian Government introduced self-isolation and lockdown measures during the initial outbreak in early 2020 and during subsequent second waves of the pandemic. Recent reports have identified that 19% of Aboriginal and Torres Strait Islander peoples surveyed were living in a house that did not meet an acceptable standard (Australian Government Australian Institute of Health and Welfare, 2019). In addition, the report noted that 20% of respondents were living in overcrowded conditions (Australian Government

Australian Institute of Health and Welfare, 2019). Further, Aboriginal and Torres Strait Islander peoples were 10 times as likely as non-Aboriginal and Torres Strait Islander people to live in social housing and were 9 times as likely to access homelessness services (Australian Government Australian Institute of Health and Welfare, 2019). The critical shortages of housing within urban, regional, and remote Aboriginal and Torres Strait Islander communities caused the capacity of families to quarantine and self-isolate adequately to be a serious concern at the outset of the pandemic (Group of Eight Australia, 2020). During the early stages of the pandemic, Aboriginal and Torres Strait Islander peoples living in urban centres were relocated back to remote communities, adding pressure to housing that was already at capacity.

The lack of appropriate housing limits the abilities of local health services and communities to control the spread of COVID-19. It also exacerbates long-standing issues of aging infrastructure, overcrowded housing, and other related issues such as hygiene and health problems and child and family well-being and safety (Group of Eight Australia, 2020). To facilitate the ability of families to effectively isolate to reduce viral spread, the taskforce recommended that an immediate supply of alternative and additional housing be supplied to remote communities (Group of Eight Australia, 2020). To ensure longer-term preparedness, it is estimated that 5500 new houses are required by 2028 to reduce the deleterious health consequences of crowded housing in remote communities (Commonwealth of Australia Department of Prime Minister and Cabinet, 2017b; Hall et al., 2020). Increasing appropriate housing was therefore an important recommendation for improving health, controlling COVID-19 infection, and ensuring long-term preparedness for future pandemics.

This recommendation was further emphasised by Moodie et al. (2020), who described that the lockdown restrictions and lack of housing are expected to exacerbate issues of overcrowding and family violence. In turn, this is predicted to lead to increased mandatory reporting of children's exposure to violence (Moodie et al., 2020). Considering the historical over-policing in Aboriginal and Torres Strait Islander communities, and the increased police presence amidst the COVID-19 crisis, Moodie et al. (2020) emphasise that young Aboriginal and Torres Strait Islander people will be at a greater risk of experiencing police harassment. Therefore, effective intervention to establish adequate housing for families and support for the compounding effects of lockdown measures was emphasised as an essential measure to safeguard the livelihoods of Aboriginal and Torres Strait Islander youth (Moodie et al., 2020).

Maintain COVID-19 Public Health and Clinical Responses

Public health responses to COVID-19 are integral to controlling and supressing the spread of any virus or pandemic. Yet, unless these responses address inequity, they are unlikely to reduce the disproportionate risk of pandemics to Aboriginal and Torres Strait Islander peoples and are likely to result in significantly poorer health and economic outcomes for Aboriginal and Torres Strait Islander peoples (Bond & Whop, 2020). To maintain advocacy for an equitable public health agenda, the taskforce recommended that the ATSIAG be maintained until full recovery from COVID-19 is achieved in Australia (Group of Eight Australia, 2020). Relatedly, it was recommended that accurate public health messaging by and for Aboriginal and Torres Strait Islander peoples is frequently communicated to the Aboriginal and Torres Strait Islander public during recovery, to enable strong health literacy (Group of Eight Australia, 2020).

Acquiring timely and specific data is integral to understanding how the pandemic impacted and continues to impact Aboriginal and Torres Strait Islander peoples with regard to their health and well-being (Power et al., 2020). However, data relating to the rates and impact of COVID-19 on Indigenous peoples globally are scarce, and data that are collected are often not separated by ethnicity (Power et al., 2020). With this in mind, the taskforce recommended that efforts be made to monitor Aboriginal and Torres Strait

Islander COVID-19 cases and related epidemiological data (e.g., data on infection rates, hospitalisation, and death, and the social, economic, and health impact) and to communicate this information publicly (Group of Eight Australia, 2020). The taskforce also emphasised the need to evaluate the impact of COVID-19 on the SEWB of Aboriginal and Torres Strait Islander peoples. Aboriginal and Torres Strait Islander-led and culturally safe research that considers the social, political, and cultural determinants of health will provide important information for effectively responding to future pandemics (Group of Eight Australia, 2020).

Implement Aboriginal and Torres Strait Islander Health Workforce Review

The taskforce recommended that long-term and sustainable initiatives are required to build the local health workforce capacity (Group of Eight Australia, 2020). Health workforces in Aboriginal and Torres Strait Islander communities often depend on staff from interstate and overseas (Group of Eight Australia, 2020). The outbreak of COVID-19 and the subsequent travel restrictions, lockdown measures, and quarantine requirements exacerbated staff shortages among already under-resourced health services (Group of Eight Australia, 2020). The taskforce explicated the critical need for a temporary surge of workforce support should any COVID-19 outbreaks arise in communities (Group of Eight Australia, 2020). To establish local capacity, the taskforce strongly advised that NACCHO, as the national authority on Aboriginal and Torres Strait Islander comprehensive primary healthcare, initiate a Health Workforce reform in partnership with State, Territory, and Commonwealth governments (Group of Eight Australia, 2020). It is imperative that the reform process considers how to retain and increase the interstate and overseas workforce (Group of Eight Australia, 2020). Reform processes should endeavour to increase Aboriginal and Torres Strait Islander Public Health and Infectious Disease expertise to assist State and Federal Health Departments as a senior Public Health Group (Group of Eight Australia, 2020).

23.5 The Impact of COVID-19 on Mental Health and an Aboriginal and Torres Strait Islander Recovery Plan

The COVID-19 pandemic is expected to have long-term and lasting effects on SEWB and the mental health of Aboriginal and Torres Strait Islander peoples (Dudgeon, 2020; Milroy, 2020; Milroy et al., 2020). The downstream impacts of the pandemic resulted in the temporary closure of businesses, unemployment, and social isolation. For Aboriginal and Torres Strait Islander peoples, gathering with family and community and engaging in cultural activities on Country is immensely important to maintaining SEWB (Gee et al., 2014). However, unintended consequences of the pandemic restrictions, such as restrictions on regional travel and limits on the size of gatherings, diminished the ability and opportunities for Aboriginal and Torres Strait Islander peoples to connect to family, community, culture, and Country in this way (Milroy, 2020). These factors are expected to exacerbate many of the preexisting health inequalities related to the social, historical, and political determinants of health, placing Aboriginal and Torres Strait Islander peoples at a higher risk of experiencing trauma, mental illness, economic distress, and burnout in the enduring effects following the pandemic (Power et al., 2020). For Aboriginal and Torres Strait Islander peoples, mental health and concepts of healing and recovery are viewed holistically, as described by the SEWB Framework (Commonwealth of Australia Department of Prime Minister and Cabinet, 2017a; Gee et al., 2014; Social Health Reference Group, 2004; Zubrick et al., 2014). Therefore, pandemic recovery responses for Aboriginal and Torres Strait Islander peoples and communities must consider this holistic view of well-being.

To determine and address the specific mental health and well-being needs of Aboriginal and Torres Strait Islander peoples during the COVID-19 pandemic and recovery, the University of Western Australia's Poche Centre for Indigenous Health convened a working party of Aboriginal and Torres Strait Islander research leaders, Aboriginal and Torres Strait Islander mental health experts, representatives from Aboriginal and Torres Strait Islander health organisations, Elders, and allies with a background in Aboriginal and Torres Strait Islander mental health and SEWB (Dudgeon et al., 2020). The working party collaborated during two months over iterative virtual roundtable meetings that prioritised Aboriginal and Torres Strait Islander peoples' voices and community needs, between which new participants were invited to contribute their expertise. Minutes and drafts were shared for feedback, and a final set of recommendations was published and distributed (Dudgeon et al., 2020). These comprehensive and evidence-based recommendations formed the *National COVID-19 Pandemic Issues Paper on Mental Health and Wellbeing for Aboriginal and Torres Strait Islander Peoples* (Dudgeon et al., 2020) and they are summarised next.

23.5.1 Recommendation 1: The Right to Self-determination

Consistent with the *Roadmap to Recovery* report (Group of Eight Australia, 2020), self-determination was also a central recommendation advised by this working party (Dudgeon et al., 2020). Mainstream mental health services often lack Aboriginal and Torres Strait Islander representation and culturally safe service provision (Davidson, 2014; Larkin, 2006). In Australia, the Aboriginal Community Controlled Health Services (ACCHSs) represent an excellent demonstration of self-determination and provide equal, or better, healthcare, access, and culturally appropriate service provision compared to mainstream services (Finlay & Wenitong, 2020; Mazel, 2016; Panaretto et al., 2014). Ensuring that Aboriginal and Torres Strait Islander peoples are appropriately supported to lead the mental health recovery responses for Aboriginal and Torres Strait Islander peoples will ensure culturally safe and responsive services that meet their needs.

The working party advised that a national Aboriginal and Torres Strait Islander SEWB Consortium for COVID-19 be established to lead Aboriginal and Torres Strait Islander-specific policy responses and ensure consistency between national and local planning (Dudgeon et al., 2020). The working party emphasised the imperative to fund Aboriginal and Torres Strait Islander organisations and the ACCHO sector to lead, develop, and implement Aboriginal and Torres Strait Islander-led recovery initiatives to address the needs of peoples and communities (Dudgeon et al., 2020). Additionally, the working party highlighted the need for increased presence of Aboriginal and Torres Strait Islander representatives in the management of the pandemic, in the immediate, short, and long term. A further recommendation was that a cultural governance and evaluation strategy (Australian Government Productivity Commission, 2020) be employed when developing and implementing any legislation that may affect Aboriginal and Torres Strait Islander peoples during and following the pandemic (Dudgeon et al., 2020). This broader recommendation is in line with priority reform one of the *National Agreement on Closing the Gap* which outlines the commitment of formal partnerships and shared decision making with Aboriginal and Torres Strait Islander peoples and communities (Australian Government, 2020). This commitment from all governments needs to be implemented in the recovery from COVID-19.

23.5.2 Recommendation 2: The Health and Mental Health Workforce

A lack of access to culturally safe mental health services continues to be a persistent barrier to improving the mental health of Aboriginal and Torres Strait Islander peoples (Davidson, 2014; Dudgeon et al., 2020; Prentice et al., 2017). Additionally, local mental health and SEWB services are often chronically under-resourced and under-accessed, and sparse or nonexistent (Davidson, 2014; Productivity Commission for the Steering Committee for the Review of Government Service Provision, 2020). Since the

COVID-19 outbreak, mental health and SEWB services in Aboriginal and Torres Strait Islander communities are under increasing demand from increased psychological distress from the ongoing effects of the pandemic (Dudgeon, 2020; Dudgeon et al., 2020; Fitts et al., 2020; Indigenous Allied Health Australia, 2020). Additionally, issues around lack of access and limited staffing have been exacerbated by travel restrictions and complexities around the transition to telehealth for Aboriginal and Torres Strait Islander communities (Fitts et al., 2020).

To address the mental health care needs in Aboriginal and Torres Strait Islander communities, the working party called for needs-based funding to support the development and increase the capacity of culturally responsive services (Dudgeon et al., 2020). Building the community-controlled sector (particularly, health, housing, early childhood, and disability sectors) was a commitment outlined in the *National Agreement on Closing the Gap* and should be implemented to facilitate cultural safety and improvements in mental health and well-being (Australian Government, 2020).

In addition, the rapid upskilling and training of mental health staff was emphasised by the working party as a key action to enable community services to build a local workforce (Dudgeon et al., 2020). Workforce development must be consistent with the *National Aboriginal and Torres Strait Islander Health Workforce Strategic Framework 2016–2023* (Australian Health Ministers' Advisory Council, 2017). To address the shortage of mental health services and a SEWB workforce in remote communities, workforce development should include online training that facilitates equitable remote education (Dudgeon et al., 2020). In addition to upskill and training efforts, the development of long-term education and employment models must be prioritised that establish a community-based, Aboriginal and Torres Strait Islander-governed, mental health workforce (Dudgeon et al., 2020). The working party advised that formal recognition of Aboriginal and Torres Strait Islander knowledge, abilities, and skills, including SEWB and cultural healing, is central to community-based workforce development (Dudgeon et al., 2020). Finally, the working party emphasised that the non-Aboriginal and Torres Strait Islander mental health workforce must be culturally responsive and appropriately qualified to work effectively with Aboriginal and Torres Strait Islander patients (Dudgeon et al., 2020).

23.5.3 Recommendation 3: Social and Cultural Determinants of Health

Social and cultural determinants have a significant impact on the health and well-being of Aboriginal and Torres Strait Islander peoples (Commonwealth of Australia Department of Prime Minister and Cabinet, 2017a; Gee et al., 2014). Effective pandemic recovery responses must therefore address the social and cultural determinants of health. As described earlier, social determinants of health include income, employment, education, food security, and access to housing; cultural determinants of health include racism and discrimination, and protective factors, including connection to mind, body, family, community, culture, land, and spirit (Gee et al., 2014). For Aboriginal and Torres Strait Islander peoples in Australia, access to their land and waters, community and family cohesion, and the ability to engage in cultural and spiritual practices are also integral cultural determinants of SEWB (Zubrick et al., 2014). The increased rates of unemployment, restrictions, distress, and uncertainty arising from the COVID-19 pandemic have amplified pre-existing risk factors of the social and cultural determinants of health, and protective factors from cultural activities have been restricted (Power et al., 2020). Therefore, recovery responses aimed at reducing risk factors and increasing protective factors is critical.

First and foremost, the working party advised that access to essential human needs, including adequate housing, water, food, and energy, must be ensured for all, with priority given to those who reside in bushfire and other disaster-affected regions (Dudgeon et al., 2020). Another important priority was to facilitate creation of jobs and the continuity of work, by developing services and infrastructure that addresses community needs and builds community capacity, and the local workforce (Dudgeon et al., 2020). Finally, COVID-19 mental health and well-being recovery responses must address the specific needs of groups including: the elderly, young people, LGBTQI + SB, women's and men's groups, and individuals with disabilities or experiences of child abuse, family violence, imprisonment, or homelessness (Dudgeon et al., 2020). Finally, the working party advised that a COVID-19 SEWB Consortium be convened to consider the effects of the pandemic on Aboriginal and Torres Strait Islander peoples and use the information gathered to inform the development of methods to bolster the protective cultural determinants of SEWB (Dudgeon et al., 2020). One way to support cultural determinants of health and strengthen SEWB in the short term would be to promote cultural cohesion through the funding of local initiatives and Aboriginal and Torres Strait Islander-specific online community events. In the long term, community-led, strengths-based SEWB programs that encourage peoples' reconnection with Country, culture, and community are needed to ensure community healing, empowerment, and resilience (Dudgeon et al., 2020).

23.5.4 Recommendation 4: Digital and Telehealth Inclusion with Immediate Attention to an Aboriginal and Torres Strait Islander Helpline

Before the pandemic, access to adequate healthcare was a significant difficulty for Aboriginal and Torres Strait Islander peoples, particularly in rural and remote regions, because of pre-existing disparities in the health system. COVID-19 lockdown restrictions forced mental health services to adapt to alternative models of service delivery, particularly telephone and online platforms. The COVID-19 pandemic poses a distinctive opportunity to build and implement innovative, sustainable, equitable, and effectual models of digital mental healthcare for Aboriginal and Torres Strait Islander peoples (Dudgeon et al., 2020). Emerging research has shown that telehealth can be an effective alternative model of care for Aboriginal and Torres Strait Islander peoples and increases accessibility to care in remote and rural communities (Caffery et al., 2017; Smith et al., 2019). However, digital mental health may worsen pre-existing issues with access, as a result of digital exclusion, predominantly in rural and remote regions where the digital infrastructure is lacking or rudimentary (Dudgeon et al., 2020). Therefore, it is critical that telehealth and digital mental health (eMH) models of care are evaluated to identify and address access issues and build stronger models in the longer term (Dudgeon et al., 2020).

To address issues of need, cultural safety, and access, the working party first advised that an immediate investment be made to establish a helpline for Aboriginal and Torres Strait Islander peoples. Further, increased funding for scholarships in telephone counselling for Aboriginal and Torres Strait Islander health workers was recommended (Dudgeon et al., 2020). A second priority outlined by the working party was the need to build and improve digital capacity and infrastructure across all Aboriginal and Torres Strait Islander communities (e.g., ensuring that communities have reliable access to the Internet). Additionally, there is a need to further evaluate eMH services/tools to establish their cultural safety and clinical efficacy for Aboriginal and Torres Strait Islander peoples in the context of the COVID-19 pandemic (Dudgeon et al., 2020). However, to facilitate the long-term sustainability of such tools and ensure that they are culturally safe, the working party advised that in the longer term, services and tools for Aboriginal and Torres Strait Islander peoples and communities should be developed, tested, and validated by Aboriginal and Torres Strait Islander SEWB and mental health professionals (Dudgeon et al., 2020).

23.5.5 Recommendation 5: Evaluation that Includes Indigenous Data Sovereignty

For Aboriginal and Torres Strait Islander peoples, cultural context is intrinsically linked to SEWB and holds great relevance to mental health. Mainstream models of mental healthcare are often grounded in Western epistemologies and practices that deemphasise the importance of cultural context. Consequently, mainstream mental health models are often not appropriate for Aboriginal and Torres Strait Islander peoples and hold little benefit to improving SEWB (Dudgeon et al., 2020). It is therefore imperative that all services for Aboriginal and Torres Strait Islander peoples are developed and maintained using the guiding principles of the SEWB framework, data sovereignty, and Indigenous governance (Carroll et al., 2020; Commonwealth of Australia Department of Prime Minister and Cabinet, 2017a; Dudgeon et al., 2020; Social Health Reference Group, 2004). When services are not developed in this way, the services and their funding agencies must be accountable for their role in the health and well-being outcomes of Aboriginal and Torres Strait Islander peoples (Dudgeon et al., 2020).

As outlined earlier, current issues relating to data quality and data sharing about Aboriginal and Torres Strait Islander clients by mainstream services need to be rectified, consistent with priority reform four in the *National Agreement on Closing the Gap* (Australian Government, 2020). This recommendation reflects Indigenous data sovereignty principles that emphasise Aboriginal and Torres Strait Islander control over data that are collected about Aboriginal and Torres Strait Islander peoples, to ensure the collective benefit of obtaining such data (Carroll et al., 2020). Current data relating to COVID-19 infection rates as well as the short- and long-term impact of the pandemic on Indigenous peoples worldwide are lacking (Power et al., 2020). Yet, these are the very data that are essential to building evidence towards the impact of disaster risk and resilience in Indigenous communities and, in turn, justifying needs-based funding and culturally responsive mental health models of care (Power et al., 2020). Aboriginal and Torres Strait Islander-led research is best placed to understand and examine the impact of COVID-19 among Aboriginal and Torres Strait Islander peoples and communities, including both encouraging and difficult experiences (Dudgeon et al., 2020). By developing an evidence base through data collection on COVID-19, established on the core principles of Indigenous data sovereignty, Aboriginal and Torres Strait Islander communities can build necessary information to safeguard Aboriginal and Torres Strait Islander peoples from future pandemics and other disasters.

23.6 The Continuity of COVID-19: Where to from Here?

Since the establishment of the *Roadmap to Recovery* report (Group of Eight Australia, 2020) and the *National COVID-19 Pandemic Issues Paper on Mental Health and Wellbeing for Aboriginal and Torres Strait Islander Peoples* (Dudgeon et al., 2020), the COVID-19 pandemic is ongoing. In July 2020, Melbourne experienced a second wave of the virus, leading to several months of enforced lockdown (Maiden, 2020). Further, in the subsequent months, during the Christmas period, a viral cluster in Northern Beaches, Sydney, led to the lockdown of this area and several nearby suburbs (Noble & Oliveri, 2020). Fortunately, a COVID-19 vaccine is now available in Australia, and the rollout of the vaccines has received support from primary healthcare, including ACCHOs (ABC News, 2021). Despite this, health experts warn that the ongoing economic and social instability associated with the pandemic, and its detrimental impact on the mental health of all, will persist for many years to come (Savage, 2020).

For Aboriginal and Torres Strait Islander peoples, pre-existing inequalities in health and well-being have already been exacerbated by the pandemic and its associated policies because of shortages of housing, lack of access to culturally responsive health and mental health care, enforced isolation, and disrupted cultural practices. The health gap between Aboriginal and Torres Strait Islander and non-Aboriginal and Torres Strait Islander peoples will inevitably widen if governments do not act in line with the response plans advised by Aboriginal and Torres Strait Islander taskforces, advisory, and working groups, who represent the voices of Aboriginal and Torres Strait Islander communities. The recent annual *Closing the Gap 2020* report to Parliament further emphasised the importance of strengths-based planning, built in partnership with Aboriginal and Torres Strait Islander peoples, to close the health and well-being gap between Aboriginal and Torres Strait Islander peoples and non-Aboriginal and Torres Strait Islander peoples (Commonwealth of Australia Department of Prime Minister and Cabinet, 2020).

Perhaps these changes are part of the unprecedented social change that is happening in the Western world. For example, incidents of systemic racism and racial inequality in America sparked the widespread Black Lives Matters (BLM) protests worldwide, including in Australia, where systemic racism and institutional racism are still rife (Smale, 2020). Following the BLM protests, the Australian Psychological Society issued a statement acknowledging the historical role of psychology in contributing to "...mistreatment and the erosion of culture," but promising to stand against racism and remain committed to, and accountable for, their role in supporting Aboriginal and Torres Strait Islander mental health and SEWB (Australian Psychological Society, 2020). These events, alongside the COVID-19 pandemic, emphasise the importance of addressing not just the immediate threat of a pandemic for Aboriginal and Torres Strait Islander peoples, but to also address the longer-term social and cultural determinants of health that cause the disproportionate risk to pandemics. Addressing these determinants of health and well-being is vital to safeguarding Aboriginal and Torres Strait Islander peoples, now and following the aftermath of the pandemic.

The detrimental effects of the pandemic on mental health are predicted to continue for many years (Power et al., 2020; Savage, 2020). Therefore, responses to managing the long-term impacts of the pandemic for Aboriginal and Torres Strait Islander peoples must ensure continued investment of Government funding to these initiatives. Government funding of pandemic responses must ensure adherence to the National Strategic principles (Commonwealth of Australia Department of Prime Minister and Cabinet, 2017a; Social Health Reference Group, 2004), priority reforms in the *National Agreement on Closing the Gap* (Australian Government, 2020), Indigenous data governance and sovereignty (Carroll et al., 2020), and ethical principles (National Health and Medical Research Council, 2003), to facilitate effective, culturally safe, and responsive outcomes (National Aboriginal and Torres Strait Islander Leadership in Mental Health, 2015).

Crucially, it is well demonstrated by the actions of the ACCHOs and ACCHSs during the pandemic that self-determination is fundamental to the success of Aboriginal and Torres Strait Islander pandemic responses and outcomes (Eades et al., 2020). We have seen too frequently that irresponsible and ineffective government policies can lead to widespread public health chaos (e.g., see the ongoing effects of Trump's pandemic responses and responses in Brazil; ABC News, 2020; Ferigato et al., 2020). The pandemic has demonstrated that poor government policy has resulted in the infection, hospitalisation, and death of Indigenous peoples at a much higher rate than that of non-Indigenous peoples (Arrazola et al., 2020; Lakhani, 2021; Power et al., 2020). In Australia, Aboriginal and Torres Strait Islander-led initiatives and successful partnerships with government have enabled effective planning and responses to the pandemic and saved countless lives. With continued funding and government support to consolidate recovery plans, the ACCHOs will be empowered to continue to lead the long-term recovery from the pandemic for Aboriginal and Torres Strait Islander peoples.

Acknowledgments We acknowledge Anna-Louise Kimpton, Billy Moore, and Emily Phillips from the National Aboriginal Community Controlled Health Organisation for their support.

References

ABC News. (2020). *US surpasses 250,000 coronavirus deaths, as hospitals are overwhelmed by cases*. ABC News. https://www.abc.net.au/news/2020-11-19/us-surpasses-250000-coronavirus-deaths-covid-19/12899108

ABC News. (2021). *Indigenous communities prepare for COVID-19 vaccine rollout*. ABC News. https://www.abc.net.au/radionational/programs/breakfast/indigenous-communities-prepare-for-covid19-vaccine-rollout/13241308

Ahmed, F., Ahmed, N. E., Pissarides, C., & Stiglitz, J. (2020). Why inequality could spread COVID-19. *The Lancet. Public Health, 5*(5), e240–e240. https://doi.org/10.1016/s2468-2667(20)30085-2

Arrazola, J., Masiello, M. M., Joshi, S., Dominguez, A. E., Poel, A., Wilkie, C. M., Bressler, J. M., McLaughlin, J., Kraszewski, J., Komatsu, K. K., Peterson Pompa, X., Jespersen, M., Richardson, G., Lehnertz, N., LeMaster, P., Rust, B., Keyser Metobo, A., Doman, B., Casey, D., … Landen, M. (2020). COVID-19 mortality among American Indian and Alaska Native Persons – 14 States, January–June 2020. *Morbidity and Mortality Weekly Report, 69*(49), 1853–1856. https://doi.org/10.15585/mmwr.mm6949a3

Australian Bureau of Statistics. (2018). *Estimates of Aboriginal and Torres Strait Islander Australians, June 2016*. Australian Bureau of Statistics. https://www.abs.gov.au/statistics/people/aboriginal-and-torres-strait-islander-peoples/estimates-aboriginal-and-torres-strait-islander-australians/latest-release#data-download

Australian Government. (2020). *National agreement on closing the gap*. Australian Government. https://www.closingthegap.gov.au/sites/default/files/files/national-agreement-ctg.pdf

Australian Government Australian Institute of Health and Welfare. (2019). *Indigenous housing*. Australian Government Australian Institute of Health and Welfare. https://www.aihw.gov.au/reports/australias-welfare/indigenous-housing

Australian Government Department of Health. (2020a). *Aboriginal and Torres Strait Islander advisory group on COVID-19*. Australian Government Department of Health. https://www.health.gov.au/committees-and-groups/aboriginal-and-torres-strait-islander-advisory-group-on-covid-19

Australian Government Department of Health. (2020b). *Australian health sector emergency response plan for novel coronavirus (COVID-19)*. Australian Government Department of Health. https://www.health.gov.au/sites/default/files/documents/2020/07/management-plan-for-aboriginal-and-torres-strait-islander-populations.pdf

Australian Government Department of Health. (2020c). *Coronavirus (COVID-19) current situation and case numbers*. Commonwealth of Australia. https://www.health.gov.au/news/health-alerts/novel-coronavirus-2019-ncov-health-alert/coronavirus-covid-19-current-situation-and-case-numbers

Australian Government Department of Health. (2020d). *What you need to know about coronavirus (COVID-19)*. Commonwealth of Australia. https://www.health.gov.au/news/health-alerts/novel-coronavirus-2019-ncov-health-alert/what-you-need-to-know-about-coronavirus-covid-19

Australian Government Productivity Commission. (2020). *Indigenous evaluation strategy*. Australian Government Productivity Commission. https://www.pc.gov.au/inquiries/completed/indigenous-evaluation/draft/indigenous-evaluation-draft.pdf

Australian Health Ministers' Advisory Council. (2017). *National Aboriginal and Torres Strait Islander health workforce strategic framework 2016–2023*. Australian Health Ministers' Advisory Council. https://www1.health.gov.au/internet/main/publishing.nsf/Content/4A716747859075FFCA257BF0001C9608/$File/National-Aboriginal-and-Torres-Strait-Islander-Health-Workforce-Strategic-Framework.pdf

Australian Psychological Society. (2020). *Black lives matter: Psychologists take a stand against racism*. Australian Psychological Society. https://www.psychology.org.au/getmedia/dece6e26-f3a9-4b1a-bc55-3abdab03293d/APS-Black-Lives-Matter-position-statement-Psychologists-take-a-stand-against-racism_1.pdf

Bond, C., & Whop, L. J. (2020). *The answer to Indigenous vulnerability to coronavirus: A more equitable public health agenda*. The Conversation. https://theconversation.com/the-answer-to-indigenous-vulnerability-to-coronavirus-a-more-equitable-public-health-agenda-135048

Caffery, L. J., Bradford, N. K., Wickramasinghe, S. I., Hayman, N., & Smith, A. C. (2017). Outcomes of using telehealth for the provision of healthcare to Aboriginal and Torres Strait Islander people: A systematic review. *Australian and New Zealand Journal of Public Health, 41*(1), 48–53. https://doi.org/10.1111/1753-6405.12600

Carroll, S. R., Garba, I., Figueroa-Rodríguez, C. L., Holbrook, J., Lovett, R., Materechera, S., Parsons, M., Raseroka, K., Rodriguez-Lonebear, D., Rowe, R., Sara, R., Walker, J. D., Anderson, J., & Hudson, M. (2020). The CARE principles for indigenous data governance. *Data Science Journal, 19*(1), 43. https://doi.org/10.5334/dsj-2020-043

Commonwealth of Australia Department of Prime Minister and Cabinet. (2017a). *National strategic framework for Aboriginal and Torres Strait Islander peoples' mental health and social and emotional wellbeing 2017–2023*. Commonwealth of Australia. https://www.niaa.gov.au/sites/default/files/publications/mhsewb-framework_0.pdf

Commonwealth of Australia Department of Prime Minister and Cabinet. (2017b). *Remote housing review: A review of the national partnership agreement on remote indigenous housing and the remote housing strategy (2008-2018)* https://healthinfonet.

ecu.edu.au/healthinfonet/getContent.php?linkid=599807&title=Remote+housing+review%3A+a+review+of+the+National+Partnership+Agreement+on+Remote+Indigenous+Housing+and+the+Remote+Housing+Strategy+%282008-2018%29&contentid=33930_1

Commonwealth of Australia Department of Prime Minister and Cabinet. (2020). *Closing the gap report 2020*. Commonwealth of Australia. https://ctgreport.niaa.gov.au/sites/default/files/pdf/closing-the-gap-report-2020.pdf

Cornell, S., & Kalt, J. P. (2010). American Indian self-determination: The political economy of a policy that works. *SSRN*. https://doi.org/10.2139/ssrn.1724725

Crooks, K., Casey, D., & Ward, J. S. (2020). First Nations peoples leading the way in COVID-19 pandemic planning, response and management. *Medical Journal of Australia, 213*(4), 151–152.e151. https://doi.org/10.5694/mja2.50704

Davidson, H. (2014). Indigenous suicide: 'Prevention should focus on cultural reconnection'. *The Guardian*. https://www.theguardian.com/australia-news/2014/nov/17/indigenous-suicide-prevention-should-focus-on-cultural-reconnection

Department of Economic and Social Affairs. (2020). *Indigenous peoples & the COVID-19 pandemic: Considerations*. Department of Economic and Social Affairs. https://www.un.org/development/desa/indigenouspeoples/wp-content/uploads/sites/19/2020/04/DESA-COVID-19-Considerations.pdf

Dudgeon, P. (2020). *COVID-19 puts extra strain on wellbeing of Indigenous Australians*. https://www.news.uwa.edu.au/archive/2020062612190/regional/covid-19-puts-extra-strain-wellbeing-indigenous-australians/

Dudgeon, P., & Bray, A. (2018). Indigenous healing practices in Australia. *Women & Therapy, 41*(1–2), 97–113. https://doi.org/10.1080/02703149.2017.1324191

Dudgeon, P., Wright, M., Paradies, Y., Garvey, D., & Walker, I. (2014). Aboriginal social, cultural and historical contexts. In P. Dudgeon, H. Milroy, & R. Walker (Eds.), *Working together: Aboriginal and Torres Strait Islander mental health and wellbeing principles and practice* (pp. 3–24). Commonwealth of Australia.

Dudgeon, P., Milroy, J., Calma, T., Luxford, Y., Ring, I., Walker, R., Cox, S., Georgatos, G., & Holland, C. (2016). *Solutions that work – What evidence and our people tell us. Aboriginal and Torres Strait Islander suicide prevention evaluation project report*. The Commonwealth Department of Prime Minister and Cabinet. https://www.atsispep.sis.uwa.edu.au/__data/assets/pdf_file/0006/2947299/ATSISPEP-Report-Final-Web.pdf

Dudgeon, P., Derry, K. L., Arabena, K., Brideson, T., Cairney, S., Calma, T., Dalton, T., Darwin, L., Duarte, B., Dyall, D., Gee, G., Gibson, P., Gray, P., Groth, A., Hirvonen, T., Holland, C., Mascall, C., McPhee, R., Milroy, H., … Wright, M. (2020). *A national COVID-19 pandemic issues paper on mental health and wellbeing for aboriginal and Torres Strait Islander peoples*. Transforming Indigenous Mental Health and Wellbeing Grant, University of Western Australia Poche Centre for Indigenous Health.

Eades, S., Eades, F., McCaullay, D., Nelson, L., Phelan, P., & Stanley, F. (2020). Australia's First Nations' response to the COVID-19 pandemic. *The Lancet (British edition), 396*(10246), 237–238. https://doi.org/10.1016/S0140-6736(20)31545-2

Ferigato, S., Fernandez, M., Amorim, M., Ambrogi, I., Fernandes, L. M. M., & Pacheco, R. (2020). The Brazilian Government's mistakes in responding to the COVID-19 pandemic. *Lancet (London, England), 396*(10263), 1636. https://doi.org/10.1016/S0140-6736(20)32164-4

Finlay, S., & Wenitong, M. (2020). Aboriginal Community Controlled Health Organisations are taking a leading role in COVID-19 health communication. *Australian and New Zealand Journal of Public Health, 44*(4), 251–252. https://doi.org/10.1111/1753-6405.13010

Fitts, M. S., Russell, D., Mathew, S., Liddle, Z., Mulholland, E., Comerford, C., & Wakerman, J. (2020). Remote health service vulnerabilities and responses to the COVID-19 pandemic. *The Australian Journal of Rural Health, 28*(6), 613–617. https://doi.org/10.1111/ajr.12672

Flint, S. M., Davis, J. S., Su, J. Y., Oliver-Landry, E. P., Rogers, B. A., Goldstein, A., Thomas, J. H., Parameswaran, U., Bigham, C., Freeman, K., Goldrick, P., & Tong, S. Y. C. (2010). Disproportionate impact of pandemic (H1N1) 2009 influenza on Indigenous people in the Top End of Australia's Northern Territory. *Medical Journal of Australia, 192*(10), 617–622. https://doi.org/10.5694/j.1326-5377.2010.tb03654.x.f

Gee, G., Dudgeon, P., Schultz, C., Hart, A., & Kelly, K. (2014). Aboriginal and Torres Strait Islander social and emotional wellbeing. In P. Dudgeon, H. Milroy, & R. Walker (Eds.), *Working together: Aboriginal and Torres Strait Islander mental health and wellbeing principles and practice* (pp. 55–68). Commonwealth of Australia.

Government of Western Australia Department of Health. (2021). *Aboriginal sector communication update #12*. Government of Western Australia Department of Health. https://ww2.health.wa.gov.au/-/media/Corp/Documents/Health-for/Infectious-disease/COVID19/COVID19-Aboriginal-Sector-Communications-Update-12.pdf

Group of Eight Australia. (2020). *COVID-19 road-map to recovery: A report for the nation*. Group of Eight Australia. https://go8.edu.au/wp-content/uploads/2020/05/Go8-Road-to-Recovery.pdf

Hall, N. L., Redmond, A., Memmott, P., & Barnes, S. (2020). *Fix housing and you'll reduce risks of coronavirus and other disease in remote Indigenous communities*. The Conversation. https://theconversation.com/

fix-housing-and-youll-reduce-risks-of-coronavirus-and-other-disease-in-remote-indigenous-communities-136049

Indigenous Allied Health Australia. (2020). *Workforce response to mental health needed*. Indigenous Allied Health Australia. https://iaha.com.au/workforce-response-to-mental-health/

Lakhani, N. (2021). Exclusive: Indigenous Americans dying from Covid at twice the rate of white Americans. *The Guardian*. https://www.theguardian.com/us-news/2021/feb/04/native-americans-coronavirus-covid-death-rate

Larkin, S. (2006). Evidence-based policy making in aboriginal and Torres Strait Islander health. *Australian Aboriginal Studies, 2006*(2), 17–26.

Li, J., Huang, D. Q., Zou, B., Yang, H., Hui, W. Z., Rui, F., Yee, N. T. S., Liu, C., Nerurkar, S. N., Kai, J. C. Y., Teng, M. L. P., Li, X., Zeng, H., Borghi, J. A., Henry, L., Cheung, R., & Nguyen, M. H. (2020). Epidemiology of COVID-19: A systematic review and meta-analysis of clinical characteristics, risk factors, and outcomes. *Journal of Medical Virology, 93*, 1449. https://doi.org/10.1002/jmv.26424

Maiden, S. (2020). *Coronavirus Victoria: Melbourne makes world history crushing second wave*. news.com.au. https://www.news.com.au/world/coronavirus/australia/coronavirus-victoria-melbourne-makes-world-history-crushing-second-wave/news-story/8551d1e094b8ef0ddcd706db631f3a0e

Mazel, O. (2016). Self-determination and the right to health: Australian aboriginal community controlled health services. *Human Rights Law Review, 16*(2), 323–355. https://doi.org/10.1093/hrlr/ngw010

Milroy, H. (2020). *COVID-19: Equity and ethics in a pandemic: Indigenous perspectives*. https://www.news.uwa.edu.au/archive/2020061712163/indigenous/covid-19-equity-and-ethics-pandemic-indigenous-perspectives/

Milroy, J., Derry, K. L., & Dudgeon, P. (2020). *COVID-19: Impacts of historical, social and cultural determinants of health*. https://www.news.uwa.edu.au/archive/2020061712164/covid-19/covid-19-impacts-historical-social-and-cultural-determinants-health/

Moodie, N., Ward, J., Dudgeon, P., Adams, K., Altman, J., Casey, D., Cripps, K., Davis, M., Derry, K., Eades, S., Faulkner, S., Hunt, J., Klein, E., McDonnell, S., Ring, I., Sutherland, S., & Yap, M. (2020). Roadmap to recovery: Reporting on a research taskforce supporting Indigenous responses to COVID-19 in Australia. *The Australian Journal of Social Issues., 56*, 1. https://doi.org/10.1002/ajs4.133

NACCHO. (2020a). *Aboriginal and Torres Strait Islander Advisory Group on COVID-19, 31 March 2020*. NACCHO. https://www.naccho.org.au/news/aboriginal-and-torres-strait-islander-advisory-group-on-covid-19-31-march-2020

NACCHO. (2020b). *The Australian Government's response to the COVID-19 pandemic, submission*. NACCHO.

NACCHO. (2020c). *National Aboriginal Community Controlled Health Organisation annual report 2019–2020*. NACCHO.

NACCHO. (2021). *Aboriginal health in Aboriginal hands*. NACCHO. https://www.naccho.org.au/

National Aboriginal and Torres Strait Islander Leadership in Mental Health. (2015). *Gayaa Dhuwi (proud spirit) declaration*. National Aboriginal and Torres Strait Islander Leadership in Mental Health. https://natsilmh.org.au/sites/default/files/gayaa_dhuwi_declaration_A4.pdf

National Health and Medical Research Council. (2003). *Values and ethics: Guidelines for conduct of aboriginal and Torres Strait Islander health research*. Commonwealth of Australia.

Noble, F., & Oliveri, N. (2020). *Queues form at Sydney Northern Beaches testing clinics as thousands told to stay at home*. Nine News. https://www.9news.com.au/national/coronavirus-nsw-northern-beaches-asked-to-stay-home-as-cluster-spreads/5976cd71-a886-49ae-8ab7-fd445fc47eaa

Panaretto, K. S., Wenitong, M., Button, S., & Ring, I. T. (2014). Aboriginal community controlled health services: Leading the way in primary care. *Medical Journal of Australia, 200*(11), 649–652. https://doi.org/10.5694/mja13.00005

Parliament of Australia. (2020). *COVID-19: A chronology of state and territory government announcements (up until 30 June 2020)*. Parliament of Australia. https://www.aph.gov.au/About_Parliament/Parliamentary_Departments/Parliamentary_Library/pubs/rp/rp2021/Chronologies/COVID-19StateTerritoryGovernmentAnnouncements

Power, T., Wilson, D., Best, O., Brockie, T., Bourque Bearskin, L., Millender, E., & Lowe, J. (2020). COVID-19 and indigenous peoples: An imperative for action. *Journal of Clinical Nursing, 29*(15–16), 2737–2741. https://doi.org/10.1111/jocn.15320

Prentice, K., Blair, B., & O'Mullan, C. (2017). Sexual and family violence: Overcoming barriers to service access for aboriginal and Torres Strait Islander clients. *Australian Social Work, 70*(2), 241–252. https://doi.org/10.1080/0312407x.2016.1187184

Prime Minister of Australia. (2020). *Border restrictions*. Prime Minister of Australia. https://www.pm.gov.au/media/border-restrictions

Productivity Commission for the Steering Committee for the Review of Government Service Provision. (2020). *Overcoming Indigenous disadvantage key indicators. 2020 Overview*. https://apo.org.au/sites/default/files/resource-files/2020-12/apo-nid309865.pdf, 1448-9813 (Print), 2206-9666 (Online).

Savage, M. (2020). *Coronavirus: The possible long-term mental health impacts*. BBC. https://www.bbc.com/worklife/article/20201021-coronavirus-the-possible-long-term-mental-health-impacts

Singu, S., Acharya, A., Challagundla, K., & Byrareddy, S. N. (2020). Impact of social determinants of health on the emerging COVID-19 pandemic in the United

States. *Frontiers in Public Health, 8*, 406–406. https://doi.org/10.3389/fpubh.2020.00406

Smale, S. (2020). *George Floyd protests live updates: Black Lives Matter protesters gather around the world*. ABC News. https://www.abc.net.au/news/2020-06-07/george-floyd-protests-us-live-updates-black-lives-matter/12330128

Smith, A. C., Armfield, N. R., & Caffery, L. J. (2019). Telehealth a game changer: Closing the gap in remote Aboriginal communities. *Medical Journal of Australia, 211*(1), 43–43.e41. https://doi.org/10.5694/mja2.50208

Social Health Reference Group. (2004). *National strategic framework for aboriginal and Torres Strait Islander peoples' mental health and social and emotional wellbeing 2004–2009*. Australian Department of Health and Ageing.

United Nations. (2007). United Nations declaration on the rights of Indigenous Peoples. https://www.un.org/development/desa/indigenouspeoples/declaration-on-the-rights-of-indigenous-peoples.html

World Health Organization. (2020). *Listings of WHO's response to COVID-19*. World Health Organization. https://www.who.int/news/item/29-06-2020-covidtimeline

Zubrick, S., Shepherd, C., Dudgeon, P., Gee, G., Paradies, Y., Scrine, C., & Walker, R. (2014). Social determinants of social and emotional wellbeing. In P. Dudgeon, H. Milroy, & R. Walker (Eds.), *Working together: Aboriginal and Torres Strait Islander mental health and wellbeing principles and practice* (pp. 93–107). Commonwealth of Australia.

24 COVID-19 Pandemic in Nigeria: A Story Worth Telling from the Eyes of Social Workers

Uzoma Odera Okoye and Uche Louisa Nwatu

24.1 Introduction

The global population faces unimagined situations caused by the coronavirus (COVID-19) pandemic, which was reported in Wuhan, one of the most populous cities in China, in December 2019 (Forster et al., 2020; World Health Organization, 2020a; Yang et al., 2020). The virus spread internationally within 1 month of the first identification and was transmitted via close human-to-human contact (Huang et al., 2020). The outbreak of the virus was declared a public health emergency of international concern as well as a pandemic on 30 January 2020, and 11 March 2020, respectively, by the World Health Organization (Farzanegan et al., 2020).

One of the devastating impacts of the COVID-19 pandemic is the loss of human lives alongside some other short and long-term social, economic, and political effects. For example, the Organisation for Economic Co-operation and Development (OECD, 2020) forecasts that a long-lasting and more intensive COVID-19 outbreak is likely to drop global growth to 1.5% in 2020, which is half the projected rate of growth before the outbreak. Similarly, the International Monetary Fund (IMF) forecasts that the COVID-19 outbreak will cause a global recession in 2020 that could be worse than the one triggered by the global financial crisis of 2008–2009 (Gopinath, 2020). Sumner et al. (2020) also noted that global poverty could increase for the first time since 1990, implying that the COVID-19 poses a real threat to the United Nations (UN) Sustainable Development Goals (SDGs) for ending poverty by 2030. The World Bank (2020) believes that with the COVID-19 pandemic, many developing countries and especially in the African continent are going to face long-term consequences.

Nigeria received her shipped-in share of the novel coronavirus through an Italian consultant who arrived in Nigeria on February 27, 2020, and reported by the Nigerian Center for Disease Control (NCDC) on the 28th January 2020, being the first reported case of COVID-19 in sub-Saharan Africa (Ebenso & Out, 2020; Nigeria Centre for Disease Control, 2020a, b, c). Just as the World Health Organization predicted, the rate at which the COVID-19 is spreading in Nigeria is generating serious health concerns from the weak healthcare system (National Bureau of Statistics, 2015; WHO, 2016; Oyekale, 2017). The inadequacies and challenges that exist across the health system such as the inadequate supply of human and material resources, a low belief system in the

U. O. Okoye (✉)
Department of Social Work, Faculty of the Social Sciences, University of Nigeria, Nsukka, Enugu State, Nigeria
e-mail: uzoma.okoye@unn.edu.ng

U. L. Nwatu
Department of Social Work, University of Nigeria, Nsukka, Enugu State, Nigeria

M. C. S. Gonçalves et al. (eds.), *The Coronavirus Crisis and Challenges to Social Development*,
https://doi.org/10.1007/978-3-030-84678-7_24

new healthcare system, poor attitude of health practitioners, nonemployment of social workers in Primary Health Centres, zero levels of people's involvement, and inefficient service provision prove a very dangerous threat (Krumkamp et al., 2013; Okwaraji et al., 2012; Oyekale, 2017; Uzochukwu et al., 2018; Okoye, 2019). These issues, therefore, raise the question of the reality and ability of the Nigerian healthcare system to contain a full-blown coronavirus outbreak in the country, especially in the rural areas.

Currently, the containment of COVID-19 in Nigeria is facing many logistic, administrative, and social barriers, such as few testing and isolation centres, lack of medical equipment and personnel, especially in the area of infectious diseases, and both noninvolvement of social workers and low motivation of medical personnel (Anyika, 2014; Ibama & Dennis, 2016; Jaeger et al., 2018; Obansa & Orimisan, 2013; Titus et al., 2015). This, therefore, confirms the current reality in Nigeria where the workforce (medical/nonmedical), medical products, medical structures, technologies, and information available are all insufficient to achieve maximum health coverage and quality delivery, respectively (Eboreime et al., 2015; Oyekale, 2017; Uzochukwu et al., 2018). The fight against COVID-19 in Nigeria is also faced with challenges of low public compliance with social distancing, wearing of face masks, and constant hand-washing, probably because social workers were not involved in the required public education and awareness creation. Some traditional practitioners and pastors in Nigeria rather believe in supernatural and preternatural forces in approaching this public health issue (Benedict, 2014; Ibeneme et al., 2017; Jaeger et al., 2018).

Social workers in Nigeria are not part of the fight against the pandemic as obtains in some other parts of the world such as China, South Africa, New Zealand, and Italy. Unfortunately, the majority of the social workers in Nigeria appear not to be aware of the roles they need to play during the pandemic (Nnama-Okechukwu et al., 2020; Onalu et al., 2020), probably because the Nigerian government did not accord the needed relevance for their roles. The lack of such welfare services for vulnerable people, households, and poor individuals during the COVID-19 outbreak in Nigeria caused severe pain and economic hardship to households and poor individuals. It is against this backdrop that this chapter draws attention to the indispensable role of social workers in the period of a public health emergency. In the same vein, the responsibilities of social workers in the areas of social welfare provision and care of poor and vulnerable people stand to be relevant (Onalu et al., 2020).

24.2 The COVID-19 Experience and the Reality of the Nigerian Healthcare System

The health sector in Nigeria has been historically underfunded as it only receives 5% of the total budget rather than the 15% recommended by the Abuja Declaration of 2001 (Plan International Nigeria, 2020). Apart from underfunding, other factors such as; doctor-to-population ratio, per capita budget, percentage of budget spent on health, the teeming population of Nigeria's poor and vulnerable, and the inadequate social welfare system all contribute to the poor health condition in the country (Benson, 2020). In 2019, Nigeria (87 million) surpassed India (71.5 million) in terms of the number of people living in abject poverty (World Bank, 2020).

With increase in community transmission, the virus has infected more than 3000 people and has resulted in the death of more than 100 people in Nigeria as of May 2020. However, the total confirmed cases as of 30 November 2020 is 67,557 the Primary Health Care (PHC) Centres remain the most likely port of call for community members who develop symptoms that could be suggestive of COVID-19 (Ajisegiri et al., 2020). Unfortunately, these PHCs are poorly equipped to cope with the challenge posed by the pandemic, especially as no PHC has a social worker in its facility.

24.3 Government Response to the COVID-19 Pandemic

The Federal Government of Nigeria appears better prepared than ever before in tackling the upsurge of the COVID-19 pandemic in the country as it was among the first countries to recognize the risk and started planning ahead of the epidemic curve one week after China first reported the cases of COVID-19 (Kapata et al., 2020; Unah, 2020). The Nigerian government has undertaken numerous health, social, and economic measures to cushion the impact of COVID-19 (Dixit et al., 2020). According to the NCDC (2020a, b, c) and Africanews (2020), the government through the Presidential Task Force on COVID-19, Federal Ministry of Health, and Nigeria Center for Disease Control has been working closely in collaboration with relevant ministries, departments, agencies, partners, and other stakeholders to coordinate and review the national response strategies and implementation activities daily to effectively contain the spread of COVID-19. However, in all these efforts, social workers are still left out of the process.

24.3.1 Prior Preparedness

Before the importation of COVID-19 into Nigeria, the government established a "Coronavirus preparedness group" through its nation's leading public health agency, the NCDC, which commenced point-of-entry screening for travelers based on lessons learnt from the Ebola Virus Disease outbreak (Ajisegiri et al., 2020). The NCDC supported many states of the federation to establish Emergency Operation Centres (EOC), trained rapid response teams in all the 36 states, provided relevant public health advisory to Nigerians, shared the case-definition and preventive information with networks of national and subnational public health workers; built capacity for contact tracing and case management; and strengthened five laboratories for diagnostic capacities (Adepoju, 2020).

The World Health Organization (2020c) noted that the NCDC adopted the Polio EOC modes of operation; the NCDC activated a Level 3 Emergency Operations Centre (EOC) on 27 February 2020 (Global Polio Eradication Initiative, 2020). They also provide technical support to government agencies including NCDC and have an on-ground network of human resources including traditional and religious leaders, community mobilizers, and health workers to support the COVID-19 response. In the past 11 months (March 2020–January 2021) NCDC has supported each of the 36 states to activate testing capacity for COVID-19, further strengthening the resilience of our health system (NCDC, 2020a, b, c).

24.3.2 Lockdown Measures and a Ban on Mass Gathering

The Presidential Task Force (PTF) on COVID-19 was established to respond to the outbreak through a multi-sectoral and intergovernmental approach (Agbakwuru, 2020). To further curb the spread of COVID-19, a 5-week lockdown was imposed as of 30 March in Abuja, Lagos, and the neighboring Ogun state. Also, the Control of Infectious Disease Act was passed to further contain the coronavirus pandemic in a country of nearly 200 million (Ayeni, 2020; Olurounbi, 2020). Additional measures include a mandatory requirement to wear face masks in public spaces, massive flight cancellations and the suspension of all international flights, work-from-home by civil servants, partial closure of major food markets, ban on all religious activities, and a ban on all sporting events. In addition to all these, contact tracing and other public health measures were strengthened. NCDC has also deployed Surveillance Outbreak Response Management and Analysis System (SORMAS) to support contact tracing (Grainger, 2020).

24.3.3 Provision of Palliatives and Stimulus Packages

As part of government efforts towards encouraging the citizens to comply with the sit-at-home order and to cushion the harsh effects of COVID-19 economic realities, the federal and state governments made concerted efforts to provide palliative care in the form of food items, hand sanitizers, face masks, and other basic social care (NCDC, 2020a, b, c). The Federal Government of Nigeria expanded its social safety net, with welfare programmes in its efforts to reduce poverty and to mitigate the unintentional impacts of the partial lockdown on the livelihoods of the poor, and vulnerable households in affected states. These provisions included food rations, food vouchers, conditional cash transfers, and other forms of palliatives targeted at the vulnerable and socially disadvantaged members of society (Human Rights Watch, 2020). In May 2020, Oyo State Government, the World Bank, and Heritage Bank PLC have distributed palliative packages to more than 200 less-privileged individuals in the state; this distribution end in September 2020 (Badru, 2020). In Ondo State, the governor of the state disclosed that more than 200,000 households have benefitted from palliative distribution since the outbreak of COVID-19 (Johnson, 2020). The Central Bank of Nigeria announced the private sector Coalition Against COVID-19 (CACOVID) Relief Fund of N21.58 billion on 7 April 2020.

24.3.4 Fiscal Policy Measures

The Central Bank granted a one-year extension of the loan moratorium on principal repayments, with interest rate reduction on all intervention loan facilities; targeted credit facility to hotels, airline service providers, healthcare merchants, among others; and provided credit support to the healthcare industry (pharmaceutical companies and hospitals) (Ozili, 2020). The government also announced a freeze on loan repayments for farmers and small businesses and a reduction of the budget by NGN 1.5 trillion ($4.90 billion) (Adeshokan, 2020; Ozili & Arun, 2020). All these were the initial efforts of the government of Nigeria to both reduce the spread of the virus and mitigate the socioeconomic impacts of the pandemic on the citizens, especially the poor and vulnerable members of the Nigerian society. These government responses to an extent saved some of the citizens from the debilitating effects of hunger and starvation orchestrated by the pandemic, including saving businesses from collapsing.

24.4 Private Sector Response to the COVID-19 Pandemic

Churches and other nongovernmental organisations provided much support to communities across Lagos and the rest of Nigeria (Olubiyi, 2020). They have facilitated countless distributions of food items to some of the most deprived areas of Lagos and other areas across the country. Dozens of humanitarian organizations distributed food to ease the pains of the lockdown imposed to stop the spread of the coronavirus pandemic (Human Rights Watch, 2020; Jalloh, 2020), but only a small proportion of the population attest to receiving any support.

Non-cash donations including medical items and different varieties of foodstuff were received from different groups. Both the Christian Association of Nigeria (CAN) and the Nigerian Supreme Council of Islamic Affairs (NSCIA) supported the government lockdowns, and have worked with some local and state governments to disseminate accurate information and encourage compliance (Campbell & McCaslin, 2020). These responses from the private sector, some nongovernmental organisations as well as religious organisations, combined with government efforts contributed immensely towards improving the well-being of the most vulnerable in the country. Their contributions augmented that of the government in ensuring that the socioeconomic effects brought about by the pandemic are reduced to the barest minimum possible.

24.5 Factors That Worsened the Spread of the Pandemic and Its Attendant Socioeconomic Crisis

Regardless of these efforts by both the government and other relevant stakeholders, the country's economy was greatly overwhelmed by this pandemic as some of the support and some stimulus packages provided were reported to be insufficient and not proportional to the number of the poor masses scattered across the country. Some of the policy responses have weaknesses and loopholes that greatly contributed to the further spread of the virus and worsened the socioeconomic impacts on the people.

24.5.1 Insufficient Palliatives/Faulty Distribution Pattern

Although other countries, such as the U.S., responded to the crisis by doling out trillions of dollars as palliatives, Nigeria offered very little cash relief. The country was also further plagued by a worsening inflation rate and civil unrest/security challenges (Benson, 2020). This scourge has been exacerbated in light of emerging reports attesting to inadequacy in palliative measures (Human Rights Watch, 2020; Okojie, 2020), including the diversion of these limited resources by affluent officials (Daily Trust, 2020; Hassan, 2020). Officials in charge of the distribution of the palliatives were reported to be insincere and corrupt as they allegedly hoard the food items for their selfish interest, hence leaving the poor and vulnerable still hungry (Akinwotu, 2020).

The Ministry of Humanitarian Affairs stated that the Federal Government does not have a comprehensive list of beneficiaries of the palliatives (Obike, 2020); on the other hand, the ministry noted there is a lack of transparency, accountability, and proper planning with the scheme. Some residents of Abuja interviewed by a newspaper reporter noted that the distribution of the palliative was not done according to family size because families that had as many as 12 members got the same quantity of food as those that had only two or three members. Some of the items they received included a loaf of bread, a kilogram of rice, and two tubers of yam. Some also reported that there was a great disparity between what they were supposed to receive as lockdown palliative, as was reported on television, and what they actually received in the long run (Obike, 2020).

The whole process lacked records for spending details of both public funds and private sector donations to provide socioeconomic benefits to the country's poorest and most vulnerable people, including people living with disabilities (PWDs), no details of beneficiaries of any cash payments, cash transfers, food distribution, and other benefits during the lockdown (Socio-Economic Rights and Accountability Project, 2020).

24.5.2 Poverty

The majority of Nigerians depend on a daily income for survival (African Union, 2020; Esidene & Onyebuch, 2013; United Nations, 2020). As a result, hunger and starvation kept pushing residents to the streets against the order to stay at home, which posed a great barrier to adhering to the COVID-19 measures intended to inhibit the spread of the virus, amidst other challenges recounted (WHO, 2020b). The COVID-19 preventive measures in Nigeria appeared unfeasible and unrealistic as a result of poverty and vulnerability (Akinwotu, 2020; Daniel et al., 2020; HRW, 2020; WHO, 2020c). Many residents did not mind violating lockdown orders at the risk of contracting the virus rather than staying at home to die of hunger and malnutrition (Ukeh, 2020).

24.5.3 Illiteracy, Misinformation, and Distrust of the Government

Many Nigerians regarded the disease as a distant "white man's" infirmity that could never spread to their abode. Also, some felt that COVID-19 is a "big man disease" (i.e., disease of the highly influential persons), especially given the fact that it killed some political figures. Also, the spread of misinformation and tales regarding COVID-19 and promotion of unscientific traditional treatment within Nigeria further jeopardized the implementation of preventive measures. Some religious leaders with considerable influence created doubt among members of the public about the existence of the virus and shared conspiracy theories on its origins and the interventions (Egbunike, 2020). Also, unproven cures and interventions were regularly propagated by different groups (Ioannidis, 2020; Onyemelukwe, 2020). Unconcerned attitudes and adherence to false and superstitious beliefs by the public ensued from inadequate awareness, which further affected the level of preparedness and the proper implementation of COVID-19 protocols across the country (Reuben et al., 2020). The social media played an important role in the creation of awareness about the COVID-19 pandemic within the Nigerian population; however, it aided the spread of exaggerated, unverified, and fake news about the pandemic (Reuben et al., 2020). Some Nigerians also believed that prayer is warfare against COVID-19 spread, as this resulted in a carefree attitude from the people towards obeying the safety measures (Olapegba et al., 2020).

Since the outbreak of coronavirus in Nigeria, a good number of the citizenry believed strongly that the COVID-19 pandemic is more of a hoax than reality (Nnama-Okechukwu et al., 2020). The outright disbelief in the number of confirmed cases results in an apparent nonchalance about the pandemic. These challenges have a direct impact on the efforts to prevent the spread of the novel coronavirus in Nigeria (Onyemelukwe, 2020).

24.5.4 Unclear Directives

Movement restrictions as well as uncertainty in the lockdown rules by the federal government have led to food supply chain problems with many of the farmers at the receiving end. As commercial transportation wound down to a halt and roadblocks littered the streets, movement of food and agricultural produce proved difficult (Adeshokan, 2020). In a statement released by logistics company Kobo360, confusion over the government's directive on regulations of trucks resulted in fewer than 3000 trucks involved in the flow of essential goods pulling up for fear that if caught circulating, both the trucks and goods would be confiscated (George, 2020). The company had to call on the government to clarify the restrictions so that cargo drivers can move without harassment from security agencies, to ensure continued flow in the food supply chain.

24.5.5 Civil Unrest and Violence

In addition to the fatalities caused by the COVID-19 pandemic and an earlier Lassa fever outbreak in the year, Nigeria has also been grappling with the fatalities caused by unrest in the country's North-Eastern region. Hundreds of violent deaths were reported across North-Eastern Nigeria. In the same vein, kidnapping remained a major security challenge in the country. Unfortunately, a bad security situation never facilitates the economy of any country, and this rising rate of violence and banditry in the country became a double predicament for the government in their efforts towards containing the debilitating effects of the pandemic (Benson, 2020).

24.6 The Impact of the COVID-19 Pandemic on Nigerians

The outbreak of COVID-19 caused many poor communities in different parts of the world to face very challenging socioeconomic and livelihood consequences. With coronavirus diseases, many developing countries, especially in Africa, are going to face long-term consequences (World Bank, 2020). The COVID-19 pandemic is a real threat to all types of livelihood all over the world, but it has the greatest impact on those who are most in need of economic, social, health, and educational services. Many Nigerians belong to this group.

The most devastating impact of the COVID-19 pandemic is the negative socioeconomic impact on the livelihood of the poor (Buheji et al., 2020). Nigeria, in 2018, was announced by the World Poverty Clock to be the poverty capital of the world, with more than 40% of its citizens living below the poverty line. Therefore, a large proportion of the population lives on daily income with no savings to act as a financial buffer during the lockdown. Poor people in congested neighbourhoods were worried about how they will cope with hunger and starvation (British Broadcasting Corporation, 2020; Ozili, 2020).

The elderly, persons with disabilities, the homeless, and people working in the informal sector were hit the hardest by the pandemic (Gilaj & Ballhysa, 2020; Hekurani & Gjerani, 2020; Sinoruka, 2020). Despite advocacy for inclusion in the distribution of palliatives, women with disabilities across Nigeria were not factored into the intervention programmes by governments meant to cushion the effect of the COVID-19 pandemic (Adeyeye, 2020). Although the poor and small businesses have been at the centre of advocacy for government relief, it seems that persons with disabilities have been left out. Many of them reported that it was very difficult and frustrating to get palliatives or financial support during the COVID-19 lockdown (Lazarus & Oluwole, 2020). Globally, the coronavirus pandemic has had an especially harsh impact on people with intellectual and developmental disabilities and so they need special support (Thomas, 2020; Johns Hopkins University, 2020). The scale of the current economic downturn is the worst since the Great Depression, according to the IMF (Omole, 2020). Furthermore, as the global economy plummets, exceeding the Great Recession of 2007–2009 (Gopinath, 2020; IMF, 2020), mass layoffs, including cuts in paychecks and unemployment, have ensued in Nigeria.

Some states across the country do not have state-wide 3 G mobile access, so students in the final year of secondary school who are about to take their senior school certificate examinations had their lessons through the radio (Ayeni, 2020). Before the COVID-19 outbreak began, Nigeria already had a weak and underdeveloped digital economy. There were few universities or schools that offered a full educational curriculum online from start to finish. Nigerian schools, universities, and educators could not put coursework online so that students quarantined at home do not have to miss out on key aspects of their education while school is closed or when students cannot get to school. This loss affected the students as many of them could not learn during the entire period of the lockdown.

There was also an increase in sexual violence against women and children all over the country. For instance, between January and May 2020, Nigeria's Inspector General of Police reported that the force arrested 799 suspects associated with 717 rape cases (Olufayo, 2020). According to Ejiofor (2020), the restrictions in movement, loss of income, isolation, overcrowding, and high levels of stress all contributed to the increase in sexual violence in different homes as the stay-at-home order made it difficult for victims to stay away from the perpetrators. Apart from sexual violence, Umokoro (2020) reported an increase also in reported cases of other forms of domestic and gender-based violence, which was attributed to the forced proximity occasioned by the lockdowns.

24.7 The Nigerian Social Welfare System and the Place of Social Work Amidst the COVID-19 Pandemic

Nigeria does not have a national social welfare programme that offers assistance to all individuals and families in need such as healthcare assistance, food stamps, unemployment compensation, disaster relief, and educational assistance. The consequence of not having a national social welfare programme became evident during the COVID-19 pandemic. During the outbreak, people had little to rely on, and poor citizens did not have sufficient welfare relief that could help them cope with the economic hardship (Ewalt & Jennings, 2014). This lack of such welfare services for vulnerable people, households, and poor individuals during the pandemic in Nigeria was quite glaring so that the Ministry for Humanitarian Affairs, Disaster Management, and Social Development has seen the need to develop a comprehensive welfare programme that targets real Nigerians in need and not the haphazard arrangement they are currently running (HRW, 2020).

Lack of social welfare programmes during the coronavirus outbreak in Nigeria caused severe pain and economic hardship on households and poor individuals as millions suffered hunger in Nigeria and Africa at large. Adopting the COVID-19 lockdown is never the best option for a country like Nigeria where the majority live and survive from daily earnings. As a result, many street hawkers, roadside sellers, menial workers, and all daily earners have been left with no means of survival amidst the pandemic (African Union, 2020). The order by the government to stay at home, to suspend every form of social or public gathering including the closure of markets and every commercial activity, subjected the poor and vulnerable Nigerians to the devastating effects of hunger and starvation (Abdel-Moneim, 2021; Buheji et al., 2020; Jalloh, 2020; Kalu, 2020; Roberton et al., 2020).

Social workers in some parts of the world have been ignored in this collective fight against the COVID-19 pandemic (Rasool, 2020). Social workers in Nigeria went in lockdown, unlike their counterparts in countries such as China, Italy, New Zealand, South Africa, the United Kingdom, and so many others who were part of the COVID-19 interventions and response teams (Cui, 2020; Dominelli, 2020; IFSW, 2020; Pengli, 2020; Scarnera, 2020). These social work practitioners in other countries played exceptional roles in the fight against COVID-19; unfortunately, this was not the case in Nigeria as social workers were excluded from the multidisciplinary team in the fight against the virus. The reason is because the Nigerian government has yet to pass the legal mandate for social workers to contribute in mitigating the socioeconomic impact on the poor and vulnerable during a global pandemic. Also, the fact that social work has not been professionalized in Nigeria further contributes to the exclusion of their services at the peak of the pandemic (Okoye, 2013). The roles of social workers are not valued by the Nigerian government. Social workers are supposed to be actively involved at every point in the fight against this pandemic, ranging from community sensitization, awareness creation, psychosocial counselling, referrals, and other forms of social support (Pengli, 2020; Isangha et al., 2020).

24.8 Managing Post-COVID-19: New Paths for Social Workers

Nigeria and other nations in Africa must be creative in planning their recovery in the aftermath of this pandemic if indeed there is any aftermath as infections continue to rise. The African Union (AU) estimates that, under its "realistic scenario," Africa's gross domestic product (GDP) will shrink by 0.8% in 2020, resulting in 20 million job losses across the continent (African Union, 2020). Nigeria's economy requires urgent and coordinated responses, as it was already experiencing weak growth, if the country is to avoid a prolonged recession that will wreak more havoc not just on the economy but also on social cohesion. A well-developed digital economy in Nigeria must be achieved through intense digital technology penetration. This development will to a large extent have a larger part in reducing the effect of recessions in the country and will also help in supporting economic and social activities and in the development of good healthcare systems. The COVID-19 pandemic has highlighted the need for the use of technologies and innovations to improve healthcare in Nigeria (Onyeji, 2020; Ozili, 2020) as the challenges of the COVID-19 response are a reflection of the reality of the Nigerian public health system. Although every critical measure needs to be taken in reversing the escalating trend of COVID-19 in Nigeria, ultimately one of the solutions to this crisis is positive transformation in the public health system (Plan International Nigeria, 2020).

In Nigeria and across the world, the services of a team of professionals, including social workers, are required to minimize the debilitating effects of the COVID-19 pandemic. In fact, given the bio-psychosocial focus of the social work profession, many practitioners would be instrumental in this regard (Amadasun & Omorogiuwa, 2020; Isangha et al., 2020). It is against this backdrop that social workers must be at the vanguard of promoting policy change in the context of the challenges brought about by the outbreak of the pandemic. Social workers are social engineers whose services are highly needed during social upheavals such as this pandemic (IFSW, 2020). Social workers can utilize social media platforms to sensitize and educate the public about the pandemic, attend to the psychosocial care of COVID-19 victims and their family members, participate actively in palliative distribution, and can join other healthcare practitioners in rendering help and social services to individuals and families who require psychosocial/counseling support, referral, reintegration, and other forms of social support (IFSW, 2020). Also, they can be involved in maintaining safety-inclined contacts with vulnerable clients (women, elderly, youth, physically challenged, and children) while in lockdown (Brindle, 2020); and in distribution and buying of needed goods, psychosocial counseling for the medically isolated, and the general public (Onalu et al., 2020; Pengli, 2020).

Social workers in Nigeria should strive to get proper training for the management of pandemics and epidemics for them to be well equipped in the area of needs assessment, support for vulnerable citizens, and counselling services among other important roles. This is a wake-up call for schools of social work in Nigeria to revise their curricula to reflect the realities of the public health situation in Nigeria. Social workers in Nigeria can be aware of their roles and responsibilities in a period of a pandemic through proper training during their student days; this can be realized through an all-encompassing social work curriculum that would include training on risk management and disaster control (Amadasun, 2020; Onalu et al., 2020). Social workers can assume their education roles by informing the public and policymakers about the plight of the poor and vulnerable, which is worsened by the indiscriminate allocation of palliative measures. They can provide health education to the community on the clinical features, route of transmission, and access to care. Social workers can also restate and utilize their expertise in social welfare administration (Abiodun et al., 2011; Omorogiuwa, 2020), but they can only do this if they are equipped with the requisite knowledge and skills necessary for intervention from different schools of social work across the country.

24.9 Conclusion

The COVID-19 pandemic has demonstrated the global community as close knit, sharing a homogeneous attribute of collective vulnerability to a rapidly spreading virus. So many people tried to be accustomed to the daily updates about the number of confirmed COVID-19 cases in our local communities, including its trend globally. As countries around the world closed borders to protect the local populations, social lives and affinities of the citizenry crumbled overnight, while the ever-growing pace of globalisation continued to weaken as 'de-globalisation' sets in.

In response to the impact of the COVID-19 pandemic, all mitigation strategies of the government should pay attention to the concerns of the poor, voiceless, and vulnerable members of the Nigerian society, especially the old and frail, persons with disability, homeless, women, and children. Social work education and practice in Nigeria can be enhanced through a robust social work curriculum especially as a means of getting these persons ready for future pandemics. It is believed that social workers can play an indispensable role in improving the socioeconomic conditions of people, especially the poor and vulnerable, both during and after the pandemic. Therefore, social workers in Nigeria should strive to form part of the multidisciplinary team or front-line professionals in responding to the COVID-19 pandemic in Nigeria. For this to be achieved, the government must pass the legal mandate for social work professionals to operate and be perceived as an asset to be tapped during a public/global health crisis.

References

Abdel-Moneim, A. S. (2021). Community mitigation during SARS-COV-2 pandemic: Mission impossible for developing countries. *Population Health Management, 24*(1), 6. https://doi.org/10.1089/pop.2020.0095

Abiodun, M. G., Adekeye, O. A., & Iruonogbe, T. C. (2011). Counselling services for remediating the biopsychosocial challenges of the aged in Nigeria. *Journal of Functional Management, 3*(1), 89–98.

Adepoju, P. (2020). Nigeria responds to COVID-19: First case detected in Sub-Saharan Africa. *Nature Medicine, 26*(4), 444–448.

Adeshokan, O. (2020). Coronavirus: Food insecurity fallout from Nigerians lockdown. *The African Report*. https://www.theafricareport.com/27676/coronavirus-food-insecurity-fallout-from-nigerias-lockdown/

Adeyeye, P. (2020). *Social protection for the disabled in Nigeria during COVID-19 pandemic*. Dataphyte. https://www.dataphyte.com/covid19nigeria/social-protection-for-the-disabled-in-nigeria-during-covid-19-pandemic/

African Union. (2020). *Impact of the coronavirus (COVID 19) on the African economy*. Author.

Africanews. (2020). *Coronavirus: AFDB approves $2M package for WHO's Africa response*. Africanews. https://www.africanews.com/2020/04/02/economics-of-covid-19-impact-on-africa/

Agbakwuru, J. (March 9, 2020). Buhari sets up 12 member Task Force to control Coronavirus , *Vanguard News* https://www.vanguardngr.com/2020/03/buhari-sets-up-12-member-task-force-to-control-coronavirus/

Ajisegiri, W. S., Odusanya, O. O., & Joshi, R. (2020). COVID-19 outbreak situation in Nigeria and the need for effective engagement of community health workers for epidemic response. *Global Biosecurity, 1*(4). https://doi.org/10.31646/gbio.69

Akinwotu, E. (2020, May 15). People are more scared of hunger: Coronavirus is just one more threat in Nigeria. *The Guardian*. https://www.theguardian.com/global-development/2020/may/15/people-are-more-scared-of-hunger-coronavirus-is-just-one-more-threat-in-nigeria

Amadasun, S. (2020). COVID-19 pandemic in Africa: What lessons for social work education and practice? *International Social Work*. https://www.researchgate.net/publication/341700675_COVID-19_Pandemic_in_Africa_What_Lessons_for_Social_Work_Education_and_Practice

Amadasun, S., & Omorogiuwa, T. B. (2020). *2019 coronavirus and social work: Blueprint to holistic intervention*. SAGE.

Anyika, E. N. (2014). Challenges of implementing sustainable healthcare delivery in Nigeria under environmental uncertainty. *Journal of Hospital Administration, 3*(6), 113–126. http://www.sciedu.ca/journal/index.php/jha/article/viewFile/5274/3439

Ayeni, T. (2020). Coronavirus: Nigeria's varied response to controlling COVID-19. *The Africa Report*. https://www.theafricareport.com/27773/coronavirus-nigerias-varied-responses-to-controlling-covid-19/

Badru, A. (2020, September 7). COVID-19: Oyo, World Bank, CSDA, others distribute palliatives to 200 less privileged, counsel against depression. *Vanguard*. https://www.vanguardngr.com/2020/09/covid-19-oyo-world-bank-csda-others-distribute-palliatives-to-200-less-privileged-counsel-against-depression/

Benedict, A. O. (2014). The perception of illness in traditional Africa and the development of traditional medical practice. *International Journal of Nursing, 1*(1), 51–59. http://ijnnet.com/journals/ijn/Vol_1_No_1_June_2014/5.pdf

Benson, E. A. (2020). *COVID-19: Best and worst case scenarios for the Nigerian economy*. Nairametrics. https://nairametrics.com/2020/05/19/covid-19-best-and-worst-case-scenarious-for-these-smes/

Brindle, D. (2020). I can't know the children are safe': Social workers' fear over lockdown. *The Guardian*. https://www.theguardian.com/society/2020/apr/02/children-safe-social-workers-fears-lockdown-coronavirus

British Broadcasting Corporation [BBC]. (2020). *Lagos lockdown over coronavirus: How can my children survive?* BBC. https://www.bbc.com/news/world-africa-52093343

Buheji, M., Cunha, K., Beka, G., Mavric, B., Souza, Y. L., Silva, S. S., Hanapi, M., & Yein, T. C. (2020). The extent of COVID-19 and socio-economic impact on global poverty. A global integrative multidisciplinary review. *American Journal of Economics, 10*(4), 213–224.

Campbell, J & McCaslin, J. (April 28, 2020). *How Nigeria has responded to COVID-19 so far* https://www.cfr.org/blog/how-nigeria-has-responded-covid-19-so-far

Cui, K. (2020). *Tasks and competences of frontline social workers in fighting the Covid-19 Pandemic: Stories from Chengdu, China*. The International Association of Schools of Social Work. https://www.iassw-aiets.org/covid-19/4885-tasks-and-competences-of-frontline-social-workers-in-fighting-the-covid-19-pandemic-stories-from-chengdu-china/

Daily Trust. (2020). *Nigeria: Adamawa government, APC trade words over diversion of palliative*. https://allafrica.com/stories/202004150760.html

Daniel, G., Christoph, L. R., Andres, C. A., & Haoyu, W. (2020). *The impact of Covid-19 (Coronavirus) on global poverty: Why Sub-Saharan Africa might be the region hardest hit*. https://blogs.worldbank.org/opendata/impact-covid-19-coronavirus-global-poverty-why-sub-saharan-africa-might-be-region-hardest-hit

Dixit, S., Ogundeji, Y. K., & Onwujekwe, O. (2020). How well has Nigeria responded to COVID-19. *Future Development*. https://www.brookings.edu/blog/future-development/2020/07/02/how-well-has-nigeria-responded-to-covid-19/

Dominelli, L. (2020). *Surviving COVID-19: Social work issues in a global pandemic (Child protection and welfare, social care)*. The International Association of Schools of Social Work. https://www.iassw-aiets.org/wp-content/uploads/2020/04/Child-Protection-and-Welfare -Under-Covid-Article-11-Apr-R.pdf

Ebenso, B., & Out, A. (2020). Can Nigeria contain the COVID-19 outbreak using lessons from recent epidemics? *The Lancet Global Health, 8*, e770. https://doi.org/10.1016/S2214-109X

Eboreime, E., Abimbola, S., & Bozzani, F. (2015). Access to routine immunization: A comparative analysis of supply-side disparities between northern and southern Nigeria. *PLoS One, 10*(12), e0144876.

Egbunike, N. (2020). *Nigerian pastor spreads COVID-19 conspiracies and disinformation*. https://globalvoices.org/2020/05/15/nigerian-pastor-spreads-covid-19-conspiracies-and-disinformation/

Ejiofor, B. (2020). *COVID-19: Children suffer violence during Lagos lockdown*. https://www.unicef.org/nigeria/stories/covid-19-children-suffer-violence-during-lagos-lockdown

Esidene, E. C., & Onyebuch, U. R. (2013). Economic development and mass poverty in Africa: Assessment of the Nigerian experience. *Research on Humanities and Social Sciences, 3*(1) https://www.iiste.org/Journals/index.php/RHSS/article/view/4112

Ewalt, J. A., & Jennings, E. T. (2014). The great recession and social welfare spending in the American states. *International Review of Public Administration, 19*(3), 308–323.

Farzanegan, M. R., Feizi, M., & Gholipour, H. (2020). *Globalization and outbreak of COVID-19: An empirical analysis. MAGKS Joint Discussion Paper Series*. University of Marburg.

Forster, P., Forster, L., Renfrew, C., & Forster, M. (2020). Phylogenetic network analysis of SARS-CoV-2 genomes. *Proceedings of the National Academy of Sciences, 117*(17), 9241–9243. https://doi.org/10.1073/pnas.2004999117

George, L. (2020). *How Africa risks reeling from a health crisis to a food crisis*. https://www.reuters.com/article/us-health-coronavirus-food-africa-insigh-idUSKCN2260M2

Gilaj, B., & Ballhysa, E. (2020). *The aid for isolated families: Chaos in distribution and discordance in numbers*. https://portavendore.al/2020/05/05/ndihmat-per-familjet-e-izoluara-kaos-neshperndarje-dhe-kakofoni-shifrash/

Global Polio Eradication Initiative. (2020). *Polio eradication staff support COVID-19 response*. https://www.endpolio.org/polio-eradication-staff-support-covid-19-response

Gopinath, G. (2020). *The great lockdown: Worst economic downturn since the great depression*. The International Monetary Fund. https://blogs.imf.org/2020/04/14/the-great-lockdown-worst-economic-downturn-since-the-great-depression/

Grainger, C. (2020). *A software for disease surveillance and outbreak response: Insights from implementing SORMAS in Nigeria and Ghana*. Federal Ministry for Economic Cooperation and Development. http://health.bmz.de/en/healthportal/ghpc/case-studies/software_disease_surveillance_outbreak_response/index.html

Hassan, C. (2020). *Federal government wants citizens to report diversion of palliative resources*. https://www.radionigeria.gov.ng/2020/04/16/fg-wants-citizens-to-report-diversionof-palliative-resources/

Hekurani, A., & Gjerani, E. (2020). *Coronavirus situation, insights into the elderly and families in need*. https://portavendore.al/2020/04/11/situata-e-koronavirusit-drite-hijet-e-temoshuarve-dhe-familjeve-ne-nevoje/

Huang, C., Wang, Y., Li, X., Ren, L., Zhao, J., Hu, Y., Zhang, L., Fan, G., Xu, J., Gu, X., Cheng, Z., Yu, T., Xia, J., Wei, Y., Wu, W., Xie, X., Yin, W., Li, H., Liu, M., … Cao, B. (2020). Clinical features of patients infected with 2019 novel coronavirus in Wuhan, China. *Lancet, 395*(10223), 497–506. https://www.thelancet.com/journals/lancet/article/PIIS0140-6736(20)30183-5/fulltext

Human Rights Watch. (2020). *Nigeria: Protect most vulnerable in COVID-19 response: Extended lockdown threatens livelihoods of millions*. Author. https://www.hrw.org/news/2020/04/14/nigeria-protect-most-vulnerable-covid-19-response

Ibama, A. S., & Dennis, P. (2016). Role of community health practitioners in national development: The Nigeria situation. *International Journal of Clinical Medicine, 7*(1), 511–518.

Ibeneme, S., Eni, G., Ezuma, A., & Fortwengel, G. (2017). Roads to health in developing countries: Understanding the intersection of culture and healing. *Current Therapeutic Research, 8*(6), 13–18. https://www.ncbi.nlm.nih.gov/pmc/articles/PMC5717292/pdf/main.pdf

IFSW. (2020). *Nigeria. COVID 19: Call for sober reflections and calmness*. Author. https://www.ifsw.org/nigeria-covid-19-call-for-sober-reflections-and-calmness/

International Monetary Fund. (2020). *Virus outbreak will slow global economic growth this year*. Aljazeera. https://www.aljazeera.com/ajimpact/imf-virus-outbreak-slow-global-economic-growth-year-200305013321840.html?

Ioannidis, J. P. (2020). Coronavirus disease 2019: The harms of exaggerated information and no evidence-based measures. *European Journal of Clinical Investigation, 50*(4), e13223. https://doi.org/10.1111/eci.13223

Isangha, S. O., Choi, W. M. A., & Chiu, M. Y. L. (2020). COVID-19: Where are the Nigerian social workers? *Qualitative Social Work, 20*, https://doi.org/10.1177/1473325020973336

Jaeger, F. N., Bechir, M., Harouna, M., Moto, D. D., & Utzinger, J. (2018). Challenges and opportunities for healthcare workers in a rural district of Chad. *BMC Health Services Research, 18*(7), 1–11.

Jalloh, A. (2020). *Severe hunger threatens Africa during COVID-19 lockdowns*. DW News. https://www.dw.com/en/severe-hunger-threatens-africa-during-covid-19-lockdowns/a-53212565

Johns Hopkins University. (2020). *Covid-19 poses unique challenges for people with disabilities*. Author. https://hub.jhu.edu/2020/04/23/how-covid-19-affects-people-with-disabilities/

Johnson, D. (2020, August 10). Palliatives: Over 200,000 households touched during COVID-19 in Ondo. *Vanguard*. https://www.vanguardngr.com/2020/08/palliatives-over-200000-households-touched-during-covid-19-in-ondo-akeredolu

Kalu, B. (2020). COVID-19 in Nigeria: A disease of hunger. *The Lancet Respiratory Medicine, 8*, 556.

https://www.thelancet.com/journals/lanres/article/PIIS2213-2600(20)30220-4/fulltext
Kapata, N., Ihekweazu, C., Ntoumi, F., Raji, T., Chanda-Kapata, P., Mwaba, P., & Zumla, A. (2020). Is Africa prepared for tackling the COVID-19 (SARS-CoV-2) epidemic. Lessons from past outbreaks, ongoing pan-African public health efforts, and implications for the future. *International Journal of Infectious Diseases, 93*, 233–236. https://doi.org/10.1016/j.ijid.2020.02.049
Krumkamp, R., Sarpong, N., Kreuels, B., Ehlkes, L., Loag, W., & Schwarz, N. G. (2013). Health care utilization and symptoms severity in Ghanaian children: A cross-sectional study. *PLoS One, 8*(11), e80598.
Lazarus, K. U., & Oluwole, D. A. (2020). Demographic factors, attitude and knowledge of persons with special needs towards COVID-19 in Nigeria: Implications for counselling and social policy. *Emerald Open Research, 2*, 55. https://doi.org/10.35241/emeraldopenres.13800.2
National Bureau of Statistics. (2015). *The millennium development goals performance tracking survey 2015 report*. UNDP. http://www.ng.undp.org/content/nigeria/en/home/library/mdg/NigeriaMDGsSurveyReport2015.html
Nigeria Centre for Disease Control. (2020a). *COVID-19 outbreak in Nigeria situation report*. Author. https://ncdc.gov.ng/diseases/sitreps/?cat=14&name=An%20update%20of%20COVID-19%20outbreak%20in%20Nigeria
Nigeria Centre for Disease Control. (2020b). *First case of coronavirus disease confirmed in Nigeria*. https://ncdc.gov.ng/news/227/first-case-of-corona-virus-disease-confirmed-in-nigeria
Nigeria Centre for Disease Control. (2020c). *NCDC initiates new measures for pandemic control as COVID-19 spreads to 12 states in Nigeria*. https://ncdc.gov.ng/reports/weekly
Nnama-Okechukwu, C. U., Chukwu, E. C., & Nkechukwu, C. N. (2020). COVID-19 in Nigeria: Knowledge and compliance with preventive measures. *Social Work in Public Health, 35*(7), 590–602. https://doi.org/10.1080/19371918.2020.1806985
Obansa, S. A., & Orimisan, A. (2013). Healthcare financing in Nigeria: Prospects and challenges. *Mediterranean Journal of Social Sciences, 4*(1), 221–236.
Obike, G. (2020, August 16). Battle for COVID-19 palliatives not worth the efforts. *The Nations*. https://thenationonlineng.net/battle-for-covid-19-palliatives-not-worth-the-efforts/
Okojie, J. (2020). *56% of Nigerians say palliatives not sufficient for individuals, businesses amid lockdown*. https://businessday.ng/coronavirus/article/56-of-nigerians-say-palliatives-not-sufficient-for-individuals-businesses-amid-lockdown/
Okoye, U. O. (2013). Chapter 17: Trends and challenges of social work practice in Nigeria. In V. E. Cree (Ed.), *Becoming a social worker: Global narratives* (pp. 149–157). Routledge.
Okoye, U. O. (2019). Health care social work in Nigeria. In R. Winnett, R. Furman, D. Epps, & G. Lamphear (Eds.), *Health care social work: A global perspective*. Oxford University Press.
Okwaraji, Y. B., Cousens, S., Berhanem, Y., Mulholland, K., & Edmond, K. (2012). Effect of geographical access to health facilities on child mortality in rural Ethiopia: A community based cross-sectional study. *PLoS One, 7*(3), e33564.
Olapegba, P. O., Ayandele, O., Kolawole, S. O., & Oguntayo, R., et al. (2020). *A preliminary assessment of novel coronavirus (COVID-19) knowledge and perceptions in Nigeria*. https://www.medrxiv.org/content/10.1101/2020.04.11.20061408v2
Olubiyi, T. (2020, May 12). COVID-19: The economic perspective of the pandemic in Nigeria. *Business Day*. https://businessday.ng/opinion/article/covid-19-the-economic-perspective-of-the-pandemic-in-nigeria/
Oludayo, T. (2020). *A routine activity analysis of selected rape cases during COVID-19 lockdown in Nigeria*. IntechOpen. https://www.intechopen.com/online-first/a-routine-activity-analysis-of-selected-rape-cases-during-covid-19-lockdown-in-nigeria
Olurounbi, R. (2020). Coronavirus: Nigeria's proposed COVID-19 law tears the country apart. *The Africa Report*. https://www.theafricareport.com/27969/coronavirus-nigerias-proposed-covid-19-law-tears-the-country-apart/
Omole, C. (2020). *25 prospective post-Covid-19 business trends and opportunities for Nigerians*. Financial Development and Finance. http://www.financialnigeria.com/25-prospective-post-covid-19-business-trends-and-opportunities-for-nigerians-blog-539.html
Omorogiuwa, T. B. (2020). COVID-19 and older adults in Africa: Social worker's utilization of mass media in enforcing policy change. *International Social Work, 63*, 646–650. https://doi.org/10.1177/10020872820941748
Onalu, C. E., Chukwu, N. E., & Okoye, U. O. (2020). COVID-19 response and social work education in Nigeria: Matters arising. *Social Work Education*. https://doi.org/10.1080/19371918.2020.1806985
Onyeji, E. (2020, December 18). COVID-19: How innovation in health technology can help Nigeria. *Premium Times*. https://www.premiumtimesng.com/features-and-interviews/430322-covid-19-how-innovations-in-health-technology-can-help-nigeria.html
Onyemelukwe, C. (2020). *COVID-19 misinformation and the law in Nigeria*. Bill of Health. https://blog.petrieflom.law.harvard.edu/2020/08/19/misinformation-disinformation-covid19-nigeria-law/
Organisation of Economic Co-operation and Development. (2020). *OECD Policy responses to coronavirus (COVID-19): Evaluating the initial impact of COVID-19 containment measures on economic activity*. Author.
Oyekale, A. S. (2017). Assessment of primary health care facilities' service readiness in Nigeria. *BMC Health Services Research, 17*(2), 1–12. https://bmchealthservres.biomedcentral.com/track/pdf/10.1186/s12913-017-2112-8
Ozili, P. R. (2020). COVID-19 pandemic and economic crisis: The Nigerian experience and structural causes.

SSRN Electronic Journal. https://doi.org/10.2139/ssrn.3567419

Ozili, P. K., & Arun, T. G. (2020). Spillover of COVID-19: Impact on the global economy. In *MPRA Paper 99317*. University Library of Munich. https://ideas.repec.org/p/pra/mprapa/99317.html

Pengli, C. (2020). *Social work of Chongqing University of Science and Technology volunteered to fight against the epidemic in various forms*. The International Association of Schools of Social Work. https://www.iassw-aiets.org/covid-19/4905-faculties-and-undergraduates-of-social-work-of-chongqing-university-of-science-and-technology-volunteered-to-fight-against-the-epidemic-in-various-forms/

Plan International Nigeria. (2020). *Policy brief COVID-19: The need for an inclusive approach*. Author. https://plan-international.org/publications/covid-19-need-inclusive-approach-nigeria

Rasool, S. (2020). *Social workers are an untapped resource to address the psychosocial effects of Covid-19*. https://mg.co.za/article/2020-04-13-social-workers-are-an-untapped-resource-to-address-the-psychosocial-effects-of-covid-19/

Reuben, R. C., Danladi, M. A., Saleh, D. A., & Ejembi, P. E. (2020). Knowledge, attitude and practices towards COVID-19: An epidemiological survey in north central Nigeria. *Journal of Community Health, 46*, 457–470. https://doi.org/10.1007/s10900-020-00881-1

Roberton, T., Carter, E. D., Chou, V. B., Stegmuller, A. R., Jackson, B. D., Tam, Y., & Sawadogo-Lewis, T. (2020). Early estimates of the indirect effects of the COVID-19 pandemic on maternal and child mortality in low-income and middle-income countries: a modelling study. *The Lancet Global Health, 8*, e901. https://doi.org/10.1016/S2214-109X(20)30229-1

Scarnera, A. (2020). *Coronavirus pandemic and social work in hospital: An Italian experience*. The International Association of Schools of Social Work. https://www.iassw-aiets.org/covid-19/5007-coronavirus-pandemic-and-social-work-in-hospital-an-italian-experience/

Sinoruka, F. (2020). *Roma and Egyptian Women in Albania facing a double burden to access health services*. https://www.reporter.al/grate-rome-dhe-egjiptiane-ne-shqiperine veshtiresi-te-dyfishte-per-te-aksesuar-sherbimetmjekesore/?

Socio-Economic Rights and Accountability Project [SERAP]. (2020). *SERAP asks FG, CBN to provide spending details on COVID-19 relief funds, school feeding*. Author. http://serap-nigeria.org/serap-asks-fg-cbn-to-provide-spending-details-on-covid-19-relief-funds-school-feeding.ngo/

Sumner, A., Hoy, C., & Ortiz-Juarez, E. (2020). *Estimates of the impact of COVID-19 on global poverty*. WIDER Working Paper 2020/43.

Thomas, N. (2020). *COVID-19 has disproportionately impacted those living with developmental disabilities*. CNN Health. https://edition.cnn.com/2020/08/28/health/covid-19-intellectual-development-disabilities-impact-wellness/index.html

Titus, O. B., Adebisola, O. A., & Adeniji, A. O. (2015). Health-care access and utilization among rural households in Nigeria. *Journal of Development and Agricultural Economics, 7*(5), 195-203.

Ukeh, O. (2020, April 17). Covid-19 lockdown: Between hunger and reason. *The Sun*. https://www.sunnewsonline.com/covid-19-lockdown-between-hunger-and-reason/

Umokoro, E. (2020). Amidst COVID-19 lockdown, Nigeria sees increased sexual and Gender Violence. *Premium Times*. https://pulitzercenter.org/stories/amidst-covid-19-lockdown-nigeria-sees-increased-sexual-and-gender-violence

Unah, L. (2020). *Nigeria will deal with this: High alert after coronavirus case*. https://www.aljazeera.com/news/2020/03/deal-high-alert-coronavirus-case-200301140838356.html

United Nations. (2020). *UN working to avert dual crises as COVID-19 hits hunger hotspots*. UN. https://www.un.org/en/un-coronavirus-communications-team/un-working-avert-dual crises-covid-19-hits-hunger-hotspots

Uzochukwu, B., Onwujekwe, E., Mbachu, C., Okeke, C., Molyneux, S., & Gilson, L. (2018). Accountability mechanisms for implementing a health financing option: the case of the basic healthcare provision fund (BHCPF) in Nigeria. *International Journal for Equity in Health, 17*(1), 1–16.

World Bank. (2020). *Haiti overview*. Author. https://www.worldbank.org/en/country/haiti/overview

World Health Organization. (2016). *World health statistics 2016: Monitoring health for the SDGs*. Author. http://www.who.int/gho/publications/worldhealthstatistics/2016/en/

World Health Organization. (2020a). *Pneumonia of unknown cause – China*. Author.

World Health Organization. (2020b). *WHO ramps up preparedness for novel coronavirus in the African region*. Regional Office for Africa. https://www.afro.who.int/news/who-ramps-preparedness-novel-coronavirus-african-region

World Health Organization. (2020c). *Nigeria's polio infrastructure bolster COVID-19 response*. WHO Regional Office for Africa. https://www.afro.who.int/news/nigerias-polio-infrastructure-bolster-covid-19-response

Yang, Y., Zhang, H., & Chen, X. (2020). Coronavirus pandemic and tourism: Dynamic stochastic general equilibrium modeling of infectious disease outbreak. *Annals of Tourism Research*. https://www.ncbi.nlm.nih.gov/pmc/articles/PMC7147856/

25 COVID-19 Pandemic and the Urban Poor: The Relevancy of Uganda's Social Protection Measures

Deborah Atwine and John A. Mushomi

25.1 Introduction

Pandemics are not new to sub-Saharan Africa. sub-Saharan Africa has faced pandemics before, among which is the deadly Ebola virus. The COVID-19 pandemic appeared after the Ebola virus crisis had just ended in Sub-Saharan Africa. Uganda is one of the countries that has experienced the Ebola crisis. Given this past experience with crisis, one wonders if sub-Saharan countries have drawn lessons from past pandemics to build capacity for the future crisis. Social protection programmes have always been used worldwide to achieve various objectives such as fighting poverty and hunger and increasing resilience to socioeconomic risks for vulnerable and poor populations (Abdoul-Azize & El Gamil, 2020). However, the role of social protection as a response to pandemics is still a grey area in developing countries. Although there are social protection programmes to address poverty and vulnerability, their relevancy to respond to pandemics such as COVID-19 is debatable.

The rapid spread of the COVID-19 pandemic necessitated that different measures be provided by the different countries to control the spread of the virus. These measures, implemented without taking into consideration the varying social and economic conditions of the groups of people, included strict lockdowns, curfews, quarantines, reduced working hours, and the closure of some businesses. These stringent lockdown measures affected the economic activities of many countries and increased the risks and vulnerability of people living in poverty, especially the urban poor. As a result, individuals and households that survived from hand to mouth experienced serious economic shocks that further jeopardised their livelihoods (Wilkinson, 2020). Previous studies reveal that the urban poor, who are mainly employed in the informal economy, have been hit hard economically by the COVID-19 pandemic compared to those in formal employment (Durizzo et al., 2020; Abdoul-Azize & El Gamil, 2020).

The world over, different countries responded to the pandemic by implementing social protection measures to cushion the poor and vulnerable individuals and families (Gerard et al., 2020). Social protection measures had been adopted by countries before the COVID-19 pandemic as poverty reduction strategies among vulnerable groups of people. The increased focus on social protection as a poverty reduction strategy in developing countries

D. Atwine (✉)
Faculty of Arts and Social Science, Kyambogo University, Kampala, Uganda
e-mail: koruyenje@gmail.com

J. A. Mushomi
College of Business and Management Sciences, Makerere University, Kampala, Uganda

M. C. S. Gonçalves et al. (eds.), *The Coronavirus Crisis and Challenges to Social Development*,
https://doi.org/10.1007/978-3-030-84678-7_25

emerged as a response to the global economic crisis in the late 1990s and early 2000s that largely affected the vulnerable population (Ratuva, 2019). Devereux (2016) argues that one of the functions of social protection programmes is to manage or reduce vulnerability. He emphasises that such programmes can only be effective if principles of social justice are incorporated during the design and delivery of social protection. Andrews et al. (2018) and Handa et al. (2018) affirm that social protection programmes improve household consumption expenditures and cover basic needs, promote opportunities for economic inclusion, and build household resilience to social to economic shocks. The success of formal social protection measures to mitigate poverty and vulnerability remains contentious. As a response to the COVID-19 pandemic, Hallegatte and Hammer (2020) recommend that government should use adaptive safety nets with existing social protection schemes that can easily reach the poor. This statement raises the question of whether existing social protection systems are comprehensive and adaptable to reach the majority, especially during a crisis such as the COVID-19 pandemic.

The government of Uganda focused on controlling the wide spread of COVID-19 at the expense of people's livelihoods. Social protection measures were put in place to target the urban poor, although these were surrounded by ambiguity as to whom was being targeted, and how beneficiaries were identified and offered what kind of relief. The need to investigate the relevance of the social protection measures adopted by the government of Uganda during COVID-19 pandemic and to suggest recommendations for future response to crises is proposed in this chapter. This chapter focuses on social protection measures implemented by the government of Uganda to assist the poor and vulnerable groups, particularly the urban poor during the COVID-19 pandemic. The lessons from the COVID-19 pandemic should provide a basis for building capacity to address future crises.

25.1.1 Concepts Used in This Chapter

25.1.1.1 Urban Poor

In line with assertions in this chapter, urban poverty is conceptualised as arising from commercialisation, social stress, and conflict with state authority, and to be associated with coordinated problems including social, economic, political, and environmental (Wratten, 1995). In the context of Uganda, the urban poor largely comprise the informally employed and unemployed: they are highly susceptible to social and economic risk such as that of COVID-19.

25.1.1.2 Social Protection

Social protection is a set of policies and programmes that aim at reducing poverty and vulnerability and improving resilience to social and economic risks such as sickness, disability, unemployment, and old age (Hagen-Zanker et al., 2017). Included are social assistance programmes such as social transfers and subsidies to poor households that are non-contributory (benefits are not tagged to having contributed) and social insurance programmes such as old age pensions, which are contributory (benefits are tagged to having contributed). Devereux and Sabates-Wheeler (2004) give a more comprehensive conceptualisation of social protection to include all public and private initiatives that provide income or consumption transfers to people living in poverty, protect the vulnerable against livelihood risks, and enhance the social status and rights of the marginalised—with the overall objective of extending economic benefits and reducing the economic or social vulnerability of poor, vulnerable, and marginalised people.

The social protection measures described in this chapter refer to all government initiatives to improve resilience of the urban poor against COVID-19 pandemic-related socioeconomic risks.

25.1.1.3 Social Security

The International Social Security Association defines social security as any program of social protection established by legislation or any mandatory arrangement providing for individuals with a degree of income security faced with contingencies of old age, survivorship, incapacity, disability, unemployment, or the rearing of children.[1] Social security refers to protective and preventive interventions that address risks leading to income loss and affect consumption (Ministry of Gender Labour and Social Development, 2015).

25.1.1.4 Social Assistance

The World Bank defines social assistance as part of the safety nets, referring to the non-contributory measures which provide regular and reliable support to the poor and vulnerable (World Bank, 2015). Social assistance has further been defined as the budget financed programs that address poverty and vulnerability (Barrientos, 2018).

25.2 Response to COVID-19 Crisis by the Government of Uganda

The government of Uganda responded to COVID-19 by implementing public health measures to contain the spread of the virus. These measures included a nation-wide lockdown, massive testing of people in quarantine and border areas, closure of the airport and all border points, contact tracing, and social distancing (Ssali, 2020; Barugahare et al., 2020). These measures had not only social and economic implications but were also responsible for violating human rights and worsening the vulnerability of the poor. Given that most of the low-income earners in urban areas live hand-to-mouth, the lockdown measures meant that people could not earn anything at all. Food shortages and starvation became apparent, and it became necessary for the government and other nongovernment actors intervene with emergency assistance.

Closing the airport denied Ugandan citizens who were living abroad from returning home. It was criticised as a violation of human rights, especially individual liberties and freedoms (Barugahare et al., 2020). The reasons for denying Ugandans who were at the epicentre of the pandemic from returning home was the assumption that the health sector in China, for example, was better than in Uganda and thus remaining abroad was safer than returning home. Another assumption was chances of spreading the virus would be high if Ugandans who were abroad were allowed to return. Closing public transport denied a chance to those without private means to go to work and access social services, further increasing their vulnerability. Although these measures were meant to protect the public from rapid infections, they should have been instituted with some level of basic public health ethics criteria and should be balanced between benefits and burdens on the population (Kass, 2001).

Public mandatory quarantine was also one of the measures instituted in response to COVID-19 pandemic. All people arriving from high-risk countries were required to be quarantined for 14 days at a cost of 100 US$ per day. This mandate was later revised in response to the public outcry about the unaffordable quarantine cost. Subsequently, relatively affordable private quarantine places and free government facilities were put in place.[2]

Physical and social distancing was another measure adopted by the government to control the spread of the pandemic. To this end, the government suspended all transport. To implement this measure, the government suspended public transport and later public transport; banned public gatherings, and required people to stay home (Barugahare et al., 2020). To leave home, one must seek permission from government authorities such as Resident District Commissioners. These restrictions were implemented without exceptions for people with health emergencies such as pregnant women, HIV/AIDS-positive people, and people with sickle cell disease. Restriction on transport limited access to social services, especially healthcare and informal social support from relatives and friends. The social isolation weakened the informal social protection from extended family, community,

[1]https://ww1.issa.int/.

[2]https://www.hrw.org/news/2020/03/19/ugandans-trying-get-home-forced-pay-covid-19-quarantine.

and neighbourhood. Inherent values of informal social protection such as sharing, solidarity, and reciprocity were threatened or ignored, moreover, among the urban poor who largely depend on informal social protection in the absence of formal social protection. With each family isolated, and struggling for its own survival, there was almost no support from informal support systems. Banning of social gatherings has enfeebled the emotional and physical support that is important during difficult times.

The lockdown measures were introduced on 18 March 2020 when Uganda had only two cases. Ugandans thus were prohibited from leaving their homes, apart from a few who were providing essential services such as food markets, health services, supermarkets, banks, pharmacies, those working with water and electricity companies, security companies, and garbage collection. All other nonessential services were closed, with devastating economic implications for the lives of the people, especially the urban poor who live hand to mouth. Most of these poor are food vendors, motorcycle riders, taxi operators, street vendors, and others who derive their livelihood by daily earning. These households had no access to formal social assistance and depended on informal social assistance, which was also overstretched during lockdown. One of the characteristics of such households is having many dependants, mostly children who are not covered by social protection. A disruption in household income causes food insecurity and increased vulnerability to chronic poverty.

Dafuleya (2020) argues that all countries were affected by the COVID-19 pandemic, but those with institutionalised social assistance coped better because they relied on domestic resources and responded faster. Uganda lacks institutionalised social assistance not only for the urban poor but for the entire population. The existing social assistance for the elderly is largely funded by donors, targets rural districts, and excludes cities and municipalities. The response from government that was in the form of food distribution to the poor was largely provided from donations and took more than a month to reach the poor.

The economic downturn caused by COVID-19 has already had an impact on formal social protection. As organisations downsize, laid-off workers struggle to survive in the absence of unemployment benefits in Uganda. Contributions towards insurance and provident funds are equally curtailed.

25.3 Social Protection During Pandemics

Poverty eradication in all its forms remains a key global agenda, and the focus of sustainable development goal (SDG) 1. Social protection has been earmarked as one of the targets to achieve SDG 1 (poverty eradication) and SDG 10 (reduced inequalities) (United Nations, 2015). As such, many countries have implemented social protection policies in a bid to reduce poverty and vulnerability. The COVID-19 pandemic has compounded the vulnerability of those without access to formal social protection and exposed the inadequacy of states' social protection systems to respond to covariate risks (Razavi et al., 2020). It is worse in low-income countries where social protection still limited. The global crises have devastating effect on poverty levels on developing countries where social protection systems are limited and weak (McCord, 2010). The crises negatively affect the already weak economies in developing countries and diminish hope for expanding social protection to the affected populations. The novel COVID-19 has destabilised people's livelihoods and poses a challenge to both high- and low-income countries. There is a need to build capacity and preparedness to respond to future crises, which requires governments to implement adaptive social protection programmes before, during, and after crises. Although some social protection measures and programmes were put in place in Uganda during the lockdown, there is anecdotal evidence about their relevancy to the actual needs of the urban poor.

The urban poor in Uganda are among the most vulnerable yet the least covered by formal social protection. The urban poor face particular challenges such as unemployment, a high crime rate, and escalating food prices (Adeyefa, 2016). They are largely employed in the informal economy, or self-employed in small- and medium-scale businesses that are neither registered nor regulated by the government. There are limited income data and administrative information about them, and this reduces the chances of being enrolled in formal social protection programmes (Akinboade & Adeyefa, 2018). The deserving poor end up missing social protection grants, which further increases their vulnerability.

Crises present enomous challenges to social protection because they require quick mobilisation of resources which must be implemented in a timely manner to prevent negative consquences (Mateo-Perez et al., 2015; McCord, 2010). Marzo and Mori (2012) define crises as covariate shocks that can lead to catasptrophic economic and social stresses on a country's population and can arise from economic problems, natural disasters, pandemics, and conflicts.

Despite the inherent potential of crises to cause damange to social, economic, and political systems, very few countries and organisations have proper risk management plans to cope with such eventualities. Moreover, crises present in different ways and are sarrounded by much uncertainity. Marzo and Mori (2012) attribute this uncertainity to diversity of crisis in terms of origin, channels of transimission, and impacts. Faulkner (2001) posits that current crisis management methods are insufficient to cope with increasing crises and disasters, necessitating alternative frameworks that classify shocks according to severity, probability, type of event, and level of uncertainty and developing tools for each of these shocks.

Conventional social protection methods such as social assistance, social insurance and informal risk sharing meachanisms may be inadequate to avert the massive risk (Marzo & Mori, 2012). The need to prioritise instituting emergency assistance to crises is paramount today than ever before because crises affecting livelihoods seem to be on the increase with globalisation. Globalisation that leads to interdependency between countries and communities, fuels the crises because when one country is affected, the rest are equally affected (Marzo & Mori, 2012).

The World Bank resolution to expand social protection as a response to the global economic crisis of 2008–2009 speaks volumes about the importance of social protection as a response to crises. In June 2012, during the International Labour Organisation (ILO) conference, the global community consented to national social protection floors. Social protection floors require that states should provide a basic form of social protection that guarantees income security sufficient to live, through pensions, in cash or in kind, to vulnerable groups such as the elderly, persons with disabilities, the unemployed or employed poor; and ensure access to essential goods and services such as health services, primary education, housing, water, and sanitation (Bachelet & Office, 2012). Social protection floors were envisaged to prevent poverty and vulnerability by responding to social and economic shocks. Different states have since implemented different social protection policies and programmes depending on their financial capacity and commitment to their pledge.

Despite the pledge to adhere to social protection floors, the coverage of social protection in sub-Saharan Africa in still miserably low and is inadequate not only during crises but also in the absence of covariate risks. The case in Africa is not different from Bangladesh, where 50% of the population's vulnerability is induced by poverty rather than by risk (Azam & Imai, 2012). The COVID-19 crisis is a test to states' commitment to these social protection floors. States with more comprehensive social protection may cope better during a crisis than those with limited social protection. Mateo-Perez et al. (2015) revealed that communities with better social services show lower levels of poverty and social exclusion both during and after a crisis. This finding implies that, although crises overburden the existing social protection systems, an existing comprehensive social protection provides a favourable ground for a crisis response. The COVID-19 pandemic is therefore an eye-opener to building capacity and preparedness to guarantee minimum income security and basic services during a crisis. The situation further points to the need for countries to mainstream social protection in disaster preparedness policies and programmes.

McCord (2010) argues that social protection responses to crises that have been implemented have been limited to ad hoc regressive interventions such as generalised food subsidies rather than pro-poor interventions. De Vogli (2014) and McCord (2010) argue that responses to crises tend to focus on economic stimulation and austerity programmes rather than on the actual cause of a crisis, further exacerbating inequities. De Vogli (2014) recommends that governments and international institutions should abandon the neoliberal ideology prioritising global markets and the Gross Domestic Product (GDP) and focus on fair and just means to human and health improvement. A social justice paradigm is advocated in this context to promote equality and reduced vulnerability.

25.4 Social Protection Policies and Programmes in Uganda

Social protection in Uganda, as in many developing countries, is perceived as a catalyst for enabling beneficiaries to live secure and dignified lives by directly reducing poverty and vulnerability. Uganda has made reasonable improvement in expanding social protection programmes to the poor and vulnerable population. Among other poverty reduction programmes, social protection policies and programmes have been used to prevent individuals and households from sliding into poverty and to improve the resilience to risks of the poor and vulnerable groups of people.

Social protection is well stipulated in the Constitution of the Republic of Uganda under the laws that address risks and vulnerabilities. It is also consistent with other national policies and planning frameworks. The government of Uganda pledges the responsibility to guarantee social protection to the population and social assistance to vulnerable groups of people by age, social class, location, disability, disaster, or unemployment to promote equity (Ministry of Gender Labour & Social Development, 2015). The Constitution of the Republic of Uganda under the national objectives (objective XIVb) stipulates that all Ugandans shall enjoy rights and opportunities and access to social services such as education, healthcare, clean and safe water, shelter, and decent work, adequate clothing, food security, and pension and retirement benefits. However, in reality, only a very small segment of the population has access to social protection despite the majority being vulnerable to poverty. For example, the coverage of formal social protection in Uganda stands at about 5.7% of the entire total population.[3] Formal social protection focuses on the formally employed and leaves more than 90% of the informally employed and unemployed Ugandans without any formal social protection. The urban poor largely comprise the informally employed and unemployed, and they are highly susceptible to social and economic risk such as COVID-19. There is neither social assistance nor any emergency policy in place specifically targeting the urban poor.

According to Uganda's national social protection policy, social protection comprises two pillars: social security as well as social care and support services (Ministry of Gender Labour & Social Development, 2015). Social security is composed of social assistance in the form of direct income support that is non-contributory and social insurance that is contributory. On the other hand, social care and support services are services meant to provide care, support, protection, and empowerment to the vulnerable who are unable to care for themselves. The purpose of social assistance is to provide regular and predictable cash and in kind transfers as a relief from deprivation to the vulnerable individuals and households. Although the majority of Ugandans is vulnerable to poverty, there is hardly any formal social assistance apart from the Social Assistance Grant for Empowerment (SAGE) programme. The SAGE programme was introduced in 2010 and was meant to provide direct income support to the elderly who are 65 years and older, and vulnera-

[3]Uganda National Population Council annual performance report, 2019; http://npcsec.go.ug/wp-content/uploads/2013/06/2019-SUPRE.pdf.

ble households.[4] Despite progress made by the SAGE programme, it still excludes many elderly because of the recent government decision to extend age eligibility from 65 to 80 years.

Formal social protection in Uganda focuses on the formally employed. Uganda's social protection policy has been criticised for being largely westernised by donor influence, western-oriented curricula, and poorly conceived policies and theories (Bukuluki & Mubiru, 2014). As such, it is dominated by contributory social protection and less social assistance. Formal social protection in Uganda includes Public Service Pension Scheme for government employees (PSPS); the National Social Security Fund (NSSF) for employees in the private sector and parliamentary pension scheme. The overall goal is to safeguard workers and guarantee decent livin upon retirement, but not to the urban poor who are largely informal sector workers.

Uganda implements other social protection initiatives embedded in government programmes such as orphans and vulnerable children programmes, community rehabilitation programme for persons with disability, school feeding programme, and livelihood investment support for youth and other adults, among others. However, these initiatives are limited in scope and coverage, are ad hoc, and are not provided under an integrated and unified policy framework.

Given the foregoing, there is need to strengthen social assistance if poverty and vulnerability are to be tackled while leaving no one behind (UNDP, 2019). Uganda spent only 0.48% of its GDP on social assistance in 2012, translating into US$ 8.53 per person per year (UNDP, 2019). This is inadequate to have meaningful impact on the poor and partly explains the continued existence of poverty and inequalities in Uganda. Dafuleya (2020) argues that the fact that social assistance in most African countries cannot be enforceable, as a legal right for all the vulnerable, and that there are no clear and transparent national wealth redistribution channels, means that social assistance is devoid of a rights perspective. In Uganda, dispensing social protection is not mainstreamed in government plans and policies. It continues to be implemented depending on availability of resources and implemented on an ad hoc basis.

[4]Vulnerable households were later scraped off because of lack of clear data about household income.

25.5 Non-state Social Protection

Formal social protection in Uganda is limited, and the majority rely on non-state social protection mechanisms. Non-state social protection is in two categories, namely, formal social protection and informal social protection. The former is provided by nongovernment organisations, formally registered and regulated by government and operating with clear policies and guidelines. The latter is based on extended family and kinship, community, and neighbourhood arrangements deeply rooted in cultural norms and values, and based on principles of compassion, equality, human respect, dignity, solidarity, and reciprocity (Ruparanganda et al., 2017; Kaseke, 2013; Mpedi & Darimont, 2007). These mechanisms have evolved with time, and communities have come up with their own measures and resources to safeguard themselves against livelihood risks. Common among these are mutual aid groups such as burial associations, rotating savings, and credit associations. They are based on balanced reciprocity (direct exchange) and formed with the purpose of enhancing the economic and psychosocial welfare of members.

The activities of informal social arrangements are neither registered nor regulated by government but are characterised by complex and well-developed cultural institutional arrangements that guide their operations (Calder et al., 2014). It is on the basis of these values and norms that social and economic risks are shared in the community. The concept of ubuntu, which is considered a pan-African philosophy, puts collective needs above individual needs and requires every member to be responsible not only for their own needs but also the needs of others (Twikirize & Spitzer, 2019). Informal social assistance is important in times of adversity, such as food insecurity, sickness, death, old age, and unemployment. Assistance can be in form of small handouts such as sharing foodstuffs as well as large ones such as sharing harvests with the needy (Dafuleya, 2020).

The efficiency of informal social assistance has declined because of social economic changes brought about by globalisation, urbanisation, HIV/AIDS, natural calamities, and pandemics (Oduro, 2010). These external factors have rendered informal social assistance incapable of handling covariate risks such as COVID-19 because all members are exposed to the same risk at the same time and none is in a position to help the other. Although relatively well-off households may cope better, they may lack capacity to help needy households as they focus on their own survival. Stavropoulou et al. (2017) affirms that informal social assistance produces unequal power relationships and are incapable of handling covariate risks, have difficulty in handling change, and place an disproportionate burden on women.

Nongovernmental organizations (NGOs) have been operating in Uganda for decades. They have increased in operation since 1986 because of an enabling political environment and willingness by the government to incorporate them in a national strategic plan (Makara, 2003). By 2010, there were more than 7000 registered NGOs in Uganda and operating both at national and international level. NGOs have had a fundamental role in provision of social services such as health, education, water and sanitation, relief services in case of disasters, micro-credit services, and general poverty alleviation. Despite their increased presence and their noble role, there is no policy that complements them and enables their operations; rather, they work under inhibiting and stifling government control (Asingwire et al., 2014). They are uncoordinated, and each operates independently of the other. As such, their assistance is fragmented, ad hoc and uncoordinated, and their impact is hardly felt. A study by Asingwire et al. (2014) in Uganda revealed that much as non-state actors in social protection address members' vulnerabilities, almost half (47%) of the beneficiaries reported not having their pressing needs met.

The previous discussion recap is that existing non-state social assistance schemes are helpful and relied upon by many in Uganda. Capacity to respond to social protection during a pandemic such as COVID-19 still remains a challenge for Uganda and is perhaps a similar scenario in many African countries. There is no policy to coordinate them; their operations are scattered, and they work independently of each other. There is a need for an integrated emergency action plan that coordinates all stakeholders for improved service delivery.

25.6 Uganda's Emergency Assistance During COVID-19

Uganda's social protection is still limited to a few, and there is no existing social assistance for the urban poor. Thus, assistance was ad hoc, without clear financing policy and operations procedures. The government relied heavily on loans and local donations from nongovernment organisations. The government responded to the COVID-19 pandemic with public health measures and social protection measures, albeit in selected areas in the country. The limitation to the social protection approach was a focus on the city while leaving behind small towns where most of Uganda's poor populations reside. Social protection measures included food relief for the urban poor, suspending disconnections for utilities during lockdown, suspending recovery and selling mortgaged property during lockdown, suspending closing down businesses for nonpayment of taxes and eviction of tenants for nonpayment of dues (Ssali, 2020). However, the relevance of these measures to effectively address the needs of the urban poor is worth discussing. Understanding the relevance of these measure is key to developing the capacity for future crises and pandemics.

25.6.1 Food Relief

The government took up the responsibility to distribute donations to poor households. Donations from state and non-state actors were given to the urban poor in the form of food and other relief items including mattresses, blankets, water containers, and soap. However, the process of distribution excluded most of the potential beneficiaries. The government allocated a supplementary budget of approximately US$ 250 million and, of this amount, about US$ 80 million was allocated to relief response to COVID-19 (Anguyo, 2020). The move for government to be the sole distributor of relief items excluded other non-state actors that would have filled the gap for social assistance during the crisis. Other towns and municipalities across Uganda were never considered for government food relief, which also raised concerns about the selection criteria. A study on the implications of the coronavirus disease (COVID-19) pandemic on household income and food security in two East African countries, Kenya and Uganda, using online survey data from 442 respondents found that the proportion of food-insecure respondents increased by 44% in Uganda. National social security schemes were less likely to mitigate respondents' income shock during the COVID-19 period. It is recommended that future government responses should focus on structural changes in social security by developing responsive packages to cushion members pushed into poverty by such pandemics, while building strong financial institutions to support the recovery of businesses in the medium term and ensuring the resilience of food supply chains (Kansiime et al., 2020).

With no clear records about incomes of people in urban areas, delivering social assistance relied on information provided by local council leaders, who decided who should get assistance based on their personal judgment. The assumption was that local council leaders would be fair enough and distribute food according to need. This assumption implied that the emergency response negated the social justice approach as it was based on whether one had acquaintance with the relief providers.

25.6.2 Suspending Disconnections of Utility Bills and Eviction of Tenants

This measure was also a social assistance measure implemented during lockdown.[5] As part of the interventions to promote hand-washing, the president of Uganda gave a directive, at the height of the COVID-19 outbreak, to the water body (National Water and Sewerage Corporation) not to carry out any water disconnections during lockdown to avoid failure to practice hand-washing that could ensue as a result of limited water supply (Ainamani et al., 2020). Suspending disconnections of utility bills without a waiver on service fee and value-added tax increased the debt for the urban poor. The government, which is the main provider of essential services such as water and electricity, neither waived off nor reduced taxes on utility bills. These charges were instead carried forward and have now accumulated to nonredeemable levels. Although this directive was in good faith, water users would still need to clear their water bills at an appropriate time when they get money. Further, the presidential directive not to evict tenants during lockdown without giving an alternative to landlords assumed that landlords have other sources of livelihood apart from their houses.

25.7 Conclusion

Shocks or crises can exacerbate inequalities, and so can policy responses to mitigate the impact of these crises or shocks. The responses to the COVID-19 crisis could be a setback to various equalities, including gender and income (Ragasa & Lambrecht, 2020).

The response to the most vulnerable in Uganda left much to be desired. There was need for a flexible and adaptable plan to assist the urban poor. The government response should have been made available at national, sub-national, and community levels.

This lack points to a need for distinguishing social assistance from emergency assistance at all levels. The former is largely based on rights and freedoms that are espoused in Uganda's Constitution.

Response to the COVID-19 crisis in Uganda was not based on any existing guiding policy on response to emergencies. It was a convenience-based approach with limited or no information on

[5] The independent newspaper, https://www.independent.co.ug/govt-halts-land-evictions-during-covid-19-lockdown/.

the grassroots. Focusing on Kampala, Uganda's capital city, and ignoring other towns was done with no justification, hence negating the social justice principle in social protection. As of this date, vulnerability statistics relevant to social protection will be required for reliable information to guide social protection. There is a need to establish a specific database to guide social protection for the most vulnerable for now and in case of future emergencies. This goal could be achieved through strengthening community surveillance to maintain social protection during emergencies.

The neoliberal economy approach applied by the government of Uganda in response to the COVID-19 crisis, without safety nets covering the urban poor, might not suffice in response to crises and safeguards for the most vulnerable in society.

The provision of food relief was an attempt to respond to the needs of the vulnerable, especially in the city and other surrounding areas. However, its inadequacy revealed gaps in the country's disaster relief response in a context of poverty, which highlights the need for social safety nets for the most vulnerable in society, even in a liberalised society.

References

A. U. UNDP. (2019). *The state of social assistance in Africa*. Author. https://www.africa.undp.org/

Abdoul-Azize, H. T., & El Gamil, R. (2020). Social protection as a key tool in crisis management: Learnt lessons from the COVID-19 pandemic. *Global Social Welfare*, 1–10.

Adeyefa, S. A. (2016). Determinants of food insecurity among the urban poor in the city of Tshwane, South Africa. *Journal of Economics, 4*(2), 101–114.

Ainamani, H. E., Gumisiriza, N., & Rukundo, G. Z. (2020). Mental health problems related to COVID-19: A call for psychosocial interventions in Uganda. *Psychological Trauma Theory Research Practice and Policy, 12*(7), 809.

Akinboade, O. A., & Adeyefa, S. A. (2018). An analysis of variance of food security by its main determinants among the urban poor in the city of Tshwane, South Africa. *Social Indicators Research, 137*(1), 61–82.

Andrews, C., Hsiao, A., & Ralston, L. (2018). Social safety nets promote poverty reduction, increase resilience, and expand opportunities. In K. Beegle (Ed.), *Realising the full potential of social safety nets in Africa*. World Bank. https://doi.org/10.1596/978-1-4648-1164-7_ch2

Anguyo, I. (2020). *The politics of food relief in Uganda's COVID-19 era. Africa at LSE.* London School of Economics and Political Science. https://blogs.lse.ac.uk/africaatlse/2020

Asingwire, N., Muhangi, D., Namara, R. B., & Kemigisa, M. (2014). Governance, performance and sustainability of non-state social protection services in Uganda. In *Advancing research excellence for governance and public policy in Africa*. PASGR. http://www.pasgr.org/wp-content/uploads/2016/10/

Azam, M. S., & Imai, K. S. (2012). Measuring households' vulnerability to idiosyncratic and covariate shocks – The case of Bangladesh. In *Research Institute for Economics and Business Administration, Kobe University, Japan (Discussion Paper Series)*. https://www.rieb.kobe-u.ac.jp/academic/ra/dp/English/DP2012-02.pdf

Bachelet, M., & Office, I. L. (2012). *Social protection floor for a fair and inclusive globalization*. International Labour Office.

Barrientos, A. (2018). The informational basis of emerging social assistance in low and middle-income countries. In A. Barrientos (Ed.), *The informational basis of emerging social assistance in low- and middle-income countries. GDI Working Paper 23.*

Barugahare, J., Nakwagala, F. N., Sabakaki, E. M., Ochieng, J., & Sewankambo, N. K. (2020). Ethical and human rights considerations in public health in low and middle-income countries: An assessment using the case of Uganda's responses to COVID-19 pandemic. *BMC Medical Ethics, 21*(1), 1–12.

Bukuluki, P., & Mubiru, J. (2014). *The status of social security systems in Uganda* (1st ed.). Konrad-Adenauer-Stiftung. https://www.kas.de/

Calder, R., Tanhchareun, T., & Crescent, J. M. (2014). *Informal social protection: Social relations and cash transfers*. Commonwealth of Australia. https://www.dfat.gov.au/

Dafuleya, G. (2020). Social and emergency assistance ex-ante and during COVID-19 in the SADC region. *The International Journal of Community and Social Development, 2*(2), 251–268.

De Vogli, R. (2014). The financial crisis, health and health inequities in Europe: The need for regulations, redistribution and social protection. *International Journal for Equity in Health, 13*(1), 1–7.

Devereux, S. (2016). Social protection for enhanced food security in sub-Saharan Africa. *Food Policy, 60*, 52. https://doi.org/10.1016/j.foodpol.2015.03.009

Devereux, S., & Sabates-Wheeler, R. (2004). *Transformative social protection*. IDS.

Durizzo, K., Asiedu, E., Van der Merwe, A., Van Niekerk, A., & Günther, I. (2020). Managing the COVID-19 pandemic in poor urban neighborhoods: The case of Accra and Johannesburg. *World Development, 137*, 105175.

Faulkner, B. (2001). Towards a framework for tourism disaster management. *Tourism Management, 22*(2), 135–147.

Gerard, F., Imbert, C., & Orkin, K. (2020). *Policy brief: Social protection response to the COVID-19 crisis: Options for developing countries*. ECONFIP.

Hagen-Zanker, J., Mosler Vidal, E., & Sturge, G. (2017). *Social protection, migration and the 2030 Agenda for Sustainable Development*. ODI.

Hallegatte, S., & Hammer, S. (2020). *Thinking ahead: For a sustainable recovery from COVID-19*. World Bank. https://Blogs.Worldbank.Org/Climatechange/Thinking-Aheadsustainable-Recovery-COVID-19-Coronavirus

Handa, S., Daidone, S., Peterman, A., Davis, B., Pereira, A., Palermo, T., & Yablonski, J. (2018). Myth-busting? Confronting six common perceptions about unconditional cash transfers as a poverty reduction strategy in Africa. *The World Bank Research Observer, 33*(2), 259–298.

Kansiime, M. K., Tambo, J. A., Mugambi, I., Bundi, M., Kara, A., & Owuor, C. (2020). COVID-19 implications on household income and food security in Kenya and Uganda: Findings from a rapid assessment. *World Development, 137*, 105199.

Kaseke, E. (2013). *Informal social security in Southern Africa*. A paper prepared for the SASPEN and FES International Conference on Social Protection for those working informally.

Kass, N. E. (2001). An ethics framework for public health. *American Journal of Public Health, 91*(11), 1776–1782.

Makara, S. (2003). *NGOs in Uganda: Their typologies, roles and functions in governance*. Centre for Basic Research Kampala. http://www.Ids.Ac.Uk/Ids/Civsoc/Final/Uganda/Uga6.Doc

Marzo, F., & Mori, H. (2012). *Crisis response in social protection*. World Bank. https://openknowledge.worldbank.org/

Mateo-Perez, M.-A., Martinez-Roman, M.-A., & Domenech-Lopez, Y. (2015). Social services in times of economic and social crisis: The case of Spain. *Revista de Cercetare Si Interventie Sociala, 50*, 96.

McCord, A. (2010). The impact of the global financial crisis on social protection in developing countries. *International Social Security Review, 63*(2), 31–45.

Ministry of Gender Labour and Social Development. (2015). *The Uganda national social protection policy*. http://socialprotection.go.ug/national-social-protection-policy-3/

Mpedi, L. G., & Darimont, B. A. (2007). The dualist approach to social security in developing countries: Perspectives from China and South Africa. *Journal of Social Development in Africa, 22*(1), 9–33.

Oduro, A. D. (2010). Formal and informal social protection in sub-Saharan Africa. In *Accelerating the world's research*. https://d1wqtxts1xzle7.cloudfront.net/

Ragasa, C., & Lambrecht, I. (2020). COVID-19 and the food system: Setback or opportunity for gender equality? *Food Security, 12*(4), 877–880.

Ratuva, S. (2019). *Back to basics: Towards integrated social protection for vulnerable groups in Vanuatu*. *Crawford School of Public Policy*. The Australian National University. https://openresearch-repository.anu.edu.au/

Ruparanganda, L., Ruparanganda, B., & Mupfanochiya, A. T. (2017). Traditional social security systems in the face of urbanization: Lessons from a rural community in Buhera District of Zimbabwe. *International Journal of Humanities and Social Science, 7*(2), 214–220.

Razavi, S., Behrendt, C., Bierbaum, M., Orton, I., & Tessier, L. (2020). Reinvigorating the social contract and strengthening social cohesion: Social protection responses to COVID-19. *International Social Security Review, 73*(3), 55–80.

Ssali, S. N. (2020). Gender, economic precarity and Uganda Government's COVID-19 response. *African Journal of Governance & Development, 9*(1.1), 287–308.

Stavropoulou, M., Holmes, R., & Jones, N. (2017). Harnessing informal institutions to strengthen social protection for the rural poor. *Global Food Security, 12*, 73–79.

Twikirize, J. M., & Spitzer, H. (2019). *Social work practice in Africa*. Fountain Publishers.

UN. (2015). *Transforming our world: The 2030 agenda for sustainable development*. United Nations, Department of Economic and Social Affairs.

Wilkinson, A. (2020). Local response in health emergencies: Key considerations for addressing the COVID-19 pandemic in informal urban settlements. *Environment and Urbanization, 32*, 503.

World Bank. (2015). *The state of social safety nets*. Author. https://openknowledge.worldbank.org/bitstream/handle/10986/22101/9781464805431.pdf

Wratten, E. (1995). Conceptualizing urban poverty. *Environment and Urbanization, 7*(1), 11–38

26 Social Work as an Unwitting Enabler of Oppression and Disenfranchisement of the Masses: A Freirean Analysis of Social Workers' Perspectives on the Government of Zimbabwe's COVID-19 Response

Victor Chikadzi and Ajwang' Warria

26.1 Introduction

Social work is a profession that is concerned with enhancing the welfare of individuals, groups, and communities. In its early years, social work was largely concerned with and focused on the welfare of individuals. During these early years, the profession had a paternalistic orientation in which individuals were seen as being responsible for causing their own problems by their lack of moral uprightness. Thus, the profession's focus was on helping individuals to adjust to their environment by finding ways to cope with any given context or circumstances. The assumption of this early orientation of social work was that there was something wrong with the individual and no attention was given to the contextual and environmental factors that lead to social distress. However, over time, the focus of social work began to shift from individual malfunction alone on awareness of how the environment affects individuals' functioning began to proliferate.

Kurevakwesu (2017) supports the work that social workers engage in in Zimbabwe to advance developmental agendas even though the profession is not being given the dignity and worth it deserves. However, Muchanyerei (2017) criticises Zimbabwean social workers for being silent, for being absent at the periphery of social change and social justice, and questions their commitment, preparedness, and readiness to actively engage in Zimbabwe's political discourse. The migration of Zimbabwean social workers because of social, political, and economic challenges as some of the main reasons for leaving the country has been reported in several studies (Chogugudza, 2018; Mangena & Warria, 2017; Willet & Hakak, 2020). This chapter considers the role of social workers in the context of COVID-19 in advancing the social change and social justice mandates of the profession. Using critical theory in social work, this chapter argues that social work practice in Zimbabwe should be (re-)awakened to support its clients facing structural injustices. First social work and its social justice mission are revisited. Next, social work, politics and the social justice nexus are interrogated. Third, Paulo Freire's work as it relates to

V. Chikadzi (✉)
Department of Social Work, University of Namibia, Windhoek, Namibia
e-mail: victorchic@gmail.com

A. Warria
Department of Social Work, University of the Witwatersrand, Johannesburg, South Africa
e-mail: Ajwang.Warria@wits.ac.za

M. C. S. Gonçalves et al. (eds.), *The Coronavirus Crisis and Challenges to Social Development*
https://doi.org/10.1007/978-3-030-84678-7_26

social work is presented. Next, the methodology is highlighted, and this is followed by the presentation and discussion of findings. Finally, an overview of the implications of findings for critical social work practice in Zimbabwe is provided.

26.2 Social Work and Its Social Justice Mission

The early focus in social work can be traced to the influence of psychology, and the shift to the focus on the environment can traced to the influence of sociology. Case work in the early years was heavily influenced by the work of Mary Richmond in the nineteenth century, when concern for solving individual problems was dominant. On the other hand, the environmental focus can be traced to Jane Addams, who was instrumental in pioneering the settlement house movement whose focus was largely on environmental fixes to human problems. To bridge this historical interest, the person-in-environment focus was born. This stage allowed social workers to holistically assess a client's situation looking at both individual and environmental factors causing psychological, social, and economic distress (Kam, 2014; Popple & Leighninger, 2008; Segal et al., 2007).

The environmental focus that was influenced by Jane Addams led to the birth of social work's social justice mission. Thus, since the nineteenth century, social work has always had a steadfast commitment to social justice. The social justice orientation of social work has led to ceaseless efforts by social workers to focus on structural changes within society to birth a social order that is devoid of discrimination, marginalisation, and disenfranchisement of the poor, minority groups, and the vulnerable in society. This commitment to social justice has never been more relevant for social work than it is now. Inequality and poverty have become so rampant within the twentieth century that the poor, who are largely the clientele base of social work, find themselves in precarious situations and circumstances that cannot be helped through psychological fixes. Yet, it seems that social work practice that is responsive and true to the social justice mission is becoming a rarity. Increasingly, many scholars are noting with concern that social work is abandoning its social justice orientation. Factors such as professionalisation and changes within the socioeconomic and political sphere have been blamed for moving social work away from its social justice mandate (Kam, 2014; Ferguson, 2008; Olson, 2007; Solas, 2008). Casework is increasingly becoming the dominant mode of intervention despite the fact that the root causes of most problems require structural changes in the environment, which calls for a commitment to further the social justice mission of social work rather than treating symptoms of social dysfunction through individualised intervention methods (Specht & Courtney, 1994). Worryingly, Kam (2014) notes that although there has been much scholarly debate within the profession around the diminishing attention of social work's social justice mission, discussions on possible remedies have been minimal.

Social justice concerns itself with how society's goods, burdens, and opportunities are distributed (Rawls, 1971; Miller, 1976). As the world continues to gravitate towards a neoliberal consensus, the gap between the rich and poor continues to increase. Economic vulnerabilities are much more widespread, and the retreat of the welfare state in many countries is eroding social protection measures, which are the last line of defence against poverty. This hostile socioeconomic and political environment has become a breeding ground for poverty and a myriad of other social ills (Ferguson, 2008; Nikku, 2019; Conneely & Garrett, 2015): this is largely the context in which social work finds itself.

Notably, the joint statement by International Federation of Social Workers (IFSW) and International Association of Schools of Social Work (IASSW) in 2004 calls for social workers to remain true to the profession's commitment to social justice. In the joint statement, it was stated that "social workers have a responsibility to promote social justice, in relation to society generally, and in relation to the people with whom they work and social justice means challenging negative discrimination, recognising diversity, distributing resources equitably, challenging unjust policies and practices and working in solidarity" (IFSW & IASSW, 2004, pp. 2). Although the call to remain committed to social justice as part of the core mission of the profession is clear, many social workers are increasingly finding themselves working in constraining environments. These occupational settings make it nearly impossible for them to influence change at the structural level, leading to the abandonment of the social justice and social change mission, both of which have been the hallmark of the profession for decades.

O'Brien (2010) notes that in social work there is no universally agreed position on the application of social justice in practice despite the concept being a key premise upon which the profession was founded. There may be agreement about the common dimensions of social justice such as socioeconomic restructuring through policy and political reforms to ensure equitable distribution of resources and opportunities (O'Brien, 2010; Solas, 2008; Craig, 2002; Rawls, 1971; Miller, 1976), but many social work practitioners are not clear about how to operationalise this in their day-to-day practice Not much attention has been given in social work scholarship to guiding the translation of social justice principles and values into daily practice (Craig, 2002).

26.3 The Social Work, Politics, and Social Justice Nexus

Social work and politics are inseparable entities that have to be integrated (Nikku, 2019). Despite the obvious link between the social work profession and politics, social workers seem keen to avoid being seen as political (Pawar, 2019). The apolitical stance is, however, not practical and sustainable, as it would signal abandoning the social justice mission that is integral to the social work value system. At both the individual and professional level, social workers cannot escape the political nature of life itself. Thus, political neutrality has no room in professional practice. To this end, "for social workers, it is not only the case that the personal is political; the professional is political as well" (Chu, 2009, as cited by Chu et al., 2009, p. 293). Authentic social work practice cannot therefore escape or avoid the political.

Despite the professional being political for social work, many social workers find themselves trying to adopt an impossible apolitical stance (Pawar, 2019). Across the globe, social work practice contexts have been largely impacted by neoliberalism, which has led to the dearth of macro practice. The neoliberal rearrangement of social services is eroding social work's ability to influence macro-level social change, a development that is leading to the de-politicisation of the profession (Nikku, 2019; Conneely & Garrett, 2015). In such a context, it is impossible to be pro service users and pro social work without being anti status quo. Any practice that is devoid of attempts at social change while working in an oppressive system that breeds and maintains socioeconomic marginalisation, poverty, and inequality is an abnegation of the profession. It is a stance that fulfils Specht and Courtney's (1994) characterisation of social workers as unfaithful angels because of their abandoning of the social justice mission as a key premise of social work.

The joint statement from IFSW and IASSW (2004) on the definition of social work shows a conscious recognition of the political nature of the social work profession and that its goals of attaining social justice and social inclusion can only be achieved by social workers working at the macro level to effect structural change within their practice contexts. This joint statement calls for the active involvement of social work in both social and political action that promotes socio-economic development, particularly for the marginalised population groups. Across the globe, the neoliberal onslaught is eroding the ability of social workers to remain true to the social justice mission. Chu et al. (2009) note that the moral and political base of social work is being threatened, and this is equally true for developing countries because of the politicised nature of the environments within which social workers operate. The call for social work to return to its social justice mission (Nikku, 2019; Conneely & Garrett, 2015; Chu et al., 2009; Reisch, 2002; Specht & Courtney, 1994) is important. However, it is has become even more pressing for social work scholars and practitioners to grapple with finding clarity on how this can be practically translated into practice.

26.4 Freire and Social Work

Paulo Freire is arguably one of the most popular educators of the twentieth century, and his work continues to influence the world beyond the classroom, across many academic disciplines and civil society. Freire's work is very relevant for social work, now more than ever before. The insights from his body of work are useful in helping to inform how social work responds to the socioeconomic and structural challenges of our time. Although an educator and not a social worker, Freire worked with social workers during his lifetime and his ideas have enjoyed widespread acceptance in social work, particularly among social workers who subscribe to the critical and radical social work traditions. Freire enjoyed a close connection with social workers and was a guest at several social work events and conferences. Freire interacted with many social workers in their capacity as his students, associates, and friends. His ideas continue to influence social work both in social work education and in practice settings, community work practice in particular (Moch, 2009).

Carroll and Minkler (2000) note that in the last decade of his life, Freire made a deliberate effort to spread his ideas to social workers given his close connection to the profession over his lifetime. Freire realised the close connection of social workers to the grassroots, and he hoped to hone and promote in them the qualities of activism (Carroll & Minkler, 2000). Today, many social work activists are guided by his ideas in their praxis. Hegar (2012) notes that Freire should occupy a position of prominence in social work consciousness given the congruence of his educational philosophy and the principles of social work. Consistent with the social work goal of creating social change, Freire was a revolutionary who saw the structural transformation of society as the end goal (Carroll & Minkler, 2000). Freire's writings show that he loathed co-option and placatory practice, which sought to preserve rather than alter the status quo. In his work, Freire advocated for structural change that would bring about a fairer, socially just, and equitable economic order for the poor, that is, a similar mandate of social work (IFSW, 2010; NASW, 2008). Below we discuss several of Freire's ideas that we will use as the lenses through which we analyse the discourse of social workers in this chapter.

26.4.1 Critical Consciousness

One of the most popular ideas for which Freire is known is that of critical consciousness. He worked to achieve critical consciousness in his work with various groups of people in society. It is a concept and a quality that refers to the ability to authentically reflect on the issues and questions of the day and understand the root cause and complex process that sustain and maintain any given status quo. For social workers and their clientele base, critical consciousness is the in-depth comprehension of how personal, social, economic, and political factors interact and affect the way society is organised and functions. For Freire, this understanding is crucial, as he argued that we cannot correctly fix that which we do not understand. Accordingly, critical consciousness is the genesis of progressive action towards genuine and progressive change. For Freire, critical consciousness is necessary not only for the practitioner but also for the people with whom the practitioner seeks to partner in changing their situation. It is a process of birthing a new way of thinking and perceiving reality, and with this understanding people become unrestful in pursuing action to change unfavourable conditions (Freire, 1970).

26.4.2 No Room for Neutrality

Gibson (1999) notes that Freire viewed all forms of education not as neutral but as, rather, a call to action. With the rampant social ills, poverty, inequality, authoritarianism, and disenfranchisement of many people in society, it is hypocritical to claim neutrality. Gibson (1999) further argues that Freire's thinking lays bare the partisanship of those who claim to be neutral in the face of injustice. As Freire (1970, as cited in Carroll and Minkler (2000, p. 28) argues, "claiming neutrality does not constitute neutrality; quite the contrary, it helps maintain the status quo." For Freire, social workers cannot maintain neutrality in the face of dehumanisation but must act with decisiveness and choose to pursue change that leads to humanisation, failing which one assumes a position in favour of the status quo (Carroll & Minkler, 2000).

26.4.3 Praxis

In his address to social workers Freire notes that progressive social workers must be capable of demonstrating praxis in their daily work. By praxis, Freire refers to the need to harmonise thought and actions, which he saw as being bound together. Thought informs action (practice) and what we learn in the course action (daily practice) must in turn inform our thinking. In praxis, there is reciprocity between thinking and action, and each process informs the other in a continuous process of advancement and action towards liberation (Moch, 2009).

26.4.4 Critical Curiosity

Freire also argued that the social worker must nurture, develop, and grow "a permanent critical curiosity toward the world in himself, but also to do so in those with whom she or he works" (Moch, 2009, p. 95). As Moch (2009) argues, Freire was of the view that social workers ought to always question things and not accept anything passively. He notes that people in the world are increasingly conditioned towards passive pedagogy, what he termed "a pedagogy of the answer, and not a pedagogy of the question" (p. 95). The notion of the pedagogy of the question is critical in both social work education and practice. It forces social workers to remain relevant to the people they serve by avoiding the imposition of their own reality and worldview. When we avoid providing answers to what has not been asked, we not only avoid the imposition of our reality on other subjects but we are also forced to seek what their questions of the world are. This view is compatible with the social work value of beginning where the client is and allowing them the right to self-determination.

26.4.5 Social Workers Must Be Competent

Consistent with the social work ethic, which dictates that one should not practise in an area beyond one's competence, Freire argued that one cannot be a progressive social worker without being competent. He argued that efforts towards transforming the world and advocating for social change requires, and can only be achieved by, social workers who are competent. Tied to the notion of critical curiosity discussed above, Freire argued that social workers should have rigour in their work and should use scientifically valid methods in understanding how society is structured and functions. From this base, one can then work to attain social change (Moch, 2009).

26.4.6 Impatient Patience

Freire also introduces us to a very important notion of impatient patience as a key quality that all progressive social workers ought to have. Impatient patience for Freire is the quality of being able to have an end goal in mind, which one immediately gets to work achieving. However, in pursuit of the goal, a social worker who possesses the quality of impatient patience knows that 'Rome wasn't built in a day.' Accordingly, one is careful to work progressively towards the realisation of a goal in a manner that is realistic and demonstrates awareness of constraints and correctly estimates abilities and possibilities. The notion of impatient patience is contrasted to pure impatience, which denotes a state in which one seeks to achieve change 'overnight', negating all the insurmountable hurdles in the way. Such efforts inevitably lead to failure and frustration, as "pure impatience forgets that in history, one does what is possible and not what one would like to do" (Moch, 2009, p. 96).

26.4.7 Understanding of the Limits of Social Work Practice

Closely linked to the idea of impatient patience is the need to understand the limits of social work practice. Freire argues that a progressive social worker understands that not all things which are desired can be attained and that social work has its own limits in terms of what can be done. Thus, in every practice setting, progressive social workers should reflect on the limits of their practice. This awareness is critical: for Freire, those limits can be "social, ideological, cultural, political, and historical" (Moch, 2009, p. 97).

26.5 Methods

This chapter uses secondary data that were gathered from a WhatsApp platform which was set up to inform, harmonise, and coordinate social work interventions in Zimbabwe during the current COVID-19 crisis. Permission to use the data was obtained from the group administrator, and ethical clearance was given by the University of Namibia under protocol number DEC-HSS/02/04/2021. The WhatsApp platform comprises more than 200 social workers who joined the group voluntarily. Several topics are discussed daily on the group, and these professional conversations by social workers offer rich insights into the attitudes and thinking of many social workers regarding their ideological, moral, and professional positions on diverse issues pertaining to social work practice. Varied perspectives and group dynamics are apparent in this WhatsApp group. The prevailing discourse on the WhatsApp platform about the way the government is responding to the COVID-19 crisis and the role of social workers offers interesting lenses through which to understand the role of social work in the post-colonial developmental reversal in Zimbabwe.

Using thematic data analysis, purposively selected topics and texts from the dialogical exchanges among social workers are analysed according to Freirean principles. The selected texts are indicative of the beliefs and professional standpoints of different social workers on given topics, and these views are juxtaposed and critiqued against the ideas of Freire. As already discussed in the preceding sections, Freire's ideas have had a profound impact on social work. He is a role model to many social workers who seek to advance social change in society. His ideas represent a rejection of placatory and oppressive practice in social work. In this regard, the use of Freirean lenses in analysing the conversations yield rich insights on the ideological and moral position of social work and social workers within a given context. It should, however, be noted that the selected texts are not exhaustive or representative of the views of all social workers in Zimbabwe and thus cannot be generalised.

26.6 Presentation and Discussion of Findings

26.6.1 Suppression of Critical Views

One of the common daily patterns that is obvious on the WhatsApp platform is that whenever critical questions are raised that may lead to the government being criticised, the issues are hardly ever discussed in an authentic way. Responses to uncomfortable problem-posing questions are normally delivered in the form of sharp and hostile rebukes whose intent is to silence any "critical dissent dialogue" (Ledwith, 2016, p. xi). The selected parts of the following dialogue show how questions that are posed are suppressed before honest dialogue can begin. Subsequently, most people hold back, and in the long run this begins to promote a culture of silence amongst social workers whenever uncomfortable issues are raised. Yet, it is in discussing these uncomfortable questions that critical consciousness can be awakened among social work practitioners. Such consciousness is the basis for future collective action in advocating for change.

Participant 1 (P1):[1] *What has Zimbabwe independently done towards COVID-19?*

P2: The sad thing is even us black Zimbabweans don't cherish or appreciate our own success or potential.

P3: The samples do not represent a nationwide prevalence of the virus. Fears are in rural areas as well; many assume (they are not positive) but have not been tested.

P5: So far even America is still to test a representative sample.

P2: We Zimbabweans have done very well. It's a shame we don't acknowledge some of the positives that we have done as we tend to focus more on what hasn't been done. A common phenomenon amongst majority Zimbabweans. Very good at pointing at the bad and pathetic at pointing out the positives. I stand to be corrected on this one. I can write a book about some great strides that Zimbabwe has done so far which may have helped curtail the prevalence or transmission of COVID-19.

P4: The World will never cherish everything black…

P1: I am sorry I regret to say Zimbabwe has 'independently' done nothing as a nation towards COVID-19.

P4: 1. Zimbabwe sealed its borders with fewer than 10 cases.
2. We are quarantining despite the challenges.
3. We are testing slow though but better than others.
4. We are donating to beef up our own ailing healthcare system.

The foregoing exchanges were prompted by some social workers who were raising concerns over what they saw as negligent efforts from government in responding to the COVID-19 pandemic. When these concerns were raised, they were not discussed. Instead, the dialogue descends into a lambasting of those who had raised the concerns. A question on what government is independently doing apart from donor efforts is 'greeted' by a response that characterises Zimbabweans as unappreciative and negative towards their own government. When P3 raises a concern around the fact that the samples that government had taken were not representative of the national demographics and geographic segmentation, P4 responds with a false equivalence by claiming that even America has not done that. His reasoning is a defensive position that is aimed at silencing the critical voices that are raising concern about the government's COVID-19 response efforts. Bringing America into the discourse is meant to justify the failures of government that were so glaring. Thus, in the reasoning of P4 the government's poor response in failing to widely test is justifiable because America was yet to do the same. This remark negates the difference in context and constitutes an acceptance of what is bad simply because it is being done elsewhere. P4 escalates the issue and makes it a racial one despite the fact that all participants in this dialogue are black and he completely digresses from engaging with what has been asked.

In the foregoing dialogue, the social worker who asks the question is showing an inquisitive attitude and engages in what Freire termed the pedagogy of the question. In Freire's view, social workers ought to always question things and not accept anything passively. Thus, by questioning the government's response efforts, the social worker is showing a consciousness that is expected of social workers in pursuit of their social justice mission. The responses from fellow practitioners, however, are an attempt to silence the pedagogy of the question and force the social worker and other participants to adopt a culture of silence and passive pedagogy that simply accepts what is, without question (Moch, 2009)

[1] P = Participant and the numbers are used to distinguish the participants.

The attempt to silence fellow colleagues is indicative of what Freire termed horizontal violence. Social workers who are supposed to be acting in solidarity are turning against each other. What is more shocking in this case is that at the time of this dialogical exchange, nurses and doctors were being forced to work without protective clothing, government hospitals did not have oxygen ventilators, and government pharmacies had no stocks of essential medication. The frontline workers were being paid meagre salaries that were barely enough for them to afford transport, food, and accommodations because of the collapsed economy. Zimbabwe is a nation endowed with an abundance of natural resources, yet due to rampant looting, corruption, and poor governance, the health sector and other sectors of the economy are in a state of decay. There is, therefore, a clear lack of critical consciousness on the part of fellow practitioners who are taking defensive positions that force fellow practitioners to be appreciative of the lame efforts of government when there is a glaring lack of competence and accountability on the part of government. Social workers are supposed to be instruments and advocates of social change and not instruments of social control, as reflected in the thinking of the social workers who sought to silence the dialogue.

In the last part of the preselected dialogical exchange above, P4 raises the issue of donations being made as part of justifying that government is doing something. This thinking negates the fact that government has enough resources to adequately fund the healthcare sector without having to extend the begging bowl. Such donations and the other issues that P4 raises in defence of the lame efforts of the government of Zimbabwe indicate a failure to realise what the philosopher Engels called "false generosity," which are efforts that do not take people out of their misery but only sustain them while continuing to trap them in a cycle of deprivation and desperation. As this dialogue continued, the social workers who were raising questions began to hold back, and the conversation was dominated by those that were defending the unjust status quo. This clearly points to a failure to engage in reflective praxis as social workers. Assuming a compliant posture in the face of such poor governance is not reflective of social workers who are true to their social justice mission. Social workers have to challenge the oppressive structures and systems that breed vulnerability, poverty, and marginalisation and should not be found defending such injustice. To do so is to actively participate in social control and domination of the deprived masses—an injustice indeed.

26.6.2 'Political Neutrality'

In the following dialogical exchange, P6 had raised some key issues that could not be defended, but P2, who tended to quickly assume a defensive position on all matters that exposed the government's lack of responsiveness, is quick to want to silence any discussion on the matter. The responses of P2 betray the fact that deep down he knows all is not well in the manner in which the government of Zimbabwe is handling the COVID-19 pandemic response efforts, yet he is quick to want to silence any discussion that exposes the government.

P2: These may be valid issues of state expenditure and misplaced prioritisation in governance whose attempt to dissect may lead to some unnecessary and unhelpful political discussions. Which will tarnish the status and ethos of this group. So, I suggest we steer away from politics or maybe reserve that for other groups.

P6: So we are not allowed to address political issues in this group?

P2: My understanding is that purpose of this group is to discuss COVID-19-related challenges and solutions. But I will let … answer that one.

P6: We are not discussing politics, my question is asking as to the nexus between COVID-19 response and our political environment because in whatever way we avoid being political about the virus, it is political in every sense from decision making to implementation. Hence, I am seeking clarity as to the rules of the group and I am sure, the elders will assist me as to whether that is allowed in here.

P7: We have legal policy addressing some of the much debated issues, bringing out to debate what is within the policy, I think it is more professional, to avoid friction.

It is clear from the dialogue above that P2 is trying to silence P6 by insinuating that the matters he raised are political and therefore should be avoided. P2 is making a false assumption that COVID-19 matters can be discussed in a manner that is devoid of political content. P6 calls him out on this and shows P2 that it is not possible to deal with matters of service delivery without being political. P2 is pushing for a false position of political neutrality in the group, something that is not possible for social workers. This false position of political neutrality is in essence of a tacit defence of government's failure, and he actively attempts to silence any discussion that exposes the state by hiding behind the need to be politically neutral.

For Freire, there is no room for neutrality in the practice of social work. The imagined structure of what society should be and the change that social workers conceptualise in their minds and seek to achieve in practice is itself a political dream. The pursuit of social change as a goal of social work practice makes political neutrality impossible (Moch, 2009). In other words, for Freire, a social worker cannot assume a position of neutrality in practice. One is either for or against a particular status quo. In a situation of an unjust status quo, social workers have to be pro-people and anti-establishment. At any given point in practice, one is either an instrument of social change or social control, and political neutrality is therefore a myth. Silence itself assumes one is actively taking a position. Thus, as Moch (2009) notes, for Freire, social workers, just like educators, are not neutral agents in their daily practice. This thinking has far-reaching implications for how social workers ought to approach their daily practice. It is a position that is consistent with the notion that the personal and the professional are both political (Chu et al., 2009).

Social workers do not operate in a vacuum; rather, the space and practice terrain of social work is politically charged. An overwhelming majority of social workers find themselves operating in contexts where their daily practice is directly and indirectly influenced by the politics of the day through government policies and programmes dictating what can and cannot be done. Resource distribution which speaks to issues of social justice is not a politically neutral endeavour. It is the politics of the day that determines what social workers earn how the profession gets to be recognised, and the resources at their disposal to fulfil their mandate. Most social work clients have problems whose root causes can be traced to societal structures and politics (Chu et al., 2009; Reisch, 2002; Shamai & Boehm, 2001; Kingdon & Thurber, 1984). In this regard, it is not possible to pursue the social justice mission of social work without being political in the practice of social work. Chu et al. (2009) note that social work is itself a political vocation given that the practice of advocacy and push for social change as part of fulfilling the social justice mission of social work involves pushing for reforms that challenge the entrenched political interests in an effort to shift the balance of power. In this regard, there exists a clear nexus of social work and politics that is evident in the social justice mission of the profession. Similar concerns are noted by Reisch (2002), who notes that the daily practice of social work inescapably impacts the political order and processes. It is therefore impossible to be politically neutral as a social worker. Daily practice in service of clients inevitably leads to political action as social workers seek to promote the interests of their marginalised client groups. Any attempt to be politically neutral is a tacit abandonment of the profession's social justice mission, which is at the core of its value base (Chu et al., 2009; Reisch, 2002).

Lastly, Pawar (2019, p. 15) notes that "social work needs to rethink its non-political and non-religious neutral stand." He argues that social workers must be able to understand how local politics work in their sphere of practice and be able to competently engage political players in order to influence political decisions for the benefit of their clientele groups. Similar concerns around the assumed non-political stance of social work were raised by Chu et al. (2009, p. 288), who noted that "there is a risk of collective amnesia in the social work profession, resulting in a repression of its critical and political nature." To this end, the scholars argue that social work has to critically engage with the politics of the day and this by can be achieved through ensuring that personal values are aligned to professional values.

26.6.3 Horizontal Violence

In the selected dialogue extracts following, the context was that a social worker had encountered a case of a service user who needed special medication after an animal bite. All government hospitals in the country were phoned to try and find the medication, but no hospital pharmacy had such medication in its stock. Faced with a desperate life-and-death situation the social worker wrote a letter to a nongovernmental organisation (NGO) seeking funds to urgently procure the medication from a private pharmacy. The price was prohibitively expensive for the service user; at the same time there was nothing the government could do. The service user managed to get help as a result of this timely and effective intervention by the social worker. However, the letter that the social worker wrote was later leaked to the media, and journalists used the case to expose the rot in state hospitals. The dialogue below shows some of the views of social workers with regard to the letter that a fellow colleague wrote.

P8: Now I get worried when my former student drafts a letter like this, especially the stubborn truth which says "there is no medication in all government hospitals." With social media, this letter can go far and journalists may find a big story in it.

P9: It's already flooded on Twitter and activists are criticising the government left, right, and centre.

P10: Mwana wangu veduwee [It's my former student]; she is visually impaired.

P8: It happens; we learn from our mistakes.

P11: Social workers, is it our duty to expose government?

P12: She is a real hero, the government must be exposed, she was doing her job professionally…that's Social Work.

P13: For me, she should have appealed for assistance but that part saying "there is no medication in all government hospitals" should have been left out.

These dialogue excerpts are deeply shocking and worrying. One would not expect to find such thinking among social workers. The dialogue clearly shows a case of horizontal violence in which a fellow social worker who has just done a splendid job in saving the life of a service user finds herself under attack from fellow social workers for writing the truth. It was the truth that the medication that was needed by the service was not available in all state hospitals countrywide. Yet, some fellow social workers were more worried about protecting the image of the government rather than celebrating the good work of a fellow colleague and showing appreciation for a life saved. It was even more deplorable that a fellow colleague pleaded on behalf of the social worker in question by saying she is visually impaired. This remark was meant to evoke sympathy for the social worker, but P10 is rather displaying blatant ignorance and prejudice against people living with disability. Firstly, being visually impaired had nothing to do with the matter at hand. Secondly, the mention of visual impairment assumes that the letter she wrote, which was being characterised as wrong although it was right and progressive, had been because of her condition.

It is worrying that while many social workers in Zimbabwe claim to be change agents, some are conducting themselves in a manner that is contrary to the ethos of social justice. In line with the notion of praxis, Freire argues that the primary virtue of a progressive social worker is the ability to ensure congruence between what one says and what one does. Freire notes that there is usually a chasm between what is said and what it done, and it is often difficult to bridge this gap. Talking is much easier but following up with corresponding actions is hard. A failure to harmonise the two is a failure of praxis. Talking in a progressive way while acting regressively in some aspects of one life means that one is not a progressive practitioner. Thus, vices such as prejudice, horizontal violence and discrimination—all which manifest in the dialogue excerpt above have no room in progressive social work. In Freire's view, the failure to harmonise thought and action, words and practice, shows incoherence that negatively affects progressive pedagogy in social work practice and education (Moch, 2009).

An attack on a fellow practitioner who had gone out of her way to save the life of a service user in the name of protecting the name of the government does not constitute progressive social work practice; this clearly shows a lack of critical consciousness. Instead of advocating for structural changes at the government level to ensure that hospitals are adequately equipped, some practitioners find themselves on the side of the 'oppressive forces,' which in itself constitutes a defence of the status quo. This in essence is a betrayal of social work's social justice mission. Borrowing from Freire, several social work scholars have noted that a critical social worker has to be committed to conscientisation to be awake and to awaken those experiencing oppression. Critical conscientisation awakens social workers and service users to the structural factors that impact their lives negatively. A critical social worker ceases to engage in practice that defends an unjust status quo. Social workers who practice critical conscientisation become true agents of social change in that they foster in themselves and others the capacity to fight for their own emancipation (Leonard, 1993; Carroll & Minkler, 2000; Hegar, 2012) rather than actively defend injustice, as is evidenced in the dialogue above. Although the dialogue is not representative of the views of all social workers, it is worrying that many remained silent on the platform and only a few dissenting voices were evident. The foregoing dialogical exchange points to social workers as part of the problem rather than the solution.

26.6.4 Oppressive Practice

The context of the following dialogue is that a grandmother was arrested after police found 71 children at her homestead. It was reported that she was using her dilapidated dwelling place as a makeshift childcare facility. These children had their own families but would come to the grandmother's place during the day. Most children were there because she provided them with meals during the day.

P14: Reason for arrest?

P15: Running an unregistered residential childcare facility as provided in the Children's Act.

P16: Came across this heart-breaking situation yesterday and today I am reading on social media that the police have arrested this Gogo [grandmother] and her helpers. I really can't understand why. Does anyone have info on this, otherwise it sounds like a miscarriage of justice for community care model.

P17: Guys what does the law say? Childcare facilities should be registered with Department of Social Welfare.

P16: But this was not a childcare facility: this was old women with a heart to care for children and other people brought children to her. When I saw this I actually thought a developmental model would be used here help this definitely less literate women formalise her care because that was her call also for government to help her take the children from her to formalised care.

P18: Are you a qualified social worker or you are still aspiring to be one?

P19: It's illegal what she was doing. Ignorance has no place in Zimbabwe Laws!

P20: I think you really need to go through the Children's Act for Zimbabwe.

P16: We should always balance the letter of the policy and the spirit of the same law. I will not be surprised some children will see themselves back to Gogo with those impoverished circumstances she has there.

The foregoing dialogue reflects the fact that many of the social workers involved in this exchange were concerned about the welfare of the 71 children who were found at the grandmother's home, which had become a makeshift childcare facility. On the surface of it, the social workers are right to justify the arrest of the grandmother, given that taking care of 71 children under squalid conditions at a time when the risk of the spread of the COVID-19 virus was high is rather 'irresponsible.' P16 shows concern and is not in agreement that the grandmother in question should have been arrested. He agrees that something urgent needed to be done to secure the safety of the children. However, he disagrees with the arrest of the grandmother who was operating the makeshift care facility. This heated debate went on for 3 days. Fewer than five social workers disagreed with the arrest of the grandmother, while many supported the arrest and many more remained silent on the matter. When P16 insisted on defending the grandmother, his credentials as a social worker were questioned and he was asked to go and read the Children's Act.

The foregoing dialogue exposes the narrow approach to practice that social workers adopt in their daily practice. It is concerning that the focus is on the narrow interpretation of the law rather than the underlying issues. P16 shows critical consciousness in that he agrees that the children were in danger but disagrees with the arrest of the grandmother who was taking care of the children. A deeper analysis of the context of this sad story revealed that these children were in danger of hunger from the chronic poverty in the area. The grandmother in this instance is a hero of her community who is providing a necessary service without which the health and well-being of many children would have been compromised. So why arrest her? Social workers who are true to their social justice mission should be asking the deeper questions. Why are these children living in chronic poverty? If the parents of these children are willing to have their children cared for under such squalid conditions, what is the likely condition of their own homesteads? If the grandmother stops feeding these hungry children, who will feed them? Where have the police and social workers who came to close the place been all along? What prevention and early intervention initiatives were put in place? Where are the so-called formal social protection systems to cushion children and vulnerable families from hunger, especially in a country with a more than 90% unemployment rate and a broken economy? With all the exploitation of mineral wealth and other productive economic activities, why is the government failing to proactively provide adequate care for vulnerable families and children? Beyond looking at the narrow provisions of the law that criminalised the grandmother's care efforts, the foregoing are some of the questions that a social worker operating from an anti-oppressive framework ought to ask. Critically conscious social workers should have held the position of their colleague P16, which was to push for the urgent removal of these children because of the vulnerability of their circumstances while also showing gratefulness to the grandmother for her care work effort rather than support her arrest.

26.7 Implications for Critical Social Work Practice

In the select dialogue excerpts just presented, most of the professional points of view and moral positions adopted by social workers are rather worrying and paint a picture of a profession that seeks to maintain rather alter the unjust status quo. The positions held by many social workers in the foregoing dialogue demonstrate how social work has become an instrument of social control rather than social change. It shows a failure to understand the root causes of suffering, deprivation, and marginalisation. In the end, we focus on dealing with symptoms of the problem and fail to confront the deep-seated structural issues that engender the suffering of the masses.

The COVID-19 pandemic has made the social and economic vulnerabilities confronting the poor more glaring. However, for many people in developing countries, such as Zimbabwe, which is the context of this chapter, this has largely been the everyday reality for many years, with many people living at the margins of the mainstream economy. These socioeconomic challenges require a sociopolitical solution. The malfunctioning is located within the environment rather than in persons. Such a situation requires that social work respond to its social justice mission and find ways to confront the unjust socioeconomic order currently prevailing. Sadly, social work remains largely rooted in a therapeutic posture that focuses on individual psychosocial (mal)adjustments rather than on changing the environment that breeds vulnerability and social ills. Increasingly, the social justice commitment of social work is being lost (Chu et al., 2009; Margolin, 1997). The dialogue excerpts presented above show that Specht and Courtney (1994) and Muchanyerei (2017) were right in their characterisation of social workers as unfaithful angels for abandoning the profession's social justice mission. They note a concern about social workers increasingly drifting towards clinical social work and pathologising service users instead of focusing on policy reforms and structural changes that tackle the root causes of many social maladies. Similarly, social work is criticised for neglecting to focus on helping the poor, who have historically been the core concern of the profession (Figueira-McDonough, 2007). If this is the case, should social workers be given enough space to engage in work they believe in (Kurevakwesu, 2017) if in doing so they take on the position of the oppressor?

What remains clear from the dialogue excerpts presented here is that there is still much work to be done for social work in Zimbabwe to (re-) awaken critical consciousness among social workers, without which the profession will continue to be an unwitting instrument of oppression and social control in the hands of the state. Without being true to the profession's social justice mission, social work will only serve a legitimation function through what the philosopher Engels called "false generosity" (Ledwith, 2016, p. xiii), and we end up providing help that does not take people away from their misery but only barely sustains them while allowing them to remain trapped in a cycle of deprivation. Social workers should be torchbearers. We need reflective praxis as social workers, rather than assuming a compliant posture. In other words, social work must actively challenge oppressive structures and systems that breed vulnerability, poverty, and marginalisation. More importantly, there is a need for collective action and thinking within the profession. If social work is guided by a common value base and set of principles, there is no reason why social workers should be engaged in horizontal violence. As noted by Chikadzi and Pretorius (2011), when there is a leaking tap, there is a need for social workers to think not only about mopping the floor, but also ways to close the tap.

26.8 Conclusion

This chapter analysed perspectives of social workers as reflected in WhatsApp conversations. Using a Freirean lens, we found that the social workers' perspectives were varied, but mostly reflective of false generosity, placatory practice, and activism devoid of transformative praxis.

To this end, and in conclusion, social work has to remain true to its social justice mission and focus on tackling the underlying causes of suffering, deprivation, and marginalisation. Social work can be a tool for and vehicle to drive social, political, and economic agendas for development. However, for this to be possible, social workers have to go beyond treating individual symptoms and be true agents of social change through transformative praxis. Social workers have to actively work at the political and policy-making levels to influence how social work responds to the socioeconomic challenges of the day. In this regard, the reading and understanding of Freire is critical for social work practitioners who seek to engage in authentic and liberating praxis and who are true to their calling. There are many lessons to be learnt from the COVID-19 crisis. For social work practice and education in the third world context, COVID-19 is a secondary crisis that has simply unmasked the unequal global arrangements of capital that make poor people in the Global South more vulnerable to global calamities. Poverty remains the main challenge facing populations in the Global South. It is only through confronting economic marginalisation that social work will become relevant and impactful. In this regard, the works of Freire can provide social workers with practical and conceptual tools to tackle structural forces that bread inequality and socioeconomic marginalisation.

References

Carroll, J., & Minkler, M. (2000). Freire's message for social workers. *Journal of Community Practice, 8*(1), 21–36. https://doi.org/10.1300/J125v08n01_02

Chikadzi, V., & Pretorius, E. (2011). Unhelpful help: The social work profession's response to mass poverty in South Africa. *Social Work/Maatskaplike Werk, 47*(3), 225–269.

Chogugudza, C. (2018). *A critical analysis of the recruitment and experiences of overseas Zimbabwean social workers in the UK*. Unpublished PhD Thesis, Royal Holloway, University of London, London.

Chu, W. C., Tsui, M. S., & Yan, M. C. (2009). Social work as a moral and political practice. *International Social Work, 52*(3), 287–298.

Conneely, E., & Garrett, P. M. (2015). Social workers and social justice during a period of intensive neoliberalization: A preliminary investigation from the Republic of Ireland. *Journal of Progressive Human Services, 26*(2), 126–147.

Craig, G. (2002). Poverty, social work and social justice. *British Journal of Social Work, 32*(2), 669–682.

Ferguson, I. (2008). *Reclaiming social work: Challenging neo-liberalism and promoting social justice*. SAGE.

Figueira-McDonough, J. (2007). *The welfare state and social work: Pursuing social justice*. SAGE.

Freire, P. (1970). *Pedagogy of the oppressed*. Continuum.

Gibson, R. (1999). Paulo Freire and pedagogy for social justice. *Theory & Research in Social Education, 27*(2), 129–159. https://doi.org/10.1080/00933104.1999.10505876

Hegar, R. L. (2012). Paulo Freire: Neglected mentor for social work. *Journal of Progressive Human Services, 23*(2), 159–177.

IFSW. (2010). *Global agenda on social work and social development*. Author. http://www.ifsw.org/cm_data/110301_GlobalAgenda_en.pdf

IFSW & IASSW. (2004). *Ethics in social work: Statement of principles*. Author. http://www.iassw-aiets.org/archive/ethics-in-social-work-statement-of-principles/

Kam, P. K. (2014). Back to the 'social' of social work: Reviving the social work profession's contribution to the promotion of social justice. *International Social Work, 57*(6), 723–740.

Kingdon, J. W., & Thurber, J. A. (1984). *Agendas, alternatives, and public policies*. Little, Brown.

Kurevakwesu, W. (2017). The social work profession in Zimbabwe: A critical approach on the position of social work on Zimbabwe's development. *Afro Asian Journal of Social Sciences*. http://www.onlineresearchjournals.com/aajoss/art/232.pdf

Ledwith, M. (2016). *Community development in action: Putting Freire into practice*. Policy Press.

Leonard, P. (1993). Critical pedagogy and state welfare: Intellectual encounters with Freire and Gramsci, 1974–1986. In P. McLaren & P. Leonard (Eds.), *Paulo Freire: A critical encounter* (pp. 155–168). Routledge.

Mangena, C., & Warria, A. (2017). The challenges experienced by Zimbabwean social workers practising in Gauteng townships. *Social Work, 53*(2), 250–265.

Margolin, L. (1997). *Under the cover of kindness: The invention of social work*. University Press of Virginia.

Miller, D. (1976). *Social justice*. Oxford University Press.

Moch, M. (2009). A critical understanding of social work by Paolo Freire. *Journal of Progressive Human Services, 20*(1), 92–97. https://doi.org/10.1080/10428230902878285

Muchanyerei, B. (2017). Apathy or fear? The role of social workers in Zimbabwe's political discourse. *African Journal of Social Work, 7*(2), 60–64.

NASW. (2008). *Code of ethics*. http://www.socialworkers.org/about/Ethics/Code-of-Ethics-English

Nikku, B. R. (2019). Empowering people: Role for political social work in South Asia. *International Social Work, 62*(2), 877–891.

O'Brien, M. (2010). Social justice: Alive and well (partly) in social work practice? *International Social Work, 54*(2), 174–190.

Olson, J. J. (2007). Social work's professional and social justice projects: Discourses in conflict. *Journal of Progressive Human Services, 18*(1), 45–69.

Pawar, M. (2019). Social work and social policy practice: Imperatives for political engagement. *The International Journal of Community and Social Development, 1*(1), 15–27.

Popple, P. R., & Leighninger, L. (2008). *The policy-based profession: An introduction to social welfare policy analysis for social workers* (4th ed.). Pearson.

Rawls, J. (1971). *A theory of justice*. Harvard University Press.

Reisch, M. (2002). Defining social justice in a socially unjust world. *Families in Society, 83*(4), 343–354.

Segal, E. A., Gerdes, K. E., & Steiner, S. (2007). *An introduction to the profession of social work: Becoming a change agent* (2nd ed.). Thomas Books/Cole.

Shamai, M., & Boehm, A. (2001). Politically oriented social work intervention. *International Social Work, 44*(3), 343–360.

Solas, J. (2008). What kind of social justice does social work seek? *International Social Work, 51*(6), 813–822.

Specht, H., & Courtney, M. (1994). *Unfaithful angels: How social work has abandoned its mission*. The Free Press.

Willet, L., & Hakak, Y. (2020). The immigration of social workers: From Zimbabwe to England. *International Social Work*. https://doi.org/10.1177/0020872820962206

27 The Professional Practice of the Brazilian Social Worker: Problems About the Impacts of the COVID-19 Pandemic

Evelyn Secco Faquin, Líria Maria Bettiol Lanza, Eliezer Rodrigues dos Santos, Fabrício da Silva Campanucci, and Carolina Camilo da Silva

27.1 Introduction

As we conclude this text, Brazil totals more than 300,000 deaths from the COVID-19 pandemic and mobilises scientific, social, and political efforts, among others, both external and internal, to confront it. Brazilian social workers are among the professionals whose professional practice has been redimensioned by the pandemic context, considering that public and private social services are the largest employers of these professionals. Social Service has been institutionalised as a profession intervening in social policies since the 1930s. It is considered a liberal profession, with a regulatory framework, such as the Code of Ethics of the Social Worker; the Law of Regulation of the Profession, and Class Councils that supervise and guide this exercise; however, hegemonically these professionals are wage earners. Nevertheless, it is still an area of knowledge in Brazil, within the applied social sciences, consolidated by its contributions to the production of knowledge in the country.

Similarly, we have identified Social Service productions, such as the study by Negri et al. (2020), which analysed the documents published by the entities representing the profession about the skills and attributions of the practice in the pandemic context; other studies and approaches to the debate are found in Moreira et al. (2020), as well as in Pereira and Cronemberger (2020), reflecting the context of professional work from reports of experiences in the health, education, socio-juridical, social assistance, and social security areas.

Even so, there are still difficulties in controlling the pandemic, leaving Brazilian society in a perpetual state of exposure and fear. The effects on everyday life (Narvai, 2020) are felt in a general way, also, in social work. Thus, the objective of the chapter is to discuss the impacts of COVID-19 on the professional exercise of social workers in their various sociooccupational spaces. We have chosen impact research, based on the self-assessment of the informant subjects, aiming at contributing to the debate within the profession, as well as producing scientific evidence (Mota & de Souza Kuchenbecker, 2020) which demonstrates how the work performed by

E. S. Faquin (✉) · L. M. B. Lanza
Department of Social Work, State University of Londrina (UEL), Paraná, Brazil

Researcher Program in Social Work and Social Policy, State University of Londrina (UEL), Paraná, Brazil

Social Work and Health: Training and Professional Practice, State University of Londrina (UEL), Paraná, Brazil
e-mail: evelynsecco@uel.br

E. R. dos Santos · F. da Silva Campanucci · C. C. da Silva
Social Work and Health: Training and Professional Practice, State University of Londrina (UEL), Paraná, Brazil

M. C. S. Gonçalves et al. (eds.), *The Coronavirus Crisis and Challenges to Social Development*,
https://doi.org/10.1007/978-3-030-84678-7_27

Brazilian social workers was affected during the COVID-19 pandemic.

The impact research implies knowing the direct effects of an action, of public and private programs and projects (Cotta, 1998; Fabiani et al., 2018). In contrast to other forms of evaluation, it attempts to analyse the cause-and-effect relationship. Hence, we start from the assumption that the pandemic context has reaffirmed the social determination of health that, according to Souza (2020), we can only understand and intervene from capitalist social relationships.

Based on this scenario, this qualitative research with quantitative resources dared to cover the entire national territory. The data collection process was carried out through an online questionnaire produced on the Cognito forms platform structured in two blocks: general profile, and specific questions about the impact of the COVID-19 pandemic. This was subdivided by topics so as to 'maintain' the focus of the interviewee in each requested area by creating a 'context' so that the fluidity of the answers could facilitate their understanding and reduce the time invested in the act of answering, to minimise dropouts in the data collection process. The system's architecture was designed so that it could be accessed by both smartphones and computers, with contrasting colors, intuitive scrolling, and buttons for answers of adequate size for typing to avoid errors produced by involuntary touches. A pre-test was conducted by the team with participants from the city itself. The link to the questionnaire was made available to a number of groups, trade associations, educational institutions, and personally, via messaging app and email, between December 2020 and February 2021. No structural corrections were necessary during the data collection period, although this format makes it possible.

Self-assessment is common in the healthcare field, even considering its limitations, such as its subjective character (Barros, 2008), but it also represents the possibility of capturing, through its subjects, their perceptions and relationships established with the proposed object of study. A total of 201 responses were obtained, including all five Brazilian regions, with higher representativeness in the South and Southeast regions. In terms of informants, 85.3% have been/were working in the year 2020, of whom 88.5% were women. The average acting time was 12 years, with a standard deviation of 9 years; 68% were acting in social assistance policy, only 2 being managers.

As for the target public, its heterogeneity characterises basic and territorialised services, according to the 1988 constitutional guideline for social policies, in particular the public policies of health, social assistance, and education. In relationship to the labor bond, 55.8% are statutory (social workers with public bonds), and the 30-h working week has been predominant (55.1%). The majority are not unionised (55.1%) and do not engage in activities linked to the representative instances of the profession (51.3%), such as ABEPSS (Brazilian Association of Education and Research in Social Work), CFESS (Federal Council of Social Work), and CRESS (Regional Councils of Social Work). The latter was the location responsible for the greatest participation, as 42.3% of them informed their participation in these spaces. The average salary, considering the valid answers, is R$4400.00 (approximately U$813.00), and the most mentioned benefits received were the health plan and the food voucher. In Brazil, there is not a minimum wage for social workers, configuring a labor market with low and discrepant wages, which can be questioned from the perspective of gender relationships, in which patriarchy, as a dominating system, is still active in the world of labor. Historically, in Brazil, women workers receive lower salaries than men, even in equal positions.

Based on the theoretical reference that sustains the study, the following variables were chosen to measure the impact: working conditions; relationship with managers/employers; work–family relationships; and health conditions, taking into account gender and class as determinants. Because it is mainly a female profession, the issue of care is considered as women's attribution, as we have noticed that nearly 57% of the informants declared that the impacts on their work–family relationships are medium (28.8%)

or high (28.8%). As such, for 33.3% of informants, the impact on mental health was rated high. The sexual division of labor raises the problem that these are workers who have accumulated functions beyond their paid work, which have been worsened by social isolation measures, such as the closing of schools and daycare centers.

The main arguments of the study were divided into three sections. In the first section, we start from the critical debate concerning the Brazilian scenario and the institutions that are central to the organisation and control of the COVID-19 pandemic as the locus of professional exercise. In the second part, we outline a sociohistorical perspective of Brazilian social service and its current professional prospect. Next, we present some impacts in the professional exercise from the self-assessment of the informants disclosing the real and concrete conditions in which these workers have been acting in the aforementioned context. Finally, we present our major findings.

27.2 Constitutive Aspects of the Sanitary, Political, Economic, and Social Scenario in Brazil

The arrival of COVID-19 in Brazil in the first quarter of 2020 impelled the country into the biggest health and social crisis of our generation. The Brazilian sociopolitical scenario had already been undergoing a serious crisis, the most significant points being the fall of the first female president and the election of a conservative president supported by an anti-democratic motto. Brazil had already been submitted to a process of continuous recession since the past decade, which has been sustained by neoliberal premises, and deepened by the governments since 2016, which rooted the abyssal social inequality and did not move the country into the promised growth curve.

Analysis of the aspects of living conditions before the pandemic revealed that regressions have occurred in almost all social indicators, which show a quick decrease in income and purchasing power for the populations of working-age and retired people as well as the most vulnerable, causing increasing poverty, inequality, and exclusion, at work and in income, and in pension and welfare protection. This decrease was combined with the institutional degradation of citizenship and decrease in the supply of public goods and services, in quantity and quality, that are fundamental to the social needs of the majority of the population, such as health and education. Also, violence and uncertainty have increased, leading to a significant reduction in the social well-being of the majority of the population, which has already been far from reasonable, compared to countries in the same condition and with the abundance of Brazil (Castro, 2020, p. 62).

It is worth pointing out that in Brazil, the social security system includes both contributory policies (social security) and noncontributory policies (social assistance and health), which is a hybrid system. Yet, the perspective of universal access is inconclusive, given the counter-reforms directed at social policies as a whole, based on the dismantling of everything that is public and state run, which reached its peak in 2019 with the social security, administrative, and tax reforms. The idea was to shield the country from an international crisis, reduce obligatory state spending, and make room in the budget to stimulate the economy.

This encouragement was given by attacking basic rights that would guarantee the survival of the working class and with financial contributions to capital, especially foreign capital; in other words: a guarantee of maintaining the privileges at the expense of reducing the rights historically won by workers. The new element here is the speed at which the system has been dismantled since 2019 and the political apathy that resulted from the alienating structures of subordinate bourgeois democracy and globalised capital, whose permanent legitimacy crisis was accentuated in the COVID-19 pandemic (Souza, 2020).

Given these circumstances, the necessary restrictive measures adopted to fight the new coronavirus pandemic deepened the economic recession and were decisive in increasing the impoverishment of the population. The informants of this study were invited to analyse the economic impacts on themselves and their families: 6.4% pointed out that they had a reduction in salary and 12.1% claimed that these salary changes had a high impact on their working conditions. We also investigated whether the COVID-19 pandemic period impacted family income. To this question, 38.4% answered that there was a reduction in family income and 2.5% stated that it was necessary to hire caregivers to accompany their children while they were working. Such hiring needs also impacted the economic condition of the subjects who reported the survey.

The motto of the new campaign [...] was "the economy can't stop," and, lately, "I take the risk of the deaths" (Silva, 2020, p. 108, author translation). However, more vigorous responses were required to keep alive the class that made its living from the sale of its labor force. In the face of the pandemic, this led to the emergency aid provided by the Federal Government. The objective was to provide the population who had their income source interrupted with the amount of 200 reais, which does not correspond to 20% of the minimum wage. This amount was questioned by the opposition and adjusted to 600 reais for a 3-month period, and was reduced by 50% in subsequent months. The guarantee of emergency aid for 2021 was only given in March, and the amount can range from R$150 to R$375. It should also be pointed out that the great number of individuals who have accessed this amount demonstrates how deep and worrying is the impoverishment of the working class in Brazil.

Moreover, because the revenues of all federative entities had considerable losses, the President of the Republic was compelled to financially assist states and municipalities because of the political and administrative decentralization in several public policies; among them, the most demanded in this pandemic period were social assistance and public health. In April, the Supreme Court gave autonomy to states and municipalities to manage the coronavirus crisis, yet these officials found themselves in greater economic and social distress and were incapable of managing the crisis on their own. This financial contribution was also the focus of negotiation of the current government, as its allocation was conditioned to political support and the wage freeze of city workers until 2021, which articulates his attacks on public services and promotes his administrative reform.

The economic, social, and political assumptions are linked to health strategies in this pandemic moment. In response to the latter, the President of the Republic has aligned himself with the negationist/neoliberal thinking. On one hand, he denies the seriousness of the pandemic, positioning himself against social isolation, in the wake of U.S. President Donald Trump, and supports the use of chloroquine and hydroxychloroquine as a way to combat the disease; on the other hand, he does not work on the implementation of the Brazilian Unified Health System (SUS).

The SUS is the ideal space for virus containment and pandemic relief, and a robust and powerful system in terms of population healthcare. It could be a fundamental instrument in the fight against COVID-19 and in mitigating the effects of the virus. Consequently, it would relieve the economic crisis, which dismantles the argument that puts health and economy as opposing and excluding sides. The history of dismantling the SUS, however, goes back to its own inception in the 1988 Federal Constitution (DeMatos, 2020). These elements have proven to be completely ineffective in times of pandemic, when state action and massive investments in healthcare are required.

The battle against the pandemic in Brazil experiences a lack of basic elements of public management: planning and political commitment. The first item is caused by the Executive's inability to govern; the second is manifested by the third replacement of the Minister of Health.

Any political leader who wished to overcome the crisis in a humane and respectful manner would invest in strengthening the SUS. What has been happening is a dismantling of the current system which has, contradictorily, attacked the health system countless times, politicising its existence and repeatedly breaking down its structures. The most recent attacks were the promise to revoke more than 100 mental health-related ordinances, which weakens the anti-manicomial campaign, and the current experience of a complete lack of mass vaccination plans for the Brazilian population in the face of the imminent approval of vaccines against COVID-19.

As this text was being written, one of Brazil's capitals was entering the worst crisis experienced so far by a collapsed health system and the depletion of oxygen for mechanical ventilation, causing deaths in an entire wing of the University Hospital of Manaus on 15 January 2021, a fact that was widely reported in the main Brazilian media and social networks.

It is within the scenario outlined here, of changes, uncertainties, and deepening of the crisis, that social work inserts itself and builds its professional identity, as described in the next section.

27.3 Brazilian Social Work: Organization and Direction

Social work in Brazil is supposed to be conceived from the responses given by the State and society to the social question and its expressions. Since its genesis (1930s), the category has been assuming heterogeneous positions in accordance with historical contexts, either by approaching conservationists (with religious and charitable actions), or with the intention of rupturing (based on Marxist historical-dialectic materialism) by acting from the perspective of rights. In this way, the profession in Brazil assumes a dynamic aspect, which seeks to be remade according to sociohistorical determinations (Yazbek, 2016).

The social meaning of the profession has been built by the theoretical debate in the academic sphere and by the revision of regulations, which has legitimised it in the labor market, such as the 1993 Code of Professional Ethics for Social Workers, Law 8662/1993, and the 1996 Curricular Guidelines, both of which form the basis of the Social Work Ethical-Political Project.

The Law 8662/1993 regulates the profession in the country and establishes the exercise of the profession, besides the registration in the professional council and payment of annuity. It establishes the competences and private attributions of the social worker, such as elaboration, evaluation, implementation, and execution of several social policies that can be linked to the public administration, companies, entities, and popular organizations.

The current Code of Ethics, in turn, establishes the principles that must be observed in the exercise of the profession, such as the uncompromising defense of human rights, the respect for freedom, the refusal of any form of discrimination, and the position in favor of equity and social justice.

In Brazil, social workers are recognised as professionals registered in the social-technical division of labor, being paid workers who have a professional project. The Ethical-Political Project of social work does not refer only to the legislation indicated: it is also possible to identify the political dimension of the profession, which acts in the contradictory movement of the capitalist order and imprints a social direction on the actions (Netto, 2006).

This project conducts the professional exercise by the principles of diversity, equity, and social justice, expansion and consolidation of citizenship, universalisation and equality in access to goods and services, as well as the positioning in favor of workers and the participation of users (Netto, 2006), who hold the hegemony of the professional category through the representative bodies of the professional category. In the Brazilian context, the understanding that professional exercise is expressed through the articulation of the theoretical-methodological, ethical-political, and technical-operational dimensions is hegemonic, and they are inseparable from each other.

Overall, it is demanded of the social worker to comprehend the expressions of the macro-societal context present in everyday professional life, as well as the limits and possibilities of exercise when confronted with the need to provide answers of an ethical-political and technical-operational nature, theoretically and methodologically based (Iamamoto, 2009b).

To build these responses, social workers need, according to DosSantos (2016), to act in a conscious and realistic way as they are taught in the theoretical-methodological field about employing institutions; to understand the universal determinants and particularities of the expressions of the social issue and how they express themselves in a unique way when presenting the demands of the subjects who request assistance; to be theoretically competent in understanding the movement of reality, deciphering the possibilities of intervention in this stage of the capitalist economy; and being able to decode the new expressions of the social issue.

As far as the ethical-political field is concerned, DosSantos (2016) indicates that ethical competence is necessary to build the practice in the direction of the principles foreseen in the Ethics Code and to politically position itself in favor of democratic institutions. Thus, professionals in this area must understand that the exercise of the profession is imbued with political implications, being tensioned by class struggle (Iamamoto, 2011). The technical-operative dimension holds instruments, techniques, procedures, and strategies used by social workers to build responses to the demands posed by the population and employing institutions, the contact and proximity with the people who demand their actions being inherent to the profession.

Based on data made available by the CFESS (Federal Council of Social Work)/CRESS (Regional Councils of Social Work) group, as of September 2020 there were 199,622 professionals with active registration. The last survey on the profile of social workers in Brazil, promoted by the CFESS/CRESS set, was held in 2004 and, according to Iamamoto (2009a), more than half the social workers in the country worked in state institutions, with statutory ties, followed by private companies and nongovernmental organizations (NGOs), in actions of management and execution of social policies, such as formulation, planning, evaluation, in Councils of Rights and others. Most of them were active in social assistance, followed by children and adolescents, health, and the elderly, among others. It is important to highlight the expansion of multi-professional teams in which they are inserted, mainly in areas such as social assistance, health, education, and sociolegal, achievements from the 1988 Federal Constitution and other regulations. Currently, the legal conquests established by the struggle and organisation of social movements have provided more interference from the State in facing the expressions of the social issue, object of the social worker's practice.

On the other hand, the counter-reform of the post-constituent Brazilian state, the deregulation of labor rights, and the tendency to mercantilise social policies, have directly interfered in the work of these professionals and in their working conditions, causing the closure of some fields of action, depriving professionals of labor rights, and overburdening workers and establishing fierce competition among them.

In 2015, a document (updated in 2018) was published by the CFESS/CRESS group, which expresses the flags of struggle to be defended by social workers and reinforces the importance of professional exercise based on their private competences and attributions as a worker's right, as well as access to decent working conditions. As for the beneficiaries of the services, the defense of the supremacy of social needs at the expense of economic profitability is foreseen, which implies the expansion of the allocation of resources for social security policies, being health, welfare, and social assistance. In this sense, it considers the defense of social policies as universal and of State responsibility, elaborated in a participative and democratic way (Federal Council of Social Work [CFESS] and Regional Councils of Social Work [CRESS], 2015).

In the following topic, we discuss how this practice has been constructed in the sociopolitical and economic context, as well as in a pandemic context.

27.4 Impacts on Professional Practice in Pandemic Times: Idiosyncrasy and Loneliness

What are the impacts of the COVID-19 pandemic on the work done by Brazilian social workers? What effects has the work–family–institution–health articulation brought about for all these workers? What protection did they receive considering the various sociooccupational spaces?

To answer such questions, we would like to state that our way of socialising with other people, as well as our work relationships, have brought several orders of challenge to the professional exercise of social workers. Of the professionals who took part in this survey, 66% declared that there have been changes in their work processes and 80.1% declared that the functioning of the services in which they work has been altered, indicating that the pandemic context has directly or partially affected their performance in regard to medium and high impacts.

As a result of the context instigated by COVID-19, social workers are now being required to assume unusual contexts related to global health, human mobility, state responses to demands posed by contamination, and public health protocols, in addition to having to promptly adopt new institutional norms. We can affirm, beforehand, the presence of a gap in the discussions on emergencies and public calamity in the process of training Brazilian social workers, even though the care and defense of the interests of the population contained in these contexts are regulated as an ethical obligation. The subject is not even considered in the curricular guidelines for undergraduate courses in social work.

To handle the countless impacts of the pandemic on their professional practice, Brazilian social workers have received general guidance from the Federal Council of Social Work (CFESS), which works together with the Regional Councils of Social Work (CRESS) to discipline, orient, regulate, inspect, and defend the professional practice of the social workers in the country. Among the documents published were three Resolutions: one Normative Orientation; two Notes; and one Legal Opinion on issues involving the professional exercise of social workers in the current situation.

In the manifesto published on 23 March 2020 and widely distributed among social workers, the Federal Council guided professionals to negotiate with their supervisors on the possibility of rotation, escalation, suspension, or maintenance of activities as well as on the most appropriate form of assistance in each situation, aiming at fulfilling sanitary guidelines and protecting the health of the professional and the user (Federal Council of Social Work, 2020b).

These guidelines, although pertinent, raise some questions that connect the pandemic context with the demands of the labor world: Are workers open to negotiate with their managers? Are there enough teams to provide for escalation? Do the services have the necessary equipment for working remotely, protecting the professionals and users? What is teleworking? How do we organise it? When maintaining the relationship with users, as the intervening nature of the profession is expressed mainly through physical contact, how do we create a bond through telephones and Internet? What about users who do not have access to technologies? How to establish the practice with a perspective to expand access and collectivise demands? How to handle the fear of contamination and the "abandonment of users" with the necessities of closing down or reducing the potential of social services?

These and so many other doubts and challenges were certainly remarkable in professional exercise in 2020. The territorial extension of Brazil and the different levels of propagation of the disease in states and municipalities caused the sanitary guidelines, as well as compliance with the respective guidelines, to present successive changes. The professionals who participated in this survey pointed out that some services were closed; others emphasised telework and maintained face-to-face care assuring adequate distance, demanding the mandatory use of masks and hand hygiene with 70% alcohol; there were discrepancies in the attendance hours, in the dismissal of risk group workers in different periods, and in the suspension of face-to-face collective activities.

When questioned about the support of professional entities for work performance during the pandemic, only 30.7% of participants declared themselves satisfied. Among the professionals dissatisfied with the support offered, 23% indicated that they do not feel supported and 30.1% stated that they feel partially supported.

Impacted by the pandemic, services and work procedures have been adapted. The main changes in professional practice and in the functioning of the services highlighted by the subjects of this research illustrate the challenges faced by professionals when following health guidelines without violating their Code of Ethics and failing to meet institutional goals. Such situations challenge the professional category and places it among the principles, attributions, and professional skills and recommendations on ways to prevent and contain COVID-19.

Among the main changes in professional practice, that is, *the implementation of social services by telephone and face-to-face care with doors and windows open, with distance of at least 2 m, the use of masks and the use of alcohol*, 70% were marked by more than half of the subjects, 53.2% and 51.2%, respectively. As for the changes in the operation of the services, we highlight *the suspension of collective activities*, declared by 65% of the professionals; *the reduction of home visits*, indicated by 47.4%; *the suspension of in-person care and remote care*, indicated by 36.5% of the subjects; and *the reduction of face-to-face care with priority to remote care*, remarked by 32.6% of the social workers.

Thus, the professionals, with greater frequency, used actions of individual and collective character for direct attendance to the users having, as main instruments of intervention, interviews, home visits, meetings, and thematic groups, as subsidies even for the construction of reports and social opinions (Trindade, 2012). In this direction, it was the social workers' responsibility to face dilemmas related to the reduction of the mobilization potential caused by the pandemic, that is, the impossibility of meetings and gatherings, in a context where the only channel was the digital environment. In the face of a process of greater demand for social services, pointed out by 51.9%, intensification of demands placed by the user population, indicated by 69.8%, and the beginning of service to new audiences, reported by 35.8%, needed to incorporate in their daily lives technological resources, such as computers and cell phones with access to the worldwide web. In addition, it was necessary to expand the control of information systems as a means of contact with users, and transform resources that were once auxiliary into essential. Thus, it is a paradox: on one hand, the dismantling of the protection system and, on the other, the need for its expansion. According to 69.2% of the participants, these aspects generated work overload, causing medium and high impacts to the professional exercise.

The pandemic context has deeply affected the planning, execution, and evaluation of professional actions as social workers have had to adapt to constant changes in health regulations and guidelines. The loss of the territorial potential of social services is notorious, because most of the regulations indicated the establishment of telework or the reduction of face-to-face care, with home visits and collective actions being prohibited, requiring new strategies for either face-to-face or remote care.

The guidelines regarding federal benefits, especially emergency assistance and benefits of continued delivery, were marked by 60.8%. Others reported guidelines and dispensation of municipal benefits (55.1%), mainly basic food items, benefits linked to temporary vulnerability, personal documentation, and institutional reception of all orders; modifications in the functioning of social services (58.9%); elaboration of reports (64.1%); situations referring to the reduction of family income and unemployment (51.2%); articulation with the social services network (47.4%); and issues arising from the intensification of family conflicts and domestic violence (36.5%). The greatest demand was for emergency assistance, a temporary benefit proposed to meet the needs of the unemployed and self-employed workers who were affected by the economic paralysis, which shows the impact on the lives of Brazilians and especially on the economic condition that was generated by the pandemic. However, the high demand for BPC (continued benefit), which has a low-income criterion, as well as for the Bolsa Família, a Cash Transfer Program that aims to fight poverty and establishes conditionalities regarding the access and continuity of the benefits that are aimed at the public served by the social assistance policy, shows that the economic and social problems did not arise with the pandemic: even before it, the living conditions of Brazilians were no longer satisfactory.

As identified by the CFESS, the most significant difficulties of the professional category in this context, especially in health and social assistance policies, have been "ensuring working conditions in the face of precariousness, the absence of PPEs, the intensification of demands and the fragility of working relationships" (Federal Council of Social Work, 2020c, p. 3; author translation). Although 67.9% of professionals have received PPE from their employers, 20.5% responded that they do not feel safe with the equipment and another 33.3% feel only partly safe. Among the reasons for the insecurity of more than half of the professionals, 14.7% indicated that the quantity supplied is not enough, 12.82% doubted the quality of the product, 12.1% distrusted the effectiveness of the products, and 4.4% complained about the discomfort and pain caused by the use of PPE.

The Legal Opinion No. 05/2020-E deals specifically with the lack of personal protective equipment (PPE) for social workers and points out the appropriate legal measures. The document clarifies that the responsibility to define which are the essential services and workers is that of the health authorities and that "it is the responsibility of the employer to provide the PPE necessary for the exercise of the working activities" (Legal Opinion CFESS No. 05, 2020-E, p. 7). Therefore, it is the responsibility of employers to comply with the legal determinations of the competent bodies and to protect workers. However, considering that 20.5% of the subjects did not receive PPE from their employers, it can be stated that the latter are not fulfilling their responsibilities.

Another significant impact of the pandemic has been the increase in labor costs for working women and men who are working in the telework modality, causing "the intensification of the exploitation of wage labor and economy for the employing institutions" (Federal Council of Social Work, 2020c, p. 5; author translation).

It should be noted that the gradual process of implementing remote work has been abruptly intensified. This accelerated introduction of information and communication technologies (ICTs) has had a direct impact on work processes, especially with regard to the relationship with other professions and the user population and the ethical and technical conditions of professional practice (Federal Council of Social Work, 2020c)

By means of the guidelines published in 2020 the Federal Council emphasised the exceptionality of remote services and made it more flexible to provide services with "closed doors," which guaranteed the confidentiality of the information passed on by the population using the services. The obvious need for this flexibility created yet another challenge for professionals: to protect themselves and the population of users from contamination and to follow their ethical principles, guaranteeing the right of the user to have their information kept confidential.

When questioned whether the pandemic context had caused ethical implications, 34.6% said yes, 35.8% said they believed that the ethical implications were partial, and only 12.8% said they did not perceive ethical implications arising from the changes we are experiencing. The reasons most highlighted by the informants about the difficulties of complying with the Ethical Code were the realisation of open-door services to meet sanitary orientations (48.7%); the difficulty of performing educational and reflective activities through remote work (40.8%); and the need to make social evaluations at a distance in specific situations, such as in the case of people in home isolation or affected by COVID-19 (33.9%).

The necessary search for new knowledge, which is essential in this context, has generated medium and high impacts to the professional exercise (73%), indicating that, for the most part, this journey was a solitary one, as they did not receive institutional training. Consequently, they had to acquire knowledge about transmission, symptoms, and necessary care (48%), about benefits offered, and about the use of new technologies (52.5%). A part of the participants (37.8%) also reported the need to improve knowledge already acquired, given the context's particularity. This report reaffirms the historical characteristics of the profession that accompanies the movement of reality and is influenced by it, as well as the requirement to remain in the process of training based on new knowledge and/or resuming the theoretical contribution already seen previously, as was also demonstrated by the responses. The lack of training offered by the employers, which was necessary for the performance in that space, generated a series of problems for the professionals, making the improvement of their actions an individual responsibility. Thus, the professionals end up studying beyond their working hours, compromising the time that would be dedicated to their personal life, increasing the financial expenditure to have access to new knowledge, not to mention not being able to count on the institutions to promote continued education.

27.5 Final Considerations

The conducted survey intended to produce data that were not the result of the hypothesis associated with the more general picture of the work in Brazil, but which objectively encompassed the impacts related to the professional exercise according to the opinion of the informants.

Brazil's political and economic scenario, worrying in itself, has been intensified by a multifaceted crisis during the past decade, which was deepened with the arrival of COVID-19, highlighting the weaknesses of our institutions. The lack of coherent leadership on the part of the Federal Executive made combat action ineffective and without guidelines that could contain the pandemic, requiring the intervention of the Federal Supreme Court to prevent further deaths. Consequently, in addition to the deaths, we have had severe impacts on the Brazilian economy.

Considering the objective of problematising the impacts of the COVID-19 pandemic on the work of social workers in their various socio-occupational spaces, we found that the profession in Brazil, since its beginnings, has assumed a dynamic characteristic, following the historical processes and demands arising from society. From the conjuncture analysis, it directs the qualification and the professional exercise in a critical way, considering the theoretical-methodological, ethical-political, and technical-operative dimensions, which, combined, provide the recognition of the social worker as a professional able to handle the social problems caused by class division and the characteristics of a country marked by profound social inequality.

The changes arising from the COVID-19 pandemic took place under the massive withdrawal of funding from Brazilian social services, in which one major impact is the lack of adequate human resources, among them social workers. The dismantlement of the public social service infrastructure has resulted in workers being held accountable, forcing them to seek training, pay for their PPEs, and face their work process in a solitary manner.

The survey reaffirmed the precarious working conditions of the social worker, showing that the awareness of these professionals has had a high impact on their own living conditions by reducing salaries, changes in their work processes, and the entire pandemic context which has also had a high impact on the mental health of these workers.

Despite such an adverse context, it was possible to identify through this research that Brazilian social workers are daily reaffirming their commitment to the quality of the services provided to the user population, seeking new intervention strategies in terms of approaching them, and new ways of transferring information and orientations linked to norms and rights, thereby reconstructing their professional practice. It is important to reaffirm that most social workers, even without the support of their employers (public or private), have developed a continuous search for qualification and access to content that has allowed them greater competence in the analysis of the pandemic situation, proposing and carrying out actions that come and meet the (new and historical) needs of the population at this time.

The paradox inherent in the professional exercise of social workers as a result of the pandemic signals that the population using social services has been affected as much or even more than the professionals. Therefore, Brazilians continue to demand more comprehensive social policies, proper services with working and assistance conditions, universality of access, and the State's commitment to public health.

References

Aquino, E. M., Silveira, I. H., Pescarini, J. M., Aquino, R., Souza-Filho, J. A. D., Rocha, A. S., et al. (2020). Medidas de distanciamento social no controle da pandemia de COVID-19: potenciais impactos e desafios no Brasil. *Ciência & Saúde Coletiva, 25*, 2423–2446. https://doi.org/10.1590/1413-81232020256.1.10502020. https://www.scielo.br/pdf/csc/v25s1/1413-8123-csc-25-s1-2423.pdf

Barros, M. B. D. A. (2008). Inquéritos domiciliares de saúde: potencialidades e desafios. *Revista Brasileira de Epidemiologia, 11*, 6–19. https://doi.org/10.1590/S1415-790X2008000500002. https://www.scielo.br/pdf/rbepid/v11s1/01.pdf

Brasil. (2012). *Código de ética do/a assistente social. Lei 8.662/93 de regulamentação da profissão* (10th ed.). Conselho Federal de Serviço Social.

Castro, J. A. (2020). Bem-Estar Social Dos Brasileiros E A Pandemia do Coronavírus: Ruim e Vai Ficar Pior. In D. Castro, D. D. Seno, & M. Pochmann (Eds.), *Capitalismo e a Covid-19: um debate urgente* (pp. 56–64) http://abet-trabalho.org.br/wp-content/uploads/2020/05/LIVRO.CapitalismoxCovid19.pdf

Conselho Federal de Serviço Social. (2020a). *Serviço Social contra a Covid-19 (Coronavírus)*. Author. http://www.cfess.org.br/visualizar/menu/local/covid-19-coronavirus

Conselho Federal de Serviço Social. (2020b). *CFESS Manifesta. Os impactos do Coronavírus no trabalho do/a assistente social*. Author. http://www.cfess.org.br/arquivos/2020CfessManifestaEdEspecialCoronavirus.pdf

Conselho Federal de Serviço Social. (2020c). *Teletrabalho e Teleperícia: orientações para assistentes sociais no contexto da pandemia [Nota]*. Author. http://www.cfess.org.br/arquivos/Nota-teletrabalho-telepericiacfess.pdf

Conselho Federal de Serviço Social & Conselhos Regionais de Serviço Social. (2015). *Bandeiras e Luta do Conjunto CFESS-CRESS*. CFESS. http://www.cfess.org.br/arquivos/FolderBandeiradeLutas-Livreto.pdf

Cotta, T. C. (1998). Metodologias de avaliação de programas e projetos sociais: análise de resultados e de impacto. *Revista do Serviço Público, 49*(2), 103–124. https://doi.org/10.21874/rsp.v49i2.368. https://revista.enap.gov.br/index.php/RSP/article/view/368/374

DeMatos, M. C. (2020). A Pandemia de Coivd- 19 e o Trabalho De Assistentes Sociais na Saúde. In A. Loie, I. Stampa, & R. L. R. Gomes (Eds.), *Para Além da Quarentena: Reflexões Sobre Crise e Pandemia* (pp. 235–349). Mórula.

DeOliveira Figueiredo, M. C., Sena, A. P. M., Costa, L. M. B., Junior, A. A. F., Lima, J. J. A., Dias, L. R. D., et al. (2020). Notas sobre os impactos da pandemia do coronavírus no trabalho dos/as assistentes sociais. *Revista Interfaces: Saúde, Humanas e Tecnologia, 8*(3), 775–784. https://doi.org/10.16891/2317-434X.v8.e3.a2020. https://interfaces.leaosampaio.edu.br/index.php/revista-interfaces/article/view/859/pdf

DosSantos, C. M. (2016) Do conhecimento teórico sobre a realidade social ao exercício profissional do assistente social: desafios na atualidade. In: M. L. Deoliveira e Silva Serviço Social no Brasil: história de resistências e de ruptura com o conservadorismo (pp. 265–285). : Cortez

Fabiani, P., Rebehy, S., Camelo, R., Vicente, F. J., & Mosaner, M. (2018) *Avaliação de impacto social: metodologias e reflexões [artigo]*. Instituto para o Desenvolvimento do Investimento Social – IDIS. https://www.idis.org.br/wp-content/uploads/2018/05/Artigo_Avaliacao_Impacto_Social_06.pdf

Helioterio, M. C., Lopes, F. Q. R. D. S., Sousa, C. C. D., Souza, F. D. O., Pinho, P. D. S., Sousa, F. N., & Araújo, T. M. D. (2020) Covid-19: Por que a proteção de trabalhadores e trabalhadoras da saúde é prioritária no combate à pandemia? *Trabalho, Educação e Saúde, 18*(3), 1–13. https://doi.org/10.1590/1981-7746-sol00289. https://www.scielo.br/pdf/tes/v18n3/0102-6909-tes-18-3-e00289121.pdf

Iamamoto, M. V. (2009a). Os espaços sócio-ocupacionais do assistente social. In *Serviço Social: Direitos Sociais e Competências Profissionais* (pp 341–375). CFESS/ABEPSS.

Iamamoto, M. V. (2009b). As dimensões ético-políticas e teórico-metodológicas no Serviço Social Contemporâneo. In A. E. Mota, M. I. S. Bravo, R. Uchoa, V. Nogueira, R. Marsiglia, L. Gomes, & M. Teixeira (Eds.), *Serviço Social e Saúde: formação e trabalho profissional* (4th ed., pp. 161–196). Cortez, OPAS, OMS, Ministério da Saúde.

Iamamoto, M. V. (2011). A herança conservadora do Serviço Social: atualização e busca de ruptura. In M. V. Iamamoto (Ed.), *Renovação e Conservadorismo no Serviço Social: ensaios críticos* (11th ed., pp. 17–39). Cortez.

Lei nº 8. 662, de 7 de junho de 1993. (1993). *Dispõe sobre a profissão de Assistente Social e dá outras providências*. CFESS. http://www.planalto.gov.br/ccivil_03/leis/l8662.htm

Maciel, F. B. M., Santos, H. L. P. C. D., Carneiro, R. A. D. S., Souza, E. A. D., Prado, N. M. D. B. L., & Teixeira, C. F. D. S. (2020). Agente comunitário de saúde: reflexões sobre o processo de trabalho em saúde em tempos de pandemia de Covid-19. *Ciência & Saúde Coletiva, 25*, 4185–4195. https://doi.org/10.1590/1413-812320202510.2.28102020.

https://www.scielo.br/pdf/csc/v25s2/1413-8123-csc-25-s2-4185.pdf

Moreira, E., Gouveia, R., Garcia, J., Acosta, L., Botelho, M., Rodrigues, M., et al. (2020). *Em tempos de pandemia: propostas para a defesa da vida e de direitos sociais*. UFRJ, Centro de Filosofia e Ciências Humanas, Escola de Serviço Social.

Mota, D. M., & de Souza Kuchenbecker, R. (2020). Considerações sobre o uso de evidências científicas em tempos de pandemia: o caso da COVID-19. *Vigilância Sanitária Em Debate: Sociedade, Ciência & Tecnologia (Health Surveillance under Debate: Society, Science & Technology), 8*(2), 2–9. https://doi.org/10.22239/2317-269x.01541. https://visaemdebate.incqs.fiocruz.br/index.php/visaemdebate/article/view/1541/1146

Narvai, P. C. (2020). Covid-19 no Brasil: incúria, medo, ceticismo e resistência popular. *Revista da Boitempo, 35*(2), 125–130.

Negri, F. L., DosSantos, M. T., & Krüger, T. R. (2020). *Atuação da/o assistente social em face da pandemia da covid19: orientações técnicas elaboradas pelo conjunto cfess/cress [artigo]*. Comitê SUAS/SC – COVID19: em defesa da vida.

Netto, J. P. (2006). A construção do projeto ético-político do Serviço Social. *Serviço Social e Saúde, 4*, 141–160.

Netto, A. R. Z., Vivan, J. B., Costa, K. C., Pegoretti, M. L., Piccolo, F., & Maeyama, M. A. (2020). Uma análise das recomendações governamentais brasileiras no enfrentamento da pandemia da Covid-19 a partir das evidências disponíveis. *Brazilian Journal of Health Review, 3*(3), 4735–4759. https://doi.org/10.34119/bjhrv3n3-064. https://www.brazilianjournals.com/index.php/BJHR/article/view/10284/8613

Ornell, F. E. L. I. P. E., Schuch, J. B., Sordi, A. O., & Kessler, F. H. P. (2020). Pandemia de medo e COVID-19: impacto na saúde mental e possíveis estratégicas [editorial]. *Revista Debates in Psychiatry*. http://www.ufrgs.br/ufrgs/noticias/arquivos/pandemia-de-medo-e-covid-19-impacto-na-saude-mental-e-possiveis-estrategias

Parecer Jurídico CFESS n. 05/2020-E. (2020). *Ausência de Equipamentos de Proteção Individual – EPI para assistentes sociais. Medidas jurídicas cabíveis*. http://www.cfess.org.br/arquivos/Cfess-ParecerJuridico05-2020-E-EPI.pdf

Pereira, S. L. B., & Cronemberger, I. H. G. (2020). *Serviço social em tempos de pandemia: provocações ao debate*. EDUFPI.

Santos, J. A. F. (2020). COVID-19, fundamental causes, social class and territory. *Trabalho, Educação e Saúde, 18*(3), 1–7. https://doi.org/10.1590/1981-7746-sol00280. https://www.scielo.br/pdf/tes/v18n3/0102-6909-tes-18-3-e00280112.pdf

Silva, L. C. (2020). Neoliberalismo em xeque, mais qua vez. In D. Castro, D. D. Seno, & M. Pochmann (Eds.), *Capitalismo e a COVID-19* (pp. 101–114).

Souza, D. D. O. (2020). A pandemia de COVID-19 para além das Ciências da Saúde: reflexões sobre sua determinação social. *Ciência & Saúde Coletiva, 25*, 2469–2477. https://doi.org/10.1590/1413-81232020256.1.11532020. https://www.scielo.br/pdf/csc/v25s1/1413-8123-csc-25-s1-2469.pdf

Teixeira, C. F. D. S., Soares, C. M., Souza, E. A., Lisboa, E. S., Pinto, I. C. D. M., Andrade, L. R. D., & Espiridião, M. A. (2020). A saúde dos profissionais de saúde no enfrentamento da pandemia de Covid-19. *Ciência & Saúde Coletiva, 25*, 3465–3474. https://doi.org/10.1590/1413-81232020259.19562020. https://www.scielo.br/pdf/csc/v25n9/1413-8123-csc-25-09-3465.pdf

Trindade, R. L. P. (2012). Ações profissionais, procedimentos e instrumentos no trabalho dos assistentes sociais nas políticas sociais. In C. M. D. Santos, S. Backx, & Y. Guerra (Eds.), *A dimensão técnico-operativa no Serviço Social: desafios contemporâneos* (pp. 69–102). Editora UFJF.

Uchôa-de-Oliveira, F. M. (2020). Saúde do trabalhador e o aprofundamento da uberização do trabalho em tempos de pandemia. *Revista Brasileira de Saúde Ocupacional, 45*, 1–8. https://doi.org/10.1590/2317-6369000012520. https://www.scielo.br/pdf/rbso/v45/2317-6369-rbso-45-e22.pdf

Weinberg, M., & Banks, S. (2019). Practicing ethically in unethical times: Everyday resistance in social work. *Journal Ethics and Social Welfare., 13*, 361. https://doi.org/10.1080/17496535.2019.1597141

Yazbek, M. C. (2016). Prefácio. In M. L. DeOliveira (Ed.), *Serviço Social no Brasil: história de resistências e de ruptura com o conservadorismo*. Cortez.

28 Front-Line Social Workers' Practices Under the Political and Sanitary Crisis in Chile

Taly Reininger, Gianinna Muñoz Arce, Cristóbal Villalobos Dintrans, and Ignacio Wyman

28.1 Introduction

The first confirmed case of COVID-19 in Chile was identified on 3 March 2020. The virus propagated at an alarmingly rapid rate, leaving the government scrambling to rapidly impose sanitary restrictions to stop the virus's spread. What began as social distancing and sanitary guidelines quickly evolved into one of the longest lockdowns on an international scale, with zones of the country under lockdown for more than 6 months. The social and economic impacts of the virus and subsequent sanitary measures have led to a considerable increase in unemployment, housing loss, food insecurity, poverty, violence, and mental health issues (Jiménez et al., 2020; Vergara et al., 2020). These devastating effects have disproportionately affected households living in situations of vulnerability, leading to a substantial increase in inequality in the country as well as unveiling the ineffectiveness of Chile's social protection system (COES, 2020).

The State's response to the social and economic impacts of the virus has been a series of reactionary and focalised aid measures. Growing civil unrest stemming from the lack of access to food led to the "Alimentos para Chile" (Food for Chile), a State-organised nationwide distribution of food packages to vulnerable neighborhoods. Vulnerable families were also the target population of a three-month emergency income plan, a plan quickly extended in both amount and duration in response to harsh critiques from opposition parties and civil society. Other State measures included a financial aid package for the middle class, an employment protection law, parental medical leave, and a legal amendment allowing individuals to withdraw from their pension funds (COES, 2020). New social programs were also developed targeted at specific populations such as the homeless, children, and older adults (Escuela de Trabajo Social UC-Centro de Autoformación Cívica, 2020). Despite the implementation of such an eclectic assortment of measures, the actions of the State have been deemed inadequate in protecting citizens from the economic and social impacts of the virus (Gutiérrez, 2020; Pérez-Roa, 2020).

Front-line social workers, defined as professionals directly involved in the implementation of social policies (Muñoz Arce, 2018), have been largely absent from the discussions in regard to the aid measures enacted. Their voices are particularly relevant, as front-line social workers are those actors who experience, interpret, translate, and ultimately re-design social policy, thus often

T. Reininger (✉) · G. M. Arce
Department of Social Work, Universidad de Chile, Santiago, Chile
e-mail: tal.reininger@uchile.cl

C. V. Dintrans · I. Wyman
Centro de Estudios de Políticas y Prácticas en Educación (CEPPE-UC), Pontificia Universidad Catolica de Chile, Santiago, Chile

M. C. S. Gonçalves et al. (eds.), *The Coronavirus Crisis and Challenges to Social Development*,
https://doi.org/10.1007/978-3-030-84678-7_28

representing the state in interactions with citizens (Lipsky, 2010; Muñoz Arce, 2018; Tummers, 2013; Weinberg & Banks, 2019). Considering the important role of front-line social workers in the implementation of social programs, questions arose as to how social programs had adapted to the current context of sanitary restrictions and lockdowns. Furthermore, considering the precarious employment conditions of essential front-line workers during the pandemic internationally (Nyashanu et al., 2020), plus the historical precarious conditions of front-line social workers in Chile (Muñoz Arce, 2018), the need arose to examine whether employment conditions had worsened. To explore these questions from the perspective of front-line social workers, a sequential explanatory mixed-methods study was undertaken between the months of June and October 2020. This chapter presents the findings from this study.

The chapter begins with a brief contextualisation into Chile's social and political context before the arrival of COVID-19, followed by a section analysing the implementation of social programs in Chile and its impacts on front-line social workers. A third section presents the study's methodology, followed by a results and discussion section that presents the study's main findings. The chapter concludes with a discussion of the challenges social work faces in the current and future context.

28.2 Chile's Political and Social Climate Pre-COVID-19

In October 2019, mass civil protests erupted in Chile, bringing the country to a standstill. What began on 7 October as student-led protests against an increase in public transportation fares quickly evolved into massive organised fare evasions that exploded on 18 October with violent clashes with police and the destruction of various metro stations. The government's response was to immediately enact a state of emergency, impose a curfew, and harshly persecute all those suspected of committing violent acts during the demonstrations. Nevertheless, and contrary to the government's projections, the repressive measures implemented only fuelled greater discontent amongst the population. The student-led protests had resonated with many, specifically with deeply ingrained perceptions of systematic injustice, inequality, exclusion, and anger towards a corrupt and abusive elite (Güell, 2019). Although Chile had experienced mass student-led protests in the past, this time the movement amassed a broad range of supporters embracing a diversity of causes (Villalobos, 2021). Citizens who took to the street waved signs signalling that "Chile despertó" (Chile awoke) and "No son 30 pesos son 30 años" (it is not 30 pesos but 30 years). A common thread that unified the vast array of demands was a discontent with the neoliberal model forcibly implemented during Augusto Pinochet's 17-year dictatorship and maintained during the subsequent 30 years of democracy (Somma et al., 2020). Social workers and social work organizations such as the National School of Social Workers, and its local chapters, as well as the Assembly of Self-convened Social Workers, participated actively in protests as well as holding meetings to discuss and suggest necessary structural changes to the neoliberal model (Morales, 2021).

The neoliberal model imposed during the dictatorship in Chile produced lasting economic, political, and cultural impacts (Hall & Lamont, 2013). These impacts included the privatization of national industries and public services (including health, education, and pensions); rising levels of inequality; the rise of technocracy and managerialism; and the ascent of meritocracy, individualism, and competitiveness as cultural ideals (Rodriguez, 2020). Privatisation reforms had a direct impact on the provision of social services, creating a dual system in which the poor received inadequately funded public services while those who had the means received private care. Social policies in turn were primarily targeted to the poor through means-tested social programs (Larrañaga, 2010; Raczynski, 1995).

Since the return to democracy in 1990, social policy had undergone a substantive change. On one hand, social spending was notably increased, leading to the creation of new administrations (ministries, undersecretaries, institutes, and services) and the development of new social programs aimed at specific populations such as children, young people, older adults, women, indigenous people, and the disabled. At the same time, foreign organisations, which during the dictatorship had provided funding for alternative social programs, began to withdraw, leading to the demise of many civil society organizations and the adaption of others (Moyano & Garcés, 2020). As a consequence of these changes, most social programs in Chile began to operate through a public bidding framework organised by the State, thus promoting outsourcing. This outsourcing (defined as the delegation of responsibility for social services by the State or civil society organizations and private entities in some cases) has resulted in a substantive transformation of both working conditions and the ways in which social programs are implemented in Chile (Basualdo & Morales, 2019), being the front-line social workers are among the actors most affected by these outsourcing processes (Muñoz Arce, 2018).

The conditions of front-line social workers in Chile can be defined by three characteristics. In the first place, and mainly the result of outsourcing, there is a tendency to exacerbate the principles of competition between organisations. This sense of competition has not only inhibited the possibility of sharing and consolidating learning regarding the implementation of social programs but has also produced uncertainty and instability in employment conditions. This uncertainty and constant competition have been identified as factors that produce high levels of stress and burnout in front-line professionals (Sánchez & Villarroel, 2017; Schöngut-Grollmus, 2017; Bilbao et al., 2018; Muñoz Arce & Madrigal, 2018).

A second characteristic caused by the dynamics of competition and uncertainty mentioned previously are high turnover rates, especially in regard to front-line social workers (Iturrieta, 2017). Front-line social workers are often hampered by low wages and high workloads, lack of material resources and infrastructure, weak supervision and advisory systems, and few spaces to reflect on the implementation process itself, leading to instability in implementation teams (Muñoz Arce, 2020).

Finally, the outsourcing of social programs, by its very nature, has deepened the gap between the design and implementation of social programs. Thus, social programs follow a top-down logic in which design and evaluation are undertaken at a centralised state level whereas implementation remains the responsibility of civil society organisations and private entities. Under this framework, the professional teams that implement social programs are rarely heard by those making policy decisions at central levels, while the program designs emanating from these central levels often lack meaning or relevance for those front-line professionals who are implementing the programs (Muñoz Arce, 2018; Picasso-Rizzo & Andrade-Guzmán, 2019).

Although these characteristics have tended to be maintained throughout the period of the Chilean post-dictatorship (1990–2019), the pandemic caused by COVID-19 can be understood as a moment of break that could maintain, deepen, or transform these characteristics. Analysing these aspects is precisely the objective of this chapter.

28.3 Methodology

To explore the impact of COVID-19 on front-line social workers and the implementation of social programs, this study utilised an explanatory sequential design. This design was chosen to explore quantitative results in greater depth (Creswell, 2015). During the first quantitative phase of the study, an online survey was disseminated through a collaboration between the Department of Social Work at the University of Chile, the National School of Social Workers, and the Chilean Association of Schools of Social Work (ACHETSU). Each organization sent out emails and invited individuals to participate by posting information on the study on their websites and other social networks. The survey was available online between 10 June and 14 July 2020. A total of 872 individuals completed the survey; however, only 652 responses were included in the analyses, to focus solely on front-line social workers who were implementing social programs before the start of the pandemic. Respondents hailed from all Chile's 16 regions, concentrated primarily in the Metropolitan, Biobío, and Valparaiso regions. The survey was answered mainly by women (82.8%), of whom 49.7% were 34 years of age or younger. In addition, 15.5% stated that they had completed post-graduate studies. In regard to employers, the highest percentage of respondents indicated working in municipalities (43.6%), followed by companies or private foundations (21.7%), public institutions with central administration (20.7%), and lastly NGOs (14%); 76.7% indicated working full-time and about 50% earned between $700,000 and $1,100,000 Chilean pesos a month. (For full sociodemographic characteristics, please see Table 28.3 in the Appendix.)

For the second qualitative phase of the study, 42 semi-structured interviews were conducted with social workers who completed the survey and had indicated an interest in participating in interviews. COVID-19 restrictions meant all interviews were conducted using Zoom. Participants were sent informed consent forms before interviews providing details on the study. All interviews were held between August and October of 2020. Interviews were transcribed verbatim and analyzed using thematic analysis (Braun & Clarke, 2006).

28.4 Results and Discussion

The results presented in this section correspond to results in regard to changes in the employment conditions of front-line social workers and to changes in the implementation of social programs caused by COVID-19. The results are organised into two sections: employment conditions and program changes.

28.4.1 Employment Conditions

Table 28.1 shows the descriptive results of changes in front-line social workers' employment conditions. Nearly 75% of front-line social workers who responded to the survey reported perceiving a greater or much greater workload than before the pandemic. Findings from interviews corroborated these results, with social workers elaborating on the different reasons their workloads increased during lockdown. The following quote from a social worker employed in education illustrates how working from home during lockdown blurred the boundaries between work and home:

> The workload has been excessive, too much. There has been no general respect regarding the schedule. It is understood … it is misunderstood that the fact that you are at home means that you have to work until … or they can call you perfectly at 8, at 9 at night. (…) If one does not set the limits, the truth is that it is very difficult to be able to do everything. (Female, Education, Valparaiso Region).[1]

This lack of separation between work and home caused by lockdown measures has been identified as particularly problematic for women, who often assume greater care responsibilities in the household, care responsibilities that have increased exponentially from school and child-care center closures for sanitary measures (Power, 2020). Juggling work and care responsibilities has been especially difficult for many of the social workers interviewed, especially those with young children. The increased stress brought about by these extraordinary circumstances are additional factors to take into consideration relative to the already high burn-out and stress levels of front-line social workers in the country (Sánchez & Villarroel, 2017; Schöngut-Grollmus, 2017; Bilbao et al., 2018; Muñoz Arce & Madrigal, 2018). As identified by Peinado and Anderson (2020), greater emphasis on self-care and boundary setting for front-line social workers are particularly important during these times of lockdown and social distancing.

A second factor that emerged in the interviews explaining the sensation of higher work-loads were changes in program methodology. As shown in Table 28.1, more than 80% of social workers

[1] All interview quotes were translated from Spanish to English by the authors.

Table 28.1 Changes in perceived workloads and types of changes

	No.	Percentage
Perception of workloads since lockdowns		
Less than before	72	12.4%
Same as before	76	13.1%
Greater than before	235	40.4%
Much greater than before	199	34.2%
Total	582	100%
What type of changes have programs undergone?[a]		
Communication with service users has changed to noncontact communication	514	88.2%
Physical encounters with service users have been limited	436	74.8%
Programs have been restructured or reorganised	234	40.1%
The roles or functions of the implementation team have changed	215	36.9%
Interactions with service users have been suspended	163	28%
New social programs have been developed	60	10.3%
Programs have been canceled	37	6.4%
Who assumed the costs of program changes?		
Primarily the institution	309	54.9%
Primarily the workers	211	37.5%
Primarily service users	30	5.3%
Primarily third parties	13	2.3%
Total	563	100%

[a]Survey participants could choose more than one option

reported their programs no longer communicated with service users in person, and close to 75% of social workers reported programs had limited these encounters. These changes were also observed in interviews, with most social workers indicating their contact with service users had evolved to phone calls and messaging. Interventions that were once in groups had now become individualised. The following interview excerpt from a social worker employed in school mental health explains how these changes have resulted in greater workloads:

> For example, I used to do a workshop with ten children once a week. Now I have to call each of those children individually, and not only talk to the child, also talk to the guardian. So, from there, my workload increased exponentially, because what I used to do in an hour and a half, maybe, between the driving and the planning, two and a half hours, (now) it takes me a while. At least 5 or 6 hours a week calling them by phone, trying to contact them. (Female, School mental health, Metropolitan Region)

The cost of changes in program methodologies, especially the use of technology such as phones, internet, computers, etc. from homes was also identified as problematic by front-line professionals as visualised in the following quote:

> My employer has given me absolutely nothing, let's say, to be able to move, I pay for the phone, I pay for my plan, everything, and I have spent a little more because I have needed to acquire other tools such as an external hard drive, for example, ink for the printer because I also work with my own printer and buy my own ink. (Female, Education, Valparaiso Region).

Results from the survey indicate that close to 38% of front-line social workers have assumed the cost of program changes, a preoccupying figure because these professionals already confront precarious work conditions, specifically low wages (Muñoz Arce, 2020), wages that are diminished further by the need to assume the extra costs of program changes. Technology was not the only cost front-line social workers had to assume in the pandemic, in some cases they had to provide their own protective gear once COVID-19 arrived in Chile:

I had to make one, a face shield, bought supplies at the hardware store, then my husband bought the thing here … (Female, Health, Tarapacá region).

The lack of personal protective equipment for front-line workers has been documented internationally (Nyashanu et al., 2020), indicating just how unprepared countries were for the onslaught of COVID-19, Chile being no exception.

28.4.2 Neoliberalism and Program Changes

Program changes, and particularly the decision-making processes in regard to these changes, were mostly made at centralised levels and with little participation from front-line social workers. As shown in Table 28.2, 70% of survey respondents indicated that decision making was not very participatory and changes considered mainly national guidelines or those provided by program authorities, supporting previous findings of top-down policy implementation in Chile (Muñoz Arce, 2018; Picasso-Rizzo & Andrade-Guzmán, 2019).

In reference to changes in the implementation of programs (as shown in Table 28.2), more than 50% of survey respondents indicated they perceived the changes to be moderate. However, in interviews, an interesting theme emerged from social workers who worked with families in Chile's largest poverty program (Families program), a key component of Chile's social protection system. These interviewees indicated more profound changes, specifically a shift from the program's focus on empowering families and fomenting individual responsibility to one focused on crisis assistance:

So that is the change that has occurred now because now the program has become more assistance oriented since the crisis because families are contacting us with basic needs that are not covered or, when the IFE (Emergency Family Income), there were many doubts. For this reason, now contacts are not to know if there is a training program or what project I can apply for, but rather – when are the cash transfers going to arrive, when do the family allowances expire, or when will the food box will arrive – there is an economic need so great that they have shifted the program or it has been a setback for the program. The work plans and action plans have been limited to assistance management more than with what we were working with families. (Female, poverty, Metropolitan Region)

This change in program focus is to be expected because those hardest hit by the effects of COVID-19 and subsequent sanitary measures are precisely those families who lived in situations of poverty before the pandemic (Jiménez et al., 2020; Vergara et al., 2020). These families are at a greater risk of losing employment and income, facing eviction, and experiencing food insecurity, among many other vulnerabilities. The economic and social crisis brought on by COVID-19 revealed that this program, key to Chile's social protection system, was forced to take a drastic turn from neoliberal ideals of individual responsibility, entrepreneurship, and market inclusion (Reininger & Castro-Serrano, 2020) to material crisis assistance. This shift exposed some of the cracks in the neoliberal ideological foundations of the country's social protection system and the urgent needs for reform (Cardona, 2020).

A second theme to emerge in regard to the logic behind neoliberal social policies, specifically their targeting, was the production of comparisons and resentment between service users, often times placing front-line social workers in uncomfortable positions:

…the social benefits did not reach all the users of the program, so you had to be responding to that, or why didn't the box arrive on that day, why did it arrive in that sector first and it did not arrive at mine, why did my neighbor get a gallon of gas and not me, so that makes the intervention quite complex because there is a lot of comparison and there one is like a little tied hands because you have no way to answer (…). (Female, poverty, Valparaiso Region.)

As front-line social workers represent the state in their interactions with service users (Lipsky, 2010), often such representation produces uneasiness and ethical dilemmas, especially when they do not agree with certain policy positions (Muñoz Arce, 2018; Streir & Breshtling, 2016; Weinberg & Banks, 2019). The targeting used by the State to focalise aid to those characterised as most "needy and worthy" especially in times of crises, not only produces tensions for front-line social workers, but also produces competition between

Table 28.2 Perceived participation in changes in social programs

	Number	Percentage
Perception on levels of participation in program changes		
Not very participatory, considering mainly national guidelines and/or orientations	207	39.8%
Not very participatory, considering mainly the guidelines provided by authorities (directors or coordinators) of the program	158	30.4%
Very participatory, considering mainly the opinion of professionals	112	21.5%
Very participatory, considering the opinion of professionals as well as service users	43	8.3%
Total	520	100%
How profound have these changes been?		
Slightly profound	124	21.3%
Moderately profound	317	54.6%
Deeply profound	113	19.5%
No changes were applied	27	4.6%
Total	581	100%

citizens who must demonstrate their eligibility in comparison to others. The individualised nature of aid and the competition it produces undermines social cohesion and political citizenship (Edmiston, 2018; Saad-Filho, 2016), processes that were energetically and broadly expressed during Chile's 2019 social uprising (Villalobos, 2021). Despite these hurdles, one social worker expressed how she has incorporated these processes into her interventions with families:

> I feel that currently there is something that has been overlooked in the work with families and that is strengthening social participation. In other words, whether we like it or not, nowadays, even if we are in a pandemic and in a context of social distancing, right? It is a context where social participation is really important, right? Because we are in a context of political change … in a political context that is particular, it is historical, right? It is a referendum for a new constitution, and I think that kind of thing, for example, I have been able to install in my sessions…I think that the most important people who have to participate are these people, those who have been super isolated from the system, or more than from the system, from society and culture, how it works, so I think they have many things to say and I think it is important that they motivate themselves to participate. So, I think that in my daily life I have tried to install that, which goes against what they tell me I have to do (laughs). (Female, Poverty, Metropolitan Region).

This quote not only demonstrates an overt act of resistance on the part of the social worker in following program protocols but also the historical importance of the October social uprising and the hope that it will bring about structural change. The social worker indicates that this political process requires hearing the voices of those that have too often been silenced and that social work can and should play a key role in activating political citizenship.

28.5 Conclusions

The results of this study show that the pandemic and subsequent social distancing and lockdown measures have in some cases led to greater precarity in employment conditions for front-line social workers. These professionals indicate a substantial increase in workload, be it from changes in program methodologies and/or hazy limits of work hours when working from home. Furthermore, many social workers have taken on the cost of materials needed to do their jobs from home such as paying for phones, Internet, and printer ink. As expected, the majority of program changes were taken at centralised levels overlooking the participation and valuable insights of front-line social workers. In some cases, these changes produced certain levels of unease and in others may have instigated forms of resistance linked to the social uprising of October 2019 and the hope that change is possible.

The principal outcome of the October uprising was an agreement between major political parties that called for a constitutional referendum to replace the one written during the dictatorship. This agreement materialised after almost a month of civil unrest, riots, and looting. Cities throughout the nation had experienced marches, riots, sit-ins, bikeathons, singalongs, and many other cultural manifestations of discontent with the current neoliberal system. Demonstrators included individuals from all ages, ranging from young children to older adults. Many marched against the vast inequalities in health, education, gender, and pensions and the corruption that the neoliberal model had produced. Protesters called for dignity, the recognition of rights, and for radical structural change. Political citizenship was in full force and civil society organisations were thriving and gaining strength by banding together under one larger umbrella organization (Unidad Social). Informal and formal meetings were organiszed nationwide to discuss the possibilities of a new constitution. Social workers and social work organizations such as the National School of Social Workers, the Chilean Association for University Schools of Social Work, the Assembly of Self-convened Social Workers, amongst others, actively participated in organizing such meetings, conversational spaces that were maintained online during COVID lockdowns (Morales, 2021).

The social distancing measures and lockdowns imposed in March of this year by COVID-19 have placed a difficult hurdle for the mass mobilizations that began in October of 2019. However, this does not mean that citizens' demands for change and greater equality have diminished; in fact, the devastating impacts of Covid-19 have led to greater visibility of social inequalities. On 25 October 2020, close to 80% of the population voted in favor of drafting a new constitution. A new constitution will not magically solve the historical inequalities brought on by neoliberalism, but it can however, turn over a new leaf.

What challenges does social work face in this complicated scenario of COVID-19 and social change? First, it must confront the historic precarity of employment conditions and especially those produced by the pandemic, which have led to even more precarity. This calls for organizing nationally and strengthening the voice of the national school of social workers. Secondly, social work should continue to expose the fissures and faults of the neoliberal model, be this on a micro scale in interactions with service users and/or macro level providing evidence from front-line professionals. Lastly, considering the evidence that this is not the last pandemic the world will face (Gill, 2020), social work should look ahead and innovate interventions with the use of new technological platforms.

Appendix (Table 28.3)

Table 28.3 Sociodemographic characteristics of survey participants

Variable	No.	Percentage
Gender		
Masculine	105	16.1%
Feminine	540	82.8%
Other	7	1.1%
Age (years)		
22–34	324	49.7%
35–47	255	39.1%
48–73	73	11.2%
Education		
University degree	551	84.5%
Master's and/or doctorate	101	15.5%
Principal employer		
Public institution with central administration (Ministry, undersecretary, national service, seremi's)	129	20.7%
Municipality or municipal corporation	271	43.6%
Nongovernmental organization (NGO)	87	14%
Company or private foundation	135	21.7%
Weekly work hours		
Less than 22 h	10	1.5%
Between 22 and 33 h	37	5.7%
Between 33 and 43 h	73	11.3%
44 h	497	76.7%

Variable	No.	Percentage
Flexible hours	31	4.8%
Remuneration		
$500.00 or less	82	12.7%
$500.00 to $700.00	99	15.3%
$700.00 to $900.00	215	33.3%
$900.00 to $1.100.00	128	19.8%
$1100.00 to $1300.00	68	10.5%
More than $1300.00	54	8.4%

References

Basualdo, V., & Morales, D. (2019). *La tercerización laboral: Orígenes, impacto y claves para su análisis en América Latina*. Siglo XXI Editores.

Bilbao, M., Martínez-Zelaya, G., Pavez, J., & Morales, K. (2018). Burnout en trabajadores de ONGs que ejecutan política social en Chile. *Psicoperspectivas, 17*(3), 199–210.

Braun, V., & Clarke, V. (2006). Using thematic analysis in psychology. *Qualitative Research in Psychology, 3*(2), 77–101. ISSN 1478-0887.

Cardona, B. (2020). The pitfalls of personalization rhetoric in time of health crisis: COVID-19 pandemic and cracks on neoliberal ideologies. *Health Promotion International, 36*, 714. https://doi.org/10.1093/heapro/daaa112

COES. (2020). *Informe 1. Revisión Agenda Social y Agenda COVID-19*. Observatorio de Gobierno UDP-COES.

Creswell, J. (2015). *A concise introduction to mixed methods research*. Sage.

Edmiston, D. (2018). Resistance or resignation to welfare reform? Activist politics for and against social citizenship. *Policy and Politics, 46*(3), 467–484.

Escuela de Trabajo Social UC-Centro de Autoformación Cívica. (2020). *Guía de beneficios sociales en tiempos de COVID-19*. https://drive.google.com/file/d/1RGnjnbanGQdXXBpO3chfEhsj6vbKunUl/view?fbclid=IwAR0AGHggt9Ug3Ah_eLx0NFts-6dXs94gvMTPsTn4MP49uxngtldcYhegrVjQ\

Gill, V. (2020). *Coronavirus: This is not the last pandemic*. BBC. https://www.bbc.com/news/science-environment-52775386

Güell, P. (2019). El estallido social de Chile: piezas para un rompecabezas. *Revista Mensaje Diciembre*, 10–15.

Gutiérrez, P. (2020). *Los graves problemas metodológicos y prácticos en el Ingreso Familiar de Emergencia*. CIPER. https://ciperchile.cl/2020/07/03/los-graves-problemas-metodologicos-y-practicos-en-el-ingreso-familiar-de-emergencia/

Hall, P. & Lamont, M. (2013). Social resilience in the neoliberal era. Cambridge University Press.

Iturrieta, S. (2017). Entre burbujas, sensaciones y realidades de la profesión más masificada en Chile: El trabajo social. *Cuadernos de Trabajo Social, 9*(1) 9–26.

Jiménez, A., Duarte, F., & Rojas, G. (2020). *Sindemia, la triple crisis social, sanitaria y económica: y su efecto en la salud mental*. CIPER. https://ciperchile.cl/2020/06/20/sindemia-la-triple-crisis-social-sanitaria-y-economica-y-su-efecto-en-la-salud-mental./

Larrañaga, O. (2010). *Las nuevas políticas de protección social en perspectiva histórica*. PNUD.

Lipsky, M. (2010). *Street-level bureaucracy: Dilemmas of the individual in public services (30th anniversary expanded edition)*. Russel Sage Foundation.

Morales, C. (2021). *Colectivos de trabajo social en Chile: Una posibilidad de resistencia antes el neoliberalismo*. Unpublished Undergraduate thesis, Universidad de Chile.

Moyano, C., & Garcés, M. (Eds.). (2020). *ONG durante la dictadura*. Ediciones Universidad Alberto Hurtado.

Muñoz Arce, G. (2018). The neoliberal turn in Chilean social work: Frontline struggles against individualism and fragmentation. *European Journal of Social Work, 22*(2), 289–300.

Muñoz Arce, G. (2020). Trabajo interprofesional en Chile. *Revista Rumbos TS. Un espacio crítico para la reflexión en Ciencias Sociales, 21*, 87–108.

Muñoz Arce, G., & Madrigal, J. (2018). Trabajo interprofesional en Chile: Neoliberalismo y la producción de subjetividades profesionales críticas. *Intervención, 8*(2), 4–22.

Nyashanu, M., Pfende, F., & Ekpenyong, M. (2020). Exploring the challenges faced by frontline workers in health and social care amid the COVID-19 pandemic: Experiences of frontline workers in the English Midlands region, UK. *Journal of Interprofessional Care, 34*(5), 655–661.

Peinado, M., & Anderson, K. (2020). Reducing social worker burnout during COVID-19. *International Social Work, 63*(6), 757–760.

Pérez-Roa, L. (2020). *Por qué tenemos que seguir promoviendo el endeudamiento como único medio para asegurar los ingresos de los hogares?* CIPER. https://ciperchile.cl/2020/07/10/por-que-tenemos-que-seguir-promoviendo-el-endeudamiento-como-unico-medio-para-asegurar-los-ingresos-de-los-hogares/

Picasso-Rizzo, F., & Andrade-Guzmán, C. (2019). Desafíos para las políticas e intervenciones sociales en el contexto sudamericano. Reflexiones en materia de relación pública-privada y encuentro entre implementadores/as y sujetos de intervención. *Revista de Ciencias Sociales, 28*(42), 32–51.

Power, K. (2020). The COVID-19 pandemic has increased the care burden of women and families. *Sustainability: Science, Practice and Policy, 16*(1), 67–73.

Raczynski, D. (1995). Focalización de programas sociales: lecciones de la experiencia chilena. In C. Pizarro, D. Raczynski, & J. Vial (Eds.), *Políticas económicas y sociales en el Chile democrático*. CIEPLAN/UNICEF.

Reininger, T., & Castro-Serrano, B. (2020). Poverty and human capital in Chile. The processes of subjectivation in conditional cash transfer programs. *Critical Social Policy*. https://doi.org/10.1177/0261018320929644

Rodriguez, J. P. (2020). *Resisting neoliberal capitalism in Chile: The possibility of social critique*. Palgrave Macmillan.

Saad-Filho, A. (2016). Social policy beyond neoliberalism: From conditional cash transfers to pro-poor growth. *Journal of Poverty Alleviation and International Development, 7*(1), 67–93.

Sánchez, M., & Villarroel, R. (2017). Tensiones en la Intervención Social: (des)encuentros en la relación Estado-ONG. Estudio de caso sobre ONG que opera la política social de infancia. *Revista Trabajo Social, 91*, 1–16.

Schöngut-Grollmus, N. (2017). Ensamblajes socio-técnicos para la producción de intervenciones psicosociales en un programa del Servicio Nacional de Menores de Chile. *Psicoperspectivas, 16*(3), 41–51.

Somma, N., Bargsted, M., Pavlic, R., & Medel, R. (2020). No water in the oasis: The Chilean spring of 2019–2020. *Social Movement Studies*, 1–8. https://doi.org/10.1080/14742837.2020.1727737

Streir, R., & Breshtling, O. (2016). Professional resistance in social work: Counterpractice assemblages. *Social Work, 61*(2), 111–118.

Tummers, L. (2013). *Policy alienation and the power of professionals: Confronting new policies*. Edward Elgar.

Vergara, F., Encinas, F., Aguirre, C., Trufello, J., & Ladrón de Guevara, F. (2020). *Ciudad y COVID-19: Desigualdad socio espacial y vulnerabilidad*. CIPER. https://ciperchile.cl/2020/03/25/ciudad-y-covid-19-desigualdad-socio-espacial-y-vulnerabilidad/

Villalobos, C. (2021). Una continuidad discontinua. Análisis retrospectivo del 18-O a la luz del ciclo de protestas juveniles en el campo educativo. In S. Alé, K. Duarte, & D. Miranda (Eds.), *Saltar el torniquete. Reflexiones desde las juventudes de octubre* (pp. 41–47). Fondo de Cultura Económica.

Weinberg, M., & Banks, S. (2019). Practicing ethically in unethical times: Everyday resistance in social work. *Journal Ethics and Social Welfare., 13*, 361. https://doi.org/10.1080/17496535.2019.1597141

Part III

Outlook: Looking Ahead Beyond the Pandemic

29 Time for New Epistemological Inquiries, the Global South, and Resilience in the Time of COVID-19

Lars Bedurke

29.1 We've Run Out of Air

In 2020, young Chilean mass protesters adopted a paraphrased version of a song by Víctor Jara as one of the mottos: "The right to breathe in peace."[1] That year, 2020, might as well be branded "The year we ran out of air." And not only because of the health crisis that is inherently linked to the annihilation of the rainforests—the lungs of the planet—but because of the breathtaking speed of recent events and the material breathlessness of the millions of people who have died at the hands of the virus we call SARS-CoV-2. In record time, countries and institutions in the Global North (GN)[2] developed concepts to prevent the expansion of the virus, while well-off individuals acquired excessive amounts of basic commodities and hygiene products and essentially emptied their local stores. Conversely, in the Global South (GS), containment measures and massive hoarding were not an option. Because most of the Southern Hemisphere is familiar with financial crashes, coup d'états, natural disasters, and epidemics, this new crisis was not met with as much surprise and concern as in the North. What can we learn from the South in this context? This chapter intends to adopt a different epistemic perspective, one that does not exoticize nor romanticize the South, but that weaves a narrative where the Southern struggles and experiences are acknowledged as sources of knowledge. This acknowledgment implies asking ourselves some questions: How do we live and how does our life affect others? How does it affect the breath of the planet? Is it possible for us to obtain knowledge and wisdom produced in the peripheries, outside the established centers? Is it possible that those centers of knowledge production ceased to be central long ago? How can we face life challenges while curbing and stopping the imperial modes of life, and choosing different ways of living?

29.2 Learning from the Virus

The COVID-19 pandemic has taught us many things. In a short span of time, a series of events yielded important lessons for humanity. It all seems to have started with a virus that originated in China, which traveled the Earth at a tremendous speed. Although Wuhan is a 10-h flight away from Milan, it was in Italy where the virus caused worldwide panic, attracting the world's attention, and the horrific images of Lombardy

[1] Originally "El derecho de vivir en paz" [The right to live in peace].

[2] For a further discussion on the terminology used in this chapter, see https://www.e-ir.info/2020/07/03/the-global-south-as-a-political-project/.

L. Bedurke (✉)
Brot für die Welt, Berlin, Germany
e-mail: lars.bedurke@brot-fuer-die-welt.de

M. C. S. Gonçalves et al. (eds.), *The Coronavirus Crisis and Challenges to Social Development*, https://doi.org/10.1007/978-3-030-84678-7_29

that traveled the world made people aware of what was happening. The pictures of military trucks filled with coffins, driving through the streets of Bergamo in March 2020, preceded similar snapshots from Guayaquil, Manaus, and New Delhi. Once again, we learned that we live in an interconnected world where diseases can disseminate at full speed.

Instead of breaking with imperial visions, this interconnectivity, this globalization, this perennial movement of people and commodities have perpetuated them. This vision is noticeable in aspects such as racism: the SARS-CoV-2 virus contributed to creating a global fear of people who "looked Chinese." To "look Chinese," a person did not have to belong to that huge country nor have ever been there. Any person who looked East Asian was exposed to rejection because of their facial features. Additionally, the narratives surrounding the origins of the virus set the scene for the construction of a racist discourse. The query was not focused on the correlation between the current development model and the pandemic, nor on the relationship between the deforestation of rainforests, the subsequent reduction of habitat of wild fauna, and the zoonotic transmission of this coronavirus to humans. Discussions focused mostly on the allegedly exotic food tastes of the Chinese. And the expanse of the crisis was reduced to a narrative of archaic food tastes that were foreign for the Western mind and which gave way to a terrible pandemic.

Although the hoarding of toilet paper may have become a mere anecdote in countries such as Argentina or Germany, it was also the grim prelude to the war for masks,[3] in which shipments of masks were "hijacked" by powerful countries at airports. But the tipping point has undoubtedly been the GN's appropriation of vaccines. By February 2021, more than three quarters of the vaccines had been administered in the 10 countries that account for 60% of the gross world product. Meanwhile, in about 130 countries, with a total population of 2.5 billion people, not a single dose had been administered.[4]

Another central aspect that shows it is essential to learn from the consequences is that recipes for facing the contemporary and future challenges are not static and cannot only come from the GN. It is essential for Northern countries to get rid of their *white paternalistic* attitude of being representatives of the South and ruling its bodies. Their impossible-to-follow proposals are forms of epistemic violence. And a crisis as significant as the one we are currently experiencing cannot be faced only with solutions designed in the North. For instance, the initial suggestions of physical distancing, hygiene, and voluntary isolation may very well be followed in Berlin, New York, and Tokyo. However, they cannot be as easily enforced in Luanda, the refugee camp of Moria, or Manila. How are we supposed to isolate a person who lives with their extended family in one of the large marginal urban neighborhoods of the South? How can a person wash their hands when 2.2 billion people do not have access to clean water, and 673 million people lack basic sanitation services?[5] How can 60% of the world's population stay home when they live in the informal economy?[6] What are the financial implications of the pandemic for families from the GS, especially from Central America[7] and the Philippines,[8] who depend on the remittances sent by their relatives living abroad?

[3]Coronavirus: US accused of 'piracy' over mask 'confiscation' (2020, 04.04) BBC, https://www.bbc.com/news/world-52161995 Accessed 01 May 2021.

[4]Yamey, G. (2021, 24.02) Rich countries should tithe their vaccines. https://www.nature.com/articles/d41586-021-00470-9 Accessed 01. May 2021.

[5]Drinking-water (2019, 14.06) World Health Organization. https://www.who.int/news-room/fact-sheets/detail/drinking-water. Accessed 01 May 2021.

[6]Press release. More than 60% of the world's employed population are in the informal economy (2018, 30 April) International Labour Organization. https://www.ilo.org/global/about-the-ilo/newsroom/news/WCMS_627189/lang%2D%2Den/index.htm. Accessed 01 May 2021.

[7]Remittances represent around 21.4% of the GDP in El Salvador; 20% in Honduras; 12% in Guatemala; and 11.3% in Nicaragua. https://www.gob.mx/cms/uploads/attachment/file/567288/Anuario_Migracion_y_Remesas_2019_Segunda_Parte.pdf. Accessed 01 May 2021.

[8]According to the official statistics of the Philippine government, there were 2.2 million Filipinos working under

How did Southern countries face the crisis? One of their first strategies implied counting hospital beds, ventilators, and medical and support staff. The figures were, and still are, discouraging and distressing. But they are just the tip of the iceberg, because the same could be said of masks, gloves, beds, budgets, and staff. It is undeniable that structural adjustment programs have eroded the investment in public health. Consequently, the health infrastructure has been decimated, health workers have sought more lucrative jobs elsewhere, and the implementation of fees for healthcare services has forced some sectors of the population to forego health services.[9] While a social state that promised a better future even for the poorest members of society was being built in Europe, structural adjustment created a new kind of poverty. The lesson is that the COVID-19 crisis has affected the weakened South particularly violently because of its underfunded health systems and the economic adjustment policies designed in the Global North.[10]

Another important lesson we have learned is that not everyone has lost out in this pandemic. The profits of online solutions and Internet companies have increased at a particularly unusual rate. A significant characteristic of the time we are living in is that social distancing and isolation are not expected to be enforced by corporations. Making people work in crowded places, the lack of sufficient governmental regulations, and a generalized indifference have characterized the pandemic. All of this was observed in the large infection chains in Lombardy as well as in the meat-producing regions in Germany.[11] It is no secret that Germany's initial 600 million Euro contribution to the worldwide COVAX initiative[12] is almost laughable compared to the 9 billion Euro bailout granted to the airline Lufthansa.[13]

Based on a series of lessons, it can be confidently argued that the measures designed by the GN to face the COVID-19 pandemic are mostly not applicable to the GS. It is a fact that the North's historical policies (structural adjustments, foreign debt, free trade agreements, protectionist policies) have violently jeopardized the South, particularly in the case of the crisis caused by this pandemic. It should be taken into consideration that these measures are not only inadequate, but they have also clearly shown to be erratic, have required permanent adjustments, and have ultimately failed to break with the rationales of what has largely driven this cataclysm. This poses a significant question: Which forms of social organization attest to the effective resilience of the most vulnerable people in the context of the current pandemic?

29.3 Approaches for Finding a Solution

29.3.1 The Collectivity

It is essential that we turn our attention to a series of concepts and realities that could give us clues regarding how to survive in the current circum-

contract abroad, especially in vulnerable fields, such as domestic work, or in affected sectors, such as the maritime sector. https://psa.gov.ph/statistics/survey/labor-force/sof-index. Accessed 01 May 2021.

[9] Timon Forster, Alexander E. Kentikelenis, Thomas H. Stubbs, Lawrence P. King. Globalization and health equity: The impact of structural adjustment programs on developing countries. *Social Science & Medicine*, Volume 267, 2020. https://doi.org/10.1016/j.socscimed.2019.112496. Accessed 01 May 2021

[10] Franco-Giraldo A, Palma M, Álvarez-Dardet C. Efecto del ajuste estructural sobre la situación de salud en América Latina y el Caribe, 1980–2000. *Rev Panam Salud Publica*. 2006;19(5):291–299. https://www.scielosp.org/article/rpsp/2006.v19n5/291-299/. Accessed 01 May 2021.

[11] Ziady H., Halasz St., Kottasová I., (2020, 27. June) The giant meatpacking company at the heart of Germany's new coronavirus hotspot. CNN. https://edition.cnn.com/2020/06/22/business/meat-plant-germany-coronavirus-outbreak/index.html. Accessed 01 May 2021.

[12] Press Release (2021, 19. February) Foreign Minister Maas on the global fight against COVID-19. https://www.auswaertiges-amt.de/en/newsroom/news/maas-covax/2443492. Accessed 01 May 2021.

[13] Sweney M., (2020. 25. May.) Lufthansa agrees €9bn bailout with German government. The Guardian. https://www.theguardian.com/business/2020/may/25/lufthansa-9bn-bailout-german-government-coronavirus-flights. Accessed 01 May 2021

stances. Indubitably, one of these aspects is well-being. Are there ways of obtaining well-being that go beyond consumption? Are there more environmentally friendly and socially conducive ways to obtain satisfaction and find a greater meaning in life and a sense of belonging? Are happiness and well-being based on individual experiences or should they be based on collective notions? If we take it to be the latter, much could be learned from the indigenous communities and organization strategies of the GS. If we want to find answers or at least learn about different solutions and proposals that arise elsewhere, beyond white European or North American intelligibility, we could turn our eyes to the collective constructions produced at the margins, in the "anti-spaces" of this world.

The indigenous communal organization strategies can provide certain clues. It is essential to acknowledge that, to create resiliency, indigenous communities have opted for organization models. Among them we can find communal assemblies, the organization of communal work, the governance of (ancestral) knowledge, and the addition of their worldview (cosmovisión) to their everyday endeavors. This view also applies to the sustainable use of natural resources, understanding them not as endless resources whose exploitation is based on a vision of uncontrolled growth, but as goods that are carefully and moderately harnessed. In many cases, communal organization is noticeable in the creation of commissions or assemblies, especially those that promote a communal consensus and vision. The organizational level of indigenous communities in terms of communal work, assemblies, and family ties is remarkable. And the argument is not that urban European or North American societies should adopt the rural indigenous ways of living, but that ancestral knowledge should be valued. We should look into their deep understanding of the ecosystems they inhabit, because it could help us rethink the Western premise that natural resources need to be capitalized. Valuing indigenous ways of knowing and thinking is essential; and this argument does not stem from a faux traditionalism but from the fact that indigenous communities have experienced processes of perennial change, just like any other society. If we want to part ways with white supremacy and dominance, it is critical that we acknowledge the existence of other ways of seeing, reading, and building the world.

Latin American indigenous communities face a very wide range of issues, but at least three broader aspects can be mentioned. First, the crisis of political systems (along with their legitimacy crises and a substantial loss of trust in them), which is characterized by corruption and an almost absolute lack of representation of native populations. Second, the growing violence and insecurity that affects their communities, although not exclusively. Third, another fundamental aspect is the constant threat to natural resources, such as subsoil minerals, water sources, wooded lands, territories, and even the wind in mountain and coastal regions. Amid these complexities, spaces of active and purposeful resistance have been created to safeguard life in the communities. These experiences serve as space for organizing political participation and promoting the deepening of democracy; in fact, profoundly democratic alternatives are drafted and designed there, within the margins of a logic imposed by colonial mentality. And it is important that the future begins to be built considering these alternatives that fluctuate between "utopia and realism." It should be emphasized that there may be contradictions or diversity in these proposals, and that indigenous peoples also have heterogeneous worldviews. But when we study these modes of coexistence, we can understand how worldviews and organization modes go hand in hand and produce strength and momentum to "disrupt and sabotage the projects of domination," without it seeming "like an essence that should be maintained, that should be protected from contamination by external forces, or an archaic form of the past".[14] Moreover, these processes also allow indigenous movements to

[14]Tzul Tzul, Gladys (2017), "Sistemas de gobierno comunal indígena: la organización de la reproducción de la vida." ("translated by author") In: https://horizontescomunitarios.wordpress.com/2017/01/16/apantle1/. Accessed 01 May 2021.

obtain enough legitimacy with their communities and facilitate their work being built on solid grounds.

29.3.2 Safeguarding Life

Now we know that the destruction of forest areas will be irrefutably linked to the expanse of the pandemic, and we can confidently state that the destruction of this habitat intrinsically implies the destruction of the "lungs of the planet," and that the global CO_2 absorption capacity decreases every day. Although it is essential to point out that the destruction of the planet's lungs implies the direct destruction of the lungs of living beings, it should also be noted that Latin American indigenous communities have built a countermodel to resist the colonial mode of life based on the exploitation of resources. One third of rainforests in Latin America are protected by different indigenous peoples who have historically preserved their biodiversity by using their resources sustainably; this translates into 815 million acres of forest areas in the region, which is at least nine times the area of Germany. Unfortunately, there is heavy pressure to exploit these forests, exerted not only by China, but also by Europe and North America. According to the World Wildlife Fund (WWF), Germany's import of soy, palm oil, beef, wood, cocoa, and other products contributes on its own to the destruction of about 106,000 hectares of forest each year.

A study conducted by the Fund for the Development of the Indigenous Peoples of Latin America and the Caribbean (FILAC)[15] confirms that reaffirming and revitalizing indigenous cultures and their ancestral knowledge are essential for preserving forests and life. Recent studies such as this one show that communities with traditional knowledge are better at forest conservation. The effort of indigenous communities is going to be essential for recovering health and recovering as a society in the post-pandemic period. What is particularly relevant about these experiences is that the indigenous communities themselves have determined their own measurements and forms of organization, thus contributing to the planetary well-being and to building a narrative that contradicts the inescapable need to exploit natural resources. And the same has been observed during the pandemic, from self-quarantines and self-generated medical processes, to the closure of territories; the responses have been varied, but they have always been characterized by these processes, which are based on the communities' own participation systems. An example of how resiliency is built and of the extent to which indigenous peoples must adapt can be observed in the Yagan community. This group from the south of Chile has used the prolonged lockdown to extensively teach the youngsters about its ancestral practices and promote that these practices become part of a more resilient modality in critical times.[16]

29.3.3 When Subalterns Organize Themselves

It is possible to find a series of proposals that originate in the large urban centers of the Global South, be it in Johannesburg, Sao Paulo, or Manila. Young people and women organize themselves and create new forms of action and knowledge that go beyond the familiar but ineffective solutions of the GN. The considerable disruptions experienced by the Southern populations contrast with the resiliency developed in marginalized communities. How can Latin America be described, then, after the first year of the pandemic? Poverty and inequalities have increased, economies collapsed, and, after the first vaccines became available, corruption came swiftly behind. In 2020, many health ministers in the region stepped down. We cannot put aside the problems of a young generation that has few chances of completing school and even less of

[15] http://www.fao.org/americas/publicaciones-audio-video/forest-gov-by-indigenous/en/. Accessed 01 May 2021.

[16] Blanco-Wells, G., Libuy, M., Harambour, A., et al. Plagues, past, and futures for the Yagan canoe people of Cape Horn, southern Chile. *Maritime Studies* **20**, 101–113 (2021). https://doi.org/10.1007/s40152-021-00217-2. Accessed 01 May 2021.

finding a dignified job. Women have been particularly affected because poverty, migration, and violence against them have increased. It is not an overstatement to claim then that the health crisis has become a humanitarian crisis as well.[17]

Even so, are things mostly tragic and despairing in the Latin American panorama? The pandemic came at a very turbulent time for Latin America; despite the safety recommendations, there have been massive demonstrations in Argentina, Chile, and Colombia. At first, it was hard to conceive protests taking place during the health crisis. The Bolivian elections and the sweeping victory that allowed the MAS party to return to office; the victory of Argentinian women when the pro-abortion law was passed; the emphatic victory in the Chilean referendum to revoke the constitution written during the military dictatorship; the removal of the transitional government in Peru; and the large number of votes obtained by left-wing candidates in the Ecuadorian elections paint a clear picture of an active and combative continent. If we wished to analyze who has played a significant part in Latin American social movements, we could identify some historically marginalized groups, such as organized young people and women, especially in Argentina, Mexico, Chile, and Peru. But it is impossible to observe these struggles without also considering the increasingly visible part indigenous populations are playing.[18]

Contrary to expectations, collective struggles have intensified during the pandemic. In 2020, there was a boost in the use of social media, given that militant struggles knew they urgently needed to create networks and modes of immediate action. It should also be noted that sensibility in the face of corruption also increased considerably; in fact, what is now known as "Vacunagate"[19] some years ago would not have even made it to a footnote. The violent irruption of the virus in personal and collective lives, as well as the uncertainty of the future, have contributed to making the population aware of the importance of not overlooking corruption of any kind. The immediate response of the Peruvian youth to the violence exerted by the transitory government of Manuel Merino—which took the lives of two young people—shows that the tolerance toward governmental violence and corruption has indubitably decreased. Merino's government did not last a single week in power. In Colombia, Mexico, Guatemala, Paraguay, and Costa Rica, social protests have escalated as well, stirred by different causes, such as political violence in Colombia, corruption in Guatemala, and women's struggles in Mexico. Despite the current crisis of unimaginable proportions, Latin America has mobilized beyond the obvious. In fact, during the regional elections in Brazil, President Jair Bolsonaro also experienced some backlash.

Certainly, some movements in Latin America are also of ambivalent character, and not all narratives successfully turn struggles into social movements. The specific circumstances in some regions have allowed politicians such as Daniel Ortega in Nicaragua, Nicolás Maduro in Venezuela, or Nayib Bukele in El Salvador to either expand their power or at least violently hold on to their power through the use of force.

In contrast, in 2020, for the first time in 60 years, Cuban officers had to converse with young people about their specific demands regarding freedom of speech and artistic freedom. Latin America is in motion: the organization of its communities does not necessarily stem from a set of ideological demands, but is a consequence of social discontent, especially as women, young people, and indigenous groups have positioned themselves as a subject of rights.

[17]The *Lancet*. Editorial. 396(10261):1463, November 07, 2020. https://www.thelancet.com/journals/lancet/article/PIIS0140-6736(20)32328-X/fulltext. Accessed 01 May 2021.

[18]Turkewitz, J., Villamil, S.A., Biles, J. (3 May 2021). Indigenous Colombians, facing new wave of brutality, demand government action. https://www.nytimes.com/2020/10/24/world/americas/colombia-violence-indigenous-protest.html. Accessed 01 May 2021.

[19]Romo, R. (18 February 2021). A chronicle of scandal foretold: Vaccine furor highlights long history of misconduct by elected officials in Peru. https://edition.cnn.com/2021/02/18/americas/peru-vaccine-scandal-analysis-latam-intl/index.html. Accessed 01 May 2021.

29.3.4 The Hispanic Paradox

If we look north of the Rio Bravo, we may understand how Latin American people manage to survive in challenging contexts, in increasingly worse socioeconomic circumstances, regardless of whether they live in the north or south of the continent. In the United States of America, scholars have observed and studied a phenomenon called *the Hispanic paradox*. An example of this paradox in action is that the Hispanic population in the U.S. has better health rates than white people, who are financially more privileged. Despite living in poverty and experiencing social exclusion, the rates of suicide, alcoholism, and drug overdose are below average in this segment of the population.

In the era of COVID-19, we have witnessed other signs of this paradox. The pandemic has had a violent effect on this already marginalized population, especially on people who do not have health insurance or who have an irregular migratory status.[20] From the very beginning, solidarity networks were established, whether they were spontaneously created groups, Hispanic churches, or existing organizations. There is plenty of evidence, especially in the U.S., confirming that both formal and informal solidarity and mutual support networks have significant effects on the recipients' survival and quality of life during challenging seasons. And these are not inspiring or anecdotical examples, but actual processes that safeguard life itself. In fact, the life expectancy of Hispanic people in the US is 81.8 years, exceeding that of white people.[21] Despite former President Trump's racist discourse, which considered Latinos an imminent danger, by naming them drug dealers or violent threats, mutual solidarity, accompaniment, and the premise that "No one should be left on their own" contribute to creating resilience. We can observe this model all throughout the Americas, whether in neighborhood organizations, groups of women, or indigenous communities. The precarious situation of many people forces them to depend on direct and active solidarity from organized collectives. It is the case of soup kitchens run by neighbors, or of the Uruguayan network "Contagiando Solidaridad" [Spreading Solidarity], which was created a week after the pandemic was declared, in March 2020. It was a joint effort of several trade unions, and it consists of 30 soup kitchens that depend on the support of neighbor organizations and individuals. This kind of network is not new but is merely an expression of the so-called "unionized pots," which usually emerge in times of financial crisis or natural disasters. And it is possible to find this kind of neighborly form of solidarity all throughout Latin America. Collective responses to catastrophes have played a decisive part in the construction of resiliency, and in many cases, they have been the most effective strategy to combat adverse situations. There are innumerable examples of this, such as the spontaneous organization of the Mexican youth after the earthquakes that took place in September 2017, in Mexico City. Back then, they organized food and medical supply chains, and even rescue actions.

Another aspect of the pandemic that is particularly significant is the hastened production of knowledge in the GS. There has been a rapid and wide production of texts, as well as a thorough criticism of the system that has led Latin America to collapse. Many studies have provided alternatives to current development models, and the production of virtual anthologies about the pandemic has been prolific.[22]

If we observe the processes surrounding the COVID-19 pandemic, we can state without a

[20]Andrade, A., Biles, J. (2020). Latin American immigrants in New York face Covid-19 crisis (2020). https://nacla.org/covid-latin-american-immigrants. Accessed 1 May 2021.

[21]Kristof, N. (27 June 2020). June now is a time to learn from Hispanic Americans. https://www.nytimes.com/2020/06/27/opinion/sunday/hispanic-americans.html. Accessed 1 May 2021.

[22]The extensive production of texts and discussion posts on the pandemic becomes notably evident at N-1 Edições, a Brazilian publisher. Essays and short stories, among other things, are published under the hashtag "Pandemia Critica." The majority of contributions originate in countries of the Global South and are accessible free of charge on the website. https://www.n-1edicoes.org/textos. Accessed 01 May 2021.

doubt that some of the actions implemented to stop the spread of the virus have been erratic and eruptive. Many decisions have been taken spontaneously, and their actual scope may not be entirely clear because they are disposed of and reformulated as promptly as they are taken, without being satisfactorily evaluated. We have also observed that the measures proposed by the GN correspond to contexts very different from the Southern realities. These measures are based on the premise that there is a good social security coverage, that there is an adequate health system, that people have access to basic services (such as clean water), and above all, that there is a reliable democratic margin that is noticeable in the decision-making process. This poses a relevant question: is it necessary to find solutions for the pandemic that can be adapted to the Southern contexts? We should be mostly concerned with finding solutions based on the strengths originating from the perspectives and contexts of the South. These strengths can be family ties or even informal or neighborly support networks. Moreover, we should not overlook the religious factor, which is a stronger and more substantial organizational element in the South than in the GN.

29.4 Epistemologies Are Relocating

I am hopeful that the Global South can become a center of transformation, and that marginal experiences will shed light on how to carry on with our lives, without exceptions. We should not only discuss how to reconstruct the world after the pandemic, but how we want to rebuild it as well. We should not only consider narratives that are set in the present, but also those that include the past and the future, those that are based on the premise of making the world livable in the long run.

Despite its erratic quality, the fight against COVID-19 has taken on a vertiginous speed. If we remember that the disease was particularly cruel in the early stages of the pandemic, right after the virus started spreading outside China and disseminated uncontrollably in Italy, the rest of Europe, and the U.S.—which at some point was the most affected country in the world—it is understandable that tests and vaccines were developed unusually fast. But it is also valid to ask why the response has not been as swift in the case of epidemics that mostly affect the South. The attention given to COVID-19 is quite contrasting when it is compared to the indifference surrounding the AIDS pandemic and several other modern epidemics.

If we wish to overcome this crisis, which will last longer than the presence of the virus itself, we should shift our point of view depending on our ability and desire to understand the world. In a relatively short period of time, we had to face a global disaster of unknown proportions. It was a time in which the GN set the pace, and the whole world had to follow. Meanwhile, the South, with its lack of structures and resources, was neither consulted nor included in the search for solutions. The pillage of the South was and still is the source of the region's weakness in the face of this violent pandemic. When a nation spends 1.8% of its GDP on health and 7.8%[23] on paying its foreign debt, it becomes heartbreakingly obvious how problematic indifference and constant looting have been. The inability of the GN to come up with solutions is not new and is not only characteristic of this pandemic; it is also noticeable in other failures, such as the fight against the climate catastrophe.

What could help us survive in the future? I would argue that we should at least consider certain aspects, such as looking at things from the perspective of others, without seeing the South and its experiences merely as a research subject but by getting rid of the magnifying glass of research and building an approach that stems from the experience of otherness to develop an understanding of how other worlds are possible because they emerge from other modes of think-

[23] Munevar, D. (12 March 2020). Covid-19 and debt in the global south: Protecting the most vulnerable in times of crisis. European network on debt and development. https://www.eurodad.org/covid19_debt1. Accessed 01 May 2021.

ing and living. This epistemic disobedience, to use Walter Mignolo's term, can lead us to farther places and show us the detailed realities of struggle and change, which in turn might give us a taste of what the future could look like. It might lead us far from the air-conditioned office in New York and take us on a boat through the Amazon and surprise us and make us wonder how it was possible to come all this way, with our mind set on the future of the new generations and a clear memory of how we managed to arrive safely here.

A deep self-understanding has fostered the survival of many marginal communities; in fact, indigenous groups have been able to survive because their spirituality and ancestral knowledge instill in them the strength to come through. This spirituality is undoubtedly linked to a profound knowledge of complex interrelationships, but mostly to a knowledge that diametrically opposes the Western exploitation of natural resources for profit. And that is the point: that the experiences that have been marginalized, trivialized, or even declared irrelevant become central and promote a production of knowledge that entwines different kinds of marginalization and oppression. What can we learn from the lives of stigmatized, marginalized, and oppressed people? We might obtain answers about life in general, but mostly about fostering a good life for everyone. This is about more than just coexisting inclusively. It is about doubting the conventional ways of producing knowledge. It is about inquiring where, why, and how power is underpinned, and who is responsible for it. To make changes, it is necessary to "change perspectives," especially through hermeneutical suspicion of those who have not been at the center so far. The pain, utopias, and poems of excluded communities are crucial hermeneutic mediations for the creation of new epistemic approaches. This is an epistemology based on the suffering and obstinate resistance of the groups who fight for a dignified and fair existence. And it implies placing marginalized communities at the base of hermeneutics in general.

The everyday reality of the destruction of the foundations of life forces us to come up with propositions that clearly break with the victorious attitude white Europeans have assumed toward nature, subaltern peoples, and lives that do not adjust to the moral compass of European modernity. It is not about forgetting their violent history or about hiding colonial continuities under the rug of the exoticizing enthusiasm of meeting "the other." It is time to understand and to acknowledge that the Western model is contradictory in terms of its ideals and its actual materiality. It is a model that still concentrates intellectual and cultural power on one side, and that still holds the premise of white universality against the subjects who inhabit the zone of "not being."

Clearly, other models are not perfect either, but they have guaranteed the survival of their creators, despite the adversities they face, and have fostered a fairer life for them. We must learn not to speak about other narratives, to not embrace them inclusively while we smother them; we should just sit quietly and listen. There is a great deal of hope at the margins. The Western luxury of being hopeless is not allowed there. it is as unprecedented and unimaginable as the fact that Germany took advantage of nuclear energy for 2 generations and now has to put up with its waste for about 40,000 generations.

For the planet to survive, it is essential that subalterns speak up and provide alternatives. Are we living in apocalyptic times? Are we running out of air in more ways than one? Maybe it is as Brazilian indigenous leader Ailton Krenak says:

> When we consider the prospect of a time following the here and now, we dream of a world where we, humanity, must reinvent ourselves in order to survive. We have to bring forth different bodies, different feelings, dream different dreams in order to be welcomed into this world and to dwell in it.[24]

[24]Translated by author from Krenak, Ailton. Ideen um das Ende der Welt zu vertagen., München. btb- Verlag, 2021, p. 84.

30 Decolonising Safeguarding During a Pandemic: Lessons for Research Praxis in International Social Work

Leona Vaughn, Jassi Sandhar, and Geoffrey Omony

30.1 Introduction

'Safeguarding' is a central tenet of social work practice. It is an area of law, policy, and practice that has a long-standing tradition in the provision of services, especially to children and other groups of people classed as 'vulnerable' in the UK. In simple terms, it describes attempts to anticipate, avoid, and prevent harm from occurring to children and (some) adults by the State and other organisations, most explicitly through the child and 'vulnerable adults' safeguarding legislation and protection systems.[1]

It is a concept gaining increasing momentum globally, but what is a safeguarding harm and who is vulnerable? Vulnerability in UK legislation is assumed for all people under the age of 18 years and for adults who have specific needs relating to their experience of abuse or neglect (sometimes described as 'victim' or 'survivors') or to their disability, impairment or mental health. Harm in the legal sense is regularly, and some would argue out of necessity, imagined with bounded limitations. As physical (including sexual), emotional or psychological and financial abuse or neglect. Structural harms, or social harms, such as discrimination and poverty are rarely included within safeguarding assessments (Goddard & Myers, 2017). It is clear that these ideas within safeguarding are expectant with problematic ways of conceptualisation and application.

Turning to the context of UK international research and development, safeguarding is an issue which received intense scrutiny and consideration by Government and Research Councils following high-profile incidents exposed in 2018 of sexual exploitation and abuse in Haiti by non-governmental organisations undertaking development work.[2] The scope of safeguarding in international research was consequently defined more widely than the overlapping areas of research integrity and traditional research ethics approaches, ordinarily found within (academic) research practice. The UK Collaborative on Development Research (UKCDR), an umbrella

[1] In the UK, guidance for 'Working Together to Safeguard Children' (HM Government, 2018), brings together all the statutory instruments outlining legal duties for local government authorities in child protection. For adults, safeguarding legal responsibilities are defined by the Care Act, 2014 (HM Government, 2014).

[2] See Department for International Development (DFID) Enhanced Due Diligence: Safeguarding for External Partners (2018).

L. Vaughn (✉)
Faculty of Humanities and Social Sciences, University of Liverpool, Liverpool, UK
e-mail: leona.vaughn@liverpool.ac.uk

J. Sandhar
The Goldin Institute, Chicago, IL, USA

G. Omony
YOLRED, Gulu, Uganda

M. C. S. Gonçalves et al. (eds.), *The Coronavirus Crisis and Challenges to Social Development*, https://doi.org/10.1007/978-3-030-84678-7_30

group of UK research funding councils, defines safeguarding as follows:

> "...preventing and addressing 'any sexual exploitation, abuse or harassment of research participants, communities and research staff, plus any broader forms of violence, exploitation and abuse... such as bullying, psychological abuse and physical violence'." (Balch et al., 2020)

This definition, which started as a draft in 2019 (Orr et al.) and developed further following international consultation with those involved in international development research across the global community (Balch et al., 2020), has expanded the notion of safeguarding in three key ways for research.

First, by bringing together 'prevention' of harm and action to address harms as the areas of responsibility of those involved in development research (primarily for research funders, councils, and institutions but also for individual researchers). This expression of responsibility requires proactive considerations of potential harm and forward planning for remedial actions and procedures when harm occurs, at multiple stages of the research process.

Second, by extending 'safeguarding' beyond the scope of groups who are considered to be victims (especially children and women), research is challenged to consider researchers, participants and wider communities all as potential groups to experience harm because of, or during, the research process. This is incredibly important, as a limited view of children, women and disabled people especially as being exclusively and universally vulnerable, leaves research open to making sense of this new 'safeguarding' concept in a problematic paternalistic way.[3] In terms of communities that research need to safeguard, this expanded definition can include geographical communities, such as where research takes place; communities of interest, for example trafficking survivors; or communities of identity, for example communities who share a racialised identity.

Consequently, in doing so the expanded notion of safeguarding has thirdly broadened the conceptualisation of harm. 'Harm' is imagined as action or inaction which, unintentionally, intentionally or through neglect, is experienced as harmful or violent by individuals or communities. Expanding 'harm' to go beyond what can be seen in the physical sense encourages researchers to think about harms caused through methodological, pedagogical and epistemic approaches. It also thereby allows for structural violence, such as discrimination, poverty and oppression, to be considered as harms for which research can contribute to, mitigate or actively plan to disrupt and undo.

Research undertaken within the UKCDR consultation on defining safeguarding[4] identified that the term was understood differently in various ways around the world, and in some cases not understood as a concept or literally translatable at all (Balch et al., 2020). Nonetheless, common themes of participant 'protection' and the principle of work and research 'doing no harm' emerged in the feedback. What this can be taken to indicate is that even though safeguarding as a term is arguably a new concept for research generally, the challenges for protection and avoiding harm are longstanding, systemic, and even institutionalised within research institutions and indeed in social work. These challenges have been acutely heightened in the context of the global COVID-19 pandemic.

It is important to acknowledge that this chapter's considerations of safeguarding during the COVID-19 pandemic are firmly framed by a pedagogical and epistemological understanding of structural injustice. The pandemic continues to raise questions about the power imbalance between the Global North and the Global South,

[3]See, for example, 'Contextual Risk, Individualised Responses: An Assessment of Safeguarding Responses to Nine Cases of Peer-on-Peer Abuse' (Firmin, 2018).

[4]Dr. Leona Vaughn, co-author of this chapter, was the Research Director at University of Liverpool and led this international UKCDR consultation project with Professor Alex Balch. AKN projects were part of the consultation.

and the resultant inequity in terms of access to, and the quality of, health and resources (Renton & Vaughn, 2020b). In relationship to the African continent, it also raises questions reflecting the global movement—do Black Lives Matter to research?

From the earliest stages of the global pandemic, there was an abundance of problematic assertions, particularly in relation to prioritising African nations as 'test sites' for researching and developing a vaccine. This logic was often premised on the basis of people being poor, but furthermore it was also couched in the belief of some form of biological resistance within African people to a virus which was believed to be devastating Europe in comparison to the continent (Carter & Sanford III, 2020; Vaughn et al., 2020). This not only speaks to the racist perception of the acceptable disposability of African lives during this pandemic (United Nations Working Group of Experts on People of African Descent, 2020), but it also exemplifies how risk and harm are ethnocentrically imagined and therefore corroborate this chapter's standpoint. That is, that safeguarding can, in and of itself, be harmful depending upon the positionality of those who have the power to decide who and what is risky or harmful, and to whom (Aktar et al., 2020; Bruce-Raeburn, 2018; Daoust & Dyvik, 2021; Sandvik, 2019).

This conclusion was certainly part of the reflections on the nature of the recent abuses revealed to have been perpetrated by international non-governmental organisations (INGOs) doing international social work. The events have drawn criticism for, amongst many other things, the underlying continuing legacies of the neo-colonial relationships between the Global North and Global South which have come to characterise 'development' and 'aid' in such a way that allowed for such complacency about clearly abusive practices (Munck & Kleibl, 2019):

> "Is their [Non-Governmental Organisations] lack of accountability linked to the postcolonial continuation of 'othering', which facilitates these double standards based on categorisation and differentiation, followed by subordination of the 'other'?"
> (Munck & Kleibl, 2019, p. 48)

Safeguarding therefore clearly, depending on how risk, harm, and vulnerability are perceived in this setting, has both the potential to address structural injustices, or to reify them. Especially the injustices of racism and coloniality.

The concepts of risk, harm and vulnerability, are foundational to safeguarding praxis. However, defining these concepts is an exercise of power which is often, amongst other things, imagined in ways which are gendered, ableist, racialised, and classed (Brown, 2014; Finucane et al., 2000; Gustafson & Brunger, 2014; Olofsson et al., 2014). In this way, risk as a safeguarding concept and 'risk-work' (Horlick-Jones, 2005) as a safeguarding practice can be understood to be a colonial project.

The issue that this chapter addresses, therefore, is how coloniality of thought and practice (Ndlovu-Gatsheni, 2020; Quijano, 2000, p. 545; Tamale, 2020), is a significant hazard, if not the biggest hazard, to fair and effective safeguarding within international social work research. The reality is that social work in countries categorised as 'developing', those most directly targeted by the United Nations Sustainable Development Goals,[5] is riddled with colonial logics as a legacy of both physical and psychological colonisation (Bhambra, 2020; Fanon, 1952; Hesse, 2007; Horvath, 1972; Mignolo, 2011, 2016; Munck & Kleibl, 2019; Rutazibwa, 2020). In researching international social work, or undertaking international research as part of social work, safeguarding's vulnerability to 'coloniality' is therefore elevated.

Colonial logics can manifest in how safeguarding concepts are interpreted. Exclusively envisaging risk and safety through a Western perspective; positioning Global South in the permanent role of 'risky' or 'vulnerable' and using the terms to 'other', control, subjugate or exclude, are the most obvious. More subtly, however, they appear in forms of safeguarding which are

[5]The United Nations 2030 Sustainable Development Goals (SDGs) were established in 2015 as 'a plan of action for people, planet and prosperity.' See United Nations (2015) *Transforming our World: The 2030 Agenda for Sustainable Development*.

process, policy and compliance driven, but not driven by the needs of victims and survivors; safeguarding that is focused on individual harms but not systemic harms and safeguarding that fails to address the implicit power dynamics within international development research.

In other words, colonial mentalities are issues we need to 'safeguard' ourselves from in research – they cause harm to the research, the researcher, the participants, and the wider communities. A commitment to exploring, promoting, and interrogating concepts of safeguarding is an essential part of working to achieve equity and social justice. This may be understood under different nomenclatures such as 'anti-oppressive practice' or 'anti-racist practice' but fundamentally they are the touchstones of contemporary, politically engaged radical social work (Dominelli, 1996; Lutz & Kleibl, 2020; McDermott et al., 2021; Palattiyil et al., 2019).

Indeed, as COVID-19 has exposed global structural inequalities and the unequal burdens felt by the pandemic on society's most marginalised or at-risk groups, it has also provided a unique opportunity to reassess power hierarchies, structural inequalities, and systems of oppression, from which the importance of safeguarding and decolonising international social work can be situated. However, the concept 'safeguarding' itself runs the risk of becoming both a meaningless buzzword, which is implemented by Global North scholars and practitioners and imposed on Global South partners or becoming weaponised as another neo-colonial tool that will serve to protect INGOs and not people (Bruce-Raeburn, 2018). The rush by researchers to prove the relevance of their work on international social work during this pandemic is in danger of reverting to extractive practice (Kiconco, 2020) – that is, research that bears little or no relevance and provides no benefit, or even is a disbenefit, to participants.

In this sense, safeguarding needs to decolonise conceptually and become actively anticolonial in praxis. We must ask ourselves, as researchers, how do we disrupt colonial logics in research into social work issues especially when the global crises of COVID-19 and Black Lives Matter have laid bare entrenched structural inequity, power imbalances and discrimination? How do we decolonise?

30.2 Methodology

This chapter builds on from the research project *'Enhancing Safeguarding in Efforts to Address Modern Slavery through the UN's Sustainable Development Goals'*, a University of Liverpool-led Antislavery Knowledge Network[6] (AKN) Arts and Humanities Research Council (AHRC) Network Plus initiative which ran from August 2019 to July 2020. The findings from our explorations within this project on safeguarding in the field of antislavery is used throughout this chapter to highlight lessons for how coloniality can be not only avoided, but for how better future research can be imagined.

The work explored and assessed local safeguarding practice and methods in existing AKN projects that were using arts and humanities methods to develop community-based responses to trafficking and modern slavery. Through establishing equitable partnerships and utilising a range of creative approaches, we collaboratively critiqued and expanded concepts of 'power', 'dignity,' and 'voice' that are central to understanding of safeguarding within the context of research in the antislavery and anti-trafficking field (Renton & Vaughn, 2020a). One of our project partners, YOLRED,[7] is a community-based organisation led by, and for, former child soldiers

[6]The Antislavery Knowledge Network (AKN) is an AHRC/GCRF funded project (2017–2021) led by a coalition of Universities based in Ghana and the UK. It supports research and innovative and impactful work to address exploitation and contemporary slavery in Africa using approaches from the arts and humanities. This growing network explores how approaches from the arts and humanities can address contemporary forms of enslavement by adopting a community-engaged, human rights focus that delivers development impacts: www.liverpool.ac.uk/politics/research/research-projects/akn/.

[7]Youth Leaders for Restoration and Development, YOLRED: www.yolred.org.

in Northern Uganda, and works to facilitate peacebuilding and social cohesion in the war-affected Northern region. YOLRED have partnered with AKN since 2018, and since 2019 have worked with the network to support the safeguarding project as well as develop their own internal safeguarding policies and practices. YOLRED's programmes are participatory in nature and utilise various art-based methodologies and practices; their programmes are demand-driven and place the survivors of the conflict at the heart of all activities through a process of co-design, co-facilitation, and co-production.

In common with all other research initiatives, AKN has been faced with inevitable adjustments to its planned activities and concerns about the impact of the pandemic on antislavery and anti-human-trafficking research and services. The unfolding pandemic magnified some of the issues this work had already began to reveal when we began to explore how safeguarding could be strengthened and reoriented to the needs of impacted communities in the regions we work, rather than the researchers and their institutions. In short, the coloniality of the thinking within work to 'safeguard' or protect researchers and participants from harm amplified the need for decolonising this foundational issue within collaborative and co-developed research in this field of social work/welfare.

Accordingly, with the agreement of the AHRC, funds that were originally designated for a final face-to-face event on safeguarding were redirected to AKN partners in Kenya and Uganda to carry out additional assessments on the COVID theme. This rapid assessment, based on conversations with key informants in both 2020 and 2021, focused on pandemic-related changes noted in the understanding of safeguarding; emerging or heightened risks, harms, and vulnerabilities; and impacts on the demand for or supply of services for those affected by modern slavery, human trafficking, or other forms of violence. To map out some of the increased safeguarding needs of the beneficiaries of civil society groups during the pandemic (also referred to as clients and service-users), YOLRED held a series of conversations with five civil society employees and service-providers based in Uganda, to better understand the heightened risks for social workers and their clients during the pandemic, and to also inform YOLRED's own programming and how to better serve the communities they support. These individuals represent NGOs working for war-affected individuals, refugees, marginalised women and children, and former child soldiers. The findings for this chapter are supported by this mapping and assessment.

30.3 Safeguarding Lessons in Praxis during COVID-19

This section reflects on the emerging work looking at safeguarding in international development as well as the impacts of the pandemic on communities within the Global South (Aktar et al., 2020; Bruce-Raeburn, 2018; Daoust & Dyvik, 2021; Sandvik, 2019). Assessment information may well be specific to the work of YOLRED and other small community-based NGOs, but the lessons and takeaways are transferable to other contexts of international development partnership.

30.3.1 Understanding the Concept

The burgeoning attention being afforded to principles of safeguarding of late has contributed towards the term itself being increasingly recognised by local actors in the Global South (Daoust & Dyvik, 2021). Safeguarding, although not a new consideration for many local civil society organisations (CSOs), was deemed a necessity by social workers who acknowledged the vital role of implementing safeguarding measures within their organisations, and how, when designing and putting in place new programmes or interacting with their beneficiaries, questions about how to best protect all involved are situated within this. For some, the principle of 'safeguarding' was located within, or an extension of, the long-standing 'do no harm' principle and thus is not an entirely new undertaking (Sandvik, 2019).

There are indeed limitations to the phrase, both in its operationalisation and in its ontological essence. A director of an NGO in Uganda spoke of how the concept assumes that social or humanitarian workers have the ability to make certain at-risk or socially excluded groups feel safe, even when their security has already been disrupted, and their sense of safety has been removed from them. The example was given of survivors of sexual violence who were residing in refugee camps. These individuals would have witnessed and endured a series of tragic events, so their sense of safety has to go beyond the rhetoric of ensuring they are not exploited within organisational activities. In these situations, safeguarding work was felt to be relational, prioritising restoring faith and hope in people for their immediate and future safety.

How the concept of safeguarding was understood amongst beneficiary groups was more complex. Within some community groups, all that safeguarding entails was not fully understood. Various power dynamics can influence the way individuals position themselves when they require the support of service providers. Some feel quite powerless, vulnerable, and do not fully understand their position or rights within these spaces (particularly children or minors) (Daoust & Dyvik, 2021). This ambiguity about individual rights, control, and personal well-being amongst beneficiaries is also common within Global North/Global South research projects. In YOLRED's experience, through their role as intermediary during these kinds of projects, they have found that many participants, who are often former child soldiers, will engage in research from feelings of obligation to the CSO/NGO and pressure from the international researchers. They can feel under social pressure and are often hopeful for some form of benefit (individual, family, or community). Beneficiaries become bound by power dynamics, even more so if the researcher is white. Consequently, they are neither fully comprehending their rights to be safe within these spaces nor recognising the power and control they can and should assert.

30.3.2 COVID-19 Safeguarding Impacts on Service Planning and Delivery

COVID-19 and pandemic safety measures have led to several disruptions in the provision of services from civil society groups, often hitting the most impoverished communities the hardest through increasing need for basic survival, that is, food, shelter, and clothing (Sánchez-Páramo, 2020; Valensisi, 2020). The significant increase in food prices in Northern Uganda, coupled with losses or halts in many livelihoods, has resulted in an increased number of people being unable to fulfil their most basic needs (Macdonald & Owor, 2020; Olum, 2020). The responsibilities of service providers to safeguard individuals throughout the pandemic remain, but their clients' expectations and needs have changed.

Restrictions on organisational mobility has also halted many programmes, particularly those which involve community mobilisation, a vital component of the work of organisations like YOLRED. In assessing how local communities were coping under pandemic safety measures and how they could best support them, YOLRED found that, with the socioeconomic impacts of lockdown measures, families were struggling to meet their basic needs. In response, YOLRED diverted their own funds ring-fenced for social cohesion and peacebuilding initiatives to provide critical supplies to families struggling to survive (Olum, 2020).

NGOs/CSOs reported specific issues about access to beneficiaries, further impacting their ability to deliver services:

Inability to fully assure themselves of safeguarding practices: Pre-COVID most staff within the service providers were trained on safeguarding policies and how to adhere to these standards, and most believed that their staff, as they had been working with their clients for many years and understood their unique requirements, were continuing to strongly obey these principles. However, organisations relayed that carrying out safeguarding checks on employees and how the organisation was fulfilling its safeguarding responsibilities during the pandemic had been difficult to assess. Activities were not being carried out as normal, so there was little way of exploring any changes. In terms of providing training on safeguarding during the pandemic, this was proven a challenge as all staff were working from home, often with no access to laptops or reliable Wi-Fi.

Inability to reach clients: Social distancing, restricted movement, and lack of the requisite technology, or access to technology, caused an inability to reach many clients or service users. In regular organisational activities, staff would routinely visit community groups residing in villages or remote areas so they could monitor their safety and wellbeing. The ability to manage safeguarding complaints had been affected because the regular channels or access to support systems to register complaints (i.e., civil society organisations) had become limited. A manager of one NGO stated that even if issues were reported, for example, a phone call is received from a client regarding domestic violence or harm, then you were still unable to do much about it with the lockdown and restrictions on mobility. A further example was provided, acknowledging those fleeing gender-based violence who may get stopped by the police or authorities, but would not want to disclose why they were not obeying lockdown, which would result in some sort of reprimand.

Lack of access to information on COVID: Many communities residing in villages or within refugee camps are receiving limited information on COVID because they lack access to the Internet. Official communications about the virus and staying safe are reportedly not being channelled effectively through any other methods. Hearsay, rumours, and lack of information heightened fear of the virus and often causes tension between community members.

Inability to protect individuals: Service providers, pre-COVID, were able to monitor the physical and emotional well-being of their beneficiaries, and able to provide spaces away from potential harm, for example, through moving individuals away from their communities/homes and into libraries and schools. Many beneficiaries did not have access to technology or mobiles, and so were unable to seek information about where to go should they require assistance or support. Understanding the needs of certain beneficiary groups and determining ways to safeguard them also relies on physical face-to-face and in-person assessment of emotions and reactions. Psychosocial support and counselling taking place via the phone (if it could take place at all) came with its own set of risks. It is difficult to read body language or understand if someone is in danger via a phone. For one organisation, they reported this as an issue when working with male survivors of sexual assault. Survivors are socialised to perform masculinity in a certain way, often compounded by their experiences of sexual violence, and as such may exhibit extreme anger. Their support needs, therefore, can only be accurately identified during engagement with those who are trained to recognise the signs of such mental distress. For those who are untrained in identifying these signs, and thus misinterpret responses of anger or aggression, then that relationship can become damaged very quickly and any potential to help them is lost.

30.3.3 Power Dynamics and Capacity

Where service providers had existing funding partnerships, on the whole most funders had been understanding of the change in working practices in this early stage of the pandemic. Adjustments were being negotiated by most organisations, including a shift in programme priorities, working patterns, and revised workplan outputs. One NGO director spoke of how some funders had been slightly more demanding and had required new workplans/budgets and timelines within 1 week of lockdown. This requirement presented a burden when organisations were attempting to manage their working conditions, balance simultaneous demands, and ensure that all staff were safe and able to look after their families. Organisations were also involved in the urgent task of mobilising medical supplies and personal protective equipment (PPE) to clients. Having to prioritise funders' demands whilst feeling like this should not be a priority; however, it had to be accepted for fear that funding and projects would be jeopardised.

Managing new safeguarding concerns are also made more difficult when funders change priorities or impose restrictions on resource allocation. The priorities for many beneficiaries or clients change, and the most urgent needs become obtaining food for their families, medical supplies, and paying rent, but convincing funders to repurpose funds within the bureaucratic structures of international funding is challenging. Many funders during the pandemic also postponed activities consequent to their own funding uncertainties and cuts, removing grants or beginning to rearrange their funding priorities as a result of COVID, with a number wanting to explore how the pandemic was impacting various aspects of people's lives. Subsequently, local organisations not working on COVID-19-related activities are having difficulties developing new partnerships or sourcing new funds for non-pandemic-related research or activities. The situation relayed was that whilst demand for services from CSOs/NGOs had increased, the level of financial support available to them was thought to have significantly decreased, especially for smaller NGOs with less capacity to develop new proposals or spend time reaching new potential donors. This problem placed vulnerable beneficiaries at risk of further harm.

30.4 The Urgency for Decolonising Safeguarding Praxis in International Social Work and Research

In this time of COVID, when the insidious nature of inequalities and coloniality are becoming increasingly obvious, especially in North–South global relationships, international social work has a pivotal role (Lutz & Kleibl, 2020). Safeguarding has the potential to become a tool for decolonising the dynamics in international work, but, as our research shows, only if it is itself first thoroughly conceptually decolonised and then actively practised throughout the life cycle of research (Vaughn, 2020b). Avoiding harm in the design and delivery of research, especially in this context of work with trafficked and abused children and young people, means co-developing and applying anticolonial approaches to processes for research and knowledge production. This approach is of the utmost importance when it is a relationship wherein Global North researchers are undertaking research into social work in a Global South setting:

> "To ensure that risk, harm and vulnerability are locally defined and the responses are locally led, owned and sustained, Global North researchers have to be ready and willing to give up some of their power in this relationship."
> (Renton & Vaughn, 2020)

Power should not only be acknowledged and addressed through reflexive practice but should also be proactively and intentionally shared. This process of empowering is demonstrated, for example, through self-identification of risk and harm and the co-development of safeguarding practice and theory, which is shaped by and centres victims and survivors. Through our experience, we observed how the rush to deliver research to capture the 'COVID' moment or even to advance our understanding of COVID-19 and its impacts risked a very real potential for an abuse of power, even by well-intentioned actions, and for forgetting to place people's rights and dignity at the heart of the work.

The calls for 'rapid' assessments on the impacts of COVID-19 introduces funding and timeline pressures that potentially jeopardise or undermine ethics and principles of fairness and 'doing no harm' in research. COVID-19 restrictions on international travel, for example, have seen an increase in projects utilising virtual fieldwork, which requires the use of technology to obtain data. Online/virtual interviews may have benefits, such as being cost- and time effective and more environmentally friendly, but also have disadvantages (Vaughn, 2020a). Free and informed consent for involvement is a prerequisite of ethically sound research; the participant should understand what the research is about and how it benefits them. This concept can lack clarity when it is virtual. In addition, the most marginalised, impoverished, or remote communities who do not have access to adequate technology, or do not possess the digital skills and knowledge required to engage in virtual projects, will inevitably become absent from future research (Sah et al., 2020). Therefore, the populations who are in greatest need of the potential positive outcomes of COVID-19-related research are those least likely to be able to access these projects.

Many marginalised or vulnerable groups generally appreciate when researchers engage in slower-paced research and come to know them and their culture over a long period of time. Carrying out virtual fieldwork could indicate a lack of commitment or unwillingness to wait until post pandemic to carry out the research project. Even if gatekeepers or interlocutors are able to provide these technologies on behalf of potential participants, it is likely to feel artificial, distressing, or uncomfortable as they would not have carried out research through these mediums previously. It particularly may not work when trying to build trust and rapport with communities. In YOLRED's case, for example, their beneficiaries may not feel comfortable engaging in an interview with someone, particularly someone unfamiliar to them, via a screen, as the human interaction or face-to-face comfort is not there as would be with a physical presence.

Participatory or action-based work or research is advocated as empowering methodological approaches and practices for working with vulnerable communities (Gustafson & Brunger, 2014; Ruszczyk et al., 2020), but clearly this can be a challenge with pandemic safety measures. The need to safeguard against problematic research practices being reintroduced for the sake of expediency is paramount.

It is therefore especially important for researchers or project implementers to reflect on their own positionality, particularly their own epistemic location, and consider their actual contribution within this space. In YOLRED's experience, and amongst their beneficiaries, there remains an internalised belief in the 'white saviour'; that is, any projects or support provided by international white people (including those perceived as 'white'), that is, *mzungus*, will be, by nature, inherently good. This belief, combined with the unequal power dynamics and disparities in privilege, make it hard for local civil society organisations (and their beneficiaries) to negotiate power and the terms for how they expect to be treated. Thus, it is even more crucial for Global North actors to recognise their responsibility in challenging and dismantling these neo-colonial structures.

30.5 Results: Key Takeaways from Working in a Pandemic for Future Improvement

We identify the following key takeaways from our work during the pandemic that will assist in decolonising safeguarding for international social work research, and thus improving the quality, depth, and richness in the knowledge we produce. These results relate to research projects: (1) co-creation of safeguarding policy, (2) co-design and planning, (3) co-design and implementation, and (4) co-production, co-dissemination, and co-communication of findings.

30.5.1 Co-Creating Safeguarding Policy and Practice

There is a need for local and national communities to be involved in the drafting of safeguarding policies and procedures at the outset of considerations of research ethics and safety. This condition is of particular importance to those most impacted by abuses of power and exploitation, as without their input and ownership then the tools for safeguarding simply replicate and uphold traditional and colonial power relationships and hierarchies (Balch et al., 2020; Daoust & Dyvik, 2021). In a situation of constant change, it is acutely important to make sure responsibilities in existing research or new research partnerships are clear in respect of reporting safeguarding concerns, that the process is understood and has fair expectations of responsibility.

30.5.2 Co-Design and Project/Research Planning

The authors advocate for co-developed and co-designed methods in all North–South projects, but the necessity of such becomes heightened during situations of constant change and uncertainty, especially where local pandemic safety measures dictate how projects or research can be conducted. The increase in funding calls for international development, and COVID-19-related research is indeed attractive for many Global North researchers, who will see these as opportunities to show the relevance of their expertise on global issues such as the pandemic. However, it is also an opportunity to reframe the way North–South research projects are conducted, by giving greater agency and control to local partners and researchers, which should be seized at once. When devising COVID-19-related research, it is crucial for Global North researchers to assess their positionality and motivations, and the incentives for local communities in partner countries to be involved. Furthermore, it is also an opportunity to meaningfully address power dynamics and imbalances, by encouraging projects to be demand driven and locally led, rather than just locally-delivered or locally implemented (Kok et al., 2017). In some regions where face-to-face research is currently permitted and safe, then the absence of the Global North researcher can actually produce an environment that facilitates more authenticity in the research data (Vaughn, 2020b). This care is particularly important for the pursuit of decolonising knowledge production and uplifting local knowledge sources, and ultimately to ensure research or project agendas are not exploitatively driven by agendas of the Global North.

30.5.3 Co-Design and co-Delivery

Co-developing methods and practice will enable projects to anticipate potential risk and harm, and plan to mitigate these. Any research that involves participants sharing their lived experiences, especially those that may be traumatic, should include "insiders" (Merton, 1972) in the processes of research design, delivery, and dissemination. This increases trust and rapport among researchers, participants, and wider communities, also facilitating better safeguarding practice. Insider research partners, such as YOLRED, have a familiarity with participants, an understanding of the sensitive nature of narratives, and nuanced knowledge on what is socially and culturally accepted within a given society or community setting.

It is especially important in this period for research to be co-produced with local partners or assistants and use appropriately and ethically locally employed researchers. International researchers attempting to do research remotely with communities/groups who are already pessimistic about engaging with foreign researchers is not ethical practice. In-country researchers are more familiar and known to communities, and able to connect at a better level.

Co-production, co-dissemination, and co-communication of findings for co-benefit co-produced research needs to be more localised and involve local people, their ideas, and perspectives, but not co-opted. The local people involved in supporting the design and delivery of the study should not be forgotten nor erased in the analysis and the research 'outputs.' Analysis should be informed by local knowledge. Researchers should find a way of collaboratively producing and sharing outputs with the participants and community that are of co-benefit. The language of traditional 'outputs,' such as reports or articles, are often inaccessible to local communities and, on a practical level, require participants to have access to technology to be able to obtain or access them. Consider how co-dissemination through trusted media or radio, community groups, or cultural organisations, for example, can help to avoid further epistemic injustices against already marginalised communities.

30.6 Conclusion: An Outlook for Future Critical and Political Social Work

COVID-19, and the global shifts in conceptualising work and research practices, offer a radical opportunity to reimagine the concept of safeguarding and how it can be used as an effective tool for decolonising future research in international social work. Safeguarding measures, such as 'do no harm,' should be recalibrated to examine how future research (particularly COVID-related research) could actually 'do some good'; making a substantial contribution to working towards equity for Global South communities whilst also furthering contributions to knowledge. Research findings and outputs being co-created and communicated with local communities in accessible formats and in local languages is crucial now, more than ever. This is a time when there are heightened anxieties about the pandemic, coupled with misinformation (or even lack of information) about the virus itself. Ensuring that participants and other communities who could benefit from the new knowledge created through our research, actually have access to it is essential to the decolonisation shift.

At this time, and in all future times, to decolonise safeguarding we need to collaboratively (researcher/participant/community) think about who may benefit from our research and who may be harmed by it. We should question, for example, if our work is perpetuating stereotypes or reinforcing imbalanced power relationships, and if so, thinking about how can we implement safeguarding principles to mitigate this.

Decolonial and socially-just social work research, critical and politically-engaged, can be appropriate if it takes place in a collaborative milieu. If research projects cannot be done collaboratively throughout the life cycle of the work, then we, as researchers, have a responsibility to consider if it is right for our project to even go ahead.

References

Aktar, B., Alam, W., Ali, S., Awal, A., Bayoh, M., Chumo, I., Contay, Y., Conteh, A., Dean, L., Dobson, S., Edstrom, J., Elsey, H., Farnaz, N., Garimella, S., Gray, L., Gupte, J. Hawkins, K., Hollihead, B., Josyula, K. L., … Wurie, H. (2020) How to prevent and address safeguarding concerns in global health research programmes: Practice, process and positionality in marginalised spaces. *British Medical Journal Global Health, 5*, e002253.

Balch, A., Garimella, S., Mansaray, B., Renton, L., Smith, A., Vaughn, L (2020). *Safeguarding in international development. Research report on phase 2 international consultation & guidance*. UKCDR. https://www.ukcdr.org.uk/guidance/safeguarding-resources/

Bhambra, G. K. (2020). Colonial global economy: Towards a theoretical reorientation of political economy. *Review of International Political Economy*. https://doi.org/10.1080/09692290.2020.1830831

Brown, K. (2014). Questioning the vulnerability zeitgeist: Care and control practices with 'vulnerable' young people. *Social Policy and Society, 13*(3), 371–387.

Bruce-Raeburn, A. (30 May 2018). *Opinion: Without systemic change, safeguarding will only keep INGOs safe — not people*. Devex: https://www.devex.com/news/opinion-without-systemic-change-safeguarding-will-only-keep-ingos-safe-not-people-92854.

Carter, C., Sanford, III, E (2020) The myth of black immunity: racialized disease during the COVID-19 Pandemic. Black perspectives. African American Intellectual History Society. 3 April 2020. https://www.aaihs.org/racializeddiseaseandpandemic/.

Daoust, G., & Dyvik, S. L. (2021). Reconceptualizing vulnerability and safeguarding in the humanitarian and development sector *Social Politics: International Studies in Gender, State & Society, 00*(0), 1–24.

Department for International Development (DFID). (2018). *Enhanced due diligence: Safeguarding for external partners*. HM Government. https://assets.publishing.service.gov.uk.government/uploads/system/uploads/attachment_data/file/767037/safeguarding-external-partners.pdf

Dominelli, L. (1996). Deprofessionalizing social work: Anti-oppressive practice, competencies and postmodernism. *The British Journal of Social Work, 26*(2), 153–175. https://doi.org/10.1093/oxfordjournals.bjsw.a011077

Fanon, F. (1952). Black Skin, White Masks. Reprint. Sidmouth: Pluto Press. 2008.

Finucane, M., Slovic, P., Mertz, C., Flynn, J., & Satterfield, T. (2000). Gender, race, and perceived risk: The 'white male' effect. *Health, Risk & Society, 2*(2), 159–172.

Firmin, C. (2018). Contextual risk, individualised responses: An assessment of safeguarding responses to nine cases of peer-on-peer abuse. *Child Abuse Review, 27*, 42–57.

Goddard, T., & Myers, R. R. (2017). Against evidence-based oppression: Marginalized youth and the politics of risk-based assessment and intervention. *Theoretical Criminology, 21*(2), 151–167.

Gustafson, D. L., & Brunger, F. (2014). Ethics, "vulnerability," and feminist participatory action research with a disability community. *Qualitative Health Research, 24*(7), 997–1005.

HM Government. (2014). *The care act 2014*. HM Government. https://www.legislation.gov.uk/ukpga/2014/23/part/1/crossheading/safeguarding-adults-at-risk-of-abuse-or-neglect/enacted

HM Government. (2018). *Working together to safeguard children*. HM Government. https://assets.publishing.service.gov.uk/government/uploads/system/uploads/attachment_data/file/942455/Working_together_to_safeguard_children_Statutory_framework_legislation_relevant_to_safeguarding_and_promoting_the_welfare_of_children.pdf

Hesse, B. (2007). Racialized modernity: An analytics of white mythologies. *Ethnic and Racial Studies, 30*(4), 643–663.

Horlick-Jones, T. (2005). On 'risk work': Professional discourse, accountability, and everyday action. *Health, Risk & Society, 7*(3), 293–307. https://doi.org/10.1080/13698570500229820

Horvath, R. J. (1972). A definition of colonialism. *Current Anthropology, 13*(1), 45–57.

Kiconco, A. (2020). Speaking about violence in Sierra Leone. In A. Bunting, A. Kiconco, & J. Quirk (Eds.), *Research as more than extraction? Knowledge production and sexual violence in post conflict African societies* (pp. 10–13). Beyond Trafficking and Slavery/OpenDemocracy.

Kok, M. O., Gyapong, J. O., Wolffers, I., Ofori-Adjei, D., & Ruitenberg, E. J. (2017). Towards fair and effective north–south collaboration: Realising a programme for demand-driven and locally led research. *Health Research Policy and Systems, 15*(96), 1–17.

Lutz, R., & Kleibl, T. (2020). Rethinking international social work. *Social Extra, 44*, 247–251. https://doi.org/10.1007/s12054-020-00289-0

Macdonald, A., & Owor, A. (2020). *The view from Gulu on Uganda's food distribution and corona-politics*. LSE Blogs. https://blogs.lse.ac.uk/africaatlse/2020/06/17/the-view-from-gulu-on-ugandas-food-distribution-and-corona-politics/

McDermott, C., Stafford, J. D., & Johnson, S. D. (2021). Racial equity as a human rights issue: Field agency practices and field instructors' knowledge and attitudes. *Journal of Human Rights and Social Work*. https://doi.org/10.1007/s41134-020-00155-9

Merton, R. (1972). Insiders and outsiders: A chapter in the sociology of knowledge. *American Journal of Sociology, 78*(1), 9–47.

Mignolo, W. (2011). The darker side of western modernity. Global futures, decolonial options. Duke University press.

Mignolo, W. (2016). Sustainable development or sustainable economies? Ideas towards living in harmony and plenitude. *Dialogue Civilizations Research Institute, 2016*, 1–29.

Munck, R., & Kleibl, T. (2019). NGOs and the political economy of international development and development education: An Irish perspective. *Policy & Practice: A Development Education Review, 29*, 31–53.

Ndlovu-Gatsheni, S. J. (2020). The cognitive empire, politics of knowledge and African intellectual productions: Reflections on struggles for epistemic freedom and resurgence of decolonisation in the twenty-first century. *Third World Quarterly*. https://doi.org/10.1080/01436597.2020.1775487

Olofsson, A., Zinn, J. O., Griffin, G., Giritli, N. K., Cebulla, A., & Hannah-Moffat, K. (2014). The mutual constitution of risk and inequalities: Intersectional risk theory. *Health, Risk & Society, 16*(5), 417–430.

Olum, D. (2020). *YOLRED provides critical supplies to families struggling to survive COVID-19*. Goldin Institute. https://www.goldininstitute.org/news/9-leadership-development/888-yolred-provides-critical-supplies-to-families-struggling-to-survive-covid-19

Palattiyil, G., Sidhva, D., Pawar, M., Shajahan, P., Cox, J., & Anand, J. C. (2019). Reclaiming international social work in the context of the global agenda for social work and social development: Some critical reflections. *International Social Work, 62*(3), 1043–1054.

Quijano, A. (2000). Coloniality of power and eurocentrism in Latin America. *Nepantla: Views From South. Duke University Press, 1*(3), 533–580.

Renton, L., & Vaughn, L. (2020a). Power, dignity and voice: Enhancing safeguarding in efforts to address modern slavery. In *Anti-slavery Knowledge Network*. University of Liverpool.

Renton, L., & Vaughn, L. (2020b). *Decolonising safeguarding in a pandemic: Who has the power to define risk and harm?* Discover Society. https://discoversociety.org/2020/05/12/decolonising-safeguarding-in-a-pandemic-who-has-the-power-to-define-risk-and-harm/

Ruszczyk, H. A., Upadhyay, B. K., Kwong, Y. M. C., Khanal, O., Bracken, L. J., Pandit, S., & Bastola, R. (2020). Empowering women through participatory action research in community-based disaster risk reduction efforts. *International Journal of Disaster Risk Reduction, 51*, 101763.

Rutazibwa, O. U. (2020). Hidden in plain sight: Coloniality, capitalism and race/ism as far as the eye can see. *Millennium Journal of International Studies, 48*(2), 221–241.

Sah, L. K., Singh, D. R., & Sah, R. K. (2020). Conducting qualitative interviews using virtual communication tools amid COVID-19 pandemic: A learning opportunity for future research. *Journal of Nepal Medical Association, 58*(232), 1103–1106.

Sánchez-Páramo, C. (23 April 2020). COVID-19 will hit the poor hardest. Here's what we can do about it. Voices*: Perspectives on Development*. World Bank Blogs. https://blogs.worldbank.org/voices/covid-19-will-hit-poor-hardest-heres-what-we-can-do-about-it

Sandvik, K. B. (2019). Safeguarding as humanitarian buzzword: An initial scoping. *Journal of International Humanitarian Action, 4*(3), 1–6.

Tamale, S. (2020). *Decolonisation and afro-feminism*. Daraja Press.

United Nations. (2015). Transforming our world: The 2030 agenda for sustainable development. www.sustainabledevelopment.un.org

United Nations Working Group of Experts on People of African Descent. (2020). Statement on COVID-19: Racial equity and racial equality must guide state action. 6 April 2020. United Nations Human Rights Office of the High Commissioner. https://www.ohchr.org/EN/NewsEvents/Pages/DisplayNews.aspx?LangID=E&NewsID=25768.0

Valensisi, G. (2020). COVID-19 and global poverty: Are LDCs being left behind? *The European Journal of Development Research, 32*, 1535–1557.

Vaughn, L. (2020a). *COVID-19 and safeguarding children's rights in research. European Children's Rights Unit, Briefing Paper #8*. University of Liverpool. https://www.liverpool.ac.uk/media/livacuk/law/2-research/ecru/Briefing,Paper,8,-,COVID-19,and,Safeguarding,Childrens,Rights,in,Research-Leona,Vaughn.pdf

Vaughn, L. (2020b). Can research be anticolonial? COVID-19 race and risk. https://covid19raceandrisk.wordpress.com/2020/07/08/can-research-be-anti-colonial/

Vaughn, L., Kiconco, A., Quartey, N. K., Smith, C. S., & Ziz, I. Z. (2020). COVID-19 and racialised risk narratives in South Africa, Ghana and Kenya. In *COVID-19 ODA rapid response research project report*. University of Liverpool.

31 Participatory Photography, Ethical Storytelling, and Modern Slavery Survivor Voices: Adapting to COVID-19

Aisha Ali Haji, Rehema Baya, Emily Brady, Helen McCabe, Yasmin Manji, and Sophie Otiende

31.1 Key Findings

Conducting a truly participatory research project between partners in the Global North and Global South brings challenges in normal circumstances, yet when the COVID-19 pandemic forced our project to pause, the challenge became even more difficult. Our research project—*Survivors' Voices, Stories and Images*—intended to train survivors of modern slavery in participatory photography and ethical storytelling techniques to empower them to tell their own stories. This chapter considers how both we (the research team) and the project's survivor-participants adapted its initial project brief to conduct a successful research project in the context of the COVID-19 pandemic. As such, this chapter seeks to answer the question: How did COVID-19 impact participatory social work in Kenya, and what could be done to improve this in future?

We reflect on the adaptations made to both the workshops and the wider project outputs, and assess both their positive and negative impacts. Crucially, the shift to remote working had unanticipated outcomes that we consider key findings of this project. These results include the benefits of pooling resources with other projects; using accessible technologies; increased need for language flexibility; the challenges and potential of virtual spaces to create "community"; and the increased need for one-on-one support. Following our experience on the project, we offer the following recommendations when considering remote participatory research methods: (1) a need for flexible aims, objectives, and outputs, and (2) a need to budget for additional resources to allow for unforeseen circumstances. As with all participatory research, the need to be participant led (in this case, survivor led) is paramount. Our research shows this is still possible, with due care and flexibility, even when working remotely and in a global pandemic.

31.2 Research Context

Modern slavery is an issue that continues to have a global impact. In 2017 the International Labour Organization estimated that on any given day in

A. A. Haji
Freelance Photographer, Nairobi, Kenya

R. Baya
Freelance Writer, Nairobi, Kenya

E. Brady (✉)
Department of History, University of Leeds, Leeds, UK
e-mail: e.brady@leeds.ac.uk

H. McCabe
Rights Lab, The University of Nottingham, Nottingham, UK

Y. Manji
Clinical Psychologist registered under the Kenya Psychological Association (KPA), Nairobi, Kenya

S. Otiende
Azadi Resource Center, Nairobi, Kenya

M. C. S. Gonçalves et al. (eds.), *The Coronavirus Crisis and Challenges to Social Development*,
https://doi.org/10.1007/978-3-030-84678-7_31

2016, 40 million people were victims of modern slavery, of whom 71% were women and girls (ILO, 2017, p. 5). In Kenya, modern slavery continues to be a significant issue: the 2020 Trafficking in Persons Report labelled Kenya a Tier 2 country (U.S. Department of State, 2020), and the 2019 Global Slavery Index awarded Kenya 5/10, indicating that whilst improvements have been made there is still more that can be done in the country (Walk Free Foundation, 2019). Yet it is not just governments who are combatting the problem; NGOs make considerable efforts to support survivors of modern slavery in Kenya and the wider region. One such organisation is Awareness Against Human Trafficking (HAART). Since 2010, HAART has dedicated itself to raising awareness of, and supporting victims of, human trafficking and forced marriage. A crucial component of this work, and one frequently overlooked by governments, is empowering survivors themselves with the tools they need to serve as leaders in their communities and in anti-slavery work. As Minh Dang asserts, "treated as an afterthought, most anti-slavery efforts assume that there are no survivors in the room, or the voices and agendas of survivors are not critical to the agenda of an event, publication, or exhibit" (Dang, 2018). Within these contexts, HAART and the Rights Lab at the University of Nottingham decided to collaborate on a project entitled *Survivors' Voices, Stories and Images: Survivor-Led Empowerment Through Ethical Story-Telling and Participatory Photography*.[1]

[1]This project was funded by the Antislavery Knowledge AHRC GCRF Network+ Grant, grant number AKN00217. The project was co-led by Dr. Helen McCabe and Sophie Otiende, who is a pioneering survivor leader from Kenya. McCabe is the Rights Lab's lead on forced marriage. The UK team also included a cultural historian, Emily Brady. The Kenyan team of experts also included Aisha Ali Haji, a freelance writer and practitioner of ethical storytelling who served as Storytelling Consultant; Rehema Baya, a photographer and practitioner of participatory photography who served as Photographic Consultant; and Yasmin Manji, a therapist who worked with Otiende to ensure survivor well-being throughout the process. This team worked to create a survivor-led programme of workshops that equipped participants with the tools to both tell their own stories and take their own pictures on their own terms. For more information about the project see: https://www.liverpool.ac.uk/media/livacuk/politics/akn/AKN,Single,Page,Projects,-,Rights,Lab.pdf. We would like to acknowledge the support of Worldreader and HAART as project partners.

This project aimed to empower survivors of modern slavery through the practice of ethical storytelling and participatory photography. Adopting a survivor-led approach to these methodologies, the original intent was to run workshops to train survivors in both photographic and storytelling techniques, working in a collaborative space with other survivors, whilst maintaining space for individual reflection and activities. As such, this project marked the first meaningful combination of these two methodologies in the context of modern slavery.

In terms of participatory photography as a methodology and practice, Wang asserts that there are "three main goals: to enable people (1) to record and reflect their community's strengths and concerns, (2) to promote critical dialogue and knowledge about personal and community issues through large and small group discussion, and (3) to reach policymakers" (Wang, 1999, p.185). These goals intersect with those of ethical storytelling, which privileges ethical and survivor-led approaches to narrative. Ball asserts that ethical storytelling far beyond the production of ethical materials:

> Storytelling in advocacy can also benefit society by contributing to participatory democracy and ensuring that a diversity of voices is heard in public debate. By challenging the monopoly that privileged, well-resourced individuals and organisations often hold over public discussion and debate, storytelling creates space for the wisdom, experience, analysis and aspirations of marginalised people and communities (Ball, 2013, p. 18).

Combining participatory photography and ethical storytelling, therefore, orientates survivor participation and consent at the centre of the project, whilst privileging a 'do-no-harm' approach. As such, this project sought to intervene in existing practice to advocate for the role of survivor-led, participatory methodologies that worked across multiple modes of representation.

This chapter specifically focuses on the process of research, rather than the research findings or specific outputs produced by the project. Orientated around the experiences and insights of the practitioners, this chapter explores the practicalities of adapting a participatory research project against the backdrop of a global pandemic.

This chapter was co-written by the entire research team, and draws from monthly catch-up meetings between various members of the team and Research Assistant Emily Brady. This allowed the team to track their adaptations and reflections on the project, which are presented in this chapter.

31.3 Initial Project Aims and Expectations

The primary aim of *Survivors' Voices, Stories and Images* was to empower survivors to tell their own stories and take their own images that conveyed their experience of human trafficking. This project would produce powerful material that would not only provide an opportunity for survivors to develop skills and express themselves, but also to challenge stereotypical views of victims of human trafficking. As such, we planned to hold an initial series of workshops, in which participants would be taught storytelling and photography skills and encouraged to tell their own stories. The group of five or six survivor participants would then work within both group and individual settings to refine their skills and stories. It was originally envisioned that these stories would be the participants' own narratives, conveying their lived experience of modern slavery. Ultimately, the survivor participants would then have the option to share their work and influence policy makers. As such, the main aim of this project was to empower survivors and cultivate survivor leadership through participatory research methods. Our original plan was to publish the narratives in accessible forms and hold exhibitions of the photographs in Nottingham and Nairobi, recoding and analysing audience reactions to gauge impact and see whether our methodologies successfully helped challenge stigma, stereotypes, and lack of knowledge.

This design would have allowed us to platform and promote the work produced by survivors, whilst furthering understanding of participatory research methods. However, our plans were derailed in March 2020, when the COVID-19 pandemic made it impossible to proceed with the intended activities.

31.4 The Impact of COVID-19 on the Project

We were due to commence in-person workshops in March 2020, but the team decided we would cancel them because of COVID-19. Not only were we concerned about the health-impacts of in-person workshops (which, under existing government guidance in Kenya might still have been legally possible), we were also concerned about the ethics of proceeding. In particular, we were concerned about placing an undue burden on participants, of whether this was an appropriate time to be doing research with them, and whether the payments we were offering would act as an inducement and undermine free consent. COVID-19 led to loss of income and increased vulnerability for most survivors of trafficking, including the group that we had selected for this group. At HAART, 5 of 10 survivors whom they had worked with previously became vulnerable and in need of direct services during the pandemic.

In April 2020, however, it became apparent that the survivors recruited to this project wished to proceed. The main reason cited for proceeding with the workshops was that the activity would give them something to do during the pandemic, as they felt idle. The survivors also expressed a need for community by being surrounded by other survivors during this time. Thus, the team reconvened to determine how to do this ethically and safely—and therefore remotely. That survivor-participants in Kenya were themselves instrumental to restarting the project (and within weeks of the pandemic causing us to pause) reflects the survivor-led intentions of the research.

To conduct this research ethically and safely in a remote context, the project underwent substantial revisions. Within this chapter, we reflect on these alterations and adaptations within the context of COVID-19, and what approaches were necessary to overcome the considerable challenges posed. As such, we will highlight our individual experiences to reflect on best practice of conducting participatory research methods during a pandemic. These methods include, but are not limited to, (1) technological adaptation, (2) adaptations to the process of securing informed consent, (3) empowering survivors and ensuring well-being, and (4) managing academic outputs within a survivor-led framework.

The survivor-informed methodology employed ensured there was always fluidity built into our research programme, particularly around the structure and content of workshops, although we had set a total number and general desired set of outcomes in line with our funding and research questions. We intentionally designed the research to allow the participants to shape the content according to their own needs and aims. Nonetheless, we noticed that several significant adaptations were necessary in order to complete the project in these challenging circumstances. This section contains excerpts from monthly interviews with practitioners: the discussion of workshops will focus on the Kenya-based strand of the team, and the overall project administration and analysis of findings will focus largely on the UK-based team.

31.4.1 Adaptations Made to Workshops in Kenya

The first significant adaptation made was the shift to remote working, and holding the workshops virtually, rather than in person; this meant that consideration had to be given to the technology used, and the sizes of groups.

Delays to the project caused by COVID-19 meant that our research timetable overlapped with other work HAART were conducting with survivor-participants, in collaboration with Walk Free, a part of which involved equipping survivor-participants with mobile phones on which to collect relevant data. The Walk Free project focused on survivor leadership and making contributions to the Global Slavery Index. Therefore, on top of the workshops, these survivors also received training and mentorship on survivor leadership from Dang and Sophie Otiende. This overlap made it possible to continue with our research remotely, as it meant all our participants could be connected to each other, and to the research team, via their phones, provision of which would have been beyond our original budget. They could also take photographs with the phone's cameras and share their images easily with Photographic Lead Rehema Baya and the rest of the research team.

Participants were given an Oppo A12 smartphone, which was selected in part for its high-quality camera (13-megapixel) and for containing user-friendly features such as flash and autofocus. These smartphones were given to participants with pre-installed software that would help them attend virtual meetings (including Google Meet and Zoom), read PDF documents and versions of slide-presentations (WPS Reader), save and share their images (Google Drive), and communicate with both the project researchers and their fellow participants (WhatsApp and email). Participants were also given an individual, anonymised, email address to use for the project.

The technology used in workshops was the subject of discussion with survivors, and provided significant insight into survivor-led methodologies. Of particular note was the preference for the video-calling software Zoom. Although many academics in the UK were discouraged from using Zoom at the start of the pandemic for potential security risks, survivor-participants found the software preferable as it granted them the agency to choose, and change, their own names, or go by just their initials. They also thought that Zoom was easy to use and, because of its easy integration with Google Calendar, it was easy for them to simply click on the link on the calendar invite. Workshops were recorded, but recording did not start until all participants had changed their names to their preferred initials.

Using software with which survivors already had experience in their daily lives, such as Google services, not only made the project more accessible and user-friendly, but it also suggested a familiarity to the project wherein more academic software may have intimidated and overwhelmed participants.

Moreover, we noticed that Zoom was proving a bountiful platform for cultivating community. As academics and researchers we thought perhaps participants might experience "Zoom-fatigue," but participants embraced the ability to connect via Zoom. Otiende rightly noted, in October 2020, that perhaps we had been taking too much for granted, and that it was a sign of *all* the team's "privilege" (in her words) that we could get tired of Zoom, because we were "participat[ing] in a million webinars" as the result of COVID-19.[2] Thus, we were all already embedded in communities of fellow researchers, artists, activists, friends and family who could meet, and even increase usual activity, online. But this was not the case for our participants.

Our experience shows that to create a community you do *not* need to be in person, but can be online, so long as the commitment and support (technical and personal) is there: "There's nothing can limit you from doing exactly what you want online." There are, however, drawbacks to workshops that are conducted entirely remotely. Although born of necessity as a result of the COVID-19 pandemic, and therefore necessary to proceed with the workshops, some survivors indicated that they would have preferred in-person workshops. Feedback suggested that some survivors felt that they missed out on a sense of physical community, and that their confidence would have increased further with in-person workshops. Although there are advantages to remote working—as other survivors stated that they preferred it as it allowed them to continue working/caring for their children while in class—when safe to do so these remote workshops can be viewed as complementary to in-person interactions.

The overlap with other research involving survivor-participants, and the move to remote workshops, meant we could, and also felt we should, increase the number of participants. Our original projected number had been constrained by funding (as we would refund travel costs as well as pay participants for their time and expertise), and remote working meant more money was available. Moreover, we felt it would be unfair to exclude any participants who wanted to engage with this research as well as the work with Walk Free, and for that reason repurposed some other parts of the budget (with our funder's permission) to increase the number of participants, and the amount of hours the Kenyan team would need to work to support their work. Our number of participants increased from 5 or 6 to 16.

Having additional people in the group meant not just a wider pool of participants and materials, but a more diverse and extended community. In particular, we could include participants in more remote and rural locations: we had seen our inability to do so in the original plan as unavoidable, but a limitation. This group of 16 was separated into three smaller groups (two of 5 persons, and one of 6) according to geographic proximity: two groups in Nairobi, and one on the coast. For context, the highest case-rates of COVID-19 had been reported in Nairobi and the coastal areas around Mombasa (WHO, 2021). These smaller groups were suggested to encourage maximal participation for all survivors involved in the research.

Having a larger total group of participants than originally planned allowed for a wider sense of community, yet keeping workshops to five or six people according to geographic proximity allowed people to still actively participate in workshops without fear of being side-lined or spoken over; this also prevented survivors from feeling intimidated by speaking in front of many people.

The process of gathering informed consent was also altered from our initial plans. Whereas originally an in-person workshop would have been held in which the project would have been explained in detail, survivors could have asked questions, and ultimately would have signed a physical form, any physical interaction was deemed unsafe in the COVID-19 pandemic.

[2]Where there a direct quote from practitioners in this chapter, these are from interviews conducted with Research Assistant Emily Brady from August 2020 to December 2020. Where there are direct quotes from survivor participants, these are taken from feedback forms completed after interviews on 30 January 2021.

The research team's trained counsellor (Yasmin Manji) took on responsibility for talking participants through the project on a one-to-one basis (on Google Meet), and securing their informed consent. After having the project explained to them (including confidentiality, anonymity or use of pseudonyms, and data security), and what it would require of them made plain, and their questions about it answered, the participants were asked to type "I consent" in the chat if they did consent to take part in the research. Manji then took a screen-shot capturing the video and the chat.

Alternatively, Manji recorded phone calls with the participant in which they said "I consent" after a similar process of explanation and ability to ask, and have answered, any questions about the project. These technological adaptations to obtaining informed consent were of crucial importance to this project, as the principle of ethical storytelling in particular relies on the full comprehension and willing participation of any and all participants.

Although the project had always intended to use both group and individual sessions with survivors, as is customary in the practice of participatory photography, the COVID-19 pandemic exacerbated the need for individual, one-on-one meetings. Not only did survivors require more reassurance and feedback, they also sometimes were reluctant to admit that they did not understand a concept in group discussion. As such, the practitioners were required to offer more individual support than originally envisioned. We noticed a need for this as early as the first photography session (September 2020). Whereas in in-person workshops, there would be a chance for participants to ask individual questions with some degree of privacy, and there would be built-in elements of one-to-one supervision and feedback, this setting is almost impossible in a group Zoom session (or any online session). Participants were therefore reaching out more frequently than originally anticipated to Baya and Aisha Ali Haji (the project's story-telling expert) for further instruction, feedback, and reassurance, and Baya noted she had to be "open to communication at any time." All work with survivor-participants can involve needing to be "a bit more patient and … a bit more understanding," but this was increased in terms of taking time to explain, and support, work in the digital space. Given this experience, this was another good reason to have split the participants into smaller groups, as even in these smaller groups our experience was that people could be shy of asking questions and admitting they did not understand or needed more support in front of people who were (at least at the start) strangers. This thought applies, of course, more widely than only to work with survivors.

Because participants sometimes appeared to have understood the particular task in the workshop, but would then follow-up for detailed support and explanation one-on-one, revealing that they had not entirely understood the concept of the assignment, we also started sending personalised feedback to participants, rather than sharing general feedback in the next group workshop. This phase helped participants have a record of things they might want to consider adjusting or changing, and the feedback from experts. As Baya rightly notes "sometimes with learning you have to go through the same lesson a few times so that you're able to understand it," but this made the research much more labour intensive for the researchers than we had initially imagined.

In addition to more one-on-one sessions, we found we were required to be more flexible with language than previously thought, involving greater use of Swahili by researchers than originally imagined. Although we had this capacity in the Kenyan team, it involved making changes to the existing syllabus. More significantly, we also found it was necessary to create a programme that was very localised and relevant to the lives of the survivor-participants; this also meant significant changes had to made to the planned syllabus when workshops on story-telling had already started. The team also had to incorporate a Swahili interpreter on the calls to assist with translation, and ensure that participants who were only conversant with, or much more comfortable working in, Swahili were fully accommodated.

As such, the COVID-19 pandemic required in the Kenyan researchers to adapt the project significantly to cultivate a positive environment and culture for survivors. From technological changes, to increasing group size, to gathering informed consent, to increasing the number of one-on-one sessions, restricting the syllabus, and speaking in multiple languages, the project transformed in both predicted and unforeseen ways. This evolution extended to payments for participants; whilst we had always intended to pay for the survivors' expertise and time, we also paid additionally for the data bundles required to participate in the virtual format. These decisions and transformations were always informed directly by the survivor participants, who were vocal about what elements of the project were working and what were not. As such, the workshops in Kenya demonstrate the importance of flexibility in survivor-led participatory research practices.

31.5 Adaptations to Overall Project

Originally our project was envisioned to last 12 months, including planning, enacting workshops, and distributing findings. COVID-19 meant we had to pause the project. Our funders also kindly allowed no-cost extensions to planned projects and adaptations to respond to the global pandemic. To carry out the research, the team had to have several discussions about how to deliver this project under new circumstances.

One of the most important discussions that was held was the shifting of resources allocated to the project as a result of COVID-19. Initially, the project had budgeted to allow for two physical exhibitions, one in Kenya and one in the UK, and travel costs for team members from both the UK and Kenya to visit each other. However, as a result of COVID-19, it became apparent that completing these activities was impossible. We therefore sought approval to redistribute those costs to other areas of the project. As already mentioned, it became quickly apparent that not only could we afford to reimburse survivor participants for their time at a higher rate than previously indicated, but that we could recruit more participants as well. As such, the number of participants increased to 16 individuals. Indeed, this exceeded even our revised estimation, as our June 2020 Project Amendment document stated we hoped to increase to 10 participants. As such, we were able to platform and support more survivors than anticipated as a direct result of the shift to virtual learning in response to the COVID-19 pandemic.

Our original plans for dissemination also had to be changed in response to the pandemic. The primary output of this project remains the forthcoming Worldreader publication which, at time of this writing in May 2021, is currently being compiled. The idea that survivors could turn their stories and images into a readily accessible publication had been one of the foundational components of this project. Partnering with Worldreader importantly allows these stories to be shared with people across the world in a highly accessible fashion. Not only do Worldreader host many texts in languages other than English (including Swahili), their e-reader platform is designed to be accessible from almost any mobile phone, and is entirely free to readers (and without advertisements). Their aim is to encourage reading across the globe by providing interesting and accessible reading material. Our partnership with Worldreader means the stories produced by participants can be shared with a global public audience, not just with other practitioners and academics, and in a wide range of countries in both the Global South and Global North where survivors of human trafficking often face marginalisation and stigma, including some of the countries where people are from or are now living. Kenya has experienced human trafficking and exploitation.

Our initial plan involved analysing data from Worldreader about where these stories were being read, and general demographic information about who was reading them and how they were engaging with them. In part, this was aimed at empowering our participants by showing them concrete evidence of other people engaging with their work; in part, it was aimed at showing NGOs, policy makers, and academics who work with survivors that narratives generated through ethical story-telling techniques could have global impact, and to therefore encourage their adoption. COVID-related delays have meant we have not yet uploaded the narratives to Worldreader, and so we have not been able to analyse any data to date, but this remains a core part of our ongoing research in this area.

As it is an e-reader, our plans to publish with Worldreader were unaffected (apart from how quickly we thought we could have finished narratives to share with them) by COVID-19. However, other key outputs such as a physical exhibition and conference papers were effectively derailed by the pandemic. Thankfully, in the case of this project, the survivor-led nature of the outputs meant that flexibility had been a cornerstone of the outputs suggested. Thus, we were able to adapt to the shifting circumstances to devise an alternative plan for outputs that remained impactful.

For example, members of the team have been able to present collaboratively at a range of different online events. Importantly, members of the team from Nottingham and from Nairobi have been able to present together, which would have been more difficult (not least because much more expensive) before the pandemic. This is an important benefit of the shift to more online events caused by the pandemic, particularly regarding access to dissemination events for researchers and scholars in the Global South (and access to their research and expertise for researchers, practitioners, and policy makers in the Global North).

In addition, we are in the process of designing an online exhibition, which will mean our outputs have an even wider reach than the original plans for exhibitions in Nottingham and Nairobi. A website need never "close" (unlike a physical exhibition), making it accessible to people in multiple countries and time zones. And although some people will be barred from accessing it because of a lack of access to technology (such as smartphones, laptops, or an internet connection), our survivor-participants will be able to see the exhibition, and show it to family and friends, via the phones they received as part of the project itself. Moreover, we can more easily track interaction with and reaction to the photographs online, as well as record anonymous demographic data automatically through the software. This ability has great advantages for our research into the impact of the work produced by participants in our project, and how members of the public engage with it, and with what results.

By adapting to the shift to virtual spaces, therefore, new opportunities for impact and engagement can be embraced. Crucial to this are notions of flexibility, which are built into the methods we chose to use. It has been exciting for the whole team to see where participants wanted the project to go. Of course, our methods mean researchers have to cede control of the project, which undermines the usual power dynamic in research between "the researcher" and "the researched." In our case, too, this involved ceding power from a research institution in the Global North to survivor-participants in the Global South, which also makes it an interesting case study in what can be possible in terms of challenging hierarchical relationships and legacies of colonialism. Our project has proven our initial hypothesis that ethical story-telling and participatory photography could both be used, in tandem, as part of meaningful work with survivors of modern slavery and human trafficking to give them control of their narratives. COVID-19 aside, it has also shown that deliberately flexible and participant-led methods can be powerful tools in doing research in a changing, and often uncertain, world—we hope with wider application than only the context of human trafficking in Kenya in the COVID-19 pandemic. It has also shown what is possible for research teams from institutions with very different histories; geographic locations; and financial, social, and political statuses when working together in a participatory and deliberately co-operative manner.

31.5.1 Positive and Negative Consequences of Adaptation

The impact of COVID-19 on this research project cannot be understated, yet these impacts were not consistently negative. Indeed, the COVID-19 pandemic response generated innovative research practices both to support, and at the request of, the survivor participants. International collaboration became easier than ever before, as presenting remotely via online events became easier than previously, and everyone became much more proficient with MS Teams, WhatsApp, and Zoom (and such technology because ubiquitous). On the project itself, the decision to change our outputs and the impact of the Kenyan travel ban meant that there was more space for participants in the project, and made it more accessible to participants. Crucially, the project provided a space for survivors to connect with each other and cultivate a community. At a time when many survivors of human trafficking were isolated, and cut off from their regular support networks, this project provided a safe space for survivors to tell their own stories, take their own images, and develop new skills. Indeed, people who may have otherwise been unable to travel (even with financial support) because of issues such as childcare could now participate in the project.

It is important to note, however, that the challenges posed by the COVID-19 pandemic were on occasion negative, and subsequent adaptations were not universally successful. Indeed, we as a team worked within a considerably volatile and stressful time to complete this project, and some additional burdens and disappointments were inevitable. One particular consequence of the shift to virtual learning was that more pressure fell on the HAART strand of the project than originally intended. This shift included extra costs such as translation, editing, and increased numbers of one-on-one meetings, and increased technical support in terms of giving feedback on photographs and writing samples, exacerbated by the increase in participants from 5 or 6 to 16. Although the Rights Lab strand of the project offered additional administrative assistance where possible, the burden of most extra work fell on the Kenyan team because of their geographic location, expertise and confidentiality agreements with participants. The research team were all working on this project part time, and everyone experienced increased pressures in their professional and personal lives from COVID-19. If we were to re-plan the programme, we would change our proposed timeline accordingly, allowing for a longer period of time for producing the artistic outputs, and gathering data for later analysis about their impact. Whilst the HAART team succeeded in delivering a series of workshops that empowered and engaged survivors, we have learned that future projects of this nature should ensure that, in survivor-led projects, additional funds should be set aside to ensure that any additional work that is required can be accommodated.

31.6 Conclusion and Considerations for Future Projects

In the case of our project, the decision to proceed with the research in a virtual space was at the direct request of the survivor participants. As such, the survivor-led nature of the project meant that we were able to proceed with this core value intact despite disruption from COVID-19. With the flexibility of the team, and the adaptability of our project's funders, we were able to deliver a project which, although not what was originally intended, managed to keep consistency with the original ideals of the proposed research. At the core of this project was a dedication to ethical practice and survivor well-being, which informed the decision-making process. Our project shows it is possible to successfully conduct ethical research even remotely and during a global pandemic, and this conclusion should have important implications for future research.

However, we noted that there were several unexpected costs of working remotely, including the increasing need for survivor support in one-on-one contexts. This need could have been better reflected in the initial re-budgeting of this project and is something needing careful consideration for future research. This said, our ability to work remotely had other budgetary implications, not least on travel to and from Kenya, and within Kenya, and this also has implications for future research. Our project shows that collaboration and regular meetings are made easier by using remote technologies (such as Zoom, Teams, and WhatsApp), as well as highlighting the need for a sense of "community" among researchers and participants. This sense can be created using technology and software (e.g., WhatsApp groups), but there is no real substitute for meeting in person, and existing personal relationships between members of the research team, and between participants and key members of the HAART team, were vital in ensuring the continued running of the project and allowing us to be flexible as this was based on a strong sense of mutual trust.

The potential of virtual workshops to be an alternative to physical practice, when conducted with proper infrastructural support, may widen participation as never before. However, within the context of this project, we have seen both the advantages and disadvantages to a remote context, and thus we hope that this project will pioneer a way forward that combines both the best, and safest, aspects of both physical and virtual workshops.

In terms of challenging international social work, our project demonstrates that trusting local experts and taking the lead from those participating in your research is fundamental to best practice. Participatory research naturally complements this approach. Our key recommendations for those seeking to run a similar project in future would be the following:

1. Have an open conversation with funding bodies about expectations in survivor-led projects, especially as pertains to outputs. Likewise, prepare to be flexible with your own anticipated outputs.
2. Ensure that funding is allocated to cover unanticipated additional costs, especially as pertains to direct participant engagement.
3. If possible, look to pool resources with other projects with similar aims.
4. Establish a regular means of communication and accountability with the wider team.

There is no easy roadmap to a successful survivor-led research project, particularly when challenged by the impact of COVID-19, but the adaptability and resourcefulness of the team and, crucially, the survivor participants in this project resulted in the production of original material that makes a significant intervention in the field of participatory research studies and in conducting participant-led social work and research in the Global South. Social work of this nature has the potential to empower and strengthen local communities as we move to "build back better" post-pandemic, and achieve all the Sustainable Development Goals (including, but not limited to, ending modern slavery, forced labour, and forced marriage).

References

Ball, R. (2013). "When I tell my story, I'm in charge:" Ethical and effective storytelling in advocacy. *CLC Fellowship Report 2013*. http://ssrn.com/abstract=2689990

Dang, M. (2018). Survivors are speaking, are we listening? *Walk Free: Global Slavery Index, 2018*. https://www.globalslaveryindex.org/resources/essays/survivors-are-speaking-are-we-listening

International Labour Organization and Walk Free Foundation. (2017). Global estimates of modern slavery: forced labour and forced marriage. https://www.ilo.org/wcmsp5/groups/public/%2D%2D-dgreports/%2D%2D-dcomm/documents/publication/wcms_575479.pdf

U.S. Department of State. (2020). Trafficking in persons report, 20th edn. https://www.state.gov/wp-content/uploads/2020/06/2020-TIP-Report-Complete-062420-FINAL.pdf.

Walk Free Foundation. (2019). Country Data: Kenya. *Global Slavery Index*. https://www.globalslaveryindex.org/2019/data/country-data/kenya/

Wang, C. C. (1999). Photovoice: A participation action research strategy applied to women's health. *Journal of Women's Health, 8*(2), 185–192.

World Health Organization. (2021). *Kenya situation*. World Health Organization. https://covid19.who.int/region/afro/country/ke

32 Social Work in the Time of a Pandemic: COVID-19 and the Need for Resilience-Critical Thinking

Anna Pfaffenstaller
and Jacques Love Babatoundé Zannou

32.1 Introduction

At the beginning of 2020, the whole world was, and still is, violently shaken by the spread of COVID-19. No nation expected it and the international political system underestimated it. Because humanity is organized into nations, the national feeling has prevailed over this virus. The planetary solidarity that is so much advocated by the United Nations (UN) is relegated to the background, in spite of the fact that the Global South cannot do much against the virus without the help of the Global North. Numerous states, under the active or passive umbrella of supranational organizations, are trying to control the situation by imposing restrictive measures on its citizens. Social work, whose primary task is to help people in social difficulties, is struggling to fulfil this mandate. At the same time, the capitalist system is at an impasse with the COVID-19 pandemic. A critical look at it and especially at social work, which is an important instrument of social case management, is the goal of this chapter.

We argue that social work must help human beings to get out of a precarious or crisis situation without imposing solutions from the capitalist system. Rather, the focus should be on helping clients to concretize their own envisaged solutions to feel up to the challenges that are inherent in human nature, combined with the demands of a capitalist society. With this in mind, we first explore the basics of resilience and the need for a resilience-critical approach in social work. Based on the assumption that social work must be resilience critical, we then show that social work has to integrate the thoughts of critical theory and postmodernism to help its clients to free themselves from the yoke of capitalism. This need is particularly relevant in times of crisis such as the COVID-19 pandemic, which social effects will serve as an example in this chapter. On the basis of these remarks, we develop further thoughts on the implementation of resilience critique in the practice of social work.

32.2 Resilience Critique and Social Work in Times of COVID-19

Social work is massively affected by the COVID-19-pandemic and "has an essential frontline role in the fight against the spread of the virus through supporting communities protect themselves and others through physical distancing and social solidarity" (IFSW, 2020).

At the same time, the concept of resilience is more popular than ever in times of COVID-19.

A. Pfaffenstaller (✉)
University of Bamberg and KSH München University of Applied Sciences, Munich, Germany

J. L. B. Zannou
Universität der Bundeswehr München, Abomey-Calavi, Benin

M. C. S. Gonçalves et al. (eds.), *The Coronavirus Crisis and Challenges to Social Development*
https://doi.org/10.1007/978-3-030-84678-7_32

Not for nothing is resilience often referred to as the key concept of the twenty-first century (Bröckling, 2017, p. 1). The concept of resilience is not only used in popular advice literature, but also often in the professional context of social work. Particularly in times of COVID-19, there is an appeal to sustain one's own resilience, and reference to the need to develop further resilient "competences" in times of crisis. The term resilience describes the ability to withstand stressful circumstances and events and is a positive antonym to vulnerability (Gabriel, 2005, p. 207). Masten (2011) describes resilience as "the capacity of a dynamic system to withstand or recover from significant threats to its stability, viability or development" (p. 494).

Because of the existing challenges and threats, resilience varies in both time and space (Gabriel, 2005, p. 207) and is not a completed process (Bröckling, 2017, p. 3). From the start, we want to clarify that we are not against resilience. On the contrary, it is an important protective factor in life and in the work with clients it is helpful to look at this topic for their own development. Nevertheless, we wish to take a critical look at the circumstances in which the concept of resilience is used and implemented, because it is not without problems. As authors from the Global North and Global South, respectively, we have come to the following explanations after an intensive and critical discussion about resilience.

According to a critical understanding of resilience, people learn from childhood a fundamental acceptance of the world in which they live and try to meet the demands of society despite objectively worse starting conditions. A critical analysis of the causes is not intended, but rather a flexible adaptation to the circumstances of life (Graefe, 2019, pp. 128–129). Reflections and publications on such a critical understanding of resilience exist for a longer time, but they are less discussed in the practice of social work. In this context, *medico international* (2017) critically described resilience as a panacea for crises, conflicts, and problems. The present interpretation of the concept of resilience perceives it as part of the neoliberal hegemony in which social responsibility is shifted to the private sphere (Gebauer, 2017, p. 17).

Thus, risky environmental conditions are not changed, nor are individuals, organizations, and communities moved to critically question and change circumstances. The measures have aimed at adapting people to the risks and increasing their resilience rather than reducing burdens and their destabilizing and destructive consequences (Bröckling, 2017, pp. 3–7). The important and necessary critique and transformation potentials of the conditions are concealed by this. In times of COVID-19, this crisis mode becomes even more apparent, as it is about system preservation instead of change and development. The concept of "systemic-relevance" leaves the system itself unquestioned and makes it difficult to question the system. Thus, in times of COVID-19, it is primarily about securing the imperial way of life and not about transformation (Graefe, 2020).

At this point, the concept of systemically relevant groups, to which social work belongs, can be discussed (DBSH, 2020).

32.2.1 A Brief Resilience-Critical View of Social Work and Its Systemic Relevance

"Part of the concept of resilience is that 'systemic relevances' are discussed, but at the same time the real causes of systemic crises are not sought. These crises appear as unavoidable side effects of economic growth and development" (Graefe, 2020, author translation). After several months of the COVID-19 pandemic, no sustainable changes are evident for system-relevant groups (e.g., care professions), which were often vociferously called for at the beginning of the pandemic. In contrast to other systemically relevant occupational groups facing similar difficulties, the field of social work remains invisible in the public discourse and receives little attention. This lack also affects the vulnerable clients of social work, who are particularly affected by COVID-19 (DBSH, 2020). The pandemic particularly affects those who are already living in poverty with limited resources. The associated interactions will have a massive impact on social work in the coming years. The virus reveals the existing social injustice and inequality at the national and international levels and reinforces them in a dimension that is not yet foreseeable. In the medium and long term, this will make a future more likely in which the pandemic state of emergency is made permanent and the population is trained to remain and become resilient, that is, to adapt more and more flexibly to changing circumstances (Graefe, 2020).

Social work that does not critically reflect on resilience concepts, as stated earlier by Graefe (2020), is at risk of understanding and implementing resilience as a constant adaptation of the clients to crises and ongoing challenges, even in times of COVID-19. This risk is also relevant for social workers and the organizations in which they work, as they are often faced with similar challenges in the context of resilience and adjustment. However, a critical discussion of the concept of resilience brings numerous dilemmas and difficulties for the profession of social work (e.g., mandates, financing). According to our understanding of social work, system relevance does not mean maintaining the social system in its current form and supporting an unreflective understanding of resilience. It is rather about changing it by criticizing the system from the inside and acting in a resilience-critical way, so that social justice and social transformation are possible (DBSH, 2020).

32.3 Thoughts for Social Work in Times of COVID-19 and Beyond, Incorporating Critical Theory and Post-Modernism

Based on the previous remarks, we share ideas and thoughts of resilience-critical social work in times of COVID-19 and beyond, which will serve to develop professional reflection and practice. Among other things we will refer to critical theory and post-modernism.

First, we have to recognize that many crises are natural, such as COVID-19. They are sometimes abused by world systems such as capitalism and neoliberalism to be influential and seminal. As the COVID-19 pandemic develops, people, especially in the Global North, are protesting against lockdowns and related measures. What is the reason? A simple lack of resilience or a lack of space to be resilience critical? The protesters want to deal with the pandemic independently and in their own way. The governments are implementing measures against the COVID-19 virus to which the citizens are expected to adhere. In the Global South, especially in Sub-Saharan Africa, there are similar protests: first, because people do not believe the virus exists; and second, because they have to earn their daily wage, and governments can barely manage to feed them in lockdowns. Thus, social work is confronted with very different backgrounds, opinions, and mindsets when working with its clients, and these become even more apparent in the context of COVID-19.

So, how are constructive criticism and resilience critique expressed in times of COVID-19? We understand critique as a constitutive component of human practice (Jaeggi & Wesche, 2009, p. 7) and, following Foucault (1997), "the art of not being governed or better, the art of not being governed like that and at that cost" (p. 29). Critique is about "a certain way of thinking, speaking and acting, a certain relationship to what exists, to what one knows, to what one does, a relationship to society, to culture and also a relationship to others that we could call, let's say, the critical attitude" (Foucault, 1997, p. 24).

With this understanding of critique, we make the following remarks on resilience-critical social work. Our intention is to critically reflect on existing circumstances and to ask how a different understanding of resilience and social transformation can be implemented together.

32.3.1 Social Work from the Top and Related Difficulties During the COVID-19 Pandemic

Social work evokes on the one hand that people are able to be social and on the other hand that they have social needs. Independent of the angle from which one considers social work, one has to understand social being as concurrent social contracts between people to achieve together individual and collective goals, particularly with regard to exigencies. This understanding of social being often operates at the local level or on a small scale. Today, social being remains mostly under state control in the form of a political social contract that: refers to processes by which everyone in a political community, either explicitly or tacitly, consents to state authority, thereby limiting some of her or his freedoms, in exchange for the state's protection of their universal human rights and security and for the adequate provision of public goods and services (UNDP, 2016, p. 9).

To what extent does the state fulfil its duties under the social contract to its citizens? Institutionalized social work can be seen as an instrument of policy to achieve welfare towards people; and it somehow tries. Such social work operates from the top down, making it accountable to the state, and when the state is in trouble so is social work. For example, the COVID-19 pandemic is a crisis situation that demonstrates the limits of social work dependent on government. At the beginning of COVID-19, several governments experienced a debacle in dealing with the pandemic. In this way, social work and health care also faced great difficulties under circumstances that were complicated anyway. Why?

One reason for this situation is, according to Khella (1982, as cited in Engelke et al., 2014, p. 426), that social work does not practice a continual critical analysis with its state, communal, churchly, or free responsible bodies. It simply submits to its sponsors. So this form of social work is called 'social work from the top', whereas Khella makes a plea for a 'social work from the bottom up'. For him, 'social work from the bottom up' is a constructive approach. It is "a practice-oriented antithesis to therapeutic immobilism, pedagogical pessimism, charitable approaches, and subcultural orientation" (Khella, 1982, p. 32, as cited in Engelke et al., 2014, p. 423; author translation). Thus, the spread of COVID-19 is primarily from the bottom up, so it should ideally be managed from the bottom up. Therefore, the practice of social work is always two sided: it strives to solve a problem of an individual case and/or a social group and pays attention to the inclusion of the affected people in the cohesion of society as a whole and in history-changing practice (Engelke et al., 2014, p. 426).

So how can it be surprising that institutionalized top-down social work is struggling with the pandemic, when it has to change the way of working, as do all institutionalized organizations (job centers, schools, universities, social services, or hospitals)? Our societies are replete with exigencies, whose challenges become overstraining and depressing in the long term. We argue for a different understanding of resilience that takes into account the resilience-critique elaborated earlier. A resilient citizen refrains from the dominant system and comes over to the people, who understand the importance of social interpersonal relationships.

We need to take up the critical reflection of social work "to encompass an awareness of how assumptions about the connection between oneself and social context/structure can function in powerful ways, so that awareness of these assumptions can provide a platform for transformative action" (Fook, 2015, p. 441).

32.3.2 No Resilience-Critical Social Work without Critical Thinking Canons

Therefore, we will explore the main traditions of critical thinking such as postmodernism and critical social theory. These two critical thinking canons have something in common: they fight epistemologically and heuristically "the dominant groups who are attempting to exploit society for their own interests" (Borg et al., 1995, p. 124). Although the contents of these theories are very abstract and complex, it is indispensable to delve into them, if one searches for "related perspectives on the shortcomings of positivism as well as new ways to theorize and study contemporary societies" (Agger, 1991, p. 105). The positivist thinkers succeed in building societies in which people live in permanent fear, subordinate themselves and see everything as predetermined and irreversible. This is particularly noticeable in times of crisis, where the real victims are the oppressed and barred. No one wants to publicly take responsibility for an ongoing crisis. Positivism, whose expressions are capitalism, neoliberalism, Eurocentrism, neocolonialism, fetishism, sexism, etc., pushes a collective responsibility. "In particular, capitalism deepens false consciousness, suggesting to people that the existing social system is both inevitable and rational" (Agger, 1991, p. 108).

This is the reason why there is no space for a resilience concept, where the people can determine and place themselves how they want to survive vicissitudes and crises. However, most citizens do not demand this space at all. They blindly believe in capitalism and the existing system. Many countries underestimated COVID-19 at the beginning and faced massive deaths and overloads. Who will die most? The mortality at the global level mainly affects the lower and middle layers. What tragedy could be seen in sub-Saharan Africa if demographic and climatic circumstances, among other factors, did not work against the virus? Black Africans, in exaggerated terms, would be eradicated from the Earth because they are not economically strong enough to fight COVID-19, especially as the rich countries are struggling with economic and social problems in the course of COVID-19 and are barely providing any support measures.

An example of this is how the world politics capitalistically implements the development of vaccines against COVID-19, which are now approved in various powerful countries. The vaccinations are carried out on a global level in a capitalistic way: people in the Global North are vaccinated first. In addition to high-risk groups, priority is given to system-relevant health workers and imperial system guards. Then, world politics will support people from the Global South to receive vaccinations on capitalist principles. This scheme illustrates the existing world system, as already stated by Agger (1991). Social work instead pursues the goal of social justice and social transformation, which requires an internationally connected social work that advocates solidarity and distributive justice. The existing dependencies and capitalist entanglements must therefore be questioned in a resilience-critical way. For this purpose, it is essential to develop critical assumptions and practices in social work.

In contrast to positivism, which thinks "one can perceive the world without making assumptions about the nature of the phenomena under investigation … [and] experiences the world as rational and necessary, thus deflating attempts to change it" (Agger, 1991, p. 109), critical theory "attempt to develop a mode of consciousness and cognition that breaks the identity of reality and rationality, viewing social facts not as inevitable constraints on human freedom (…) but as pieces of history that can be changed" (Agger, 1991, p. 109).

It can be seen how relevant this is for social work, especially when people are confronted with distress and need. If people are educated or socialized in a resilience-critical way, they would be more able to evade the capitalist consequences and act more confidently and independently against crises such as the COVID-19 pandemic. This effort would be even more successful if the state promoted a capitalism-critical resilience concept through social workers.

Social work has to critically reflect the demands of the system and look for vicinity to its clients, who often need support and protection. So social workers must work with clients together to find out which practical approach is promising – top-down or bottom-up. "By making connections between the personal and structural, and emphasizing the importance of communication, critical social theory points to how a critical reflection process might help us forge bridges between our own experience and that of others to bring about desired social changes" (Fook, 2015, p. 446).

When a system that is supposed to give us social care and healthcare is struggling or failing, social work must be resilience-critical and capitalism-critical. A different understanding of resilience can become effective in the first step when everyone has learned to get through distress and need without expecting much from the dominant system, and if they do then as a homogeneous group of individuals who come together to achieve the same goals: survivability and solidarity. In this way, a decentralized, multilayered or bottom-up approach is necessary. This is what postmodern theorists suggest. They: examine the social world from the multiple perspectives of class, race, gender and other identifying group affiliations, … refuse the totalizing claims of grand narratives … [and distrust] radicals and radicalism, preferring the decentered knowledges available not only to a central knowledge commissar but also to people who engage with the world from the irreducible perspectives of their own experience (Agger, 1991, p. 116).

A government drawing on critical theory and postmodern ideas can renounce power and constraints to overcome COVID-19. Postmodern resilience is what makes people responsible and freely engaged citizens, even in times of crisis. We also argue for such an understanding in social work.

32.4 Ideas for the Development of Resilience-Critical Social Work in Times of Crisis

Social work in times of crisis will be successful if it operates according to postmodern views and critical theory.

For effective social work, we have to compromise between the center-dominant system and the native homogeneous communities. For this, we advocate for a social work that works on a local level and must be connected internationally. The focus should not only be on the mutual exchange of social problem situations and the related problem-solving approaches between the Global South and the Global North (Lutz & Kleibl, 2020, p. 4). We also need to develop concepts for action that integrate a resilience-critical view into the practice of social work at the local and international level. On the one hand, it must be questioned to what extent social work acts in a resilience-uncritical way. In this context, it is important to develop solutions for and with the clients and organizations that include a resilience-critical attitude at all levels. On the other hand, it is important to find out what contribution social work can not only make in acute phases of crises and the time beyond, but also preventively on a resilience-critical basis. For this, postmodernism and critical theorys can be used as a basis for reflection. Social work must also position itself much more politically and publicly. From our discussion, we can deduce reflexive questions for a professional social work practice, which can be further developed:

- What is our understanding of resilience as an organization and individuals? How can we implement resilience-critical aspects in our work with clients and at the organizational level?
- How is the organization in which I work structured? Top-down or bottom-up? What does this mean for my daily work and the resulting challenges?
- How can we create and rethink social work from a resilience-critical perspective?
- How can we translate the core ideas of postmodernism and critical theory into our everyday practice?
- Are there opportunities for exchange and networking with other organizations that are engaged in resilience critique as well as postmodernism and critical theory?
- What public and political positions are necessary for resilience-critical social work, not only in times of crisis?

These questions are incomplete and are intended mainly as inspiration for discussing resilience critique in social work.

At present, the focus is primarily on coping with acute crisis situations. The measures against COVID-19 often lead to severe contact restrictions up to a complete break-off of contact in the work with clients, while at the same time there is increasing need and less available resources. For social work this means in the time of COVID-19 and the time beyond:

1. ensuring that the most vulnerable are included in planning and response.
2. organizing communities to ensure that essentials such as food and clean water are available.
3. advocating within social services and in policy environments that services adapt, remain open and pro-active in supporting communities and vulnerable populations.
4. Facilitating physical distancing and social solidarity.
5. As a profession, advocating for the advancement and strengthening of health and social services as an essential protection against the virus, inequality, and the consequent social and economic challenges (IFSW, 2020).

This scheme also includes overcoming and reducing obstructive bureaucratic structures in social work to provide the best possible support for the clients who need help most urgently. COVID-19 also opens up a broad platform for conspiracy theories, right-wing populism and fake news. As critical social workers, it is important to take COVID-19 seriously and take a clear stance against it, irrespective of whether one is acting from the top or from the bottom.

Furthermore, it is important to mention that social work professionals are confronted with numerous ethical dilemmas during the COVID-19 pandemic. For example, Banks et al. (2020) and Truell and Crompton (2020) provide many examples and show how these are dealt with. For social work, it is necessary to deal with the potential long-term consequences of COVID-19 and to change professional critical social work in a powerful way. From the point of view of resilience-criticism, there is a need for further critical reflection on the ethical dilemmas and underlying difficulties as well as a critical discussion of the role of social work in times of COVID-19 and in a capitalist world system in general. This can help to develop new perspectives and a more differentiated understanding of social work as a profession.

We conclude in relationship to our understanding of critical resilience discourses, critical theory, and postmodernism, that the existence of people in the social environment should be determined by them. Therefore, it cannot be about the unreflective adaptation of resilience to increasingly severe crises. Social workers should act according to this self-determined existence. Or as Graefe (2019) writes, it is about" *not* adapting and resigning ourselves to the world we live in, but on the contrary, insisting that we can change it – not because we are fully sovereign and rational *or* because we are exposed, powerless, and unknowing, but because 'we' are both: autonomous *and* dependent, vulnerable *and* (nevertheless) able to act, unknowing *and* rational" (pp. 195–196, author translation).

32.5 Conclusion

In summary, there is a lack of critical discussion of the current understanding of resilience and the related challenges in social work, especially in times of crisis. This lack of understanding has a stabilizing effect on the system and can lead to unreflective adaptations of social work practice. In particular, social work from the top has to deal with difficulties in the COVID-19 pandemic due to its structuring. The implementation of a resilience-critical stance is necessary at the national and international levels if social work is to achieve greater social justice and transformation. We argue that resilience-critical social work must be holistically critical. This means being critical with the system in which social work is embedded; being critical in working with clients and colleagues; and being critical with one's own professional understanding of resilience. This can be implemented in the first steps with the help of reflections on postmodernism and critical theory as well as the listed questions.

References

Agger, B. (1991). Critical theory, poststructuralism, postmodernism: Their sociological relevance. *Annual Review of Sociology, 17*, 105–131. http://www.jstor.org/stable/2083337

Banks, S., Cai, T., de Jonge, E., Shears, J., Shum, M., Sobočan, A. M., Strom, K., Truell, R., Úriz, M. J., & Weinberg, M. (2020). *Ethical challenges for social workers during Covid-19: A global perspective*. International Federation of Social Workers.

Borg, D., Brownlee, K., & Delaney, R. (1995). Postmodern social work practice with aboriginal people. In R. Delaney & K. Brownlee (Eds.), *Northern social work practice* (pp. 116–135). Lakehead University Centre for Northern Studies.

Bröckling, U. (2017). Resilienz. Über einen Schlüsselbegriff des 21. Jahrhunderts. https://www.soziopolis.de/beobachten/kultur/artikel/resilienz

DBSH. (2020). Soziale Arbeit während der Corona Pandemie – Who cares? https://www.dbsh.de/media/dbsh-www/redaktionell/pdf/Sozialpolitik/2020/05052020_DBSH_Kampagne_Stellungnahme_Who_cares.pdf

Engelke, E., Borrmann, S., & Spatscheck, C. (2014). *Theorien der Sozialen Arbeit. Eine Einführung*. Lambertus Verlag.

Fook, J. (2015). Reflective practice and critical reflection. In J. Lishman (Ed.), *Handbook for practice learning in social work and social care: Knowledge and theory* (pp. 440–454). Jessica Kingsley.

Foucault, M. (1997). What is critique? In S. Lotringer & L. Hochroth (Eds.), *The politics of truth* (pp. 22–82). Semiotext(e).

Gabriel, T. (2005). Resilienz: Kritik und Perspektiven. *Zeitschrift für Pädagogik, 51*(2), 207–2017. https://doi.org/10.21256/ZHAW-3318

Gebauer, T. (2017). Fit für die Katastrophe. Ein neues entwicklungspolitisches Modewort verhindert Ursachenbekämpfung. In Medico International (Ed.), *Fit für die Katastrophe? Kritische Anmerkungen zum Resilienzdiskurs im aktuellen Krisenmanagement* (pp. 13–22). Psychosozial-Verlag.

Graefe, S. (2019). *Resilienz im Krisenkapitalismus. Wider die Logik der Anpassung*. Bielefeld: transcript.

Graefe, S. (2020). Schlägt die Stunde der Resilienz? Luxemburg online. https://www.zeitschrift-luxemburg.de/corona-schlaegt-die-stunde-der-resilienz/

IFSW. (2020). Updated information on IFSW and COVID-19. https://www.ifsw.org/updated-information-on-ifsw-and-the-covid-19-virus/

Jaeggi, R., & Wesche, T. (2009). *Was ist Kritik?* Suhrkamp-Verlag.

Khella, K. (1982). Sozialarbeit von unten. Praktische Methoden fortschrittlicher Sozialarbeit. Hamburg.

Lutz, R., & Kleibl, T. (2020). Internationale Soziale Arbeit neu denken. *Sozial Extra, 44*, 247–251. https://doi.org/10.1007/s12054-020-00289-0

Masten, A. (2011). Resilience in children threatened by extreme adversity: Frameworks for research, practice, and translational synergy. *Development and Psychopathology, 23*(2), 493–506. https://doi.org/10.1017/S0954579411000198

Medico International. (2017). *Fit für die Katastrophe? Kritische Anmerkungen zum Resilienzdiskurs im aktuellen Krisenmanagement*. Psychosozial-Verlag.

Truell, R., & Crompton, S. (2020). *To the top of the cliff – How social work changed with COVID-19*. International Federation of Social Workers.

UNDP. (2016). Engaged Societies, Responsive States: The Social Contract in Situations of Conflict and Fragility. Concept Note April 2016. United Nations Development Programme and the Norwegian Peacebuilding Resource Centre (NOREF). https://www.undp.org/content/dam/undp/library/Democratic%20Governance/Social_Contract_in_Situations_of_Conflict_and_Fragility.pdf

33 A Social Work and Social Development Perspective on the Need to Decolonise African Economies in Light of the COVID-19 Pandemic: Lessons for Africa

Victor Chikadzi

33.1 COVID-19: A Health Crisis with Devastating Economic and Social Consequences

The COVID-19 pandemic has had devastating effects on the healthcare systems of many nations globally, with concomitant ripple effects on the social and economic dimensions of human life and livelihoods (Nicola et al., 2020). van Barneveld et al. (2020) note that the COVID-19 pandemic is an unprecedented humanitarian crisis that has altered the global order in a way that is likely to have a lasting impact. In a world that has increasingly become connected and integrated, the impact of the COVID-19 pandemic goes beyond the health consequences. The global lockdown first implemented in China and swiftly spread across the globe severely impacted both the global production and consumption of goods and services. Millions of jobs were affected by the disruption of global supply chains (Fernandes, 2020).

There has been a birthing of the 'new normal,' and it is unlikely that the old order will return even beyond the crisis. The pandemic is causing disastrous worldwide health, social, and economic impacts. The impact of the crisis is worsened by the fact that the global order is currently dominated by global capitalism, which has weakened the ability of many countries in the Global South to adequately respond to the crisis. Under the neo-liberal order, the primacy of markets rather than the state is championed, giving rise to a global economic order in which the policy autonomy and response capabilities of nation states, especially those considered to be still developing, is largely compromised and decimated (Midgley, 1995; O'Brien, 2013).

It is estimated that the COVID-19 economic crisis will plunge about half a billion people into poverty, and for the first time since 1990, global poverty is expected to rise. Sub-Saharan Africa is already affected by many other social and economic crises, such as political instability, high levels of inequality, and poor healthcare systems. As such, the current COVID-19 will have an added effect on these areas (Filho et al., 2020).

The current global economic and social order has proved to be unsustainable. A birthing of a new global economic order is needed. In this regard, social work has to add its voice in informing a developmental framework that will usher in a more just, equitable, inclusive, and sustainable global economic ecosystem. A status quo in which millions of people are left vulnerable to the vagaries of global markets without adequate

V. Chikadzi (✉)
Department of Social Work, University of Namibia, Windhoek, Namibia

M. C. S. Gonçalves et al. (eds.), *The Coronavirus Crisis and Challenges to Social Development*,
https://doi.org/10.1007/978-3-030-84678-7_33

social protection is simply unjust and tragic. A more just global economic path informed by the ideals of the social development approach is possible, and social work practitioners are better placed to partly inform this path.

33.2 Poverty and Social Work

More than any other profession, social work has largely been directly and indirectly concerned about poverty. A majority of social work clients come from the economically marginalised population groups; poverty is a major root cause of many pathologies and social dysfunction amongst social work clients. Despite the material and financial circumstances of people largely accounting for the major reasons why they come into contact with social services, social workers are yet to find solutions to address poverty and economic deprivation at a macro scale. Most interventions by social work practitioners and agencies largely focus on helping individual circumstances while negating the structural factors the breed poverty and make it an acceptable norm in the first place (Becker, 1997; Davis & Wainwright, 2005).

Davis and Wainwright (2005) further note that the services that social work clients receive may be responsible for sustaining the poverty experienced by social work service users. In their analysis of the response of social work to mass poverty in South Africa, Chikadzi and Pretorius (2011) conclude that social work is complicit in sustaining poverty amongst social work service users by adopting a poverty management posture rather than poverty eradication, largely because most social work interventions address the symptoms of poverty rather than tackling its root causes. Social workers do seem to have an awareness of structural and institutional factors that cause deprivation and disadvantage amongst the masses, but it seems that thus has far it has been beyond the remit of social work to craft policy and practice interventions which address the underlying structural factors that lead to poverty.

Davis and Wainwright (2005) argue that a poverty-conscious approach to social work practice is necessary. They note that such an approach should be centred on ensuring that social work practitioners have an understanding of the structural and institutional causes of poverty and the manner in which it affects people at a personal level. Many critics, especially in academia, have rightly championed the need for social work practice that addresses the structural issues connected to social ills such as poverty (Chikadzi & Pretorius, 2011; Lombard, 2008; Midgley, 1995); however, many are yet to put forward alternative and plausible models of intervention to realise this ideal.

Current social work practice needs to be understood from the standpoint of the current dominant global capitalist economic order. As the world has almost completely gravitated towards neo-liberalism, poverty is hardly seen through the lenses of structural disadvantage; instead the dominant view is that individuals are responsible for their own situation. Within a neo-liberal framework, which is the dominant context within which most social work practice takes place, poverty is seen as being unconnected to economic distribution of goods and services and the state is seen as not being responsible. When state intervention does occur, it is minimal and temporary (Lawson & Elwood, 2014). The very core features of neo-liberalism make it difficult for social work to operate within this economic framework.

33.3 The Social Development Approach: An Antithesis to Neo-liberalism

Social development has been touted as one of the most progressive approaches suited to remedy the problems of underdevelopment that have become commonplace in most emerging economies particularly in Sub-Saharan Africa. As an approach, social development holds much promise from a theoretical standpoint especially when one reads the scholarly rhetoric around the approach. Social development has its roots in Keynesian economics. Richard Maynard Keynes was a British economist whose ideas where most influential during the great depression. The central notion in Keynesian economics is the idea that state intervention in the economy is desirable and necessary. Keynes believed that centralised state planning was key in guarding against, as well as protecting citizens from, market excesses. Further, state intervention is seen by Keynesian economists to be key in directing development in an equitable and inclusive manner that ensures all people can actively participate and benefit from the productive economy (Midgley, 1995).

33.3.1 Social Development Is an Approach That Goes Beyond the Narrow Confines of Social Work

There are varied definitions of the social development approach, but scholars are largely in agreement on its central features or characteristics. On closer analysis of these features of the social development approach, one realises that its implementation is beyond what is possible for social work and social workers alone. Although significant literature on the social development approach has been advanced by social workers, there has been a hesitance in acknowledging the limits of social work and social workers insofar as the realisation of the approach is concerned. From looking at the characteristics of the social development approach, one realises that its goals are much broader and extend beyond the narrow confines of what is practically possible for social work and social workers. Following is a discussion of the characteristic features of the social development approach.

33.3.2 Social Development Is Interventionist

One of the key defining features of social development is the idea that it is interventionist. The idea of interventionism in the social development approach as noted earlier is linked to Keynesian economic thought. Interventionism in Keynesian economic thought centres on the notion that state intervention in the directing of inclusive socio-economic development is necessary and inescapable. This thinking is contrary to neo-liberalism, which argues against state intervention in economic development. Under neo-liberal thought, state intervention leads to market dysfunction that would ultimately make people suffer. Markets are seen as the primary channel through which people should locate the resources for livelihood. It is believed that markets are capable of self-regulation. As such the state has to adopt a hands-off approach. The only role of the state countenanced under neoliberalism is that of making rules and regulations that are favourable for the functioning of the market. Such favourable regulation allows for markets to thrive, and it is assumed that when the markets thrive this automatically leads to the trickledown effect. However, proponents of the social development approach argue that the trickledown effect is a myth given that many countries continue to experience widening poverty and inequality in their populations despite attaining notable economic growth (Midgley, 1995; Patel, 2005).

Looking at the notion of state interventionism, one realises that it is an undertaking requiring political intervention beyond the professional boundaries and traditional confines of social work. At best, social work practitioners can try to advocate for policies that favour state interventionism. However, they hardly have direct influence over such an undertaking.

33.3.3 Social Development Is Multisectoral

Another key characteristic of the social development is that it is multisectoral. In other words, social development cannot happen if the key sectors of the economy do not work in a coordinated manner which ensures integrated service delivery (Gray, 1997; Midgley, 1995). The idea of multisectoral arrangements can only be realised through collective planning and coordinated service delivery that harmonises approaches and resource pooling. In African countries, this requires that different ministries have to work together, not just on an ad hoc basis but in a thoroughly thought-out manner. This ideal is easy to talk about but nearly impossible to realise.

33.3.4 Social and Economic Development Are Interlinked Aspects

An equally important feature of the social development approach, according to Midgley (1995), is the idea that social and economic aspects of development cannot be separated. In other words, there is a need to harmonise social and economic development at the planning level. Activities that are designed to bring economic development have to be planned in a manner that automatically leads to social improvement in the population. Similarly, social welfare initiatives should not only be consumptive but must directly and indirectly lead to economic benefit. In this regard, social policies have to directly contribute to the empowerment and strengthening of human capacities for self-reliance; this allows beneficiaries to become productive and contributing citizens rather than mere consumers (Midgley, 1995). On closer analysis of this key feature, one also realises that a harmonisation of social and economic aspects of development can genuinely be achieved on a macro scale through state planning rather than isolated micro-level efforts of social workers and their agencies, even though efforts at those levels is equally critical. In this regard, the implementation of the social development is beyond social work. As soon as this fact is acknowledged, social workers will be in a better position to define a more practical and achievable agenda for the profession that allows it to contribute meaningfully to the realisation of social development.

33.3.5 Social Development Is Universal and Inclusive

Another distinguishing feature of the social development approach is that it is said to be inclusive and universalistic (Gray, 1997; Midgley, 1995). Thus, unlike traditional social welfare approaches that target the needy and vulnerable, social development is targeted at macro-level development, which benefits all segments of the population. For example, improvements in healthcare and education at a policy and practice level will benefit not only disadvantaged groups but all people in the population. While social workers have been claimed to be at the forefront of 'implementing' the social development, most social work interventions are largely targeted at the poor and marginalised within society. Thus, most efforts remain largely remedial and curative, barely scratching the surface of authentic social development practice.

The foregoing discussion clearly shows that social development is best realised through politics rather than professional commitments of social work alone. Without directly influencing the politics and policies of the day in any given context, it would be fraudulent for social work to claim this approach. Its realisation can only come about as a result of cross-sectoral arrangements underpinned by centralised state planning and coordination. Proponents of the social development approach need to clearly articulate ways through which such arrangements can become possible.

Social work clients are largely victims of unjust economic arrangements born out of bad politics. As argued, the current neo-liberal trajectory, which is nearly universal in its application, has led to the creation of structural and institutional disadvantages that trap many people in poverty. Social development is an approach that rejects neo-liberal economic thinking (Midgley, 1995). It is therefore paradoxical for social workers to claim to be implementing the social development approach while operating in a state dominated by neo-liberal economics and with a welfare sector characterised by a residual approach. The two approaches cannot coexist.

33.4 Rethinking Social Development: Lessons for a Post-COVID-19 Socioeconomic Agenda for Africa

The introductory part of this chapter was focused on discussing the impact of the COVID-19 pandemic with a bias on African economies. The discussion showed that emerging economies around the globe are the most affected economically and will take time to recover. The COVID-19 crisis has a human cost to it beyond health fatalities. The economic disruption caused by the pandemic will plunge more than half a billion people into poverty (Filho et al., 2020). The crisis is a wakeup call for developing countries in Africa to rethink their development trajectory. It is also a time for social work to reflect on its complicity role as an instrument of the state within global neo-liberal economic arrangements. Social work is arguably a profession that has for long been focusing on supporting the poor in state-directed ways that largely maintain the poor in their poverty and keep them disenfranchised. Social development is an approach that holds much promise; however, social workers need to rethink their thinking of this approach. This section discusses several lessons that can be gleaned from the COVID-19 crisis to inform a post-COVID-19 socioeconomic agenda for Africa. The lessons are as follows.

33.4.1 The Current Global Economic Arrangements of Neo-liberalism Are Not Sustainable and Are Incompatible with Social Development

The major lesson to be learnt from the current COVID-19 crisis is the realisation that the current global arrangements of neo-liberalism are simply not sustainable, especially for developing economies. van Barneveld et al. (2020) note that ever since the crisis started it has become apparent that neo-liberalism as a political and economic regime is simply not sustainable, given its negative impact on the economies, health, and social well-being of people especially in developing nations. Based on neo-liberalism's prescription of markets as the panacea to all human problems, the dismantling of the state's role in economic and social planning has left many countries with limited capacity to manage the crisis. The global arrangements of capitalism, which have been made possible by the rapid pace of globalisation, have led to a situation wherein countries now specialize in producing products and services according to their inherent capabilities and comparative advantage (Mason, 2017). These market arrangements which happen on a global scale lead to a reduced role of the state in directing economic development as multinational corporations take the lead role in determining the global economic arrangements. This undermines and erodes the autonomy and ability of the states to determine domestic economic policy especially on industrialisation. Such neo-liberal arrangements have served to ensure that African countries remain trapped in the role of global suppliers of raw materials and other basic primary products while the first world specialises in sophisticated industrial production and value addition of African commodities.

Desai (2019) notes that "in the dialectic of uneven and combined development that drives them, dominant capitalist nations seek to create and maintain the unevenness of world capitalist development that favours them (p. 1054)". It is clear that the neo-liberal prescription of non-state involvement in global economic arrangements does not apply to first world governments. This is a prescription that largely applies to emerging economies and is clearly indicative of the uneven power relations. In reality first world governments retain state autonomy in regulating markets when it is in their interest to do so while denying the same privilege to developing countries. Social development is largely anchored in the notion that state intervention in economic planning and market regulation is necessary. Thus, social development is not compatible with neo-liberalism as it is not possible to achieve social development objectives under neo-liberal economic arrangements. Social work and social workers in Africa need to be conscious of this reality. A post-COVID-19 social development agenda for Africa should be centred on reclaiming state sovereignty in determining the economic direction of states. Such economic planning needs to be focussed on ensuring that economic arrangements serve the interests of the majority of people rather than the capitalist interests of the elite classes in society as is currently the case. This is an agenda that social work can contribute to but will certainly not be able to drive it alone.

33.4.2 Globalisation Has Its Advantages But Makes Africa Vulnerable

Another key lesson to be gleaned from the current pandemic is a fact commonly known, that despite the many benefits of globalisation; in its current format it hurts African economies. Millions of people in African countries live on the margins of the mainstream economy because of the adverse effects of exploitative global economic arrangements (Mutenheri & Kokorwe, 2020; Rodney, 1972). The ease with which African countries can import finished goods and services from advanced nations undermines the ability of Africa countries to build local industrial capacity for production of such goods (Kanu, 2020). This reliance on developed economies leaves Africa vulnerable. In the face of the COVID-19-induced closure of national borders, the globalisation project has been crushed, and countries are looking inwards and becoming protectionist. The whole global supply chain has been disrupted, leaving many African countries with dire shortages of life-savings goods and services. African countries need to rethink the makeup of their economies and ensure that in future disasters, which are inevitable, they are able to manage better and protect their citizens. van Barneveld et al. (2020) posit that the COVID-19 events have largely exposed why it is irresponsible for governments to follow a neoliberal path which has led to the decline of industrial production in critical sectors. van Barneveld et al. (2020) further argue that countries need to ensure that they operate strategic sectors which will enable them to cope with future disasters that may lead to the disruption of global processes.

Developed countries have also clearly demonstrated that in the face of a catastrophe the first and foremost commitment will be to their countries rather than pushing for global solidarity and collective action (van Barneveld et al., 2020). Such narrow nationalistic interests leave Africa vulnerable and desperate. The very nations responsible for pushing economic policies that undermine the state capacity to respond while privileging the role of markets have shown the obvious need for strengthened state capacity to regulate markets, especially in times of catastrophes. Scholars such van Barneveld et al. (2020) and Chowdhury and Jomo (2020) note that there was a failure to show global leadership in responding to the pandemic and the leading economies looked inwards to the narrow nationalist priorities. The message sent out by such nationalistic responses should be clear for Africa and other emerging economies: 'you are on your own in times of crisis so better be prepared.' It would be very irresponsible on the part of developing countries to fail to heed such a clear message. Economic reform in the post COVID-19 dispensation is an imperative for Africa. Without these higher-order actions, social workers will continue to work on interventions that keep the poor poor and maintaining them in their disenfranchised positions. It is at the political level that such high-impact changes can be realised.

Globalisation cannot be undone and is indeed necessary, but the global social and economic arrangements need revisiting. As already argued in the first section of this chapter, Africa will struggle to recover from the COVID-19 pandemic. There is a real possibility that more lives will end up being lost from economic vulnerabilities than by fatalities caused by the virus. Africa, and Sub-Saharan Africa in particular, has for years been faced with an even more lethal 'virus' of poverty. It affects more people than those who will die from the current pandemic. It is therefore key for African economies to realise the need for urgency in reimagining and recreating new economic models based on self-reliance and people-centred principles rather than the current economic models that are designed to carter for the needs of first world economies. Social work in Africa has a key role in informing the post-COVID-19 socioeconomic order. We need to amplify our voice by providing insights that will lead to the creation of a more just and humane society anchored on the preservation of human dignity and cultivation of human capabilities for self-sustenance. The social development approach, if implemented in its authentic form, can indeed lead to a fair socioeconomic order. Thus, it is important for social workers to distinguish the social development approach from the current welfarist practices that have been claimed to be social development when in reality its low-level actions keep the poor dependant and vulnerable.

33.4.3 African Countries Need to Delink from the Global Economy

Since the COVID-19 pandemic began, 10 billionaires increased their wealth by $400 billion, and the wealth of many more people from developed nations has dramatically increased during the period of the pandemic (Neate, 2020). It is 'immoral' that close to half a billion people face starvation and suffering while an insignificant portion of the wealth that is in the hands of the world's richest persons is enough to avert such unnecessary suffering. Indeed, African countries have been recipients of, and continue to receive, global aid flowing from rich nations. However, it should be noted that most such aid is largely used in consumptive ways and takes away the dignity of millions. It is immoral to normalise such dependence when it is possible to empower poor people to be able to sustain themselves. The donor aid trap has to be avoided, and this can only happen if Africa begins to wean itself from its reliance on first world 'benevolence.' The very same first world benefits multiple times more than the amounts they give in aid through unfair and imbalanced neo-liberal trade arrangements.

It is therefore vital that in Africa, countries should begin to think of ways to strategically delink from the global economy and initiate new post-COVID-19 economic and social arrangements. Delinking is a concept that emerged from the dependency theorists such as Emmanuel Wallerstein and Andre Gunder Frank. It is a concept predicated on two main aspects. Firstly, developing countries need to wean themselves from the parasitic economic ties that are characteristic of the current neo-liberal global economic order. Secondly, delinking focuses on the need for developing nations to assert their political independence by championing nationalistic projects that address the needs of their own people than being extensions of first world economic and political realities (Mutenheri & Kokorwe, 2020). It should be noted that delinking does not advocate for a complete break in economic and political ties; rather, it focuses on doing away with only those economic and political relationships that are exploitative and lead to chronic dependence. To this end, delinking is about building the capacity for African countries to be able to provide for their own people independent of the 'big brother nations.' Thus, although globalisation is irreversible, the dependant economic and political arrangements can be altered by building and strengthening the capacities for self-reliance by African states.

Without delinking, African countries will continue to be dependent on first world countries for even the most trivial things. Kanu (2020) notes that many African countries depend "on finished goods from Europe, America, China, etc., goods such as toothpick, face masks, ventilators, foodstuff." Africa has the capacity to feed itself and also supply the whole world with its food needs, yet Africa remains a basket case. So long the colonial ties and parasitic economic relationships remain intact, it will be difficult to build the internal capacity of African nations. Faced with crippling shortages of goods such as face masks and ventilators, some African countries have started to manufacture these life-saving goods, demonstrating the inherent potential for Africa countries to develop their own industrial manufacturing hubs. This latent potential needs to be further exploited in the post-COVID-19 dispensation and it is going to take political will. Beneficiation of raw materials and produce needs to be a key thrust for African economies in a post-COVID-19 order, creating massive job opportunities, infrastructure, and better economic returns. Further, intra-African trade needs to be aggressively promoted through improved transportation infrastructure and trade policies that enhance the ease of doing business on the continent.

33.4.4 Epistemic Delinking Is a Necessary Precursor to Economic and Political Delinking

One of the major shifts that is needed if African countries are to successfully delink their economies from the global North is to first define new social, economic, and political thought that is suited to the contextual needs of Africa rather than relying on paradigms of knowledge based on and informed by western epistemic foundations. There is need to avoid unicentrism, which obligates the global South to look at the world and understand it through Western centric paradigm. In line with decolonial praxis, it is important for African countries to attain epistemic delinking and begin to produce knowledge that is informed by multiple Afro-centric perspectives (Mignolo, 2007). Mignolo (2007) posits that a decolonial epistemic shift for the global South is needed, and its function would be to give birth to multiple epistemologies. Without this epistemic independence, Africa cannot shift towards economic and social thought that leads to its own development. In the same vein, Africa will not be able fully participate in the global material and knowledge economy without the attainment of epistemic independence that can only come about through an epistemic delink from the global north. The need for epistemic delinking that should precede the actual socioeconomic and political delinking is aptly captured by Oldekop et al. (2020), who note that "the COVID-19 pandemic has highlighted the falsity of any assumption that the global North has all the expertise and solutions to tackle global challenges, and has further highlighted the need for multi-directional learning and transformation in all countries towards a more sustainable and equitable world" (p. 1). It is therefore important for Africa, as it is indeed for all emerging economies, to promote scholarship and critical dialogue that will lead to the production of knowledge needed to inform emancipatory development and sustainable development trajectories.

33.4.5 Social Work Needs to Adopt a Radical Shift Towards a Community Development Bias to Meaningfully Contribute to Social Development

Lastly, for social work in Africa to be effective in contributing to social development and the poverty eradication agenda, a radical shift towards community development is needed. It is through local community development efforts that social work can best contribute to the fight against poverty. In the context of this chapter, community development is used to refer to any grassroots initiatives that are targeted at helping citizens to move towards self-reliance. A bias towards community development initiatives that promote self-sustenance can be one of the most effective ways to achieve social development (Midgley, 1995).

33.4.6 Address the Rural Development–Urban Divide

It is also important to note that a majority of Africa's poor reside in rural areas. Realistically, for most of the rural poor agriculture is the main and sometimes the only means of survival. However, a majority of the rural people remain landless, and where land is available, they have to rely on erratic rainfall as well as having to manually work the land as the costs of mechanised labour are exorbitant. In this regard, the land question in Africa is a reality that cannot be ignored, and social work needs to wake up to this reality if the implementation of social development is to be realised. Firstly, the rural and urban poor will have their dignity restored through land ownership. Secondly, they need to be empowered to work the land. Thirdly, they have to be linked to agricultural value chains to ensure that they benefit from fair prices for their products and are also empowered to do value addition for their produce, one of the areas that should be a key thrust for community development efforts. Rural poverty is a lived reality, and agriculture is the main escape route out of this poverty trap. It is worrying to note that there has not been much focus on this area in social work literature and social development. In the same vein, most social work services in Africa are characterised by an "urban bias" (Chambers, 1997) although the most vulnerable people are in rural communities. It is difficult to achieve authentic social development goals in Africa without addressing rural development and the land question. Western literature on social work cannot be expected to be concerned with these concerns given that Western scholars do not have such lived realities in their contexts. To this end, efforts towards epistemic emancipation and decolonisation of social work in Africa are needed. It is the African social work scholars who need to refocus the knowledge production agenda and chart a direction for social work that is grounded in Afrocentric realities.

33.5 Conclusion

The COVID-19 pandemic has shown how vulnerable Africa is in its position in a neo-liberal global order. More importantly, the pandemic has unmasked how Africa has always been faced by an even lethal 'virus' of poverty. This understanding has, however, been ignored as it hardly affects the global north and their elite counterparts in the global south who are responsible for running governments that have presided over untold suffering and widespread disenfranchisement of the masses. A rethink in approach is needed if Africa is to experience a new post-COVID-19 socioeconomic and political order that is responsive to the problems of underdevelopment. To this end, this chapter has argued for the need for Africa to delink from the global economy. This move can be achieved through enhanced state autonomy in policy making. Epistemic delinking is a prerequisite for birthing such as order. Lastly, it should be noted that by advocating for an anti neo-liberal stance the author is not necessarily pushing for a Marxist ideological position, but rather a mixed economy modelled along the social democratic ideological path would best suit African countries. This ideological position is also compatible with social development.

References

Becker, S. (1997). *Responding to poverty: The politics of cash and care*. Longman.

Chambers, R. (1997). *Whose reality counts– Putting the first last*. Intermediate Technology Publications.

Chikadzi, V., & Pretorius, E. (2011). Unhelpful help: The social work profession's response to mass poverty in South Africa. *Social Work/Maatskaplike Werk, 47*(3), 225–269.

Chowdhury, A., & Jomo, K. S. (2020). *West First policies expose myths*. InterPress Service News Agency. Available at https://www.ipsnews.net/2020/03/west-first-policiesexpose-myths/

Davis, A., & Wainwright, S. (2005). Combating poverty and social exclusion: Implications for social work education. *Social Work Education, 24*(3), 259–273. https://doi.org/10.1080/02615470500050453

Desai, R. (2019). What is to be done? The importance of Samir Amin's answer. *Globalizations, 16*(7), 1053–1061. https://doi.org/10.1080/14747731.2019.1654286

Fernandes, N. (2020). Economic effects of coronavirus outbreak (COVID-19) on the world economy. https://ssrn.com/abstract=3557504

Filho, W. L., Brandli, L. L., Salvia, M. L., Rayman-Bacchus, L., & Platje J. (2020) COVID-19 and the UN Sustainable Development Goals: Threat to solidarity or an opportunity? *Sustainability, 12*, 5343. https://doi.org/10.3390/su12135343

Frank, A. G. (1972). The development of underdevelopment. In J. D. Cockcroft, A. G. Frank, & D. Johnson (Eds.), *Dependence and underdevelopment*. Anchor Books.

Gray, M. (1997). A pragmatic approach to social development: Part 1. *Social Work/Maatskaplike Werk, 33*(3), 210–222.

Kanu, I. A. (2020). COVID-19 and the economy: An African perspective. *Journal of African Studies and Sustainable Development, 3*(2), 2630–7065.

Lawson, V., & Elwood, S. (2014). Encountering poverty: Space, class, and poverty politics. *Antipode, 46*(1), 209–228.

Lombard, A. (2008). Social work: A social partner in economic development. *Social Work/Maatskaplike Werk, 44*(2), 121–142.

Mason, J. W. (2017). *A cautious case for economic nationalism*. https://www.dissentmagazine.org/article/cautious-case-economic-nationalism-global-capitalism

Midgley, J. (1995). *Social development: The developmental perspective in social welfare*. Sage Publications.

Mignolo, W. (2007). *Delinking: The rhetoric of modernity, the logic of coloniality and the grammar of decoloniality*. Cultural Studies.

Mutenheri, F., & Kokorwe, L. F. (2020). Globalization or de-linking? Gauging the efficacy of global administration to global pandemics in the face of the novel corona virus between December 2019 and the first quarter of 2020. *Texila International Journal of Academic Research*. https://doi.org/10.21522/TIJAR.2014.07.01

Neate, R. (2020). *Ten billionaires reap $400bn boost to wealth during Pandemic*. The Guardian.

Nicola, M., Alsafi, Z., Sohrabi, C., Kerwan, A., Al-Jabir, A., Iosifidis, C., Agha, M., & Agha, R. (2020). The socio-economic implications of the coronavirus pandemic (COVID-19): A review. *International Journal of Surgery (London, England), 78*, 185–193. https://doi.org/10.1016/j.ijsu.2020.04.018

O'Brien, M. (2013). Social work registration and professionalism: Social justice and poverty – fellow travellers or discarded passengers? *Aotearoa New Zealand Social Work, 25*(3), 50–59.

Oldekop, J. A., Horner, R., Hulme, D., Adhikari, R., Agarwal, B., Alford, M., Bakewell, O., Banks, N., Barrientos, S., Bastia, T., Bebbington, A. J., Das, U., Dimova, R., Duncombe, R., Enns, C., Fielding, D., Foster, C., Foster, T., Frederiksen, T., … Zhang, Y. F. (2020). COVID-19 and the case for global development. *World Development, 134*, 105044. https://doi.org/10.1016/j.worlddev.2020.105044

Patel, L. (2005). *Social welfare and social development in South Africa*. Oxford University Press.

van Barneveld, K., Quinlan, M., Kriesler, P., Junor, A., Baum, F., Chowdhury, A., (Raja) Junankar, P., Clibborn, S., Flanagan, F., Wright, C. F., Friel, S., Halevi, J., & Rainnie, A. (2020). The COVID-19 pandemic: Lessons on building more equal and sustainable societies. *The Economic and Labour Relations Review, 31*(2), 133–157. https://doi.org/10.1177/1035304620927107

34 Critiquing Western Development Paradigms and Theories in the Age of the Coronavirus (COVID-19): An African Perspective

Ndangwa Noyoo

34.1 Introduction

In the early 1990s, the American political scientist, Francis Fukuyama, confidently declared that the ascendancy of liberal democracy around the world indeed signified "the end of history." Fukuyama's thesis, which he expounded in his book titled *The End of History and the Man*, was published in 1992. Fukuyama (1992) argued that insofar as humankind's search for ideological expression, Western liberal democracy was the ultimate ideology or political system that could not be overtaken by any other. His confidence was further extended to the belief that Western capitalism and other systems of the West were superior and thus it was inevitable that they occupied a hegemonic position in the world, because of the failure of other systems or ideologies. Thus, this thinking went on to underscore the fact that Western liberal democracy had not only surpassed other ideologies and sociopolitical systems around the world, but that it would outlast them. Furthermore, the collapse of the Union of Soviet Socialist Republics (USSR) and its satellite states in the late 1980s and early 1990s, and the supposed relegation of socialism to the historical archives, seemed to cement Fukuyama's point of view. This was not the first time that Western thoughts and systems had been taken as a fait accompli type of affair, as can be noted from the rise of developmentalism and development thought after the end of the Second World War. However, it can be argued that COVID-19 has stripped bare the presumed global omnipotence of Western development paradigms and theories in these contemporary times. Momentarily, the world's major capitalist societies have been ravaged and continue to be threatened by the COVID-19 pandemic. Arguably, Western societies have actually proved to be the worst performers in the fight against COVID-19. In particular, the United States of America (U.S.) seems to have dismally failed in this endeavour despite all the wealth and technology it has at its disposal. Notwithstanding, this was during the corrupt, racist, and infantile rule of Donald Trump. Since his defeat by Joe Biden, the U.S. seems to be doing much better in the fight against COVID-19 and has a robust vaccination rollout programme in place.

This chapter critiques Western development paradigms and theories during the COVID-19 pandemic as a way of showing how impractical development efforts, based on the former, have been in the last six decades in Africa. The discussion does this through a historical lens that casts a backward glance into Africa's recent past by trying to decipher how this continent tried to develop itself, after the fall of colonialism. In putting forward its arguments and suggestions, the

N. Noyoo (✉)
Department of Social Development, University of Cape Town, Cape Town, South Africa
e-mail: ndangwa.noyoo@uct.ac.za

M. C. S. Gonçalves et al. (eds.), *The Coronavirus Crisis and Challenges to Social Development*,
https://doi.org/10.1007/978-3-030-84678-7_34

chapter first provides a backdrop and context of development and how it was imported into Africa in the late 1950s and 1960s, after many African countries attained independence. The chapter then delineates the key conceptual and theoretical issues that inform its analysis. Thereafter, attention is turned to the pandemic and the chapter highlights how COVID-19 unfolded across the globe and afterwards in Africa. The chapter then advances the critique of Western development paradigms and theories while casting light on previous attempts that were made to develop the African continent by both the West and African countries themselves. It ends with proposals for an alternative development agenda for Africa in a post-COVID-19 era.

34.2 The Quest to Develop Africa: Backdrop and Context

After the end of the Second World War, there was an explosion of work and initiatives that aimed to answer the development question and how it related to the developing world or what was then referred to as the 'Third World.' These endeavours and efforts were, for the most, at the behest of the West. With the U.S. and Great Britain emerging triumphant over Germany and its allies, when the Second World War ended, a new global order would be shaped by the former powers. On the one hand, they established several global institutions and organisations to define and give content to this new world order. To this end, the United Nations Organisation was created in 1945 to help preserve peace across the globe. Implicitly, the UN seemed to have initially been informed by Western world views as well as Western ideologies and perspectives. However, it must be noted that as more and more newly independent nations from the Global South became members of the UN, they would vociferously champion progressive agendas related to social justice, human rights, and similar issues. Nevertheless, the creation of the Bretton Woods Institutions such as the World Bank and the International Monetary Fund (IMF) was an extension of this project. These interventions would inadvertently reinforce the notion of equating development to Westernisation, while propping up neo-liberalism as the only vehicle that could foster development. These foregoing events meant that development would be construed solely from the experiences of the West. Rapley (2007, p. 1) explains:

> In those days, development was considered largely synonymous with industrialisation. Its ultimate goal was fairly clear: to raise incomes and in the process give poor people access to the range of goods and services then widespread in developed societies. It was, in short, about getting richer or more prosperous; and prosperity was measured in dollar figures. Moreover, given the state of the industrial countries at that time, and the lessons their experiences had taught, industrialisation—and in particular, the creation of a country's capacity to manufacture finished goods—was seen as essential.

On the other hand, the said new world order was tied to Westernisation through 'development aid' which Western countries provided to the 'developing' world and, in particular, newly independent African countries. Such 'aid' had conditionalities that forced African countries to follow the trajectory of Western societies and assimilate Western traits, thinking, and so forth, into their institutions, among others. Since 'development' is something that was conceived in the West and transposed to non-Western societies, we should not lose sight of its colonial, imperialistic, and capitalist trappings. It is worthy of note that following the decline of British imperialism and the rise of decolonisation in the 1950s, a new development project emerged in a US-driven discourse. During this period, there was the emergence of the so-called 'Third World.' The 'Third World,' now known as the 'developing world,' was sandwiched between the capitalist and communist antagonists of the Cold War (Munk, 2018). To this end, development became something one party could do to another. The low level of economic development in decolonising Africa in particular was contrasted to the booming economy of the U.S., which was rapidly becoming a hegemonic power. The divide between the coloniser and the colonised of the imperial period now became the 'development–underdevelopment divide' that characterised the post-colonial period (Munk, 2018). In this regard, development was conceptualised and defined from the perspectives of the West and not from those of the developing world or Africa. Rist (1997) rightly asserts that what passes today for the truth of the history of humankind (that is, progressive access of every nation to the benefits of 'development') *is actually based upon the way in which Western society—to the exclusion of all others—has conceptualised its relationship to the past and the future*.

Thus, Western experts and institutions were preoccupied with the idea of 'modernising' the 'developing world' and Africa. To achieve this, they relied on theoretical positions of the modernisation theory. This theory, which was inspired by the ideas of Max Weber and executed by Western scholars such as Talcott Parson, Walt Whitman Rostow, and Daniel Lerner, among others, is bipolar in outlook and content, as it posits two contexts, namely, the traditional society and a modern one (Noyoo, 2015). Modernisation theory presupposes that 'backward' or 'traditional' societies have to follow the same trajectories of Western nations for them to become developed. It picks up from the biological sciences of eighteenth-century Europe that likened human society to biological organisms. Modernisation theorists saw development as an evolutionary process going through various stages and transforming all societies from traditional to modern (Noyoo, 2015). However, modernisation theory failed to capture the underlying historical and structural forces that hindered African societies from developing themselves. At the centre of Africa's so-called backwardness was its underdeveloped status, which was induced by slavery and colonialism (Dumont, 1966; Rodney, 1973; Amin, 1990). The next section presents the theoretical premise of the chapter.

34.3 Theoretical Premises of the Chapter

34.3.1 Defining Development

The main issue under scrutiny in this chapter is development. It must be borne in mind that there are many definitions and perspectives of development and what it is supposed to achieve in societies. For Himmelstrand (1994), development is a multi-dimensional concept. Thus, to understand and define development as a broad concept, one must deal with it as both an analytical concept and a method. Bellù (2011, p. 2), on the other hand, observes that in general terms development means an event constituting a new stage in a changing situation or the process of change per se. If not qualified, development is implicitly intended as something positive or desirable. Therefore, when referring to a society or to a socioeconomic system, development usually means improvement, either in the general situation of the system, or in some of its constituent elements. Development may occur by some deliberate action carried out by single agents or by some authority pre-ordered to achieve improvement, to favourable circumstances in both. Thus, development policies and private investment, in all their forms, are examples of such actions (Bellù, 2011). In many cases, development has been associated with social change. According to Leicht (2018), social change refers to the significant alteration of social structure and cultural patterns through time. In this regard, social structure denotes persistent networks of social relationships where interaction between people or groups has become routine and repetitive. On the other hand, culture signifies shared ways of living and thinking that include symbols and language (verbal and nonverbal); knowledge, beliefs, and values (what is 'good' and 'bad'); norms (how people are expected to behave); and techniques ranging from common folk recipes to sophisticated technologies and material objects (Leicht, 2018).

This chapter adopts the definition of development that was proffered by Gunnar Myrdal because it is holistic in content and outlook and seems more relevant to Africa:

> By development I mean the movement upward of the entire social system, and I believe this is the only logically tenable definition. This social system encloses, besides the so-called economic factors, all noneconomic factors, including all sorts of consumption by various groups of people; consumption provided collectively; educational and health facilities and levels; the distribution of power in society; and more generally economic, social, and political stratification; broadly speaking, institutions and attitudes—to which we must add as an exogenous set of factors induced policy measures applied in order to change one or several of these endogenous factors (Myrdal, 1974, pp. 729–730).

34.3.2 Underdevelopment

We cannot discuss development in Africa without coming to grips with the phenomenon of underdevelopment. According to Rodney (1973), all countries named 'underdeveloped' in the world are exploited by others; and underdevelopment with which the world is now preoccupied is a product of imperialist, colonialist, and capitalist exploitation. It must be noted that African and Asian societies were developing independently until they were taken over directly or indirectly by the capitalist powers. When that happened, exploitation increased and the export of surplus ensued, depriving the African and Asian societies of the benefits of their natural resources and labour. Thus, this is an integral part of underdevelopment in the cotemporary sense. Furthermore, Rodney (1973) avers that an indispensable component of modern underdevelopment is expressed through a particular relationship of exploitation by another. In this sense, underdevelopment was not a condition that was intrinsic to Africa, because it is a condition that was historically produced through capitalist expansion and imperialism.

Rodney seems to have echoed the sentiments of the progressive French scholar, René Dumont (1966), who argued that Africa's problems centred on one phenomenon, namely, underdevelopment. To him, Africa was a continent without industry, without resources of energy, and with only unskilled labour; and without modern methods of cultivation and consequently without high yields and without buying power for the products of future industries. Thus, a new vicious circle formed. Although endorsing industrialisation as a partial answer to Africa's underdevelopment, he firmly believed that agriculture was key to unlocking the continent's potential (Dumont, 1966). Agriculture's potential to catapult Africa into an age of prosperity was recognised by the eminent Egyptian intellectual, Samir Amin, as well. Amin ascribed to the notion that Africa's challenges emanated from its underdeveloped status. For him, "the ultimate reason for the failure of 'development,' more striking in this region than in any other, is that Africa has not begun its agricultural revolution, without which any development is unimaginable" (Amin, 1990, p. 8). Therefore, it can be argued that in their attempts to urge Africa to develop in a particular way, Western nations and financial organisations relied upon paradigms, theories, and models of development to legitimise their biased intentions. For newly independent African countries, there was an urgent need to move themselves out of the quagmire of inter alia: poverty, disease and illiteracy—which were direct offshoots of colonial domination. Therefore, the question that was tackled immediately after the independence of Africa's nations in the late 1950s and 1960s was: Were they the best models of development available for the task at hand? (Amaizo, 2012).

34.3.3 Paradigms and Theories

Paradigms were some of the tools relied upon by development experts and international organisations when they advised or even coerced governments and politicians of African nations to solely rely on Western perspectives of development. According to Kuhn (1962), a paradigm is a way of viewing the world, or an 'analytic lens,' similar to spectacles or a framework from which to understand the human experience. Bellù (2011, pp. 5–6) observes that countries as well as the international development community, in different periods, have privileged specific ways of achieving development, by adhering to a particular development paradigm, that is, to a defined modality or path to achieve development, based on a codified set of activities and/ or a vision regarding the functioning and evolution of a socioeconomic system. Among other things, a common definition for theory is "a systematic set of interrelated statements intended to explain some aspect of social life" (Rubin & Babbie, 2017, p. 615). King et al. (1994), as cited in Remler and Van Ryzin (2015), assert that social science theory is a reasoned and precise speculation about the answer to a research question, including a statement about why the proposed answer is correct. As can be noted from the foregoing definitions, paradigms and theories that are derived from a particular social context will mirror conditions and variables specific to such an environment. Therefore, when used to interpret the conditions of other settings such as, in this case, African countries, they fall short of proffering solutions to specific challenges existing in Africa because they are gleaned from a context that is very different to Africa.

In this sense, the West has and continues to provide its development recipes to African countries that are derived from its historical and sociopolitical context. Thus, its development paradigms and theories, which are relied upon by experts to arrive at possible solutions for African countries' development problems, are counterintuitive in most cases. In fact, it can be argued that a pernicious offshoot of the dilemma in which African countries find themselves is that they get locked into a development pathway that ultimately does not liberate them from the colonial agenda of exploitation or of underdevelopment but rather reinforces their dependent state. The former is defined as path dependence. This discussion contends that the West has locked African countries into path dependence that is inimical to its true development and for Africa to extricate itself from this pathway, it has to cast away all its borrowed development paradigms and theories, and come up with its own. In essence, path dependence describes how the reinforcement of a given set of arrangements over time raises the cost of changing them (Prado & Trebilcock, 2009). Hence:

> A simple model of path dependence would therefore emphasise three features of an arrangement: (1) an initial set of choices or random events that determine the starting position; (2) the subsequent reinforcement of those choices or events through 'feedback effects'; and (3) the degree to which switching costs may preclude good alternatives from being explored in the long run (Prado & Trebilcock, 2009, p. 351)

Arguably, path dependence has made it very costly for African countries, not in monetary terms, but in regard to being more innovative and intellectually robust, so as to come up with indigenous African paradigms and theories of development. In fact, it can be further argued that some African politicians and governments have become intellectually lazy and incompetent, over the decades, when it comes to matters of development, that they have come to see it as 'cost effective' to merely ape or parrot the West's development pursuits. The postcolonial era did not extricate Africa from the colonial clutches and subjugation it had experienced for centuries. This period only ameliorated the difficulties Africa encountered globally, whether in areas of agriculture, trade, or Foreign Direct Investment (FDI), among other things. This period has been characterised by the continued aping of the West and utilisation of this society's redundant theories as Amaizo (2012, p. 117) argues:

> Africa's economic growth and dependence since independence has been characterised by a zero-sum economic interaction with the West. This was no more than a continuation of the Centre-Periphery relationship that existed during colonial times. The result of the zero-sum game interaction between Africa and the West has been to further increase the historic unequal exchange. Economic crises marked by massive unemployment, low wages and high prices have led to dangerous migrations from the discontented continent. The problem is that the post-colonial African nations are still firmly tied to the economic theories and programmes of their erstwhile colonisers. Thus, the solutions offered by way of the West are no more than palliatives. The solution is to develop

> new theories and pragmatic solutions that derive from autonomous Africa-centred positions. This is the significance of an alternative African developmentalism.

34.4 The Structural Adjustment Programmes (SAPs) and Africa's Underdevelopment

It is important to highlight how the West had been involved in actions aimed at extorting or blackmailing Africa to follow Western development paradigms and theories. This arm twisting of African countries was in many instances operationalised by Western countries and institutions such as the World Bank and International Monetary Fund (IMF). Conditional aid and economic adjustment with conditionalities epitomised 'development aid' in this era. Hence, accepting the World Bank's advice on economic restructuring, or 'structural adjustment programmes' (SAPs), became a condition for access to concessional credit. These claimed to reflect agreement on 'good' and necessary policies between the two Washington-based Bretton Woods Institutions (BWIs) and the U.S. Treasury Department, later dubbed the 'Washington Consensus' (Sundaram & Chowdhury, 2019). Mkandawire and Soludo (1998, p. xi) rightly arrive at the following conclusion in regard to SAPs:

> For almost two decades, countries in sub-Saharan Africa (SSA) have implemented structural-adjustment programmes (SAPs), and at the threshold of a new millennium, Africa may be graduating from being a region with 'lost development decades' to becoming the world's 'forgotten continent.' After more than a decade of acrimonious debates and tonnes of evaluation reports, there is an increasing convergence of views that SAPs have not worked and that, as designed, they are grossly defective as a policy package for addressing the endemic poverty and pervasive underdevelopment of the region.

The SAPs encumbered Africa's development pursuits which were quite effective in the 1960s and 1970s in raising the quality of life of Africans. Even the Bretton Woods Institutions later admitted this fact. Sundaram and Chowdhury (2019, p. 1) point out that according to their own internal evaluations, both the World Bank and IMF have huge credibility deficits due to the policy conditionalities and advice they have dispensed to developing countries in recent decades. Taking advantage of the debt distress in many developing countries early in the 1980s, the World Bank championed neo-liberal reforms, telling countries to "privatise, liberalise and globalise" (Sundaram & Chowdhury, 2019). The IMF added 'stabilisation'—primarily cutting government expenditure to contain inflation and balance of payments deficits—to the list of conditions for countries to qualify for the BWI's financial resources (Sundaram & Chowdhury, 2019). This is the development landscape that existed in Africa when COVID-19 broke out.

34.5 COVID-19 and Development

In late 2019, it was reported in international media outlets that a new and deadly virus had been discovered in the city of Wuhan in China. It not only rendered many people ill but killed a number of them as well. By January 2020, the virus had rapidly spread across the globe. The virus was identified as the novel coronavirus (COVID-19) pandemic which is spread through the air. In January 2020, the World Health Organization (WHO) declared COVID-19 a global pandemic. Italy was the first Western nation to be decimated by the virus, with thousands of Italians falling ill and many more dying from it. This scenario was replicated in the United Kingdom (UK) and the U.S. in a short space of time. In the UK and the US, the virus exposed these countries' long-standing racial fissures and inequalities that are reproduced by these societies' socio-political and economic systems. Razai, et al. (2021) reported that COVID-19 disproportionately affected ethnic minority groups in the UK. People of black ethnicity have had the highest diagnosis rates of the virus, with the lowest rates observed in white British people. In the U.S., COVID-19 deaths were and continue to be highly disproportionately experienced by African-Americans, Native Americans and

Hispanics (Wrigley-Field, 2020). What can be discerned from the foregoing picture is that Western development, which is premised on capitalism, is not only highly exploitative but inequitable. That is why ethnic minority groups are more likely to live in urban, overcrowded, and more deprived communities and to work in lower paid jobs in the West. Many of these jobs carry a high risk of exposure to COVID-19 (Razai et al., 2021).

It is safe to assert that the failures of capitalism have been laid bare during the pandemic, which has seen major capitalist countries floundering in their responses to COVID-19. Also, individualism, which is always touted by Western development experts as something worth emulating by non-Western societies, which are also not capitalist, was seriously called into question. It was clear that in the fight against COVID-19, almost all nations had to tap into the so-called informal social networks and bonds of solidarity that are commonplace in Africa, but which have been derided by some development experts and seen as impediments to Africa's development. When taking all these issues into critical consideration, the question for Africans is this: since capitalism engendered grave inequalities in Western countries such as the U.S., where the bulk of the wealth is in few hands, why should Africa emulate the West in matters of development? Taken further: is there a middle road where African countries can blend their indigenous systems with the inherited Western systems in a more fundamental way? As the pandemic raged on in the West, where capitalism reigns supreme, it was very clear to see that poverty and inequality are also racially based. In this context, racism both shapes the social determinants of health and has its own effect on the health of ethnic minorities (Razai et al., 2021).

To understand race and health, we must understand the role of ethnicity and racism within capitalist Western societies. Here, everyday acts of interpersonal discrimination, implicit biases, and cultural and structural racism will over time lead to worse health outcomes, including higher rates of chronic diseases and lower life expectancy (Razai et al., 2021). During this pandemic, we have been reminded once more that development is about the people, as the United Nations Development Programme (UNDP) rightly pointed out in its first Human Development Report of 1995 (UNDP, 1995; Noyoo, 2020). Development is not just about stock markets, inflation rates, or economic indicators such as the Gross Domestic Product (GDP). It is about people and their value systems, their aspirations, or their hopes. It is about vulnerable populations such as people with disabilities, older persons, and orphans. Development is for and about marginalised and excluded peoples of the world. In addition, development is about collective efforts of people in sustaining their communities and societies. Interestingly enough, since time immemorial, Africans have sought to improve their living conditions collectively and not individually. Colonialism and capitalism tried to destroy this African way of life for centuries but failed as it is still existing in many parts of Africa, albeit in a diluted form. That is why the African philosophy of *Ubuntu* still exists today. It recognises the fact that people are who they are because of other people's efforts. This shows that Africans can develop properly if this approach is elevated by governments and incorporated into public policies and development models.

Presently, various vaccines are under production after the first ones were finalised in late 2020. At the time of writing, several countries in the West have already rolled out the vaccines and are vaccinating their citizens against COVID-19. However, like anything else representing capitalism, the vaccines are already commodified. Thus, the global inequalities engendered by capitalism have come to the fore with the acquisition of the vaccines, as rich countries are hoarding vaccines and poorer countries in Africa and other parts of the 'developing world' are struggling to access them. Instead of basing the rollout of vaccines across the globe on solidarity, the countries with money are not willing to share with those that are less resourced, which led to a new global phenomenon known as 'vaccine nationalism.' The 'developing world,' and particularly Africa, are at the end of the vaccines queue. As the South African president, Cyril Ramaphosa, poignantly observes: "The painful irony is that some of the clinical trials for these vaccines were carried out in Africa" (Ramaphosa, 2021). Indeed, the same pharmaceutical companies that are not willing to share vaccines with African countries would not have arrived at any antidote for the virus if Africans had not participated in their clinical trials. This reservation also applies to European nations hoarding the vaccines. However, the rich countries do not seem to worry and only seem to want Africans to be their 'guinea pigs' in clinical trials. This whole situation is based on capitalist individualism and should not be surprising to the world. This is the type of development approach that was foisted on Africans, first by the colonialists and then by the developed North in the post-colonial era. However, this type of development does not resonate with the vast majority of Africans who continue to meet their needs through the extended family system and bonds of social solidarity such as *Ubuntu*, which sees everyone's humanity expressed in others (Noyoo & Boon, 2018). During the pandemic, many Africans have tapped into these social networks to survive and care for each other. Thus, it has become abundantly clear that the African indigenous systems of social security and reciprocity are effective in alleviating the dire socioeconomic conditions wrought by the pandemic.

34.6 Africa: A Curious Case for COVID-19

Even though social distancing, hand sanitising, and washing of hands became part of African's daily lexicon, many could not do these things effectively because they were poor and lived in crammed urban informal settlements or shanty towns, where unhygienic living conditions abound. These are the dwelling places of Africa's poor who constitute the majority of its population. This situation was a time bomb ready to explode. With derelict and inexistent health and social infrastructure, and with very few health professionals, many in the West had predicted that Africa would be decimated by the pandemic. Although many Africans have died from COVID-19, the numbers are not as were predicted. When taking the aforementioned issues into critical account, it can be argued that African countries have been able to weather the COVID-19 storm differently from the well-resourced countries of the West, leading to various commentators and experts advancing conflicting theories as to why this situation came to pass. Somehow, Africans have managed to do what they know best: face adversity and death with minimal resources and ingenuity, which makes Africa unique in the world. During this health crisis Africans have fallen back on their indigenous systems of care and support, given the fact that most countries are run by inept and corrupt politicians who have used the COVID-19 crisis to plunder national resources and steal from the poor.

Perhaps COVID-19 has taught African politicians and government bureaucrats a life's lesson: to invest money in their countries' healthcare systems and personnel and not to squander taxpayers' money by flying off overseas to be treated in European, East Asian, or American hospitals. This time around, hospitals in these societies were full of COVID-19 patients and there was a travel ban in force, thus causing the African politicians and government bureaucrats to remain in their own countries and make use of their health systems. Sadly, Africa's global weak status found it at the receiving end of racist antics from Europe and, ironically, China. Many so-called scientists felt compelled to argue that Africans needed to be used as 'guinea pigs' to arrive at a cure. Some French scientists could not help themselves but blurted out on national television that Africans had to be used as 'guinea pigs.' Meanwhile, in China, Africans were being discriminated against and ill treated because of COVID-19 (Cable News Network [CNN], 2020). That is why Africa needs its own development pathway.

34.7 Proposals for an Alternative Development Agenda for Africa Post COVID-19

Since the late 1990s, there have been calls for African governments to (re)take responsibility for developing an integrated framework that tackles poverty and socioeconomic development in their countries. The shift back towards African homegrown development is based on a wide consensus (by scholars, African leaders, and their development partners) that externally crafted and imposed development programmes have largely not been successful in transforming the socioeconomic status of African countries (Okereke & Agupusi, 2015). This chapter recognises that development should not be for a privileged few, but it should be for everyone in every society. It should be taken as a human right and thus every human being has a right to development. That being said, the chapter endorses the United Nations Declaration on the Right to Development (Resolution 41/ 128 of the General Assembly of the United Nations, 4 December 1986). Article 1, Number 1 of the Declaration (United Nations, 1986) states: *The right to development is an inalienable human right by virtue of which every human person and all peoples are entitled to participate in, contribute to, and enjoy economic, social, cultural and political development, in which all human rights and fundamental freedoms can be fully realised* (emphasis added). In the case of Africa, this development should be intrinsic to African conditions and linked to the right to be left alone, that is, that others refrain from making (paternalist) interventions in Africa.

In line with Amin (1990), this chapter argues that Africa's alternative development should neither be statism nor liberalism. Second, the content and internal political and social conditions for this alternative development should be national and popular. Third, it should be implemented through South–South co-operation and through a gradual evolution of the world system towards a better balanced political and economic polycentrism (Amin, 1990). Echoing the founding president of Tanzania, Julius Nyerere, Africa's development should be premised on self-reliance. This self-reliance should cut across all facets of human endeavour. This means that Africa must have its own paradigms, theories, thoughts and so forth and not rely on outsiders' interventions. To this end, "national self-reliance is a comprehensive strategy for avoiding dependence and promoting development. It entails disengagement from the international system, restructuring of international and internal relations, and eventual re-association with the international economy" (Biersteker, 1980, p. 229).

34.8 Conclusion

This chapter critiqued Western development paradigms and theories, and made proposals for an alternative African development pathway. This task was undertaken while recognising the devastating effects of COVID-19 on Africa. The borrowed development paradigms and theories that African countries have been using for decades meant that COVID-19 found them in an already weakened position. The chapter's proposed alternative development pathway is underpinned by the idea of self-reliance, which some African countries had sought when they had attained independence in the 1950s and 1970s, but which they all abandoned in later decades. It is important to note that whenever Western systems or paradigms collapse in Africa, people turn to the indigenous ones to protect themselves from various shocks, as was exemplified during the SAPs induced socioeconomic and political crises across Africa. Furthermore, it is now evident during the COVID-19 catastrophe that indigenous systems have a crucial role in meeting the needs of Africans through networks of solidarity and *Ubuntu*. With this occurrence, this chapter proposes that African governments should seriously consider mainstreaming the indigenous systems into their policy-making processes.

References

Amaizo, Y. E. (2012). An alternative African developmentalism: A critique of zero-sum games and palliative economics. *Africa Development, 37*(4), 117–140.

Amin, S. (1990). *Maldevelopment: Anatomy of global failure*. Zed Books.

Bellù, L. G. (2011). *Development and development paradigms: A (reasoned) review of prevailing visions*. Food and Agriculture Organisation (FAO).

Biersteker, T. J. (1980). Self-reliance in theory and practice in Tanzanian trade relations. *International Organisation, 34*(2), 229–264.

Cable News Network (CNN). (2020). *French doctors' proposal to test Covid-19 treatment in Africa slammed as 'colonial mentality'*. https://edition.cnn.com/2020/04/07/africa/french-doctors-africa-covid-19-intl/index.html

Dumont, R. (1966). *False start in Africa*. Andre Deutsch.

Fukuyama, F. (1992). *The end of history and the last man*. Free Press.

Himmelstrand, U. (1994). Perspectives, controversies and dilemmas in the study of African development. In U. Himmelstrand, K. Kinyanjui, & E. Mburugu (Eds.), *African perspectives on development: Controversies, dilemmas and openings* (pp. 16–36). James Currey.

King, G., Keohane, R. O., Sidney, S., & Verba, S. (1994). *Designing Social Inquiry: Scientific Inference in Qualitative Research*. Princeton, N.J: Princeton University Press.

Kuhn, T. (1962). *The structure of scientific revolutions*. University of Chicago Press.

Leicht, K. T. (2018). *Social change*. http://www.oxfordbibliographies.com/view/document/obo-9780199756384/obo-9780199756384-0047.xml

Mkandawire, T., & Soludo, C. C. (1998). *Our continent, our future: African perspectives on structural adjustment*. Council for the Development of Social Science Research in Africa (CODESRIA).

Munk, R. (2018). Development and social change: A genealogy for an era of complexity. In G. H. Fagan & R. Munk (Eds.), *Handbook on development and social change* (pp. 1–20). Edward Elgar.

Myrdal, G. (1974). What is development? *Journal of Economic Issues, 8*(4), 729–736.

Noyoo, N. (2015). Introduction to the concepts of social development. In L. Calvelo, R. Lutz, & F. Ross (Eds.), *Development and social work: Social work of the south* (Vol. VI, pp. 27–41). Paulo Freire Verlag.

Noyoo, N. (2020). *Social policy in post-Apartheid South Africa: Social re-engineering for inclusive development*. Routledge.

Noyoo, N., & Boon, E. (Eds.). (2018). *Indigenous social security systems in Southern and West Africa*. Sun Media Press.

Okereke, C., & Agupusi, P. (2015). *Homegrown development in Africa: Reality or illusion?* Routledge.

Prado, M., & Trebilcock, M. (2009). Path dependence, development, and the dynamics of institutional reform. *The University of Toronto Law Journal, 59*(3), 341–379.

Ramaphosa, C. M. (2021). *President Cyril Ramaphosa: Opening remarks at the African coronavirus COVID-19 vaccine financing and deployment strategy webinar*. https://www.gov.za/speeches/president-cyril-ramaphosa-opening-remarks-african-coronavirus-covid-19-vaccine-financing

Rapley, J. (2007). *Understanding development: Theory and practice in the third world* (3rd ed.). Lynne Rienner.

Razai, S. R., Kankam, H. K. N., Majeed, A., Esmail, A., & Williams, D. R. (2021). *Mitigating ethnic disparities in Covid-19 and beyond*. https://www.bmj.com/content/372/bmj.m4921. https://doi.org/10.1136/bmj.m4921

Remler, D. K., & Van Ryzin, G. G. (2015). *Research methods in practice: Strategies for description and causation* (2nd ed.). Sage.

Rist, G. (1997). *The history of development: From western origins to global faith*. Zed Books.

Rodney, W. (1973). *How Europe underdeveloped Africa*. Bogle-L'Ouverture.

Rubin, A., & Babbie, E. R. (2017). *Research methods for social work* (9th ed.). Wadsworth.

Sundaram, J. K., & Chowdhury, A. (2019). *Bretton Woods institutions: Enforcers, not savior?* https://www.theedgemarkets.com/article/bretton-woods-institutions-enforcers-not-saviours

United Nations. (1986). *Declaration on the right to development adopted by general assembly resolution 41/128 of 4 December 1986*. https://www.ohchr.org/en/professionalinterest/pages/righttodevelopment.aspx

United Nations Development Programme (UNDP). (1995). *Human development report*. UNDP.

Wrigley-Field, E. (2020). US racial inequality may be as deadly as COVID-19. *Proceedings of the National Academy of Sciences of the United States of America, 117*(36), 21854–21856. https://doi.org/10.1073/pnas.2014750117

35 How Has Population Health Been Amplified Through Integrated Indigenous Community Networks? Opportunities During the COVID-19 Pandemic

Claudia Ortiz-Rico

35.1 Introduction

During the COVID-19 pandemic, indigenous peoples have applied to their organization leaders for solutions. Historically, many public health surveillance systems in Latin America have not offered systematic information categorized by ethnicity or socioeconomic status. Such absence of information on the populations limits territorial and differential planning during crises (Sachs et al., 2020).

In Colombia, all municipalities with an indigenous population have tested positive for COVID-19, representing a large proportion of individuals who undergo economic and social activities. Municipalities with the highest proportion of indigenous populations have among the highest hospitalizations and death rates from COVID-19 (Chaparro et al., 2020). This emergency deepens the social disadvantages faced by vulnerable populations, notably significant morbidity and mortality caused by preexisting inequalities (Ardila-Sierra et al., 2020; Burstrom & Tao, 2020).

Despite recognizing a multiethnic state, the government has maintained structural violence toward indigenous communities. During the lockdown to prevent the spread of COVID-19, some of these communities have experienced stigmatization and militarization of their territories (Castro et al., 2020; Observatorio Político Electoral de la Democracia, 2020). The figures for violence and death against indigenous social leaders and environmental defenders have increased in different locations with high natural wealth; moreover, the number of armed actors in ancestral territories has increased (Guimarães & Ferreira Júnior, 2020).

To promote repression and ethnic stigmatization, various authoritarian strategies that have taken advantage of the pandemic have been deployed (Ravindran, 2020). Furthermore, in emergency management, the forms of organization of the indigenous authorities have been ignored by the government, and the lack of human resources in health and social protection in the most remote places has not been considered (Fernández-Niño et al., 2020; Organización Nacional Indígena de Colombia (ONIC), 2020b). Most indigenous communities have attempted to manage the situation by applying local solidarity approaches to overcome fear. In response, the indigenous guard was strengthened as a territorial control mechanism for self-organized peacebuilding (Chaves et al., 2020; Durán Castellanos, 2020).

High levels of poverty and low levels of access to quality health and public services in Colombia

C. Ortiz-Rico (✉)
Grupo Salud ComunidUdes, Facultad de Ciencias de la Salud, Universidad de Santander, Bucaramanga, Colombia

Red GRAAL - Grups de Recerca d'Amèrica i Àfrica Llatines, Barcelona, Spain
e-mail: cl.ortiz@mail.udes.edu.co

M. C. S. Gonçalves et al. (eds.), *The Coronavirus Crisis and Challenges to Social Development*,
https://doi.org/10.1007/978-3-030-84678-7_35

limit compliance with the government's lockdown measures regarding the fulfillment of basic needs such as access to safe water, hygiene, and food. There are several preexisting inequities between the indigenous population of 1,905,617 persons and the total Colombian population of 48,258,494. For example, for these populations, access to safe drinking water is 41% and 86%, access to sewerage is 23% and 77%, energy coverage is 66% and 96%, and Internet access is 6% and 43%, respectively. Furthermore, 17.2% and 6.1% of the indigenous population and nonindigenous population, respectively, cannot read or write; only 6.7% of the indigenous population can access higher education compared to the national average of 18.8% (Departamento Administrativo Nacional de Estadística, 2018). Additionally, indigenous peoples have a higher prevalence of infectious diseases, anemia, and chronic malnutrition compared to national averages (Montenegro & Stephens, 2006).

The history of extermination, territorial invasions, and ethnocide caused by infectious diseases has strengthened the self-determination narrative that promotes a collective-care community response to guarantee the survival of their culture and languages. Moreover, for indigenous peoples, among the elder deaths in general, and deaths caused by COVID-19, imply a significant loss for their communities because these elderly individuals have leadership roles and convey traditional knowledge (Golovatina et al., 2020).

The concept of health in indigenous populations recognizes connectivity with the territory and interconnectivity among spiritual energies, the natural world, and the self. Well-being arises from the relationship with everything around each person, which leads to positive health outcomes and the exchange of knowledge. The territory and the community are an extension of the self of indigenous peoples and are structured through social networks; the loss of this connection leads to a loss of identity and lower perceived health levels (Greenwood & de Leeuw, 2007). This community concept has been an essential factor in mobilizing care networks for indigenous populations in the pandemic context, presenting an alternative to overcome inequities.

The solidarity strategies of governmental institutions are contradictory to the indigenous solidarity proposals in Latin America because institutional solidarity imposes social orders that do not benefit the majority. Likewise, the lack of social participation among vulnerable populations promotes authoritarianism. As a result, community self-organization in indigenous territories has strengthened community networks and cooperation mechanisms, thus managing individual and collective risks in regions ignored by public administrations.

35.2 Indigenous Self-Determination for Emergency Response

Indigenous organizations worldwide have requested a systematic collection of COVID-19 data disaggregated by ethnicity and the continuous presence of healthcare and social workers close to indigenous communities (Cultural Survival, 2020). In some countries, collected data for indigenous peoples are shown in the aggregate and do not identify the individual's community (Awad & Konn, 2020). This information gap is being filled by the indigenous organizations that are collecting and analyzing information to monitor the emergency (Organización Nacional Indígena de Colombia (ONIC), 2020f).

Insufficient disaggregation of national averages by ethnicity, gender, and age hide inequities and limit successful population interventions (Romero-Sandoval et al., 2017). Thus, disaggregated data allow risk management among the most vulnerable groups by improving public health planning (Krieger et al., 2020). The lack of statistical recognition of indigenous peoples limits their access to services and resources, deepens structural violence, and prevents access to culturally adapted services (Browne et al., 2016).

The 2030 Sustainable Development Goals (SDG) agenda has determined that a goal is achieved when it occurs within all groups in society. For this assessment within all groups, national indicators and data must be reported disaggregated. Disaggregated indicators allow monitoring from an equity perspective (Rasanathan & Diaz, 2016).

The Colombian government has provided the official figures of COVID-19 without disaggregation of the data by ethnicity. However, indigenous groups are organized to self-manage this information considering that Colombia has 115 surviving indigenous groups, 108 native groups, 7 migrant groups, 769 reservations, 12,000 indigenous communities, 429,000 indigenous dwellings, 535,000 indigenous families, 2 million hectares of land in ancestral territories, and 2.3 million indigenous inhabitants (Departamento Administrativo Nacional de Estadística, 2018). Hence, indigenous population data facilitate the empowerment and self-determination rights of indigenous persons (Gahman et al., 2020).

For the population census of 2018, the National Indigenous Organization of Colombia (ONIC) trained indigenous individuals to conduct the census tasks in their territories and serve the most dispersed places, using a technological tool for information capture called the Territorial Monitoring System (SMT) (Organización Nacional Indígena de Colombia (ONIC), 2020f). The prior census conducted 15 years earlier had low coverage in the indigenous territories. The SMT integrates the entire indigenous territory and monitors various populations for education, health, economic activities, natural resources, biodiversity, public policies, human rights, and georeferenced consultations. This system favors social participation, guaranteeing the human rights of indigenous peoples, and governance (Organización Nacional Indígena de Colombia (ONIC), 2020c).

During the emergency, the ONIC began issuing a bulletin with an analysis of the SMT information, reporting the expansion of COVID-19 in their territories and inviting them to adopt and strengthen all self-government measures, territorial control, cooperation between peoples, and a barter system. These bulletins also denounce structural violence, stigmatization, and human rights violations, claiming the national government a more differential approach to manage the crisis through respectful intercultural dialogue. Because of the higher recommendations of indigenous authorities in these bulletins, no reference is made to the scientific name of the SARS-Cov2 virus.

The systematic analysis in the bulletins has integrated the National Institute of Health information with SMT data. These data include populated centers locations and cases among indigenous community locations at the rural and urban levels, providing pandemic health indicators disaggregated by ethnicity. The SMT reports 50 indigenous people's organization data integrated with a network of first responders who live in Colombian ancestral territories (Organización Nacional Indígena de Colombia (ONIC), 2020d).

In low- and middle-income countries, disaggregated disease data collection presents many challenges because rural and marginalized population groups remain unserved by healthcare information systems. Usually, the underreporting of health conditions in indigenous populations reflects their marginality characteristics. Consequently, aggregated national data or global estimates homogenize territories and are inadequate for making predictions and monitoring health equity (Cookson et al., 2016).

Planning as a process is an essential element of management in any organization; however, the lack of disaggregated data has hampered this process. Public health and social work planning could be based on reliable public health surveillance systems to empower decision makers and enhance population health (Groseclose & Buckeridge, 2017). Therefore, the SMT disaggregated data are a valuable source of information to improve public health and social work practice.

Indigenous population self-planning during the pandemic has strengthened community capacities in their territories and promoted governance to continue advocating for their rights. These organizations have coordinated and agreed among themselves to deploy care plans that manage the pandemic. They also have demanded that the government implements a comprehensive long-term-care plan for the indigenous population, including ancestral knowledge in health programs.

Currently, there is an inability to address social problems and implement programs from health institutions in Colombia that allow responding to the specific needs of the population. The different strategies consolidated by indigenous groups that favor indigenous organization capillarity within their communities are not incorporated into standard social work practices. Also, social workers are not regular multidisciplinary public health team members, limiting social participation in health and social transformation. The practice of social work would fit perfectly with the effective implementation of a Community Oriented Primary Care (COPC) with a differential population focus, falling apart from the legacy of opportunistic charity and welfare. Unfortunately, there is a great void in community intervention and articulation by social workers in health and social protection systems, which weakens the social dimension of public health practices to achieve better health among populations.

35.3 Collectivity for the Amplification of Population Health

Indigenous peoples understand health from a holistic perspective and have a complex conception of the interrelationships between personal health and ecosystems, both physically and spiritually. The concept of health for indigenous communities is harmony with Mother Earth, and disease is an imbalance between the body, soul, and spirit (Lokugamage et al., 2020). Therefore, treatments are formulated by addressing these levels from a sociocultural domain with a spiritual perspective.

The spiritual and cultural order of indigenous peoples is organized based on sacred sites where life arises, allowing cultural reproduction. The health of indigenous peoples and their relationship with the environment are often harmed by policies that promote natural resource extraction for government participation in the global market. Thus, indigenous perspectives oppose mega-extractivist economies that have rendered large numbers of collectively owned sacred sites infertile and have generated imbalance on a planetary scale at the expense of all forms of life (Kauffman & Martin, 2017).

Cosmovisions and epistemologies of indigenous peoples share values such as plurality, diversity, reciprocity, and complementarity based on the collective principle that prioritizes community well-being. From a multidimensional perspective, complex indigenous thinking integrates diverse knowledge and facilitates awareness among all beings and the natural world. These visions determine the concept of harmonization and living well, which makes sense in community life and the common good. "Living well" means peace for indigenous populations, and this concept comprises harmony within the territory and living fully in the social environment (Añaños Bedriñana et al., 2020).

Indigenous organizations have approached the current international public health emergency with resilience and solidarity (Akuhata-Huntington et al., 2020). These groups have organized around a community network model based on the reciprocity and solidarity that are rooted in their traditions. Community and social networks with historical roots have enhanced their benefits through coalitions with other social movements. Fair agroecological markets have been set among their solidarity activities, namely, ancestral mechanisms such as barter and harmonization rituals (Córdoba et al., 2021).

Connection with the territory of indigenous communities has been a source of resilience during the pandemic. The collective right of self-determination allowed indigenous groups to have been better positioned to maintain isolation and adopt the restrictions imposed, participating in community decisions. In this way, it has been possible to maintain trust in their authorities and improve collective resilience in the crisis. The strong community and family ties within the indigenous community also contribute to resilience and coping with confinement and imposed isolation (United Nations, 2020).

Community networks improve their members' well-being based on reciprocity and collectivity. Reciprocity has been a fundamental organizing principle in socioeconomic indigenous life and is part of their cosmovision associated with the concept of "living well." Rituals and reciprocal exchanges guided by traditional knowledge strengthen community well-being and solidarity practices, generating high levels of self-perceived health (Córdoba et al., 2021). These strategies of indigenous communalism represent significant benefits for both collective and individual health.

During the pandemic, indigenous communities organized themselves to identify the most vulnerable community members and solve the food supply through community solidarity strategies. Also, solidarity economy strengthened barter practices, and food collections were organized for distribution among those whose need was greatest. ONIC has registered diverse collaborative care practices deployed by the indigenous guards, taking care of the transit of people through the territories to prevent the spread of COVID-19, controlling the accesses and exits of their communities, and being aware that confinement prevents contagion and helps care for others.

Even though many indigenous communities have detriments to their living conditions, those communities with better self-organization and self-determination have managed to strengthen sustainable agroecological practices and solidarity that favor food sovereignty in the context of the pandemic, maintaining the availability of food in their territories. Also, community radio mechanisms and Internet networks were strengthened to promote their ancestral knowledge and cultural richness around the world. Indigenous communities strengthen care and the sense of empathy, collectivity, solidarity, compassion, and respect for everyone and everything that surrounds them.

Similarly, cultural bonding cultivates social trust and cooperation (Tonon, 2018). Several studies have shown that social trust is directly correlated with better mental health, better self-reported general health, and less early mortality (Ehsan et al., 2019). Social trust at the individual and community level is associated with the sense of belonging and perception of solidarity, friendliness, and reciprocity. Community networks enhance the collective agency of indigenous communities based on collaboration and conciliation processes. In this way, collective capabilities are more than the aggregation of individual capabilities, allowing for establishing common goals and common goods (Murphy, 2014). Interventions to improve population health have used social trust as a prevention measure for mental illness (Fahmi et al., 2019).

In indigenous territories where public health planning has integrated with community networks, acceptance, commitment, and positive results have been generated in the indigenous populations such that they have been enacted preventively during the pandemic (Kaplan et al., 2020). Additionally, indigenous community networks have been more effective in prioritizing overall well-being. In contrast, nonindigenous populations have experienced higher proportions of food insecurity and deepening of social inequalities (Aparicio Wilhelmi, 2020). Despite the elevated morbimortality resulting from inadequate healthcare facilities, the crisis has generated less poverty in indigenous territories than in those nonindigenous: this observation is linked to solidarity and community networks that do not rely on government social assistance (Lustig et al., 2020).

Colombian indigenous organizations have deployed territorial health actions at more than 15,000 locations nationwide. They have mobilized 60,000 indigenous guards to form a sanitary cordon, combined with their traditional rituals to harmonize Mother Earth according to their concepts of relationships between health and nature (Organización Nacional Indígena de Colombia (ONIC), 2020e). Indigenous volunteers have had a leading role in the capillarity of social protection and health system in ancestral territories, assuming roles as community agents.

For medical treatments, including for COVID-19, the use of medicinal plants and ancestral knowledge has also been promoted without receiving support from the health system, even though it is a right protected by the United Nations and the biological diversity agreement. Currently, there is a lack of significant incorporation of community ancestral health agents to improve access to intercultural medicine and overcome the access gap to culturally adapted services.

The classical response of the public health system has focused on political decisions based on epidemiological models that often lack a comprehensive social component approach. This traditional public health planning ignores the complexity of the social dimensions in a given population and focuses on the political and technical components (Panamerican Health Organization, 2013). Proposals within the collective health approach try to overcome this problem, tackling the relationships between society and nature amid protective and destructive health processes. The collective health field emerges as a space of knowledge and practices of social medicine and social sciences fueled by dialogues of social justice, critical epidemiology, and social determination of the health framework, whose main objective is to transform reality through a complex multidimensional, transdisciplinary, and intercultural analysis of disease context (Breilh, 2019).

Additionally, a community-centered system can convey information with greater social trust to avoid the spread of an infodemic with the COVID-19 pandemic. The World Health Organization has defined "infodemic" as an excessive amount of information, correct or not, making it difficult for individuals to find reliable sources and reliable guidance when they need it. The existence of indigenous community networks before the COVID-19 pandemic increased the possibility of sharing reliable information and generating an effective response to the emergency. However, significantly improved long-term health outcomes would be obtained if indigenous individuals' networks were linked with health and social protection systems (Huang, 2020).

The collective health framework is much closer to understanding indigenous community health than the classical public health approach. Indigenous organizations prioritize integrating social and cultural care to achieve better health outcomes for the entire population without discrimination (Nunesa & Louvison, 2020). Thus, the pandemic has revealed that the health system's patient-centered care is insufficient and creates opportunities for a community-centered care system and COPC (Goldfield et al., 2020).

The global crisis caused by the international public health emergency has allowed us to recognize the importance of the indigenous ancestral legacy to maintain food sovereignty. In consequence, it is suggested to develop bonds of greater trust and solidarity within family and community, improving the balance between human relations and the planet, to promote new production and distribution models with greater social and environmental justice, an entire field of action for social work.

35.4 Challenges and Final Remarks

The state's role in guaranteeing its population's well-being cannot be denied for any reason and can be achieved by adequately designing public policies. Quality access to health and social protection systems must be ensured for all individuals by promoting an integrated form of sustainable human development. However, social responses in the pandemic have not recognized the unequal health capabilities of communities and individuals (Venkatapuram, 2020). The lack of mechanisms that directly guarantee marginalized population rights reproduces persistent inequalities and discrimination toward the indigenous population inherited from colonial history.

Equity in access to social institutions reduces the poverty trap, a mechanism that causes poverty to persist because of the increased inability of individuals to live life and exercise their freedoms (Ghatak, 2015). To advance equity, what must be recognized is that healthcare does not respond to the market's customary laws and must be categorized and regulated as a common good within health systems. However, the orientation of systems toward the free market impedes recognition of this common good globally. Access to healthcare as a global public good is a measure of justice within global society that is still inaccessible by marginalized populations with numerous ill-health determinants. It is essential to focus on proposals that prevent the increase of market-based power inequities worldwide.

Many indigenous individuals organized in solidarity networks have maintained food sovereignty and mitigated the adverse effects of discrimination during the COVID-19 pandemic. By contrast, government agencies worldwide have demonstrated significant limitations in responding to emergencies using an equity perspective, thus deepening social inequalities (Kabad et al., 2020). Further, the pandemic has highlighted the importance of community-based workers and interagency cooperation (Banks et al., 2020). Government institutions could look forward to alternative models such as the Open Source COVID Movement based on principles of cooperation and solidarity in Kerala State, India, which has positioned strategies to control pandemic linking universal care access with open-access research. It is essential to improve well-being outcomes mediated by trust in institutions.

The autonomous information system SMT is a remarkable collective action experience from indigenous organizations under the pandemic and a reference to mainstream society. This self-organized information system sheds light on indigenous group existence and knowledge historically neglected by institutions, resisting the domination forces to become monocultures and reaffirming their autonomy. This community surveillance system network has been a permanent task that needs to be strengthened to improve the quality of the information collected, primarily by volunteers. These disaggregated data are essential for public health planning and collective health risk management. Nevertheless, working in a coordinated manner and improving response capacity in follow-up and early-detection strategies for the timely comprehensive approach requires a more significant national government presence (Organización Nacional Indígena de Colombia (ONIC), 2020a).

Successful indigenous community organization during the COVID-19 pandemic compared with the unsatisfactory results of the Colombian health and social protection system among vulnerable populations creates an opportunity to rethink the capabilities of social response systems in emergencies and redirect them toward real solidarity systems. In this manner, it is essential to implement delayed comprehensive and intercultural primary healthcare and COPC throughout the national territory, shaping healthy environments and including rural populations. Furthermore, this indigenous organization experience encourages us to reflect on hidden workers, fundamental rights, and public services access.

Positive collective health outcomes and overall well-being have multidimensional interactions, and it is not easy to understand every component. Nonetheless, it is well recognized that principles such as solidarity and reciprocity on indigenous social networks are fundamental elements that reside in their community-based planning and positive health outcomes. The communities put shared activities at the center to guarantee the material and cultural sustenance of the community.

The conceptual approach to justice to advance equity in global health recognizes the need to strengthen the voices of the most disadvantaged populations and establish their priorities in worldwide research and resource allocation, supporting local structures and human capital (Venkatapuram, 2016) However, global health institutions have reproduced structural inequities and a global north view during the pandemic response strategy, often lacking representation of marginalized communities at the decision-making level (Büyüm et al., 2020).

This research suggests that global movements may reconsider labels such as "third world" or "developing countries" because this attitude promotes exclusion and hampers transformation. The developed economy narrative justifies the maintenance of historical extractivist economies of natural wealth protected by indigenous populations. By contrast development could be viewed from the perspective of nature's knowledge. Thus, a highly industrialized population is not necessarily at the peak of its development, recognizing that it is impossible to reach a unanimous agreement about justice as fairness (Freeman, 2016).

Additionally, increasing participation of indigenous populations in institutions and political decision-making spheres will alleviate unjust inequalities in health, improve social investment, and reduce the poverty trap. Intercultural social workers could be more effectively integrated into national institutions to exercise effective mediation with indigenous knowledge and practices (Lotta et al., 2020). It is also important to address the lack of ontological pluralisms to reimagine pluriverse and heterogeneous institutions and change dominant paradigms to identify policy priorities for well-being (Affun-Adegbulu & Adegbulu, 2020). Regrettably, some proposals to assist indigenous populations have excluded them from decision making, ignoring their immense ancestral knowledge regarding self-organization and medicinal plants (Ramírez et al., 2020).

The new planetary health field highlights that human health outcomes are multidimensional interactions dependent on natural systems. This theoretical field is also an opportunity to rethink global human forces that destroy ecosystems, even though its principal donors present contradictions. Furthermore, it should consider the ecology of knowledge and health practices that emerge from indigenous cultural systems linked to natural systems to improve global cognitive justice. The rights of nature could be recognized worldwide, and institutions may articulate with community organizations in a multiply diverse and equitable mechanism. The Bolivian experience to legally protect the natural rights of the planet is a practical approach to look forward in more extensive contexts to legislate such rights.

The planning proposals for public health and social protection services could consider, from a horizontal perspective, indigenous peoples' social participation integrating their collective narratives (Keating, 2019). Indigenous self-organization mechanisms could be viewed more as a necessary part of the future than as part of the past, and their complex thinking could help build planetary solidarity and a genuinely global civilization. The protection of biodiversity is a priority for understanding planetary interdependence and advancing social development (Castro Romero et al., 2020; Maya-Ambía, 2020). Furthermore, it is essential to translate (and share) indigenous traditional knowledge into a Western language, eliminate misconceptions, and prevent biopiracy.

Leading practices of indigenous populations such as reciprocity and self-determination processes are configured as a fundamental collective capacity to improve the relationship between freedom and social, psychological, biological, and material well-being. Collective capabilities at the heart of community practices amplify population health. Thus, public health planning and social work could benefit by incorporating indigenous complex thinking and community networks in their practices to achieve planetary intercultural population health, well-being, and empowerment in the present and future.

References

Affun-Adegbulu, C., & Adegbulu, O. (2020). Decolonising global (public) health: From western universalism to global pluriversalities. *BMJ Global Health, 5*(8), e002947. https://doi.org/10.1136/bmjgh-2020-002947

Akuhata-Huntington, Z., Foster, S., Gillon, A., Merito, M., Oliver, L., Parata, N., et al. (2020). COVID-19 and indigenous resilience. *Higher Education Research and Development, 39*(7), 1377–1383. https://doi.org/10.1080/07294360.2020.1823327

Añaños Bedriñana, K. G., Hernández Umaña, B. A., & Rodríguez Martín, J. A. (2020). "Living well" in the constitution of Bolivia and the American declaration on the rights of indigenous peoples: Reflections on well-being and the right to development. *International Journal of Environmental Research and Public Health, 17*(8). https://doi.org/10.3390/ijerph17082870

Aparicio Wilhelmi, M. (2020). Covid19 and collective rights of indigenous people. Situated resistances against the pandemic. *Revista Catalana de Dret Ambiental, 11*(2), 1–7.

Ardila-Sierra, A., Niño-Leal, L., Rivera-Triana, D., Sarmiento-Medina, M. I., & Alzate, J. P. (2020). Condiciones en la frontera sur entre Colombia y Venezuela ante la pandemia de COVID-19. *Revista de Salud Pública, 22*(2), 1–9. https://doi.org/10.15446/rsap.v22n2.86366

Awad, S., & Konn, A. (2020). *Socio-economic impacts of COVID-19*. CA.

Banks, S., Cai, T., de Jonge, E., Shears, J., Shum, M., Sobočan, A. M., et al. (2020). Practising ethically during COVID-19: Social work challenges and responses.

International Social Work, 63(5), 569–583. https://doi.org/10.1177/0020872820949614

Breilh, J. (2019). Critical epidemiology in Latin America: Roots, philosophical and methodological ruptures. In J. Vallverdú, A. Puyol, & A. Estany (Eds.), *Philosophical and methodological debates in public health* (pp. 21–46). Springer. https://doi.org/10.1007/978-3-030-28626-2

Browne, A. J., Varcoe, C., Lavoie, J., Smye, V., Wong, S. T., Krause, M., et al. (2016). Enhancing health care equity with indigenous populations: Evidence-based strategies from an ethnographic study. *BMC Health Services Research, 16*(1), 544. https://doi.org/10.1186/s12913-016-1707-9

Burstrom, B., & Tao, W. (2020). Social determinants of health and inequalities in COVID-19. *European Journal of Public Health, 30*(4), 617–618. https://doi.org/10.1093/eurpub/ckaa095

Büyüm, A. M., Kenney, C., Koris, A., Mkumba, L., & Raveendran, Y. (2020). Decolonising global health: If not now, when? *BMJ Global Health, 5*(8), 1–4. https://doi.org/10.1136/bmjgh-2020-003394

Castro, C., López Uribe, M. P., Posada, F., Castro, B., & Kishi, R. (2020). *Understanding the killing of social leaders in Colombia during COVID-19*. Armed Conflict Location & Event Data Project. JSTOR. https://blogs.lse.ac.uk/latamcaribbean/2020/10/06/understanding-the-killing-of-social-leaders-in-colombia-during-covid-19/

Castro Romero, M., Lorenzo Ruiz, A., & Melluish, S. (2020). Reimagining 'mental health' from the cosmovision of Abya Yala (Latin America). *International Review of Psychiatry, 32*(4), 299–302. https://doi.org/10.1080/09540261.2020.1782597

Chaparro, P., Zapata, H., Hurtado, I., Alzate, A., Lesmes, M. C., & Herrera, S. (2020). *COVID-19 trends in Colombian regions with the highest disease burden*.

Chaves, P., Aarts, N., & van Bommel, S. (2020). Self-organization for everyday peacebuilding: The Guardia Indígena from Northern Cauca, Colombia. *Security Dialogue, 51*(1), 39–59. https://doi.org/10.1177/0967010619889471

Cookson, R., Asaria, M., Ali, S., Ferguson, B., Fleetcroft, R., Goddard, M., et al. (2016). Health equity indicators for the English NHS: A longitudinal whole-population study at the small-area level. *Health Services and Delivery Research, 4*(26), 1–224. https://doi.org/10.3310/hsdr04260

Córdoba, D., Peredo, A. M., & Chaves, P. (2021). Shaping alternatives to development: Solidarity and reciprocity in the Andes during COVID-19. *World Development, 139*. https://doi.org/10.1016/j.worlddev.2020.105323

Cultural Survival. (2020). *Global mapping project documenting COVID-19 in indigenous communities*. https://www.culturalsurvival.org/news/cultural-survival-launches-global-mapping-project-documenting-covid-19-indigenous-0

Departamento Administrativo Nacional de Estadística. (2018). *Resultados Pueblos Indígenas. Censo Nacional de Población y Vivienda 2018* [Census data on indigenous peoples].

Durán Castellanos, M. A. (2020). Inkal Awá indigenous people: Words instead of weapons. *Revista Catalana de Dret Ambiental, XI*(2), 1–28.

Ehsan, A., Klaas, H. S., Bastianen, A., & Spini, D. (2019). Social capital and health: A systematic review of systematic reviews. *SSM Population Health, 8*(June), 100425. https://doi.org/10.1016/j.ssmph.2019.100425

Fahmi, M., Panjaitan, N. A., Habibie, I., Siregar, A. Y. M., Amarullah, G., Rahma, & Sunjaya, D. K. (2019). Does your neighborhood protect you from being depressed? A study on social trust and depression in Indonesia. *BMC Public Health, 19*(1), 1–8. https://doi.org/10.1186/s12889-019-7657-5

Fernández-Niño, J. A., Cubillos-Novella, A., Bojórquez, I., & Rodríguez, M. (2020). Recommendations for the response against COVID-19 in migratory contexts under a closed border: The case of Colombia. *Biomédica, 40*, 68–72. https://doi.org/10.7705/biomedica.5512

Freeman, S. (2016). *Rawls*. Fondo de Cultura Económica.

Gahman, L., Penados, F., & Greenidge, A. (2020). Indigenous resurgence, decolonial praxis, alternative futures: The Maya Leaders Alliance of Southern Belize. *Social Movement Studies, 19*(2), 241–248. https://doi.org/10.1080/14742837.2019.1709433

Ghatak, M. (2015). Theories of poverty traps and anti-poverty policies. *World Bank Economic Review, 29*, S77–S105. https://doi.org/10.1093/wber/lhv021

Goldfield, N. I., Crittenden, R., Fox, D., McDonough, J., Nichols, L., & Lee Rosenthal, E. (2020). COVID-19 crisis creates opportunities for community-centered population health: Community Health Workers at the Center. *Journal of Ambulatory Care Management, 43*(3), 184–190. https://doi.org/10.1097/JAC.0000000000000337

Golovatina, P., Zapata-Ramirez, P. A., Spanellis, A., Borzenkova, G., & Hernandez-Sarmiento, J. M. (2020). Engaging with indigenous communities during COVID-9 pandemic: The case of Tribugá-Choco region in Colombia. In: *ECSMID conference on coronavirus disease (ECCVID)*. Online: European Society in Clinical Microbiology and Infectious Diseases. https://www.escmid.org/research_projects/escmid_conferences/eccvid/

Greenwood, M., & de Leeuw, S. (2007). Teachings from the land: Indigenous people, our health, our land, and our children. *Canadian Journal of Native Education, 30*(1), 48. http://proquest.umi.com/pqdweb?did=144 7677771&Fmt=7&clientId=65345&RQT=309&VName=PQD

Groseclose, S. L., & Buckeridge, D. L. (2017). Public health surveillance systems: Recent advances in their use and evaluation. *Annual Review of Public Health, 38*, 57–79. https://doi.org/10.1146/annurev-publhealth-031816-044348

Guimarães, L. M. A., & Ferreira Júnior, A. (2020). Political struggles by indigenous populations in Roraima (Brazil) and the confrontation with the

Covid-19 pandemic. *Mundo Amazónico, 11*(2), 223–243. https://doi.org/10.15446/ma.v11n2.88715

Huang, Y. (2020). Tribal responses to the COVID-19 pandemic experience in the culture and health stations of Taiwanese indigenous peoples. *Journal of Indigenous Social Development, 9*(3), 224–232.

Kabad, J. F., De Moura Pontes, A. L., & Monteiro, S. (2020). Relationships between scientific production and public policies: The case of indigenous people's health in the field of collective health. *Ciencia e Saude Coletiva, 25*(5), 1653–1666. https://doi.org/10.1590/1413-81232020255.33762019

Kaplan, H. S., Trumble, B. C., Stieglitz, J., Mamany, R. M., Cayuba, M. G., Moye, L. M., et al. (2020). Voluntary collective isolation as a best response to COVID-19 for indigenous populations? A case study and protocol from the Bolivian Amazon. *The Lancet, 395*, 1727–1734. https://doi.org/10.1016/S0140-6736(20)31104-1

Kauffman, C. M., & Martin, P. L. (2017). Can rights of nature make development more sustainable? Why some Ecuadorian lawsuits succeed and others fail. *World Development, 92*, 130–142. https://doi.org/10.1016/j.worlddev.2016.11.017

Keating, C. (2019). Coloniality of knowledge, Ch'ixinakax utxiwa, and intercultural translation: The (im)pertinence of language and discourse studies. *Language, Culture, and Society, 1*(1), 141–146.

Krieger, N., Waterman, P. D., & Chen, J. T. (2020). COVID-19 and overall mortality inequities in the surge in death rates by zip code characteristics: Massachusetts, January 1 to May 19, 2020. *American Journal of Public Health, 110*(12), 1850–1852. https://doi.org/10.2105/AJPH.2020.305913

Lokugamage, A. U., Ahillan, T., & Pathberiya, S. D. C. (2020). Decolonising ideas of healing in medical education. *Journal of Medical Ethics, 46*(4), 265–272. https://doi.org/10.1136/medethics-2019-105866

Lotta, G., Wenham, C., Nunes, J., & Pimenta, D. N. (2020). Community health workers reveal COVID-19 disaster in Brazil. *The Lancet, 396*, 365–366. https://doi.org/10.1016/S0140-6736(20)31521-X

Lustig, N., Pabon, V. M., Sanz, F., & Younger, S. D. (2020). *The impact of COVID-19 lockdowns and expanded social assistance on inequality, poverty and mobility in Argentina, Brazil, Colombia and Mexico inequality, poverty and mobility* (No. 556). https://www.cgdev.org/publication/impact-covid-19-lockdowns-and-expanded-social-assistance-inequality-poverty-and-mobility

Maya-Ambía, C. J. (2020). Review of the current discussion on Covid-19 in the field of social thought. *El Trimestre Económico, 87*(348), 1233–1258. https://doi.org/10.20430/ETE.V87I348.1166

Montenegro, R. A., & Stephens, C. (2006). Indigenous health in Latin America and the Caribbean. *Lancet, 367*, 1859–1869.

Murphy, M. (2014). Self-determination as a collective capability: The case of indigenous peoples. *Journal of Human Development and Capabilities, 15*(4), 320–334. https://doi.org/10.1080/19452829.2013.878320

Nunesa, J. A., & Louvison, M. (2020). Epistemologies of the south and decolonization of health: For an ecology of care in collective health. *Saude e Sociedade, 29*(3), 1–13. https://doi.org/10.1590/S0104-12902020200563

Observatorio Político Electoral de la Democracia. (2020). *Informe de violencia contra líderes políticos, sociales y comunales* [Report on violence against political, social and community leaders]. https://moe.org.co/informe-de-violencia-contra-lideres-politicos-sociales-y-comunales/

Organización Nacional Indígena de Colombia (ONIC). (2020a). *Información para proteger la vida y los territorios*. Boletín 21 [Data to protect life and territories].

Organización Nacional Indígena de Colombia (ONIC). (2020b). *Información para proteger la vida y los territorios*. Boletín 44 [Data to protect life and territories]. Sistema de Monitoreo Territorial.

Organización Nacional Indígena de Colombia (ONIC). (2020c). *Información para proteger la vida y los territorios*. Boletín 48 [Data to protect life and territories].

Organización Nacional Indígena de Colombia (ONIC). (2020d). *Información para proteger la vida y los territorios*. Boletín 53 [Data to protect life and territories].

Organización Nacional Indígena de Colombia (ONIC). (2020e). *Informe Especial. Situación de los Pueblos Indígenas frente a la pandemia en Colombia: Aprendizajes y desafíos* [Special Report. Indigenous peoples situation during pandemic in Colombia]. https://www.onic.org.co/images/comunicados/covid19/ONIC_Informe_Situación_de_los_Pueblos_Indígenas_frente_a_la_pandemia_100_días_FINAL.pdf

Organización Nacional Indígena de Colombia (ONIC). (2020f). *Sistema de Monitoreo Territorial ONIC*. Boletín 001 [Territorial Surveillance System ONIC].

Panamerican Health Organization. (2013). Core competencies for public health: A regional framework for the Americas. In *Biblioteca Sede de la OPS* (Vol. 1).

Ramírez, J. D., Sordillo, E. M., Gotuzzo, E., Zavaleta, C., Caplivski, D., Navarro, J. C., et al. (2020). Sars-Cov-2 in the Amazon region: A harbinger of doom for Amerindians. *PLoS Neglected Tropical Diseases, 14*(10), 1–10. https://doi.org/10.1371/journal.pntd.0008686

Rasanathan, K., & Diaz, T. (2016). Research on health equity in the SDG era: The urgent need for greater focus on implementation. *International Journal for Equity in Health, 15*(1), 202. https://doi.org/10.1186/s12939-016-0493-7

Ravindran, T. (2020). When a pandemic intensifies racial terror: The politics of COVID-19 control in Bolivia. *City, 24*(5–6), 778–792. https://doi.org/10.1080/13604813.2020.1833541

Romero-Sandoval, N., Ortiz-Rico, C., Sánchez-Pérez, H. J., Valdivieso, D., Sandoval, C., Pástor, J., & Martín, M. (2017). Soil transmitted helminthiasis in indigenous groups. A community cross sectional study in the Amazonian southern border region of Ecuador. *BMJ Open, 7*(3). https://doi.org/10.1136/bmjopen-2016-013626

Sachs, J. D., Abdool Karim, S., Aknin, L., Allen, J., Brosbøl, K., Cuevas Barron, G., et al. (2020). Lancet COVID-19 commission statement on the occasion of the 75th session of the UN general assembly. *The Lancet, 396*(10257), 1102–1124. https://doi.org/10.1016/S0140-6736(20)31927-9

Tonon, G. (2018). Communities and capabilities. *Journal of Human Development and Capabilities, 19*(2), 121–125. https://doi.org/10.1080/19452829.2018.1454288

United Nations. (2020). *General assembly. A/75/185 Rights of indigenous peoples. Promotion and protection of human rights* (Vol. 75). https://doi.org/10.18268/bsgm1908v4n1x1

Venkatapuram, S. (2016). Justice and global health research. *The American Journal of Bioethics 16*(10), 46–47. https://doi.org/10.1080/15265161.2016.1214333

Venkatapuram, S. (2020). Human capabilities and pandemics. *Journal of Human Development and Capabilities, 21*(3), 280–286. https://doi.org/10.1080/19452829.2020.1786028

36 Soup Kitchens and Radical Social Work Against COVID-19 from Liberation Theology in Chile

Francisca Valdebenito-Acosta,
Paulo Álvarez Bravo, and Julio Hasbún-Mancilla

36.1 Introduction

After the return to democracy in Chile in 1990, the social fabric that had been developed in response to the civic-military dictatorship began a process of weakening as the first democratic governments aimed to eliminate the organization and popular power that had faced the authoritarianism of Augusto Pinochet's regime.

Shanty towns of the city of Santiago, such as Villa Francia and La Legua, were emblematic in the fight against the dictatorship, sharing the fact that 'worker priests' were inserted in both of these, embracing the Liberation Theology, developing a radical social work of accompaniment to empower the most oppressed people of their neighborhoods.

F. Valdebenito-Acosta (✉)
Symbolon Consulting, Santiago, Chile

Human Development and Capability Association (HDCA), Santiago, Chile
e-mail: fvaldebenito@symbolon.cl

P. Á. Bravo
Architecture and Urban Studies, Pontificia Universidad Católica de Chile, Santiago, Chile

J. Hasbún-Mancilla
Symbolon Consulting, Santiago, Chile

Department of Industrial Engineering, Universidad de Chile, Santiago, Chile

Human Development and Capability Association (HDCA), Santiago, Chile

After 30 years of apparently stable democracy with a strong neoliberal stamp and numerous 'authoritarian enclaves' (Garretón, 2003; Siavelis, 2009), in October 2019 the so-called Social Outbreak took place, which through peaceful protest, burning of subway stations, looting, and public disorder came to test and face the sociopolitical order that had dominated the country without a counterweight (Oyarzún-Serrano, 2020).

It is under this convulsive multi-crisis scenario that in March 2020 the national emergency as a result of the COVID-19 pandemic was declared, with a weak state response toward the most vulnerable sectors, causing the liberating praxis of radical social work based on Liberation Theology to return and to gain a specific weight in these sectors again. Therefore, this chapter shows a reflection based on the cases of Villa Francia and La Legua, seeking to identify radical social work practices based on the perspective of Liberation Theology that emerged in the soup kitchen of Villa Francia and La Legua as a result of COVID-19.

36.1.1 Chile 2020: Crisis of the Political-Economic Model, Constitutional Plebiscite and Pandemic

The year 2019 marks an unprecedented process in Chile: the de facto termination of the 1980 Constitution implemented by the military

M. C. S. Gonçalves et al. (eds.), *The Coronavirus Crisis and Challenges to Social Development*,
https://doi.org/10.1007/978-3-030-84678-7_36

dictatorship in Chile (1973–1989). This constitutional charter was in force from when it was promulgated in 1980 until October 18, 2019. That date marked the deepest, and most extensive and transversal, social outbreak of the past century.

On October 18 occurred the suspension of the status quo in Chile, paralyzing the means of transport, services, logistics chains, and the general operation of the country, forcing the political class through the Senate of the Republic to seek an 'Agreement for the Peace,' calling for a plebiscite organized for October 2020 to Approve or Reject a Constituent process.

The plebiscite held on October 25, 2020 had an important participation of 51% of the electoral roll, the highest since the voluntary vote was implemented in the country. The results were overwhelming: a 78.3% vote of approval and only a 21.7% rejection. Territorially, the rejection only won in 5 counties of the 346 counties that are in the whole country, and in 3 of those places 10% of the people live with the highest income; one corresponds to a military base and the other one to a small county in the affluent neighborhoods.

This crisis, which had repercussions in multiple fields, had important effects in two areas: in the way of understanding politics and in the economic activity. In the way of understanding politics, a certain replacement of political parties by movements and communities of horizontal grassroots organization is beginning to be observed; and economically, in the loss of formal jobs caused by the closure or reduction of personnel in small, medium, and large companies, as well as the reduction of the investments.

In this scenario of internal economic shock arrived COVID-19, becoming overwhelming on the national scene in March 2020, with the enactment of the State of Constitutional Exception because of the pandemic on March 18, and with the beginning of the first national quarantine on March 26, which lasted until at least September 2020.

According to the ILO report (2020), the effect of COVID-19 in the country caused a major crisis in economic activity, employment, and income. A drop in gross domestic product is projected to be between −4.5 and −5.5% for 2020; and the drop in employment of about 20% during one quarter (June–August) of 2020 translated into an increase in the unemployment rate and a strong exodus of people from the workforce: about one of three people in working age are unemployed or even a huge part of the potential workforce. Additionally, the report points out that more than one million workers were registered as employed absent, about 70% of them covered by the 'cancellation of contracts.' Formal and informal employment also declined, and the decrease mainly affected women. All these concerns translated into food insecurity in the most vulnerable sectors of the population.

36.1.2 COVID-19 and Food Safety

Food security is understood as physical, social, and economic access to sufficient, safe, and nutritious food to satisfy people's daily energy needs and food preferences (FAO, 2020). During 2020, food security in Chile was affected by the social, economic, and public health crisis.

The COVID-19 Social Survey (Observatorio Social, Ministerio de Desarrollo Social y Familia, 2020) investigated, in a statistically representative way at a national level, the social and economic consequences that the pandemic has had on the living conditions of the country's homes. This survey was carried out in two rounds, in July and November 2020, at which time a series of social work actions were being carried out, such as the soup kitchens of Villa Francia and La Legua.

The panorama showed that in July 19.4% of households nationwide presented moderate to severe food insecurity, decreasing in November to 11.5%. Specifically, in the most vulnerable, that was 40% of the population (Quintile I and II), the level of moderate to severe food insecurity approached 29.5%, decreasing to 20.4%, which meant that the recovery to cover the basic needs that the families had was very slow, as this situation has been prolonged over time.

Within the characterization of affected households, it is established that most of them are headed by women (12.4%); without complete high school education (19.3%), without occupation (21.4%), with debt (24.4%), and who have necessarily reduced their spending on food (24.3%). Additionally, 17.2% of households in this condition received the EmergLaency Family Income, so it can be inferred that this permanent support from the government has not been able to compensate for the decrease of income during that period.

36.1.3 Radical Social Work

Approaching social work in Latin America implies looking back to 1960, when the initial optimism product of the growing entry of the middle class to study a career that had concepts and methods which were direct translations of the study books of the United States; at that moment, around 1970, those previously mentioned items gave way to skepticism and disillusionment from its ineffectiveness and irrelevance toward local contexts. This experience of reconceptualization toward radical social work was marked in the region by the theoretical-methodological contributions of Liberation Theology and Popular Education, redefining the role and scope of social work, as shown in the violent detention, torture, and disappearance of social workers in Chile during the civic-military dictatorship that ruled the country from 1973 to 1990 (Ferguson et al., 2018), living a neoliberal turn in Chilean social work (Muñoz, 2018).

A central element in the turn of the teaching-learning process of social work during that period was the notion of 'conscientização,' developed by Paulo Freire as a continuous process of discovery of relationships of domination and oppression on the way to a critical consciousness (Harms-Smith, 2020). This process is what opens, through a perspective of dialogical encounter, people to a real praxis, in the sense of abandoning the status of 'objects' to become true historical subjects. This transit is carried out through praxis, which is the dialectical cycle between action and critical reflection, which means that a mere understanding of the structures of oppression is not enough, because it should also be accompanied by consistent action to mobilize individual and collective action.

Thus, Liberation Theology encouraged the practice of radical social work beyond the borders of faith-based organizations, as a foundation for the formulation of policies and practices from the perspective of people living on the margins of the world: society, based on the principles of inclusion, justice, human rights, dignity, solidarity, and emancipation (Evans, 1992; Lusk & Corbett, 2020).

36.1.4 Grassroots Christian Movements and Liberation Theology in Chile

In La Legua and Villa Francia the different experiences of radical social work have been present since their foundation, as well as the presence and influence of the liberating current of the Catholic Church, consistent with the principles of Liberation Theology. Both represent the struggle of the city's poor population for their right to housing, heirs of the most socioeconomically vulnerable social strata in the capital. In each achievement or advance toward more dignified living conditions, awareness of the process of struggle and union was fundamental. In these actions, the residents demonstrated a practical and political capacity for organization and resistance that were key elements regarding their roots and recognition, both internally and externally.

In each of these spaces, the pastoral agents who acted there did so by placing the body and its capacities in the organizations born from the people themselves, such as the popular based communities, which proliferated and sheltered hundreds of population leaders. They encouraged the demand for demanding certain law conditions and promoted a project of vindication toward social justice, equity, and human freedom, without forgetting the political dimension of the human collective, thus impacting on the local sociocultural reality. At the end of the 1960s, all these actions were systematized and founded, and presented as a new theology, typical of Latin America, known by the name of Liberation

Theology, as Gustavo Gutiérrez titled his landmark book in 1968. In that country, but also in each of the Andean countries of the American subcontinent, in Central America and in Brazil, Liberation Theology has developed theorists and scholars who encouraged its dissemination; Boff (1978), Sobrino (1982), Muñoz (1994), Comblin (1987), Trigo (1988), and Casaldáliga and Vigil (1993) are some of its initial referring people, being especially strong in Brazil and Chile. In the latter country, the strength of this true promoter of the social movement was given thanks to the fact that in those years the hierarchy of the Catholic Church was one of the most progressive ones in the region, taking the lead on issues such as Agrarian Reform, handing over unused land of the church, and promoting the activism of Catholic movements of students, workers, and peasants (Mackin, 2015).

Liberation Theology conceives practice as a constituent principle. It is there, in the so-called liberating praxis, where the preferential option of Jesus with the poor and oppressed of the earth would be embodied. It is from them and them as collective subjects, where acts of solidarity, fraternity, and transformation are assumed as a historical condition towards liberation (Castillo, 1986). The precepts of Liberation Theology, however, collided with the civil-military dictatorships that from 1964 to 1990 ravaged the region, under the influence of the United States and the National Security Doctrine, who repudiated it for considering it Marxist, pro-revolutionary, and mass activist. In Chile, the civic-military dictatorship persecuted, detained, and murdered many people of recognized affiliation to this current, among them some priests (Jorda, 2001) and religious persons.

The persecution was not only political; for example, the Congregation for the Doctrine of the Faith, influenced by the most clerical or conservative currents and Pope John Paul II himself, showed qualms, considering that Liberation Theology could, in some cases, be an ideological deviation from the legitimate option for the poor, by promoting the class struggle and by confusing the idea that the source of sin is in the structures and not in the responsibility of each human being. Despite criticism, the right part developed by the hierarchy of the Catholic Church and the marginalization of agents and pastoral actions linked to Liberation Theology not only resisted, but also in the most repressive and unfavorable moments for the popular movement it was creative, promoting demonstrations that consolidated its identity and relationship with the historically disadvantaged people always left aside by the dominant system.

36.2 Villa Francia and La Legua

Villa Francia and La Legua are emblematic shanty towns of Santiago in Chile. They were founded by people from the socio-urban edge of the capital city, large families, informal workers, and proletarians from industrial enclaves near these territories.

Both are characterized by having an eminently working-class popular social origin, and a social and political organization in favor of obtaining social and spatial improvements, which was reflected in the transformation of their territorial space, managing to provide their environment with basic infrastructure such as squares, fields, schools, clinics, and churches, and regularizing the achievement of a house of one's own.

The settlers and their families founded Legua Vieja in the early 1920s. In 1947 Nueva La Legua was added and in 1949 Legua Emergencia emerged. All three would give life to one of the best-known shanty towns in the country, whose name is associated with the fact that it is located just one league south from the Plaza de Armas (Álvarez, 2014).

Villa Francia, meanwhile, lived a more compact but also later process, its origin dates back to 1969 and it is located in the western sector of the capital city, when the current inhabitants, through a government program known as Operation Site, occupied part of the lands of the Fundo Chuchunco.

In both territories, religious, priests, or Catholic missionaries of strong influence identified with Liberation Theology settled from the beginning. They were decisive articulators of the social development of the populations, through the promotion of education, political, ethical, and cultural training. As the theologian Rolando Muñoz points out, the church should offer service to be at the service of the population, thus becoming a creative place, a shelter, and becoming a project united by community work (Muñoz, 2018). From there could emerge concrete initiatives to support the residents, from the spiritual needs to the material ones, from youth pastoral care to solidarity dining rooms.

The putsch led by Augusto Pinochet in September 1973 was a breaking point for Chile, it put an end to democratic institutions. State violence was strongly deployed in those territories that had a popular organization. La Legua and Villa Francia were considered as bastions of the left, so the forced detentions, torture, and executions directly attacked the people who participated actively in the Parishes. An example of this is the arrest and disappearance of three members of the Cristo Liberador Community in Villa Francia, and days later the arrest and torture of their priest Mariano Puga, released by intense pressure from Cardinal Silva Henríquez on the Governing Board.

The villagers and the local church responded to the circumstances with determined courage (Jorda, 2001), following the path of groups such as the Grouping of Relatives of the Detained and Disappeared (AFDD). Faced with hunger and scarcity, they organized sSoup kitchens and solidarity actions that gradually became stronger. In parallel, they fought to protect the lives of many people and became architects of resistance and denunciation, surely in a way they have never imagined before.

36.2.1 Cristo Liberador Community and the Soup Kitchen

On the day of Pentecost 2020, the base communities of the Christian Community of Cristo Liberador made the complex decision to take over the soup kitchen on Saturday at Villa Francia, thus providing coverage of at least one meal a day during the 7 days of the week to whomever required it.

This process was carried out with the agreement of the eight base communities of Cristo Liberador, and in coordination with the Territorial Assemblies and the Luisa Popular Comedor Toledo. And as it had been proposed since its founding in 1970, grassroots communities more than 50 years later continue to be part of the social net/building of the population.

This coordination with social organizations meant the ethical commitment to not accept political or business favors that proselytize solidarity during the pandemic. Therefore, the contributions in work and resources of Cristo Liberador had to come from the capacity for autonomy, organization and action that anonymously was able to reach the neighbors. In the words of one of them:

> It is the service that the Cristo Liberador Community renders in the challenge of finding the face of Christ in all the brothers and sisters who today are in need. As Matthew 25 says, because I was hungry and you gave me food, because I was thirsty and you gave me drink, you are my brother and my sister (Cristo Liberador Base Community Member)

For the Christian Community of a small chapel to have the management capacity to prepare more than 400 rations of food every Saturday for 8 months, all available community assets had to be mobilized.

36.2.2 Committee for the Defense and Promotion of Human Rights of La Legua and the Soup Kitchen

In June 2020, the members of this group decided to co-participate with other organizations from the origin of the Soup kitchen that would take place every Friday in the Nueva La Legua sector. Despite the fact that their actions and objectives are to support the victims of police repression as a result of the state intervention that this population has experienced since 2001, they understood that carrying out actions of solidarity is a constituent act with the defense and promotion of life, especially when it is backed by not having access to elemental goods such as food.

Composed of neighbors, residents, and friends from different areas of Santiago, the soup kitchen quickly filled with young people and in the majority the presence of women generated a virtuous relationship in terms of building respectful and consistent ways for the residents. The actions were carried out at the headquarters of the "Atlanta sports club" and were basically promoted by members of a rival sports club, the "Venice sports and social club." In this way, these two organizations plus the Human Rights Committee formed an active solidarity organization network.

Thanks to their organizational skills, they divided their preparations into a production group in charge of raising financial funds and supplies of all kinds, from pots to stoves to food. Another group was dedicated to buying the products that could be needed, preparing food, and serving, taking into consideration a caring protocol for COVID-19.

The service was made up of an average of 12 people who, from the day before, have been preparing food very early on Friday. At 1:00 p.m. the service begun for an average of about 200 residents, single men and women, large immigrant families, people living on the streets or on drug addiction, among others. For those who for medical reasons, or age, could not go directly, the food was left at their homes.

La Legua has a long history of solidarity among the residents. Its history is marked by poverty, the presence of criminal activities, and drug trafficking, and the institutional violence of the State, which at times has generated moments of violence and pain. In La Legua, more than 58 people were murdered during the civic-military dictatorship. The acts of love and solidarity came from the organized settlers who were supported in body and spirit by pastoral agents who also risked their lives for others, those who persist in the memory of an active, courageous, and supportive liberating church.

36.3 Method

The purpose of this chapter is to address the perception of the main actors of the soup kitchen process in Villa Francia and La Legua, both the people who worked in the organization and the neighbors who attended from May to December 2020.

For the interviews, an intentional sampling was carried out based on the following criteria: over 18 years of age; people who attended or organized the Soup kitchen weekly for at least 5 months. Ten semi-structured interviews were conducted; the arrangement of them was as follows: residents who attended the soup kitchen (3 in La Legua and 3 in Villa Francia), and organizers (2 in La Legua and 2 in Villa Francia).

Additionally, during the period studied, participant observation about the work dynamics of the soup kitchen was also carried out. Subsequently, the interviews and field notes were coded, carrying out a content analysis to find patterns in the collected data.

Participants gave their consent to publish their words, as well as identify them as part of the communities analyzed. The team, in turn, pledged to ensure anonymity and confidentiality.

36.4 Findings

In a highly segregated and classist society such as the Chilean one, spaces such as Villa Francia and La Legua show that the wealth/richness of social work from the Christian community functions as a fundamental spring over the diversity of the people who compose it, where not only people from both territories participated, but also those summoned from different social sectors of the capital.

The early and persistent existence of the soup kitchen in the pandemic, in the testimony of the pastoral and social agents who participated, expresses the rearticulation of a radical social work that reacts to the threatening of the integrity of the communities and people who make up the territory. The following are the characteristics of the practice of grassroots Christian communities during the COVID-19 pandemic.

36.4.1 Praxis Develops in the Public Space

The socio-health crisis of COVID-19 mobilized grassroots communities inspired by Liberation Theology to act in the public space in a systematic way. For years these communities, which were very active during the process of installing the families in the former Chuchunco farm, and resisting the Pinochet dictatorship, and especially during the economic crisis of 1982, once democracy was recovered, were losing ground, retreating little by little into the space of the Chapel. Therefore, although during this period the reflection on the evangelical and liberating message was always present, it was not accompanied by a systematic action in the public space by offering support and accompaniment to the most vulnerable.

> Before this COVID-19 crisis, we only did actions of an evangelical ritual type, but they were not actions that were open to the specific needs of people and communities (Organizing Team, Villa Francia Base Community).

These evangelical actions in the territory permanently and persistently allowed the deployment in the crisis, because the teaching of Liberation Theology has been latent, waiting to unfold in the emerging crises. As indicated by a collaborator of La Olla (in the Spanish soup kitchen is Olla Común (common pot), 'La Olla'), external to the base communities:

> Entering a space for community collaboration, in Chile, is not so easy, because there is no trust. Because in my case, despite the need to help, I could not find a suitable context, given that the place where I live, in my neighborhood (upper middle class), organization was not necessary. (Organizing Team, La Legua and Villa Francia)

The praxis deployed leaves the private space, and takes up the centrality of the public space, for years abandoned to the individualistic logic of consumption, recomposing a social fabric that was deteriorated by the great territorial inequity that characterizes the city of Santiago. Thus, people from different territories came together in the soup kitchen as a public meeting space for different social classes, allowing them to understand that the supposed differences that existed between them were not fundamental, and that they could work together to support the neediest neighbors of both shanty towns.

36.4.2 Networks of Trust and Collaboration as the Basis of Radical Social Work in the Pandemic

The action and critical reflection of the work process carried out allowed reconstructing and updating the links around a common problem, cementing trust within the territory and outside it, because for its realization it was necessary to rearticulate collaboration networks and to generate a contact that went beyond the local territory.

These networks of contact and collaboration that are deployed in the territory were strengthened by the broad social base that Liberation Theology still has in Chile, which reactivates its potential under a dynamic of radical social work.

This radical social work resurfaced as an experience that tends towards direct action, self-management, mutual aid and microstructural work. This is not something new in the populations, since many times the identity of these spaces has been marked by the pride of its inhabitants to rise up, despite or without the State. In effect, it is not only the absence or withdrawal of the State, but the centrality of community life attentive and close to the conditions and realities of the neighbors, which thus enhances ties, generating empathy and the hope of solving problems together as well.

> For me being here is the least I can do. I am a Christian, I believe in Jesus becoming present in the suffering people, I am a resident of this place and I see the anguish and needs of the people. What do I do for them? To be here anonymously as I think they are there for me, trying to be part of their lives too. (Villa Francia)

In this sense, the COVID-19 crisis made the difference between radical organic social work more evident, and that associated with the deployment of the State's social protection programs.

Thus, the soup kitchen was conceived as a sharing, and not as an aid, in a symmetrical perspective, making the capacities and resources available in a moment of crisis:

> We decided that we were an entity that received the sharing of people, that helping, that word, is an obligatory means of action, it is different when you share your things, your time, a plate of food, it is different to share it than to help, they are very different things. So, what we do here is take everyone's share and make it available for those most in need, our neighbors. (Organizing Team, Base Community, Villa Francia)

This plan contrasted strongly with the supports that the central government gave during the crisis, because these started from mistrust and ignorance of the reality of the people. Thus, the delivery of the food boxes in July at one of the highest peaks of the pandemic was read as something violent:

> When the government boxes were distributed, the military forces came here to deliver them, then the military entered people's houses with machine guns in hand, to deliver merchandise so that you could cook. Why did they have to enter with weapons to deliver a box with merchandise/goods? (Villager, Villa Francia)

The feeling of helplessness of the neighbors worsened with the deaths caused by the pandemic, and also because of food insecurity, with the soup kitchen being a place of support in the face of this scenario.

> Now we are five people. Me, my daughter and three children, including my granddaughter. My partner just died of COVID-19 and I miss him. I went to the office to ask for help and they did not come to see him, I went to the hospital and the same happened. He told me, 'You did everything you could' but I couldn't. Thanks to the soup kitchen I have been able to feed my family. Here I have been able to have some food because simple people, who love this town, as I love it, have given their best. (Inhabitant of Legua Vieja)

36.4.3 The Possibility of Having Transformational Spaces

One of the main lessons learned by the communities is that the active and empowered participation of neighbors in solving complex problems such as food is possible. Thus, this deployment of capabilities and teamwork on a voluntary basis is facilitated if it has a collective purpose. In this sense, the purpose of the Pot is to start from the most basic, "put the body," and associated with fraternity and sharing the experience with people, and not through indirect solidarity such as the transfer of money or species. The presence required by Liberation Theology is capable of constructing new roles, new spaces, and new alternatives, developing a physical, but not social, distancing in the context of the pandemic.

The soup kitchen configures a space for transversal collaboration where each of those who make up the community does so from their own capacities and possibilities; that is why it becomes an inclusive space in which the entire community is involved. There are those who contribute monetarily or by kindly giving a hand; the residents of the fairgrounds who on the day of their purchase reserve part of their truck to transport the vegetables and fruits; the neighbors who come the day before to clean, peel, and cut the large quantities of food for the preparation; the neighboring food handlers and chefs who give the instructions and supervise the kitchen; and the different collaborators who are in charge of preparing, serving, distributing, and cleaning the spaces.

The organization of work and permanent contact between different people (in territories and social classes) generates communication channels, which allow detecting and reacting quickly to the needs of people and communities.

The problems faced by the organization of the soup kitchen are not only technical, about how to carry it out, but also a problem of principles, which forces the participants to develop a discussion regarding common values and projects.

In this sense, the coexistence of La Olla triggers new roles and initiatives that go beyond the contingent problem of food insecurity and advance to approach the center of Liberation

Theology, which are the social structures that are the source of injustices in Chile and in all Latin America.

36.5 Conclusion

La Olla allows something decisive in the path of liberating praxis: 'seeing' without the mediation of social networks that frame information from a perspective that preserves the status quo, especially in a highly segregated and unequal society. This is how the participants and neighbors who attend transform their own references by empathizing with the others, and by managing to understand its complexity, shortening the gaps in understanding and recognition that the high socioterritorial segregation of the capital perpetuates.

From what is experienced in La Olla's day-to-day life, the approach to the causes of inequality ceases to be a theoretical construct and becomes a pain and concrete commitment for each one. It is the 'judging.' where personally and collectively not only the established powers are questioned, but also their own acting from Christian and human principles, which inspire a more just society for all.

Based on this experiential update of the problems of inequality, we seek to 'act,' because it becomes clear that action is necessary to reverse the conditions of inequality. In this way, this practice motivates during 2021 initiatives that seek not only to take charge of the contingency, but also of more structural issues of the places where the soup kitchens worked, such as access to preventive and curative health, accompaniment for the children and youth in their studies and careers, and the gaps that affect people's income generation.

Thus, the praxis of Liberation Theology enables the development of radical social work, capable of addressing inequality, no longer from a solely theoretical-evangelical and intellectual perspective from top to bottom, but from actual presence and proximity, which modifies the beliefs and capacity for action of individuals and communities, especially during periods of crisis, such as the one we have been experiencing since the outbreak of COVID-19.

References

Álvarez, P. (2014). *Legua Emergencia, una historia de dignidad y de lucha*. LDP Ediciones.

Boff, L. (1978). *Teología del cautiverio y de la liberación*. Ediciones Paulinas.

Casaldáliga, P., & Vigil, J. M. (1993). *Espiritualidad de la Liberación*. Envío.

Castillo, F. (1986). *Iglesia liberadora y política*. ECO.

Comblin, J. (1987). *El espíritu santo y la liberación*. Ediciones Paulinas.

Evans, E. N. (1992). Liberation theology, empowerment theory and social work practice with the oppressed. *International Social Work, 35*(2), 135–147. https://doi.org/10.1177/002087289203500204

FAO, IFAD, UNICEF, WFP and WHO. (2020). The State of Food Security and Nutrition in the World 2020. Transforming food systems for affordable healthy diets. Rome, FAO. https://doi.org/10.4060/ca9692en

Ferguson, I., Ioakimidis, V., & Lavalette, M. (2018). *Global social work in a political context: Radical perspectives*. Policy Press.

Garretón, M. A. (2003). *Incomplete democracy. Political democratization in Chile and Latin America*. University of North Carolina Press.

Harms-Smith, L. (2020). Epistemic decoloniality as a pedagogical movement. A turn to anticolonial theorists such as Fanon, Biko and Freire. In R. Lutz, T. Kleibl, N. Noyoo, B. Bunk, A. Dittmann, & B. Seepamore (Eds.), *The Routledge handbook of postcolonial social work*. Routledge. https://doi.org/10.4324/9780429-68728

ILO. (2020). *Chile: Impacto de la COVID-19 sobre los mercados de trabajo y la generación de ingresos*. ILO. https://www.ilo.org/wcmsp5/groups/public/%2D%2D-americas/%2D%2D-ro-lima/%2D%2D-sro-santiago/documents/publication/wcms_761863.pdf

Jorda, M. (2001). *Martirologio de la Iglesia chilena: Juan Alsina y sacerdotes víctimas del terrorismo de estado*. Lom Ediciones.

Lusk, M., & Corbett, D. (2020). Liberation theology and international social work. *Journal of Religion & Spirituality in Social Work: Social Thought, 40*(1), 92–107. https://doi.org/10.1080/15426432.2020.1848750

Mackin, R. (2015). Liberation theology and social movements. In P. Almeida & A. Cordero (Eds.), *Handbook of social movements across Latin America* (pp. 101–116). Springer.

Muñoz, R. (1994). *Pueblo, comunidad, evangelio*. Rehue.

Muñoz, G. (2018). The neoliberal turn in Chilean social work: Frontline struggles against individualism and fragmentation. *European Journal of Social Work*,

22(2), 289–300. https://doi.org/10.1080/13691457.2018.1529657

Observatorio Social, Ministerio de Desarrollo Social y Familia. (2020). *Principales resultados segunda ronda: Inseguridad Alimentaria.* http://observatorio.ministeriodesarrollosocial.gob.cl/storage/docs/covid19/Resultados_Inseguridad_Alimentaria_Covid_II.pdf

Oyarzún-Serrano, L. (2020). Chile facing the pandemic and social unrest: Crisis as an opportunity? *Latin America Policy, 11*, 320–326. https://doi.org/10.1111/lamp.12199

Siavelis, P. (2009). Enclaves de la transición y democracia chilena. *Revista de Ciencia Política*, *29*(1). Universidad de Chile. https://doi.org/10.4067/S0718-090X2009000100001.

Sobrino, J. (1982). *Jesús en América Latina. Su significado para la fe y la cristología.* Sal Terrae.

Trigo, P. (1988). *Creación e historia en el proceso de liberación*. Sal Terrae.

37 Overcoming the Socioeconomic Impacts of the Coronavirus Pandemic: Social Work Perspectives and Postcolonial Reflections from Ethiopia

Robel Afeworki Abay, Demelash Kassaye, and Tanja Kleibl

37.1 Setting the Context: The Coronavirus Pandemic, Socioeconomic Instability, and Political Conflicts in East Africa and the Horn of Africa

In the wider region of East Africa and the Horn of Africa, some 27.6 million people were already acutely food insecure, requiring urgent action across the East Africa region, before the COVID-19 crisis (FAO & WFP, 2020). According to the United Nations Office for the Coordination of Humanitarian Affairs (UN-OCHA, 2020) vulnerable households' purchasing power has sharply declined from the combined effects of reduced incomes and, in some cases, higher food prices. In addition to COVID-19, the region is facing the worst desert locust outbreak in 25 years, which is threatening the environment, food security, and livelihoods. Under the influence of the increasing global climate emergency, the region saw severe flooding in 2020, which affected nearly 1.3 million people, in addition to recovering households after the effects of recent severe droughts. The combined effect of these multiple challenges is likely to result in deteriorating food security, a nutritional situation, and potential increase in social and/or political unrest.

However, despite the worrying poverty levels in the region, most African countries are confronting the global corona pandemic by following the securitarian model of "containment" of Northern countries and the Far East. Ethiopia, just like all governments in the wider region, has imposed physical distancing and movement restrictions for the coronavirus pandemic. Movement restrictions, particularly border closures, have limited the country's access to the well-established East-African seasonal migration for agricultural labor, as well as to traditional grazing and water points for transhuman pastoralist (FAO & WFP, 2020). Such measures, combined with ongoing instability, insecurity, and the recent armed conflicts in the Tigray Region, with increased interregional and interethnic tensions, are producing massive internal population displacements (Molloy, 2021). The fact that the corona health crisis harbours additional political

R. Afeworki Abay (✉)
Department of Rehabilitation Sciences, Humboldt University of Berlin, Berlin, Germany
e-mail: robel.abay@hu-berlin.de

D. Kassaye
College of Social Sciences, School of Social Work, Addis Ababa University, Addis Ababa, Ethiopia

T. Kleibl
Faculty of Applied Social Sciences, University of Applied Sciences, Würzburg-Schweinfurt, Würzburg, Germany

M. C. S. Gonçalves et al. (eds.), *The Coronavirus Crisis and Challenges to Social Development*,
https://doi.org/10.1007/978-3-030-84678-7_37

instability and potential for armed conflicts has already been anticipated by intellectuals from Africa and the Diaspora (Ndongo Sambal Sylla, Lionel Zevounou, and Karine Ndjoko) at the early stage of the coronavirus pandemic (March, 2020; Afeworki Abay, 2020).

Beside the predicted political instability in Africa, macroeconomic challenges such as higher food prices and vulnerability to COVID-19, impacts on the agriculture exports, tourism and travel sectors (which contributes to nearly half of export earnings), are expected to cause deteriorating food security, particularly among vulnerable populations that depend on labor wages and markets. For instance, pastoralists' incomes will likely fall in response to livestock market closures, reduced demand domestically and from abroad, and increased input costs (FAO & WFP, 2020).

37.2 Attempts to Develop Epistemologies of the South

The economic scenario described here does certainly not allow for an optimistic outlook. However, this explorative article aims to broadly follow Southern epistemologies and hence focuses on silenced knowledges (Santos, 2018). Frontline social workers in Ethiopia are often considered as "absent" (Santos, 2018, p. 20) subjects in the scientific debates about socioeconomic inequalities and alternatives to the current crisis. Subjects may be conceived as useful in the front-line of services, but "absent" regarding the production of valid explanatory knowledge about the crisis. Hence, with this small study and reflection, we aim to transform "absent" subjects' knowledge into present subjects' knowledge, which we consider to be a primary condition for identifying and validating knowledges capable of explaining and changing the local and global context.

We particularly consider the so-called ecologies of knowledges, which, according to Santos (2014), are collective cognitive constructions led by the principles of horizontality (different knowledges recognize the differences between each other in a nonhierarchical way) and reciprocity (differently incomplete knowledges strengthen themselves by developing relations of complementarity among one another). Putting Santos' construction of the Epistemologies of the South and the Ecologies of Knowledges in the context of Health, Noronha, Meneses, and Nunes further state:

> [...] vocabularies and expressions of suffering, even if they do not exhaust what is at stake in addressing conceptions and experiences of life and death, violence and suffering, disease and cure, provide a convenient entry point for engaging with non-Eurocentric understandings of what counts as health, illness and disease and for pursuing the dynamics of emerging ecologies of knowledges and practices associated with care and cure. (Noronha et al., 2019, p. 2)

Departing from here, it appears of paramount importance to consider the understanding of health, illness, and disease as well as conflict and suffering from the point of view of the oppressed and to put their engagement with the pandemic into the center of the study. Furthermore, we find it useful to engage with Mwambari's (2020) assessment of the pandemic's impact on Africa more generally, which is based on a critical post-colonial reflection about the African states' economies and preparedness to confront the pandemic.

Mwambari (2020) refers to an open letter from African writers that constitutes an important reminder, a reiteration of the obvious, that the African continent must take its destiny back into its own hands:

> Adopting the securitarian model of "containment" of northern countries—often without much care to specific contexts—many African countries have imposed a brutal lockdown upon their populations; violation of curfew measures has been met with police violence. If such containment measures have met the agreement of middle classes shielded from crowded living conditions, with some having the possibility to work from home, they have proved punitive and disruptive for those whose survival depends on informal activities. (African Arguments, 2020)

Following Mwambari's assessment, specifically in relationship to the importance of recognizing local and alternative creative knowledge generated on the African continent during the current crisis (this aspect will be elaborated below based on the interviews conducted), we firmly believe that the following factors should be considered when analyzing the response to the pandemic in Africa: (1) Africa has a relatively young population (more than 60% under the age of 25); (2) the continent is already experienced in controlling other epidemic diseases; (3) potential cross-immunity from other coronaviruses; (4) the relative late arrival of the virus on the continent; as well as (5) low rates of travel and more outdoor living combined. These factors, alongside the stronger family and community level social security networks, might help to tackle the pandemic in Africa and bring some new strategic advantage to the continent over the long-term.

Indeed, more than 100 writers, researchers, and scientists from the African continent have signed the open letter (African Arguments, 2020), criticizing the way the global state of emergency, and linked to it, "containment," is being implemented in most African countries. It is well noted that countries of the Global North found themselves confronted by new types of risks and vulnerability, which uncover Northern countries strong dependency on medical infrastructure (Sumba, 2021; Afeworki Abay, 2020; Lee, 2020), and combined with that, predominantly older people's expectations, that this infrastructure should respond to their specific needs. African people, often unable to rely on their countries' health systems and on average much younger than people living in countries of the Global North, mostly responded to the corona crisis by relying on their family- and community-based social security networks (Makamo, 2020). These networks function parallel to the often-dysfunctional centralized postcolonial African state structures, which find themselves distant from their own impoverished and subalterned population (Kleibl & Munck, 2019).

37.3 Health Crisis in the Context of Colonial Continuities

In the case of Sub-Saharan Africa, history tells us, that the relatively late, but massive colonization of the African continent matters, when we look at how the coronavirus affects various African countries today. For instance, COVID-19 has emphasized the colonial continuity of huge power imbalances between the Global South and Global North. Not surprisingly, the long-standing postcolonial power dynamics contribute to the continuity of social injustice and the colonial legacies on the idea of human hierarchy (Lee, 2020), which can currently be observed in the existing unequal access to and equitable distribution of COVID-19 vaccines for the Global South. This highlights the crucial interconnections between colonialism and global inequality that are embedded in various forms of the ongoing *Necropower* that reproduces western domination and subjugation of colonial subjects in the time of COVID-19 (Afeworki Abay, 2020). These recent developments should therefore be discussed in relation to Achille Mbembe's (2019) theory of sovereignty as *Necropolitics*,[1] some human lives are worth less than others:

> the normative aspirations signalled in the choral *we are in this together* that characterised progressive political rhetoric during the Covid-19 vaccine development phase remain out of reach for a nation-state system structured around imperialism and the racialised afterlives of colonialism. As a manifestation of these hierarchies, the access gap reveals how *necropolitics at large* is a heavily contested but still deadly *modus operandi* of pandemic politics. (Sumba, 2021 pp. 4–5).

Furthermore, during the period of European colonization in Africa, germ theories of diseases were dominant in many parts of the world and pharmaceutical treatments, vaccination campaigns, and new hygienic regimes were on the rise. This led people to develop the idea that technologies could eventually control human life and its extension, leading to an increase of development funds for medical personnel in the technical services of each colonial state. However, this "benevolent" investment, according to a physician touring the Belgian Congo in the 1920s, did not stop the illnesses and debilities that the colonizers had introduced, caused, or exacerbated (Tilley, 2016).

[1] For further understanding of the concept of Necropolitics, see Mbembe (2019).

However, rejecting a purely technical or medical solution to global health management, Farmer (2004) claims that a thorough understanding of modern epidemics in the postcolonial world requires not only in-depth knowledge of history, but also insights into the contemporary political economy of development. He emphasizes the importance of a syncretic and proper biosocial anthropological understanding when trying to make sense of the 'why' and 'how' epidemics in the Global South are so strongly associated with poverty, social inequalities, conflicts, and coloniality (Sumba, 2021). As a matter of fact, colonial interventions are not just part of colonial history, but there are many examples for their ongoing impacts in many subtle modernized ways in the postcolonial moment (colonial continuity). For instance, the success reached by the African states (e.g., in Ghana, Senegal) and development of various local strategies for coping with the COVID-19 pandemic has been overlooked in the media discourses in Europe (Hirsch, 2020). Rather, Western media discourses are still focused on negative portrayal of Africa (Afeworki Abay, 2020; Ndlovu, 2018).

In effect, for economies in the Global North, whether by colonialism, by controlling the terms of international trade, or by forcing austerity programmes on postcolonial Sub-Saharan Africa, colonial subjugation still works as a well-calculated function. Looking at economic prospects in Africa, roughly 1 year into the global pandemic, and given the massive poverty levels in Sub-Saharan Africa before corona, conflict is more likely to occur on the periphery because states that have high levels of inequality and poverty are more likely become engulfed in violent conflict (Fearon & Laitin, 2003). In consequence, more and more money is wasted in investments in war and conflict, money that could be spent on healthcare, education, or infrastructure. Thus, more dependency, structural violence, and conflict are created, which lead to personal violence in what is known as a conflict trap, as already identified by Galtung (1969). Indeed, looking at the current impact of the corona pandemic in African countries, the Food and Agricultural Organization of the United Nations (FAO) and the World Food Program (FAO & WFP, 2020) warn that sociopolitical instability and levels of civil unrest in many African countries could increase as a result of corona, hence further endangering social development.

One might argue that COVID-19 has indeed brought to light that the status quo of the coloniality of power and knowledge persists (Sumba, 2021). It seems difficult for those in positions of power and privilege to recognize the global system of oppression, exploitation, and epistemic violence. It is evident that frameworks of Eurocentric discourses are interested in justifying the ever-growing inequalities in the Global South and ensuring privileges of the Global North, instead of questioning and challenging the status quo (Afeworki Abay, 2020). Therefore, tracing and addressing mechanisms of global inequality and analyzing the shifting dynamics of colonial power on racialized and subaltern communities in the Global South is indispensable for Postcolonial Social Work.

37.4 Introduction to the Development of Social Work in Ethiopia

Contemporary education in Ethiopia started after the defeat of Italy in 1941. Studies conducted to trace the time when social work education started in the Ethiopian Educational System are scant. According to Mwansa (2011), the first Schools of Social Work in Africa opened in countries such as South Africa, Egypt, and Algeria between the years 1924–1942. In Ethiopia, Social Work education started during the times of Emperor Hailesalsie's first University in 1959. It was a 2-year diploma program, which later developed into a Bachelor of Social Work (BSW) degree in 1959. Not even two decades later, the School has been banned by the Socialist Military Government of the so-called Derg, which came into power after the demise of Emperor Hailesellasie's regime in 1974. This "ban" was following the decisions of other Marxist-Leninist orientated governments in postcolonial Africa (Noyoo & Kleibl, 2020), which preferred handing over the responsibility of social service delivery to their respective mass-based organizations, such as socialist women's and youth groups (Amor, 2016). Consequently, the Derg regime disregarded the social work profession, claiming that it is a profession that sweeps away the morale and active participation of the people, hence endangering the country's sovereignty and independence. Since then, the value of social work studies and practice to confront the many social development challenges affecting the country has been reevaluated in Ethiopia, and new BA and MA courses have been established (Kebede, 2019). The reevaluation outcomes finally recommended the importance of the program to produce great number of professional social workers equipped with knowledge and skills to provide services for those in need of help. Additionally, the shift Ethiopia has made after the demise of the Socialist Military Government in 1991; from command economy to market economy and the political alteration from socialist political ideology to liberalism are also credible evidences for the reopening of various programs including social work. However, the profession struggles to find its own identity and recognition in Ethiopia, which makes its integration in the labor market and the articulation of its social justice orientation in practice difficult. It operates at the periphery of politics and society, although very close to some of the major problems that communities face in the contemporary global neoliberal era.

37.5 Effects of COVID-19 on Social Development and Social Work in Ethiopia

Ethiopia officially confirmed the first positive case of COVID-19 on March 13, 2020, and according to the available data of the World Health Organization of 21December shows that there have been 119,494 confirmed cases of COVID-19 with 1846 deaths in Ethiopia from January to December 2020 (WHO, 2020). Based on its responsibilities to ensure the provision of information regarding the pandemic and essential healthcare services, the Ministry of Health urged citizens to avoid close personal contacts, to take preventive measures such as regular hand-washing, social distancing, wearing face masks, and working from home to flatten the curve of COVID-19 (Fufa, 2020). Additionally, the government closed schools, universities, and nurseries and suspended movement both within its borders, and at international boundaries, rapid testing and quarantines have been also put in place to prevent further rapid spread of the virus (Addis et al., 2020). Despite the social effects of the pandemic which will most likely have some serious economic and social consequences in the post-pandemic world, the country has so far been managing somehow to cope with the rapid spread of coronavirus pandemic (IFSW, 2020a, b, c).

Eventually, after the declaration of WHO on COVID-19 as a global health crisis, many countries in the Global South such as Ethiopia have taken even stricter measures in accordance with the guidelines given by WHO. Yet, not much attention has been paid to the *necropolitics* of COVID-19 during the global pandemic (Lee, 2020; Sumba, 2021) due to the imperial geopolitics and existing postcolonial unequal power relationships between the Global North and South (Afeworki Abay, 2020; Ndlovu, 2018). Although the Ethiopian government has been setting up more testing labs, and prepared the health system with massive logistic and human resources, this has led to the growing concerns about the continent's ability to effectively overcome the pandemic because of existing "fragile health systems" (Hirsch, 2020). Through integrating the experience from the Global North into the nationwide preparation to develop adequate response to COVID-19, almost all public health facilities throughout the country shut down except for emergency services.

The restriction of elementary freedom of movement has increasingly been posing various challenges for economic and social participation of subaltern groups in precarious situations in central regions such as Addis Ababa but also other regions such as Amhara, Oromia, and the South Nation Nationalities Peoples Regional States are most affected by the pandemic (Addis et al., 2020). The federal government of Ethiopia, as many other African countries, has adapted the Northern securitarian model of "containment" (African Arguments, 2020), including numerous preventive measures linked to the state of emergency, including partial to complete lockdown, quarantine, awareness creation, and social protection to minimize the spread and the devastating effect of the pandemic (Molloy, 2021). However, with existing reduced infrastructures, some regions in Ethiopia have unequal access to medical treatments (Fufa, 2020). This poses additional challenge for social workers in providing adequate and professional services to communities (insufficient access to safe drinking water, sanitary and hygienic equipment, as well as the inaccessibility of information regarding the pandemic for those with relatively low socioeconomic level).

Because of the pandemic, the rising risk for sociocultural inequality of many subaltern and marginalized groups in Ethiopia leads to restricting access to participation in the societal, economic, cultural, and political activities in their communities. Countries in the Global South such as Ethiopia have been making difficult decisions to balance the demands of responding directly to the pandemic, while simultaneously engaging in strategic planning and coordinating action to maintain essential social service delivery (Fufa, 2020). The so far described complex nature of the crisis in Ethiopia and the reported rise in the number of new cases of coronavirus in combination with increased containment measures challenges social work in providing adequate services to those in need. The key barriers that prevent social work in Ethiopia from providing pandemic-related services include, but are certainly not limited to, inadequate timely access to information on COVID-19 and the lack of necessary protective measures caused by the precarious financial situations of subaltern communities (Addis et al., 2020).

As discussed earlier, the current conditions related to corona have profound impact especially on those communities living in fragile and precarious situations when it comes to maintaining their psychological well-being and mental health during and after the crisis (IFSW, 2020a, b, c). All these aspects not only aggravate the situation, including fear and uncertainty of the population (Molloy, 2021), but also influence social work preparedness and response mechanisms to the coronavirus in Ethiopia (Addis et al., 2020). Accordingly, in combination with the coronavirus pandemic, a politics of fear spreads in Ethiopia. Maintaining population trust in the capacity of the health system to safely meet essential needs in time of emergency is key to ensuring appropriate state responses to COVID-19.

As in other countries, the relevance of resilient health systems and the need for "solidarity, agility and continuity of essential services" has been emphasized in response to the pandemic in Ethiopia (Tadesse Gebremedhin, 2020). The executive and management committees of the Ministry of Health in cooperation with heads of Regional Health Bureaus have adopted guidelines on continuity of essential services for major public health programs and emergency management, which has been reflected on a weekly basis (Addis et al., 2020). As one social worker in Ethiopia pointed out, "Social workers are like doctors and nurses. We need encouragement from everyone." (Tadesse Gebremedhin, 2020).

The conditions for social work interventions that currently exist to address these barriers are very challenging. Although a sufficiently functioning social welfare system is mostly nonexistent in institutionalized settings in Ethiopia, self-organization and community-driven change is very well established.

37.6 Empirical Data on COVID-19 Social Work Responses in Ethiopia

To embed our country-level analysis into the perspectives of those working at the forefront of service delivery to the most marginalized, we carried out a small explorative research project in Ethiopia. Data pertinent to the study were gathered through expert interviews and focus group discussions in collaboration with the Social Work Department of Addis Ababa University. The interview data were analyzed using thematic analysis. The objective of the study was to highlight how community and social workers are confronting the devastating effects of the coronavirus pandemic having in mind the political, environmental, economic, and social conditions in which they are working. However, the data collection process was affected by a number of factors, the most influential being the emerging conflict in the Tigray Region, which took attention away from the socioeconomic impact of the corona pandemic and highlighted the ethnic-political tension. It created huge difficulties to interview front-line social workers, who were overwhelmed from the pandemic situation and not prepared to work under the containment regulations. Furthermore, the "digital divide" between Germany and Ethiopia and within Ethiopia was increasing, as the Ethiopian Government, based on security concerns linked to the conflict, decided to shut down Internet and mobile phone services. Hence, reaching out to social workers or their target groups, given the resources available for this spontaneous research experiment, turned even more difficult. Consequently, the focus of this project has changed from analyzing social work responses to the crisis to structural and contextual challenges that hinder the professional local social work responses.

37.6.1 Methods: Data Collection and Analysis

For the purpose of this small-scale empirical study, nine semi-structured exploratory expert interviews were conducted with social workers, nurses, and health officials. They were selected by inclusion criteria developed to identify those most close to the subject under review. Interviews focused thematically on social work responses to the coronavirus pandemic, looking specifically at social work responses to most marginalized groups, type of activities carried out as well as structural opportunities, challenges, or limitations being faced during service delivery. Our expert interviews were merited to obtain subjective perspectives of the respondents in overcoming these profoundly laid over systemic-structural challenges. The qualitative empirical data derived from semi-structured expert interviews were analyzed and interpreted using a qualitative content analysis (Mayring, 2015). The data collection proceeded after collecting the signed informed consents of all research participants.

37.6.2 Social Work in the Context of Multiple Crises: Voices of Social Workers from Ethiopia

The analysis of our empirical findings highlights not only best practices about how social work is organized in responding to COVID-19 in Ethiopia, but also the many challenges and limitations of social work in coping with the pandemic-related restrictions in providing adequate services in the context of political fragility. The empirical findings of the study show in its general picture, how even in the relative absence of material resources and low levels of institutionalized social work responses toward COVID-19, community-based approaches can contribute to successful healthcare emergency responses; this includes reframing norms of good social work practice and making sense of core aspects of their work within the politically restrictive working conditions, as the following quote exemplifies:

> The country is living as though the pandemic does not exist. The government is using it to maneuver political moves such as postponing elections and bragging about having it under control (see PM's speech at HoPR first session) he talks about how the healthcare system is doing well. (Almaz)[2]

The severe consequences of the coronavirus pandemic combined with the ongoing political processes have drawn the public's attention in Ethiopia unlike any other issues. Many subaltern communities struggle to adapt to the rapidly changing scenarios and levels of threat. Health

[2]All personal and place names are anonymized in the study to ensure the confidentiality of informants' identities.

and political emergency measures have come to disrupt everyday life. In addition to managing and trying to control internal political matters, the case of Ethiopia has shown underlying patterns of inequalities, which are the result of external macroeconomic level interventions that are clearly embedded in the global dominant capitalist production and trade system (with severe consequences on the already existing unequal structures between urban centers and rural peripheries). The following quote highlights this:

> It prioritized urban development, tourism, mining and other stuff that are not directly related to helping the people (especially those who are likely to deeply face the socio-economic impact) and to survive the multi-dimensional impact of the pandemic. (Almaz)

Regardless of the many structural difficulties that the local communities living in the marginalized socioeconomic conditions are facing, inequalities regarding healthcare systems and other basic social security issues become particularly evident during the pandemic:

> Most of the people living in the rural areas are highly affected by COVID-19. More than 10 people in minimum live in the same house together. Because they can't afford to pay for home rents unless they share it with 6–10 people. (Driba)

Beside the devastating economic consequences of the pandemic in maintaining equitable access to essential pandemic-related service delivery, social work is confronted with addressing additional challenges as like for example the issues domestic and sexual violence and other dimensions of discrimination during the pandemic, as the following statement underlines:

> There are groups who are not given equal opportunity for support. Sex workers, children, and elders received little attention in the distributions of supplies from various sources. The social work interventions need to go beyond the pandemic. For instance, the case of sexual violence caused as a result of lockdown should be addressed by fixing the law enforcement. In addition, the economic crisis should be addressed not only by providing aid but by revising the policies that benefits the marginalized groups. (Blen)

With the ever-more restrictive protection and "containment," accessing social resources such as medical or psychosocial advice, and additional protection measures, is hardly an option, especially for many vulnerable groups. Another unique finding of the study is that many forms of intergenerational, and community-based solidarity are acknowledged as an important part of community structures and religious services in Ethiopia. The ways communities with cultural and religious norms relate to each other, and can benefit from incidental acts of solidarity to support one another, is remarkable:

> It helps out to understand the extent to which people are cooperative and kind to support the people who are not able enough to get even a daily meal. The initiation from both the government and wealthy people was encouraging. (Blen)

The results of our empirical findings simultaneously highlight how both the state and social workers in Ethiopia have realized early enough to fight against the pandemic by maintaining community-based responses. However, the interview responses received and challenges observed so far rather put a stronger emphasis on the long-lasting and ongoing mechanisms of subordination emerging out of the experiences of the countries with capitalist exploitation, colonial encounters, and patriarchal structures and its consequences on marginalized groups, especially women and children in Ethiopia. A phenomenon that was only further strengthened, rather than radically questioned, during the COVID-19 pandemic so far:

> The fields of social work I believe have helped in identifying the parts of the community that is affected by the pandemic and addressing the social crisis that followed the pandemic such as the rise in sexual violence, abduction and early marriage... (Belete)

To better address the best interests of the communities during the pandemic, having in mind the specific precarious and exploitative economic situations of marginalized communities, people interviewed strongly highlighted the need to maintain and democratize access to information and substantially improve the identification of the needs of the communities. The latter would require a fundamental shift from the current emergency *modus operandi* to a longer-term alternative development vision of the country, as the following statement underlines:

> It seems essential to improve the economy of the country, delivering reliable information to the people on time, supplying face masks and reforming the disaster prevention and risk management capacity of the country. Identifying needs and prioritization of aid is very important. Planning intervention that doesn't put into consideration the needs of the community is not as effective. And the aid should make sure that the community is able to stand on its own after aid is withdrawn. (Almaz)

Although several other factors influence the effective management of the COVID-19, the findings of the study indicate that many countries in the Global South withstand the effects of health crises. In addition to overcoming the challenges caused by the pandemic, the current political tension in Ethiopia, as well as the dysfunctional development aid systems, have been affecting social workers in providing even the most basic services. Although the empirical data analysis emphasizes the reactions of community and social workers in Ethiopia as an important and potential factor in these difficult times, the complexities of the pandemic-related circumstances have enormous effects on old and new structures of inequalities. This understanding highlights the fact there is much to be done to develop future community-based social work that integrates community resources and specific needs into interventions designed to overcome challenges of health emergencies.

All in all, the data analysis has shown several complex implications for future social work research which needs to increasingly build on critical historical, political-economy and multidimensional poverty analysis having in mind postcolonial power relationships and the growing geopolitics of health management as well as the extremely limited financial resources available for applied social science research and social work practice in Africa.

37.6.3 Methodological Reflections from the Epistemologies of the South

As our empirical findings are based on an ad hoc research, we are aware that this preliminary analysis does not claim to provide a comprehensive account of the complex effects of the pandemic on social work services. It is evident that researching in the Global South is embedded in the geopolitics of knowledge and power (Mignolo, 2009, 2013; Quijano, 2000). Considering the fact that ad hoc research even goes along with more complex ethical responsibilities, we recognize that the negotiation of methodological and ethical challenges highlights the need for epistemological reflexivity, transparency (Lunn, 2014; Zhang, 2017), and imagination, "aimed at refounding the political imagination (…) to strengthen the social struggles against domination" (Santos, 2018, pp. 126–127). By acknowledging the discussed complexities and our ethical responsibilities which we see as an ongoing process of joint learning and reflection, our empirical experiences and ethical challenges opened the opportunity for an advanced discussion and a power-reflexive academic dialogue between the Global South and North as well as to "develop authentic individual responses to potentially unique circumstances" (Valentine, 2005, p. 485, cited in Zhang, 2017, p. 2). This dialogue can also be observed as a fundamental starting point in the process of decolonizing the hegemonial order of Western knowledge production, in researching *with* and not *about* the Global South. Moreover, these experiences allow researchers from the Global North to open up and be self-reflective while avoiding the frequent undervaluing of the legacy of colonialism. In this regard, we must work in the spaces of solidarity in academia, remain flexible in terms of our research approaches, and reflect on the possibilities of "epistemic disobedience" (Mignolo, 2009, p. 8) to overcome the ongoing epistemic violence in Eurocentric knowledge production in social work.

In the following section, we provide some reflections on the implications of these points for further research as a way forward based on learning from pandemic-related reactions of community and social workers in Ethiopia.

37.7 Decolonial Interventions: Discursive Construction of Vulnerability and Victimhood of Africa and the Need for Postcolonial Political Reform from Below

Analyzing the impact of COVID-19 in Ethiopia has many implications for decolonial interventions in social work including, but certainly not limited to, promoting social justice through transnational advocacy as well as maintaining power-reflexive cooperation between the Global South and North. As argued by the research participants in our exploratory research, the pandemic has highlighted the urgent need for enacting structural changes and action against social inequality and injustice in the contemporary postcolonial world, while recognizing the need for bottom-up social and political state reform that opens space for more participation of marginalized communities. This scenario shows the relevance of acknowledging the fact that countries in the Global South have their own experiences and social community systems that often provide better ways of managing the effect of COVID-19 in their own context, compared with the Northern securitarian model of "containment." Therefore, there is a need to stress the importance of overcoming the epistemic violence of Eurocentric discourses (re)producing different notions of victimhood and vulnerability in relationship to people living in countries of the Global South, particularly in Africa, by simultaneously silencing their voices and perspectives, as well as political struggles.

Touching upon the possibilities of decolonizing global power structures, the discussions of this chapter raised far more questions than we could hope to answer: for instance, how to practice social work values in a globalized capitalist world with ever-growing unequal access to basic social and health services. These questions go to the very heart of the Social Work Code of Ethics stated by the International Federation of Social Work (IFSW). Within transnational social work we therefore have to fight for social justice, dignity, and worth of the person, particularly during a global health crisis such as COVID-19 (Walter-McCabe, 2020), and seriously confront the nationalist reinterpretation of solidarity. It remains our shared belief that, during this pandemic, a greater sense of transnational solidarity and social justice is urgently needed, alongside critical engagement into the effects of development politics and the aid industry more general. Yet, these implications can only be developed into a real opportunity for renewed and strengthened transnational and postcolonial social work if we are committed to power-reflexive global solidarity. Decolonizing the notion of global is central to overcome the epistemic violence constructing vulnerability and victimhood of the Global South as an alibi, hence legitimizing economic neo-colonial interventions on the one hand (Afeworki Abay, 2020) while continuing to support an ineffective aid infrastructure on the other (Kleibl & Munck, 2019).

37.8 Conclusions for Postcolonial Social Work Research and Practice

We need to now ask ourselves what values matter most for us as social work researchers in a globalized world, and why and how do they shape our worldviews and positionalities? What values, competencies, and dispositions do we think will best serve the marginalized communities in the era of global pandemic(s)? Is anything that we are doing or saying—or anything we are NOT doing or saying—selling out our values and goals? Our exploratory research initiative has not led to the number and depth of interviews that we would have hoped for under "ideal" research conditions. In the end, we have decided to bring this joint research project to an end as from the beginning we followed the aim of supporting Southern Epistemologies, hence putting the often-silenced or absent voices of front-line social workers to the fore front. It is our duty to underline the postcolonial conditions under which social workers operate both in the Global North and the South, deeply rooted in colonial continuities. The global pandemic needs to be taken as a clear wakeup call for the social work profession to consider global hegemonic relationships as highly problematic (Kleibl & Lutz, 2020) and hence reconsider its relationship with power from a Southern Perspective, where post-colonial internal conflict is the norm and peace is the exception.

The experiences from Ethiopia show that responses to the pandemic in one context are not necessarily applicable for the specific situation of other countries' regional parts and communities, and indeed, beyond the country, as the current geopolitical structures are incompatible to such common responses and reactions to certain health emergencies such as COVID-19. More importantly, it is not only indispensable to look at the needs of the states and communities but also at their capacities and structures maintaining sustainable and effective responses to the pandemic. However, as outlined in this chapter, the world is not affected by the pandemic equally. Despite the previously existing forms of social inequalities, the rapid spread of the pandemic has been contributing to the risk of economic disparities as well as political instability across the African continent (Afeworki Abay, 2020; Sumba, 2021; Molloy, 2021). The observed increasing political and social anxiety from the armed conflicts in Ethiopia in the past few months necessitates that more efforts should be made to address not only immediate material, legal, and human capital resources but also other challenging issues such as ensuring political and social stability in a post-corona time. Even though we are aware that this is easier said than done, rethinking the long-term aid dependency of the country, which keeps its residents in a continuous situation of postcolonial economic dependency, incapable of protecting the most essential rights of subaltern groups, is an indispensable integral aspect of the decolonization process. For future research in social work, it is recommended to analyze the coloniality of knowledge (Ndlovu, 2018; Mignolo, 2013; Quijano, 2000) and to decolonize ontological and epistemological dominance of the Global North (Santos, 2018) through increased joint research with and specifically led by colleagues in the Global South, which is directly concerned with the day-to-day social struggles of the subaltern.

References

Addis, Y., Abate, D., & Ferreira, J.-B. (2020). *Societal responses and household-level determinants of coronavirus preparedness in rural Ethiopia*. https://www.tandfonline.com/doi/full/10.1080/19371918.2021.1881014

Afeworki Abay, R. (2020) Can the African Subaltern Speak? Kontinuität kolonialer Macht- und Herrschaftsstrukturen. Soziologiemagazin. https://soziologieblog.hypotheses.org/13547

African Arguments. (2020). *COVID-19: An open letter from African intellectuals to Africa's leaders*. https://africanarguments.org/2020/04/coronavirus-open-letter-african-intellectuals-africa-leaders/

Amor, A. M. (2016). *Natureza do Servico Social em Angola*. Cortez.

FAO & WFP. (2020). *FAO-WFP early warning analysis of acute food insecurity hotspots*. https://docs.wfp.org/api/documents/WFP-0000117706/download/?_ga=2.100507037.205607340.1595325541-1185675020.1594805753

Farmer, P. (2004). An anthropology of structural violence. *Current Anthropology, 45*(3).

Fearon, J.-D., & Laitin, D. D. (2003). Ethnicity, insurgency and civil war. *The American Political Science Review, 97*(1), 75–90.

Fufa, B. (2020). *Support to vulnerable people during COVID-19 pandemic in the Jimma City, Oromia Region, Ethiopia*. https://www.iassw-aiets.org/covid-19/5606-support-to-vulnerable-people-during-covid-19-pandemic-in-the-jimma-city-oromia-region-ethiopia/

Galtung, J. (1969). Violence, peace and peace research. *Journal of Peace Research, 6*(3), 167–191.

Hirsch, A. (2020). Why are Africa's coronavirus successes being overlooked? *The Guardian*. International Edition https://www.theguardian.com/commentisfree/2020/may/21/africa-coronavirus-successes-innovation-europe-us?CMP=share_btn_fb&fbclid=IwAR39KIwnVFrEvQvisongCo35MVE2_z2a2KpLFHHsNq8ESNwbQY9wzNrQ-xk

IFSW. (2020a). *Global definition of social work*. https://www.ifsw.org/what-is-social-work/global-definition-of-social-work/

IFSW. (2020b). *The social work responses to COVID-19-six months on: Championing changes in services and preparing for long-term consequences* https://www.ifsw.org/wp-content/uploads/2020/07/2020-07-01-SW-Response-to-COVID-19-Six-Months-On.pdf

IFSW. (2020c). *It is the time to replace models of nationalism and charity with new global ethical foundations: What the world can learn from international social work*. https://www.ifsw.org/it-is-the-time-to-replace-models-of-nationalism-and-charity-with-new-global-ethical-foundations-what-the-world-can-learn-from-international-social-work/

Kebede, W. (2019). Social work education in Ethiopia: Past, present, and future. *International Journal of Social, 6*(1) http://www.macrothink.org/journal/index.php/ijsw/article/view/14175

Kleibl, T., & Lutz, R. (2020). Internationale Soziale Arbeit neu denken: Zur Verschärfung Globaler Ungleichheit durch COVID-19. *Sozial Extra, 44*, 247–251.

Kleibl, T., & Munck, R. (2019). NGOs and the political economy of international development and development education: An Irish perspective. *Policy and Practice: A Development Education Review, 29*. https://www.developmenteducationreview.com/issue/issue-29/importance-feminist-development-education-through-neoliberal-times. Accessed Dec 2020.

Lee, C. J. (2020). *The necropolitics of Covid-19. Africa is a country*. https://www.thecitizen.in//index.php/en/newsdetail/index/6/18541/the-necropolitics-of-covid19

Lunn, J. (2014). *Fieldwork in the global south: Ethical challenges and dilemmas*. Routledge.

Makamo, E. (2020). Die Normalität des Risikos: Ein Kommentar zu Afrikanischen und Europäischen Antworten auf COVID-19. *Afrika Süd, 49*(3).

March, L. (2020). *Stereotypes Afrika-Bild in der Coronakrise: Afrikanische Intellektuelle fordern radikale Veränderungen*. https://www.deutschlandfunkkultur.de/stereotypes-afrika-bildin-der-coronakrise-afrikanische.1013.de.html?dram%3Aarticle_id=475654&fbclid=IwAR0_1XOR_Cz2TCQS6NrXASyVFQamhHPdexwMFC8dUodnIipVZ1uRTMZCHV4

Mayring, P. (2015). *Qualitative Inhaltsanalyse. Grundlagen und Techniken* (12th rev. and ext. ed.). Beltz.

Mbembe, A. (2019). *Necropolitics*. Duke University Press.

Mignolo, W. D. (2009). Epistemic disobedience, independent thought and de-colonial freedom. *Theory, Culture & Society, 26*(7–8), 1–23.

Mignolo, W. D. (2013). *Local histories/global designs: Coloniality, subaltern knowledges, and border thinking*. Princeton University Press.

Molloy, S. (2021). *Emergency law responses to Covid-19 and the impact on peace and transition processes: Seventh Edinburgh dialogue on post-conflict constitution-building, 2020*. International Institute for Democracy and Electoral Assistance (International IDEA). https://doi.org/10.31752/idea.2021.24

Mwambari, D. (2020). The pandemic can be a catalyst for decolonization in Africa. *Aljazeera Opinion*. https://www.aljazeera.com/opinions/2020/4/15/the-pandemic-can-be-a-catalyst-for-decolonisation-in-africa

Mwansa, L. K. (2011). Social work education in Africa: Whence and whither? *Social Work Education, 30*(1), 4–16. https://doi.org/10.1080/02615471003753148

Ndlovu, M. (2018). Coloniality of knowledge and the challenge of creating African futures. *Ufahamu: A Journal of African Studies, 40*(2), 95–112.

Noronha, D. S., Meneses, M. P., & Nunes, J. A. (2019). *Health and epistemologies of the south*. University of Coimbra, Centre for Social Studies. https://www.ces.uc.pt/ficheiros2/files/CES_Health_ESouth.pdf

Noyoo, N., & Kleibl, T. (2020). Introduction: Setting the scene for critical new social work approaches in the neoliberal postcolonial era. In T. Kleibl, R. Lutz, & N. Noyoo (Eds.), *The Routledge handbook of postcolonial social work*. Routledge.

Quijano, A. (2000). Coloniality of power and eurocentrism in Latin America. *International Sociology, 15*(2), 215–232.

Santos, B. S. (2014). *Epistemologies of the south: Justice against epistemicide*. Routledge.

Santos, B. S. (2018). *The end of the cognitive empire: The coming of age of epistemologies of the south*. Duke University Press.

Sumba, E. O. (2021). Necropolitics at large: Pandemic politics and the coloniality of the global access gap. *Critical Studies on Security*. https://doi.org/10.1080/21624887.2021.1904354

Tadesse Gebremedhin, L. (2020). *Solidarity, agility and continuity: Three cornerstones of Ethiopia's COVID-19 response*. https://www.thinkglobalhealth.org/article/solidarity-agility-and-continuity-three-cornerstones-ethiopias-covid-19-response

Tilley, H. (2016). Medicine, Empires, and Ethics in Colonial Africa. AMA Journal of Ethics. 18(7), 743–753. https://doi.org/10.1001/journalofethics.2016.18.7.mhst1-1607

UN-OCHA. (2020). *Global humanitarian response plan COVID-19—April to December 2020*. https://www.unocha.org/sites/unocha/files/GHRP-COVID19_July_update.pdf

Valentine, G. (2005). Geography and ethics: Moral geographies? Ethical commitment in research and teaching. Progress in Human Geography, 29, 483–487.

Walter-McCabe, H. A. (2020). Coronavirus pandemic calls for an immediate social work response. *Social Work in Public Health, 35*(3), 69–72. https://doi.org/10.1080/19371918.2020.1751533

WHO. (2020). *WHO coronavirus disease (COVID-19) dashboard*. https://covid19.who.int/region/afro/country/et

Zhang, J. J. (2017). Research ethics and ethical research: Some observations from the global south. *Journal of Geography in Higher Education, 41*(1), 147–154.

38 Concluding Remarks and Summation

Maria do Carmo dos Santos Gonçalves, Rebecca Gutwald, Tanja Kleibl, Ronald Lutz, Ndangwa Noyoo, and Janestic Twikirize

38.1 Introduction

This book is a collection of essays from different authors who come from various parts of the word. As editors of a book that focusses on the coronavirus (COVID-19) and how it challenges social work in its day-to-day interventions, we were acutely mindful of the need to have a diversity of thought and experience reflected in the text, even though the pandemic's outcomes were similar everywhere: sickness, misery, destruction of lives and livelihoods, new and old inequalities, and death. We thus endeavoured to represent all regions of the globe in this book, which was not easy for a number of reasons. For instance, one glaring issue that we noticed as we collated the chapters from the authors was that in the midst of the pandemic, there were parallel activities that continued unabated, from the pre-pandemic period. The former relate to inter alia, the denial and abuse of human rights by authorities in many countries across the globe. One author failed to submit his chapter as he could not finish it despite his valiant efforts to do so. Our colleague from Hong Kong was repeatedly arrested for his pro-democracy activities and stance, and therefore could not submit his chapter. Every time he asked for an extension, he would be arrested based on his political engagement. Such are just some of the challenges authors of the chapters of this book faced.

In this regard, we wish to express our gratitude to the various authors who managed to submit the chapters and stick to the publisher's deadline. We, as editors, had to also meet our own deadlines with the publisher. What this exercise sharply brought to the fore is that everyone who participated in this book project was touched by the COVID-19 pandemic directly or indirectly. We all suffered some form of loss, grief, frustration, exhaustion, or fear from COVID-19. As we went on with our writing tasks, we all equally had to manage the lived realities of lockdowns; quarantines; different "waves" of COVID-19; on-line teaching (with its attendant double workload);

M. d. C. d. S. Gonçalves (✉)
Centro Scalabriniano de Estudos Migrató, Brasilia, Brasília, Brazil
e-mail: diretora@csem.org.br

R. Gutwald
Munich School of Philosophy, Munich, Germany

T. Kleibl
Faculty of Applied Social Sciences, University of Applied Sciences, Würzburg-Schweinfurt, Würzburg, Germany

R. Lutz
Faculty of Applied Social Sciences, University of Applied Sciences, Erfurt, Germany

N. Noyoo
Department of Social Development, University of Cape Town, Cape Town, South Africa

J. Twikirize
Department of Social Work and Social Administration, Makerere University, Kampala, Uganda

M. C. S. Gonçalves et al. (eds.), *The Coronavirus Crisis and Challenges to Social Development*,
https://doi.org/10.1007/978-3-030-84678-7_38

home-schooling; bereavements of friends, family members or colleagues; loss of income; and so forth. No one who participated in this book was immune to this deadly virus' devastating effects and its aftershocks. Therefore, we the editors discussed these issues in our different planning sessions via Zoom. These are some of the practicalities and challenges related to writing a book during a global pandemic. When we began this journey of writing this edited book, the world was in a very perilous position as the vaccines against COVID-19 had not been discovered. Now we are seeing the proverbial "light at the end of the tunnel" as all of us, the editors of this book project, are now witnessing the rollout of vaccines in our respective countries: Brazil, Germany, South Africa, and Uganda, although with different availabilities due to the unequal and unjust distribution of the vaccines.

It is noteworthy that when COVID-19 initially broke out in China in late 2019 and then swept across the globe in 2020, the world was initially paralysed and did not seem to know how to respond to this novel pandemic, with dislocating effects of epic proportion. Even developed and industrialised nations, such as the United States of America (US), were caught flat footed and would go on to suffer one of the highest mortality rates in the world stemming from COVID-19, peaking at almost 600,000 deaths, as this book is being finalised. Equally, in Spain, Italy, and the UK, the colossal human losses suffered were the worst since the end of the Second World War. In this turbulent atmosphere, many political authorities and professionals were baffled and did not seem to know what to do during the first wave of the pandemic. It was even more so for the health professionals who were in the eye of the COVID-19 storm as they battled to save lives on the one hand, but also fell victim to COVID-19 on the other, with many succumbing to this dreaded pandemic and dying. Nevertheless, it was not just the health professionals who were bewildered, but also other human service professionals such as social workers who were in shock and could not immediately find ways and means to counteract the negative effects of COVID-19.

The chapters in this book have shown that not only is COVID-19 a health problem, but it also is a psychological, political, social, and economic challenge that went on to engender a plethora of social ills across the globe. The consequences of such devastation not only will be felt in years to come, but also time will be needed to decipher the social and economic costs of the pandemic.

38.2 Key Issues Emanating from the Chapters

Many issues that emerged from the book's chapters point for the need for a deep reformation of healthcare across the globe. One critical issue that was highlighted in some of the discussions was the need to revisit the notion of healthcare being a fundamental human right, as was initially envisioned in the Universal Declaration of Human Rights, when it was finalised in 1948. This thinking also sharply brought into focus the need for healthcare to be universalised in line with the Sustainable Development Goals (SDGs), specifically SDG 3: *Good Health and Well-being*. As for countries in the Global South in particular, universal health should not be an abstraction but a basic human need (*and right*). With this line of thought comes the realisation that in particular Sub-Saharan Africa is extremely laggard when it comes to social and health infrastructure. Africa is at the weakest point in regard to the provision of healthcare. Even though the global capitalist power relationships have historically and contemporarily designated Africa a subordinate role in the global sociopolitical and economic hierarchy, the challenges that Africa faces in this whole pandemic scenario are, of course, also linked to the weak political, economic, and governance systems, as well as malevolent leadership, of many countries.

The foregoing assertion is poignant as most, if not all, African leaders have a penchant for going to Europe, North America, or Southeast Asia for medical treatment when, by the same token, they neglect their country's health infrastructure. The chapters in the African segment brought forth this common theme of neglect, which is reflected in many African countries' extreme vulnerability to COVID-19. Therefore, when putting forward a post-COVID-19 scenario in Africa, it is also important to advocate for local agency, youth empowerment, and political change, so that the postcolonial myth of the African nation state based on colonial boundaries can be reimagined in local terms. For now, African leaders are to be held accountable so that they do not abdicate their responsibilities of building and maintaining health infrastructure, including safeguarding and enhancing human resources and procuring medicine and equipment for hospitals, clinics, and medical centres.

In the Latin American context, the pandemic asserted old inequities that persist in the discursive and material constructions that underlie the inequalities that still mark many of the contexts in the countries of the Americas included in the notion of the Global South. The weakening of Latino democracies represented a delay factor in the process of fighting the pandemic. Denial speeches with strong appeals against science, cuts in social support programmes, lack of articulated policies to deal with unemployment generated by the health crisis, security management based on the sovereignty of states to handle the strong migratory crisis that marks the continent, the weakening of public health systems, and the repression of democratic demonstrations linked to demands for greater efforts by the State to meet the demands of the most vulnerable segments of the population, are among others, some of the serious contexts that became more visible during the COVID-19 crisis. At the same time, as we can see in the chapters referring to Latin American countries, it is possible to identify a multitude of initiatives that arise from the process of reflection and action on these realities, led by an endless number of social workers and people who are dedicated to this field of study. In this sense, we see the stronger emergence of the perspective of "care for" and activism as a common factor that permeates initiatives aiming to face the health crisis in the continent.

Chapters from Asia and Oceania, although smaller in number, often highlighted the specific impact the pandemic has had on indigenous people's well-being, on specific policies aiming to address historical injustices as well as on local attempts to improve political governance, gender-related exclusion, and global justice. Chapters from all continents highlighted the disastrous impact the pandemic has had on people on the move, in particular forced migrants. The conjuncture of migration control with the pandemic led to an abuse of the health crisis against those that looked for protection. For many refugees, the already challenging and dehumanizing living conditions in camps have been worsened during the pandemic. Especially in the Western public discourse, the politics of confinement were ironically transformed in public health precautions.

38.3 Future Prospects for a Post-COVID-19 World

The COVID-19 pandemic represents a global inflection point that calls into question the dominant neoliberal economic development project. The health crisis exposed the accelerated process of environmental and social degradation in which we are immersed, as well as confirmed the human being as an important agent in this process. The sustainability of life makes it totally mandatory to deconstruct the notion that we can reach high levels of technological development without developing an ethical relationship with everything that lives, exists, and inhabits this planet. Our bio-nature gives us citizenship on this planet and makes us part of the ecosystem. At the same time, the challenge of sustainability calls for recognition of the profound relationship of dependence that human beings have among themselves and the responsibility to maintain life in all its senses. This awareness, from the painful experience of the pandemic, should call us to a less predatory and exploratory relationship with the world and lead us to organised, supranational and political forms of solidarity and respect of life on the planet. This hope necessarily involves sharing solutions that can help to overcome this crisis, such as the suspension of vaccine patents and supporting everyone on the planet to have the right to immunization.

38.4 Conclusion

As we conclude this book, we remain convinced about the idea of a transformed global order that is more inclusive and equitable. We argue for more synergies between human activities and their environments in this globalised world. In this regard, we stand firm for a better life for all, for which social development actors and others have to constantly fight. There is a need to engage in work and activities that expose the global social, political, and economic structures of oppression. For this book, the former undertaking remains the key responsibility of social work and social development actors across the globe, given the fact the issues they confront are not only internationally interwoven but also are political. This book examined a global pandemic that is unprecedented in the modern era. For the first time in the modern era, the existence of the whole human species was under threat in a fundamental way, and no nation was spared this scourge. It is with this understanding that we firmly believe that all countries should strive to work together to make this world a better place, because we are all interdependent.

Epilogue

Maria do Carmo dos Santos Gonçalves,
Rebecca Gutwald, Tanja Kleibl, Ronald Lutz
Ndangwa Noyoo, and Janestic Twikirize

When we were putting together the call for abstracts to this edited book, the coronavirus (COVID-19) was literally a death sentence. There was no known cure, and the only responses countries could produce were public health preventive measures, such as wearing of masks, sanitising of hands, and social distancing. The other recourse countries had was what experts referred to as the 'blunt instrument' of lockdowns, which seemed the most effective way of containing the virus and 'flattening' the proverbial curve. We were still in the first quarter of 2020 when we were conceptualising this book. Since then, much has changed. Despite the death, sickness, and misery the pandemic has brought upon humanity, various vaccines have been developed and are now being rolled out. This ray of hope that came with the development of vaccines was, and continues to be, dampened by the North–South global power dynamics, whereby those countries in the North that control the world's purse strings also determine who gets the vaccines and how these are distributed to the developing world. At the centre of this power equation are the giant Northern pharmaceutical firms that are not willing to relax their patents or intellectual property rights to allow developing countries to manufacture the vaccines. This concession would make the COVID-19 vaccines cheap and readily available to those who live in poorer nations.

Perhaps the tide is now turning, if the pledge made by the G7 nations can be trusted. At the Summit held in Cornwall, in the United Kingdom, in the second week of June 2021, the G7 nations pledged 870 million COVID-19 vaccine doses. Therefore, if the promise on this score, made by the richest nations on planet Earth, is translated into actual tangibles then the world would have turned a corner, so to speak. As the world moves into a post-pandemic era, the state of social development is at its weakest, because the pandemic negatively impacted the word's economic systems with no country being spared in the process. Unemployment and poverty rates soared,

M. d. C. d. S. Gonçalves
Centro Scalabriniano de Estudos Migrató, Brasília, Brasília, Brazil

R. Gutwald
Munich School of Philosophy, Munich, Germany

T. Kleibl
Migration and Diversity, University of Applied Sciences, Würzburg-Schweinfurt, Würzburg, Germany

R. Lutz
Faculty of Applied Social Sciences, University of Applied Sciences, Erfurt, Germany

N. Noyoo
Department of Social Development, University of Cape Town, Cape Town, South Africa

J. Twikirize
Department of Social Work and Social Administration, Makerere University, Kampala, Uganda

M. C. S. Gonçalves et al. (eds.), *The Coronavirus Crisis and Challenges to Social Development*,
https://doi.org/10.1007/978-3-030-84678-7

rendering many families and communities vulnerable. Social ills and all manner of abuse increased exponentially and again put extra strain on the social fabric of countries around the world. Not only were world systems under severe stress but the whole world also has, in a short period of time, experienced so much grief with the loss of loved ones as COVID-19 has claimed countless fatalities and continues to ravage many countries. And, despite the vaccine rollout, many countries are experiencing a third wave of the pandemic.

With so much loss, pain, and misery, the roles of human service professionals such as social workers and social development practitioners have been sharply put under the spotlight more than previously in the modern age. Although it will be important to buoy up economic systems and bolster the health infrastructure, it is the social development practitioners who must restore or strengthen the optimal functioning of individuals, families, groups, and communities in societies all over the world. Unless people are functioning optimally in their societies, there will be no economies. It is therefore imperative for national governments, all over the world, to see to it that people are able to recover from the ravages of the COVID-19 pandemic. People should also be enabled to play their requisite roles by social development practitioners: parents have to resume their functions; fathers and mothers have to resume their lives; and children as well have to honor their roles. This understanding was the reason we focused on the coronavirus crisis and the challenges it posed to global social development. No nation in the world was spared from the pandemic, and that is why we took a global and holistic view in this book, by bringing forward different insights and experiences from authors from many parts of the world.

When we started writing this book, there was only one variant of the virus emanating from China. Since then, several variants of this virus have emerged by mutation. This realisation leads to the fact that the pandemic continues to be a 'moving target' and therefore there should not be room for any complacency. Thus, we are brought to the question of global solidarity and cooperation in the fight against future pandemics. If those sections of the world that were greedy and impervious to the suffering of the world before the pandemic have not learnt anything from this global health crisis, then they will never learn anything. During this pandemic, it became crystal clear that challenges in one corner of the world can easily take on a global dimension, especially when it comes to health and matters of security. If these sections are not interested in the redistribution of wealth or making the world a better place, then they should see altruistic measures of which they could partake as a matter of their self-interest. No one was immune from death, sickness, suffering, lockdowns, and stay-at-homes. The rich, famous, and powerful were at the mercy of the virus just like those who are poor and vulnerable. Ironically, COVID-19 became the greatest equaliser in the twenty-first century, albeit in a pernicious way.

As we close this Epilogue, we reflect on the heroic efforts of all those health workers who work in hospitals all over the world, and awoke every morning, at the height of the first wave of the pandemic, to save lives. Many of these individuals did this knowing fully that they might not return to their families at the end of their shifts. Indeed, many ended up paying the ultimate price—losing their lives. The health workers reminded us of how important they were during this health crisis. They looked after the powerful and rich as well as the poor. No one was special. Everyone was treated the same. A classic example of this is that of the British Prime Minister, Boris Johnson, who had nonchalantly gone about his business, shaking hands and dismissing the pandemic in the early days of COVID-19. He later tested positive to the virus and was eventually admitted to the intensive care unit. With his life hanging by a thread, the healthcare workers nursed him back to life. He would admit after recovery that if it were not for the healthcare workers and the National Health Service (NHS), he would have probably died. We also reflect on the heroic efforts of the people who in 'normal' times are not noticed by their societies. The essential workers, who are the garbage removers, bus and train drivers, those individuals who keep our cities clean and keep our electricity on, law enforcement officers and firefighters who keep us safe, and many others, showed us how fickle are some highly paid professions. Although these unsung heroes and heroines are paid low salaries, those who are paid millions in normal times could not help their societies in any way, apart from complaining that they were suffering from 'lockdown fatigue' and were 'tired' of wearing masks.

Lastly, it is important to reflect on the state of the planet, and how the pandemic was able to show the world in a very stark way how carbon emissions and other pollutants discharged by humans from their industrial activities are actually damaging the planet. The pandemic was able to debunk the myth that climate change and global warming were not real. It was able to show how we are destroying our planet in a very simple and practical way. When the whole world went into lockdowns, satellite images showed clearly how smog had cleared in various parts of the world and how clean skies emerged after industrial activities were halted. The question is whether the world has learnt anything from this situation. Can we ill afford to engage in senseless debates about global warming and climate change when this deadly disease actually showed us how we are destroying our planet through our voracious daily appetite for wealth? Should we go back to 'business as usual'? Or can we learn from this deadly disease that we indeed need to save our planet for future generations?

Index

A

Aboriginal and Torres Strait Islander Advisory Group (ATSIAG), 268, 269
Aboriginal and Torres Strait Islander mental health and well-being, 267
Aboriginal peoples, 264
Aboriginal Recovery Plan, 271, 272
  health and mental health workforce, 272, 273
  right to self-determination, 272
  social and cultural determinants of health, 273, 274
Adaptations
  positive and negative consequences of, 379
  to overall project, 377, 378
  workshops, in Kenya, 374–377
Adaptations, to overall project, 377, 378
Adherence, 119, 128
Adversities, 105
Advocacy, 229, 230, 233, 234
Afghan refugees, 202, 204, 206
Africa
  cultural representations
    ethnography, 115
  pandemic in, 433
  post-COVID-19 socioeconomic agenda for, 393
    epistemic delinking, 396
    global economy, delink from, 395, 396
    globalisation, 394, 395
    neo-liberalism, global economic arrangements of, 393, 394
    radical shift, 396
    rural development, 396, 397
  Western development paradigms and theories, during COVID-19 pandemic, 400, 401
    COVID-19 and development, 404–406
    defining development, 401, 402
    post COVID-19, alternative development agenda for, 407
    structural adjustment programmes and underdevelopment, 404
    underdevelopment, 402
African countries
  culture of deportation, involuntary returnees in
    local communities, disconnection from, 39
    stage of life, forceful discontinuation of, 38
African Development Bank (AfDB), 88
African National Congress (ANC), 146
African refugees
  culture of deportation on, 34, 35
    legal barrier, threat of deportation as, 35, 36
    mental disorder, status insecurity and threat of deportation as, 37
    physical insecurity, 36, 37
Agency of social work, 164, 167, 169
Alcohol, 227
Algerian immigration in France, 166
Antiimmigration, 55
Antislavery Knowledge Network (AKN), 360
Anti-Torture Committee of the Council of Europe, 35
Area Development Societies (ADS), 258
Argentina
  AMBA, 174, 175
  ASOP, 174
  bed occupancy, 175
  DISPO, 174–176
  education, 176
  financial and economic crisis, 178
  internet service, 177
  isolation phases, 172
  mandatory distancing, 173
  public transport, 175
  restrictions, 173
  social justice (*see* Social justice, Argentina)
  tourism, 176
  vaccine production, 173
Arts and Humanities Research Council (AHRC) Network Plus, 360
Asia, 445
Assistive technologies, 80
AstraZeneca, 173
Asylum, 6, 31, 34, 41, 42

M. C. S. Gonçalves et al. (eds.), *The Coronavirus Crisis and Challenges to Social Development*,
https://doi.org/10.1007/978-3-030-84678-7

Attitudes, 111
  in study of coronavirus, 113–115
Australia, 3, 4, 9, 14
Autism spectrum disorder (ASD), 173

B

Bangladesh Rural Advancement Committee (BARC), 24
Bill of Rights, 149
Biometric Registry, 203
Black African attitudes, 109
Black Lives Matter, 359
Blended teaching, 138
Blunt instrument, 447
Brazil, migration
  absence of public policies, 168, 169
  Brazilian Vaccination Plan, 160
  economic analysis, 156, 157
  economic aspects, 162
  human rights, 166
  immunisation, 160
  new Migration Law, 165
  new strains of virus, 161
  normative analysis, 154, 156
  public security policies, 165
  recognition, 167
  social analysis, 157–159
  state policy, 168
  unitary concept, 168
  vaccination, 159
Brazilian Federal Constitution, 160
Brazilian social worker
  professional practice of, 323–325
    idiosyncrasy and loneliness, 328–332
    organization and direction, 327, 328
    sanitary, political, economic and social scenario, constitutive aspects of, 325–327
Brazilian Unified Health System (SUS), 326
Brazilian Vaccination Plan, 160
Broad-based black economic empowerment (BBBEE), 89
Bureau for Aliens and Foreign Immigrants Affairs under the Ministry of Interior (BAFIA), 206
Business, 102–103

C

Caixa Econômica Federal (CEF), 156
Capability approach, 88
Capitalism, 405
CARE Application, 176
CARE Nepal, 24
Catholic Committee against Hunger and Development (CCFD), 206
Central Bank of Brazil, 161
Central Business District (CBD), 59
Central Government's Supplementary Budget, 49
Chaudhury, Parul, 7, 8, 13
Child grants, 133
Children and youth in Lesotho
  blended teaching, 138
  challenges and poverty, 133
  Circle of Courage, 134, 135
  domestic violence, 135
  education, 134
  educational institutions, 137
  free primary education, 137
  gender-based violence, 136
  generosity, 140
  independence, 138–140
  married couple, 135
  residential care and homes, 136
  school, 141
  street children, 136
  unemployment in youth, 134
Chile
  front-line social workers' practices under the political and sanitary crisis in, 335, 336
    employment conditions, 338–340
    methodology, 337, 338
    neoliberalism and program changes, 340, 341
    political and social climate pre-COVID-19, 336, 337
  soup kitchens and radical social work, 421
    Committee for the Defense and Promotion of Human Rights of La Legua and Soup Kitchen, 425, 426
    COVID-19 and food safety, 422, 423
    Cristo Liberador Community and the Soup Kitchen, 425
    Grassroots Christian Movements and Liberation Theology, 423, 424
    method, 426
    networks of trust and collaboration, 427, 428
    political-economic model, constitutional plebiscite, and pandemic, 421, 422
    public space, praxis develops in, 427
    transformational spaces, possibility of, 428, 429
    Villa Francia and La Legua, 424, 425
China, 50, 347, 444, 448
Christian Association of Nigeria (CAN), 284
Chubut digital newspaper, 177
Circle of Courage (CoC), 134, 135
Citizens, 4–7
Civil society, 102
Civil society organisations (CSOs), 361
Climate change, 11, 449
Code of ethics, 327
Co-design
  and co-delivery, 366
Co-design and project/research planning, 366
Colombian Revolutionary Forces (FARC), 190
Colombian women
  armed conflict, 189
  CEDAW, 197
  challenges for social work, 195, 196
  children starvation, 188
  domestic violence, 192–194
  economic differences, 190

- equality and non-discrimination clauses, 188
- FARC, 190
- INDEPAZ, 190
- instability of labor market and discrimination, 189
- patriarchal structures, 193, 195
- poverty rate, 190
- violence prevention, 197

Colonial continuities
- health crisis in, 433, 434

Colonial logics, 359
Colonial mentalities, 360
Colonial scars, 238, 239
Colonisation, 264–266
Committee for the Defense and Promotion of Human Rights of La Legua, 425, 426
Communities
- and social work practice, 9–11

Community, 79
Community Development Societies (CDS), 258
Community mapping, 227, 229, 231
- appropriate information and relief work, initial lack of, 227, 228
- arranging livelihood documents, 230
- mental health, 231, 232
- raising funds, providing relief, and advocacy, challenges in, 229, 230
- women's and children's situation, 230, 231

Community networks, 410, 412–414
Community Oriented Primary Care (COPC), 412
Compliance, 125, 126
Constitutional Plebiscite, 421, 422
Contact tracing, 47
Coordination Platform for Refugees and Migrants from Venezuela (R4V), 203
Coping mechanisms, 105
Coronavirus preparedness group, 283
COVAX, 349
Coronavirus (COVID-19), 13, 18, 55, 443
- community resources, systems and contribution in, 127, 128
- compliance and SOPs, 125, 126
- continuity of, 275, 276
- on culture of deportation, 39
    - deportations, suspension and continuation of, 39–41
    - health risks, 41
    - lack of information and counselling, 41
- epistemological inquiries, the Global South, and resilience
    - collectivity, 349–351
    - epistemologies, relocating, 354, 355
    - hispanic paradox, 353, 354
    - safeguarding life, 351
    - subalterns organization, 351, 352
    - virus, learning from, 347–349
- Go8 roadmap, 269
    - housing supply and access, 269, 270
    - public health and clinical responses, 270, 271
    - right to self-determination, 269
- government and key stakeholder actors, 129
- health crisis, with devastating economic and social consequences, 339, 390
- implementers' interpretation and enforcement experiences, 126
- knowledge and awareness of, 122, 123
- lessons, 126
- on mental health and Aboriginal Recovery Plan, 271, 272
    - digital and telehealth inclusion, 274
    - evaluation, indigenous data sovereignty, 275
    - health and mental health workforce, 272, 273
    - right to self-determination, 272
    - social and cultural determinants of health, 273, 274
- preventive guidelines, 125, 126
- public health responses to
    - Aboriginal and Torres Strait Islander Advisory Group, 268, 269
- social work practice, implications for, 130
- South Africa
    - conceptual framework, 88, 89

COVID-19 pandemic, 3
- decent work (DW), 23
    - employment conditions and workplace rights, 23
    - social dialogue, 24
    - social protection, 23
- Nigeria, 281, 282
    - civil unrest and violence, 286
    - fiscal policy measures, 284
    - healthcare system, 282
    - illiteracy, misinformation, and Distrust of the Government, 285, 286
    - impact of, 286, 287
    - insufficient palliatives/faulty distribution pattern, 285
    - lockdown measures and ban on mass gathering, 283
    - Nigerian Social Welfare System and place of social work, 287, 288
    - palliatives and stimulus packages, 283, 284
    - post-COVID-19 management, 288, 289
    - poverty, 285
    - prior preparedness, 283
    - private sector response, 284
    - social workers in, 282
    - unclear directives, 286

Crisis relief
- in urban slum and rural communities, 224, 225
    - advocacy, 233, 234
    - community mapping, 227–232
    - Indian context, 225, 226
    - Project Jeevan Pravaah, 226, 227
    - social security provision, 233
    - strengthen local self-governance, 232, 233
    - vulnerable women, support for, 232

Cristo Liberador Community, 425
Critical and political social work
- safeguarding, decolonising, 367

Critical consciousness, 310
Cultural determinants of health, 273, 274

Cultural relativity, 115
Cultural representations
  cultural dimension
    endogenous approach, 115, 116
    ethnography, in Africa, 115
    face mask, wearing, 115
  informal economy, 116
  social inequalities, 116, 117
Culture, 109, 125
Culture of deportation, 31–34
  African countries, involuntary returnees in
    local communities, disconnection from, 39
    stage of life, forceful discontinuation of, 38
  on African refugees, Germany, 34, 35
    legal barrier, threat of deportation as, 35, 36
    mental disorder, status insecurity and threat of deportation as, 37
    physical insecurity, 36, 37
Culture of deportation
  COVID-19 on, 39
    deportations, suspension and continuation of, 39–41
    health risks, 41
    lack of information and counselling, 41

D

Dalit, 18
Decent work (DW), 22
  COVID-19 pandemic, 23
    employment conditions and workplace rights, 23
    social dialogue, 24
    social protection, 23
Decentralization, 257
Decentralized governance
  Kerala, 256, 257
Decolonization, 441
Democratic Rule of Law, 165
Deportations
  suspension and continuation, 39–41
Derg, 434
Digital inclusion, 274
Disaster capitalism, 79
District Assembly Common Fund (DCAF), 82
District of Cundinamarca, 188
Drug addiction, 227
DSD, 104
Dual economy
  South Africa, 89, 90
Dual healthcare system
  South Africa, 90–92

E

East Africa
  coronavirus pandemic, socioeconomic instability and political conflicts in, 431, 432
Ecologies of knowledges, 432
Economic Reconstruction and Recovery Plan (ERRP), 94
Economic Union of West Africa (ECOWAS), 33
Ecuador and Iran, migrants and refugees
  before and during the pandemic, 201–203
  international cooperation, 204, 205
  migration field, 203, 204
  political-social work, 207
  protecting Venezuelan and Afghan migrants, 205, 206
  social work, 207, 208
  welfare field, 204
Ecuadorian Foreign Ministry, 204
El Chubut, 178
Emergency Aid benefit, 153, 161
Emergency Assistance Program for Work and Production, 180
Endogenous approach, 115, 116
Epidemic Intelligence Service (EIS), 47
Epistemic delinking, 396
Epistemologies of the South, 432, 439, 440
Essential services, 211, 214, 215
Ethical storytelling, 372
  adaptation, positive and negative consequences of, 379
  adaptations, to overall project, 377, 378
  COVID-19, impact of, 373, 374
  Kenya, workshops in, 374–377
Ethiopia
  social work in, 434, 435
    data collection and analysis, 437
    decolonial interventions, 440
    empical data on COVID-19, 436, 437
    research and practice, 440, 441
    social development and, 435, 436
    voices of social workers from, 437–440
Ethnicity, 411
European Union's (EU), 33
Exception Visas for Humanitarian Reasons (VERHU), 203

F

Face mask wearing
  cultural representations, 115
  in Kampala, 67, 68
    data and methods, 68, 69
    determinants of knowledge, perception of risk, 69, 71
    distribution of respondents, 69
    percentage of respondents, 71
    proportion of respondents, 69
    psychosocial dimensions, 72
    psychosocial/emotional feelings, 71
    variables and knowledge, perception of risk, 69, 70
Faith-based organizations (FBOs), 105
Federal Council of Social Work, 329
Federal Law of Social Work No. 27072 of Argentina, 182
Female workers
  South Asia
    Bangladesh, 21
    COVID-19 Pandemic and Decent Work, 23
    COVID-19 pandemic, impact of, 22
    Decent Work, 22–24
    India, 20, 21
    migrant workers, impact of, 18, 19

Nepal, 21
Pakistan, 21, 22
policy response by countries, 24–26
social work, COVID-19 pandemic, and women migrant workers, 24
women migrant workers, pandemics on, 20
First wave of pandemic, 133
Fiscal policy measures, 284
Focus group discussion (FGD), 122
Food relief, 302
Food safety, 422, 423
Freire, Paulo
and social work, 310
competent, social workers, 311
critical consciousness, 310
critical curiosity, 311
impatient patience, 311, 312
no room for neutrality, 311
praxis, 311
social work practice, limits of, 312
Front-line social workers, 335
Fund for the Development of the Indigenous Peoples of Latin America and the Caribbean (FILAC), 351
Fund raising
challenges in, 229, 230

G

Gaitanis Self-Déefense Forces of Colombia, 191
Germany
culture of deportation, African refugees in, 34, 35
legal barrier, threat of deportation as, 35, 36
physical insecurity, 36, 37
status insecurity and threat of deportation as, 37
culture of deportation, African Refugees in, 34, 35
Ghana
PWD, 77, 78
economic challenges, 78–79
educational challenges, 80
emergency responses, addressing discrepancies in, 82
healthcare challenges, 80, 81
provisions, 81, 82
GINI Index, 190
Global economy, delink from, 395, 396
Globalisation, 394, 395
Global justice
strategic and meaningful solidarities for
communities and social work practice, 9–11
health responses, turning around dominance of, 3, 4
methodology, 4
migrants, refugees and citizens, 4–7
relief and systemic interventions, 12–14
women, mobility, and violence, 7–9
Global Migration Pact, 154
Global North (GN), 4, 78, 347, 366, 378, 433, 434
Global pandemic, 55–57
Global solidarity, 440
Global South (GS), 4, 78, 79, 224, 347, 354, 359, 362, 364, 367, 400, 434, 445
Global structural inequalities, 360
Global warming, 449
Go8 roadmap, 269
Aboriginal and Torres Strait Islander Health Workforce Review, 271
housing supply and access, 269, 270
public health and clinical responses, 270, 271
right to self-determination, 269
Google form, 163
Government of the Islamic Republic of Iran, 203
Grassroots Christian Movements, 423, 424
Greater Kampala metropolitan area, 68
Gross Domestic Product (GDP), 88, 97, 405
Groupe d'entraide contre le racisme envers les Asiatiques du Québec (GECREAQ), 241
GS, 349

H

Hand-washing, 122
Harm, 358
Hawk goods, 146
Health and mental health workforce, 272, 273
Health crisis
in colonial continuities, 433, 434
with devastating economic and social consequences, 389, 390
Health responses, turning around dominance of, 3, 4
Health sector
challenges in, 99, 100
Health Systems Trust, 90
Health, Justice, Law and Order sector (JLOS), 229
Hermeneutics, 193
Hindu nationalism, 233
Hispanic paradox, 353, 354
Historic and silenced traumas
vulnerability, colonial scars, and resurfacing of, 238, 239
Historical determinants of health, 264–266
Hong Kong, 443
Horizontal violence, 316, 317
Human capability
South Africa, 93, 94
Human Development Index (HDI), 89
Human rights, 77, 149, 154, 165, 166, 168

I

Idiosyncrasy, 328–332
IMF Fiscal Monitor, 181
India, 3–5, 9, 14, 20, 21
Indigenous knowledge systems (IKS), 146
Indigenous social networks
adverse effects, 415
autonomous information system, 415
collective-care community, 410
communities, 409
community-based planning, 415

Indigenous social networks (*cont.*)
  community-based workers, 415
  community organizations, 416
  community self-organization, 410
  community surveillance system network, 415
  COVID-19 pandemic, 409
  emergency management, 409
  equity, 414
  ethnicity/socioeconomic status, 409
  health, 410
  inter-agency cooperation, 415
  intercultural social workers, 416
  lack of mechanisms, 414
  lack of social participation, 410
  leading practices, 416
  medicinal plants, 416
  municipalities, 409
  organization leaders, 409
  population health (*see* Population health)
  positive health outcomes, 415
  pre-existing inequalities, 409
  pre-existing inequities, 410
  prevalence, 410
  public health, 416
  public health planning, 416
  self-determination, 410, 411
  self-organization, 416
  self-organized information system, 415
  self-organized peacebuilding, 409
  social development, 416
  social protection services, 416
  social work, 416
  sustainable human development, 414
  violence and death, 409
  well-being, 410
Indigenous social security systems, 146
Inequality, 4, 87, 97
  South Africa, COVID-19, 98
    education system, impact of, 100, 101
    health sector, challenges in, 99, 100
    vulnerable population, business shutdown on, 101
Inequities, 4
Informal economy, 116
Information and communication technologies (ICTs), 331
Institute for Peace and Development Studies (INDEPAZ), 190
Inter-American Commission on Human Rights (IACHR), 156, 194
Inter-American Human Rights System, 160
Internal economic shock, 422
International Association of Schools of Social Work (IASSW), 308
International Disability Alliance (IDA), 82
International Federation of Social Work (IFSW), 308, 440
International Labour Organisation (ILO), 82, 188, 371
International migrant, 143
International Monetary Fund (IMF), 400
International nongovernmental organisations (INGOs), 359
International Organisation for Migration (IOM), 143, 157, 204
International social work, 42
Iran-Iraq war, 203
Irregular migration, 34, 43
Islamic Republic of Iran, 202
Islamophobia, 5

J
Johannesburg Stock Exchange (JSE), 89

K
Kampala
  face mask wearing in, 67, 68
    data and methods, 68, 69
    determinants of knowledge, perception of risk, 69, 71
    distribution of respondents, 69
    percentage of respondents, 71
    proportion of respondents, 69
    psychosocial dimensions, 72
    psychosocial/emotional feelings, 71
    variables and knowledge, perception of risk, 69, 70
Kampala Capital City Authority (KCCA), 68, 211
Kenya, 380
Kerala
  COVID-19 pandemic, model state and response to, 252–254
  decentralized governance and people's participation, 256, 257
  development experience, 254–256
  Kudumbashree, 257, 258
  political mobilization of, 255
Kisenyi refugee community, 120
Knowledge, 347, 355
Korea, COVID-19
  social work
    contact tracing, 47
    economy, 48
    isolation and quarantine, 46, 47
    role of, 48, 49
    social distancing, 47
    state planning and public and private cooperation, 48
    travel restrictions, 46
    treatment, 47, 48
Kudumbashree, 257, 258
KwaZulu-Natal province, 144

L
La Legua, 424, 425
Landless Movement of Brazil, 183
Latham, Susie, 6
Latin American, 445
Latin American indigenous communities, 350
Latino migrant workers, 19
Law 13.445, 165
Lesotho, *see* Children and youth in Lesotho
Lesotho Bureau of Statistics (BOS), 134

Liberation Theology, 423
in Chile, 423, 424
Libyan Government of National Accord (GNA), 33
Livelihood documents
community mapping, 230
Livelihood Empowerment Against Poverty (LEAP), 84
Local Defense Units (LDUs), 128
Local self-governance, 232, 233
Loneliness, 328–332
Long-term lockdown, 141

M
mAbxience, 173
Maitra, Shubhada, 10
Makerere University School of Public Health Institutional Review Board (MakSPH IRB), 121
Management Plan, 268
Mandatory distancing status (DISPO), 173–175
Marginalisation, 5
Medical aid schemes, 91
Medical Schemes Act, 91
Member States (MS), 34
Mental disorder
status insecurity and threat of deportation as, 37
Mental health, 171, 181, 182, 231, 264
and Aboriginal Recovery Plan, 271, 272
digital and telehealth inclusion, 274
evaluation, indigenous data sovereignty, 275
health and mental health workforce, 272, 273
right to self-determination, 272
social and cultural determinants of health, 273, 274
Metropolitan, municipal, and district assemblies (MMDAs), 82
Migrants, 4–7
Ecuador and Iran (*see* Ecuador and Iran, migrants and refugees)
Migrants, South Africa
challenges, 143
definition, 143
living conditions, 145, 146
social workers
building resilience, 149, 150
disaster management, 148
enhancing indigenous social work practice, 150
human rights, 149
interventions, 148, 149
role, 148
xenophobia during pandemic, 146, 147
Migration, 18–20
Brazil (*see* Brazil, migration)
Ministry of Economic and Social Inclusion (MIES), 204–206
Ministry of Education and Training, 133, 134
Ministry of Health (MoH), 121
Ministry of Humanitarian Affairs, 285
Ministry of Social Development, 133, 141
Mobility, 7–9, 55–57
Mobility-based livelihoods, 59–61
Modern slavery, 371
empower survivors of, 372

N
National Association of Social Workers (NASW), 72, 214
National COVID-19 Secretariat, 138
National Decree of Necessity and Urgency 297/2020 of Argentina, 172
National Development Plan (NDP), 90, 92, 93
National Emergency Command Center (NECC), 133, 138
National Health Insurance (NHI), 93
National Health Service (NHS), 448
National Immunization Plan for the disease, 159
National Indigenous Organization of Colombia (ONIC), 411
National Institute of Health, 411
National Liberation Army (ELN), 191
National Planning Commission (NPC), 90
National Security Doctrine, 424
National Social Assistance Policy (PNAS), 163
National Social Security Fund (NSSF), 301
National Statistical Office in Colombia, 190
National University of Lesotho, 138
Necropolitics, 433, 435
Neighborhood Groups (NHGs), 258
Neoliberal model, 336
Neoliberalism, 340, 341
Neo-liberalism, global economic arrangements of, 393, 394
Nepal, 18, 21
Nigeria
COVID-19 pandemic in, 281, 282
civil unrest and violence, 286
fiscal policy measures, 284
healthcare system, 282
illiteracy, misinformation, and Distrust of the Government, 285, 286
impact of, 286, 287
insufficient palliatives/faulty distribution pattern, 285
lockdown measures and ban on mass gathering, 283
Nigerian Social Welfare System and place of social work, 287, 288
palliatives and stimulus packages, 283, 284
post-COVID-19 management, 288, 289
poverty, 285
prior preparedness, 283
private sector response, 284
social workers in, 282
unclear directives, 286
Nigerian Social Welfare System, 287, 288
Nigerian Supreme Council of Islamic Affairs (NSCIA), 284
Nominal Gross Domestic Product of Lesotho, 137
Nongovernmental organisations (NGOs), 33, 213, 302
Non-refoulement principle, 155
Non-state social protection, 301, 302
North–South global power dynamics, 447
Not One Less in Argentina, 183
Nowruz holidays, 204

O
Oceania, 445
Office of the Prime Minister (OPM), 121
One Health, 109
Online teaching, 138
Operate retail kiosks, 145
Organic Law of Human Mobility of Ecuador, 202
Organisation for Economic Co-operation and Development (OECD), 190

P
Pakistan, 21, 22
Paradigms, 402
Participatory photography, 372
adaptation, positive and negative consequences of, 379
adaptations, to overall project, 377, 378
COVID-19, impact of, 373, 374
Kenya, workshops in, 374–377
People living with disabilities (PWDs), 285
Permanent provisionality, 168
Peronism, 179
Personal hygiene, 61–63
Personal protective equipment (PPE), 128, 331, 363
Persons with disabilities (PWDs), 77
Ghana, 77, 78
economic challenges, 78, 79
educational challenges, 80
emergency responses, addressing discrepancies in, 82
healthcare challenges, 80, 81
provisions, 81, 82
Physical distancing, 297
Physical insecurity, 36, 37
Physical space, 61–63
Physical violence, 7
Pleonasm, 167
Policy, 89, 93, 94
Policy response
by countries, 24–26
Political-economic model, 421, 422
Political determinants of health, 264–266
Political neutrality, 314–316
Population health
biological diversity agreement, 413
collaborative care practices, 413
collective health framework, 414
community and social networks, 412
community-centered care system, 414
community networks, 412, 413
community radio mechanisms, 413
community solidarity strategies, 413
cosmovisions, 412
ecosystem, 412
epistemologies, 412
government social assistance, 413
indigenous communities, 412
internet networks, 413
medical treatments, 413
mental illness, 413
political decisions, 414
public health planning, 413
self-determination, 412
social and cultural care, 414
social and environmental justice, 414
social inequalities, 413
social trust, 413
United Nations, 413
Post/decolonial theories, 239
Post-modernism, 383
Poverty, 447
and social work, 390, 391
social development, 391, 392
Nigeria, 285
Presidential Task Force (PTF), 283
Primary Health Care (PHC), 282
Project Jeevan Pravaah, 226, 227
Psycho-anthropological research, 110
Psychosocial crisis, 181
Public action, 255
Public health, 409–412, 414–416
COVID-19
Aboriginal and Torres Strait Islander Advisory Group, 268, 269
Public mandatory quarantine, 297
Public policies, 163–165, 167–169
Public Service Pension Scheme (PSPS), 301
Public space, praxis develops in, 427
Public spaces, 68, 69

Q
Queensland University of Technology (QUT), 8
Queer and trans Black, Indigenous and other People of Color (QTBIPOC), 243

R
Racism, 405
Radical social work, 423
Chile, 421
COVID-19 and food safety, 422, 423
Liberation Theology, 423, 424
networks of trust and collaboration, 427, 428
political-economic model, constitutional plebiscite, and pandemic, 421, 422
Rawlsian principle of difference, 178
Refugees, 4–7, 120–122, 128, 129
Regional Councils of Social Work (CRESS), 329
Reintegration, 39
Relief and systemic interventions, 12–14
Relief work
initial lack of, 227, 228
Research practices, 367
Resilience-critical thinking
and social work, 381, 382
development of, 386–387
no resilience-critical social work without critical thinking canons, 384–386
and post-modernism, 383

systemic relevance, 382–383
top and related difficulties, 384
Robinson, Kim, 10, 11, 13
Rosenberg, Deborah, 12
Rural development, 396, 397

S
Safeguarding, 357–360
decolonising
co-creating safeguarding policy and practice, 365
co-design and co-delivery, 366
co-design and project/research planning, 356
critical and political social work, 367
international social work and research, urgency for praxis, 364, 365
methodology, 360, 361
power dynamics and capacity, 363, 364
in praxis during COVID-19, 361, 362
service planning and delivery, 362, 363
Self-assessment, 324
Self-convened by the No to La Mina in Chubut, 183
Sexual violence, 287
Single Victims Registry (RUV), 189
SIR model, 137
Sistema Único de Assistência Social (SUAS), 154
Slim Foundation, 173
Slums, 225
Small business start-ups, 105
Social and emotional well-being (SEWB), 264
Social assistance, 297
Social Assistance Policy, 163
Social attitudes, 110
Social democracy, 254
Social determinants of health, 264–266, 273, 274
Social development
and social work, Ethiopia, 435, 436
Social development approach, 391, 392
Africa, post-COVID-19 socioeconomic agenda, 393
epistemic delinking, 396
global economy, delink from, 395, 396
globalisation, 394, 395
neo-liberalism, global economic arrangements, 393, 394
radical shift, 396
rural development, 396, 397
Social development practitioners, 448
Social dialogue, 24
Social distancing, 47, 62, 297, 363
Social inequalities
cultural representations, 116, 117
Social justice, 360
Social justice, Argentina
affluent societies, 179
defense of human rights, 182
empathy, 182
inequalities, 178
justicialism, 179
nontraditional strategies, 182
peronism, 179
political economy, 179
poverty, 180
psychosocial crisis, 181
social work professionals, 182
struggle for human rights, 182
villages, 180
Social protection, 23, 296
Social protection interventions, 134
Social protection measures
Uganda, 295, 296
COVID-19 crisis response, 297, 298
during pandemics, 298–300
emergency assistance during COVID-19, 302, 303
non-state social protection, 301, 302
policies and programmes, 300, 301
Social representations, 112, 113
in study of coronavirus, 113–115
Social security, 296
Social security provision, 233
Social Service, 323
Social support, 134
Social work, 4, 24–26, 103–105, 381, 411, 412, 414, 416
Chile, 335, 336
employment conditions, 338–340
methodology, 337, 338
neoliberalism and program changes, 340, 341
political and social climate pre-COVID-19, 336, 337
Corona challenging
Korea, 45, 46
Ecuador and Iran, 207, 208
in Ethiopia, 434, 435
data collection and analysis, 437
decolonial interventions, 440
empical data on COVID-19, 436, 437
research and practice, 440, 441
social development and, 435, 436
voices of social workers from, 437–440
Korea, COVID-19
contact tracing, 47
economy, 48
isolation and quarantine, 46, 47
role of, 48, 49
social distancing, 47
state planning and public and private cooperation, 48
travel restrictions, 46
treatment, 47, 48
poverty and, 390, 391
social development, 391, 392
resilience-critical thinking and, 381–383
development of, 386–387
no resilience-critical social work without critical thinking canons, 384–386
and post-modernism, 383
systemic relevance, 382–383
top and related difficulties, 384
Uganda (*see* Uganda, social work)
Vietnam, 49–52
Zimbabwe, 307, 308

Social work (*cont.*)
critical social work practice, implications for, 318, 319
critical views, suppression of, 312–314
Freire and, 310–312
horizontal violence, 316, 317
methods, 312
oppressive practice, 317, 318
political neutrality, 314–316
politics and social justice nexus, 309, 310
and social justice mission, 308, 309
Social work practice, 9–11, 130
Social work practitioners, 9
Social work programs, mobilizing for change within, 244–246
Social work scholars engaging
in critical dialogue with racialized communities
being directly impacted *vs.* reflexive process, 240, 241
belonging, borders, and coloniality, reflecting on the question of, 246, 247
crisis, silenced traumas, and insistence of collective survival, 243, 244
deepening conditions lived, imposed, and attributed, 242, 243
historic and silenced traumas, vulnerability, colonial scars, and resurfacing of, 238, 239
methodological approach, 240
social work programs, mobilizing for change within, 244–246
vulnerability, recurrence of, 241, 242
Social workers, 225
Sociocultural norms, 125
Socioeconomic COVID-19 response
South Africa
adversities versus coping mechanisms, 105
business responding, 102, 103
civil society and Ubuntu, 102
NGOs, 103
social work intervention, 103–105
Socioeconomic response
South Africa, 92, 93
Socioeconomic status
Zimbabwe, 57–59
Solidarity, 37, 381, 386
Soup kitchen
Committee for the Defense and Promotion of Human Rights of La Legua and, 425, 426
South
epistemologies of, 432, 433
South Africa, 87
COVID-19
conceptual framework, 88, 89
COVID-19 and inequality in, 98
education system, impact of, 100, 101
health sector, challenges in, 99, 100
vulnerable population, business shutdown on, 101
dual economy, in transition, 89, 90
dual healthcare system, 90–92
human capability, during COVID-19, 93, 94
inequality in, 98
socioeconomic COVID-19 response, 102
adversities versus coping mechanisms, 105
business responding, 102, 103
civil society and Ubuntu, 102
NGOs, 103
social work intervention, 103–105
socioeconomic response, 92, 93
South Africa, COVID-19
first case, 144
first wave, 144
South African Broadcasting Corporation (SABC), 144
South African Council for Social Service Professions (SACSSP), 148
South African, COVID-19
lockdown, 145
migrants (*see* Migrants, South Africa)
South Asia
female workers in
migrant workers, impact of, 18, 19
women migrant workers, pandemics on, 20
women migrant workers
Bangladesh, 21
COVID-19 Pandemic and Decent Work, 23
COVID-19 pandemic, impact of, 22
Decent Work, 22–24
India, 20, 21
Nepal, 21
Pakistan, 21, 22
policy response by countries, 24–26
social work, COVID-19 pandemic, and women migrant workers, 24
South Korea, 45
Soviet Red Army, 202
Spaza shops, 145
Standard operating procedures (SOPs), 68, 121, 125, 126
Statistics South Africa (StatsSA), 91, 145
Status insecurity, 37
Stress, 13
Structural Adjustment Programmes (SAPs), 404
Sub-Saharan Africa (SSA), 71, 116, 295, 444
Surveillance Outbreak Response Management and Analysis System (SORMAS), 283
Survey participants
sociodemographic characteristics of, 342–343
Sustainable development goal (SDG) 1, 298, 444

T

Teaching-learning process, 423
Telehealth inclusion, 274
Territorial Monitoring System (SMT), 411
Theory of Comprehension, 193
Third World, 400
Threat of deportation, 37
THUTO portal, 138
Toleration, 35
Tong, Penelope, 11, 14
Transformational spaces, possibility of, 428, 429

Trauma counselling, 148
Trauma stress management, 148

U
Ubuntu, 102
Uganda, 68, 71, 72, 119
social protection measures, 295, 296
COVID-19 crisis response, 297, 298
during pandemics, 298–300
emergency assistance during COVID-19, 302, 303
non-state social protection, 301, 302
policies and programmes, 300, 301
Uganda National Council of Science and Technology (UNCST), 121
Uganda, social work
challenges, 214
effect of covid-19 lockdown, 216–218
epidemics and emergencies, 214
implications, 221
methods and sources of data, 214
missed opportunities and missing links by excluding social workers, 219
nonessential services, 214–216
positive contributions during covid-19, 218, 219
positive outcomes and opportunities, 220
UK Collaborative on Development Research (UKCDR), 357, 358
Umkhonto we Sizwe Military Veterans Association (MKMVA), 146
UN Refugee Agency, 202
Underdevelopment
Africa, 404
Unemployment, 447
Unequal opportunities, 90
Unified Health System (SUS), 159
Unified Social Assistance System (SUAS), 164
Unionized pots, 353
Unitary concept, 168
United Nations (UN), 381
United Nations Development Programme (UNDP), 89, 405
United Nations High Commission for Refugees (UNHCR), 143, 157
United Nations Population Fund (UNFPA), 157–158
United Nations Sustainable Development Goals, 359
Universal Declaration of Human Rights, 444
Urban laborers' crisis, 253
Urban poor, 295, 296
US Immigration and Customs Enforcement (ICE), 206
Utility bills
suspending disconnections of, 303

V
Venezuelans, 153–159, 161
Vietnam
social work, 49–52
Villa Francia, 424, 425
Village Health Teams (VHTs), 128
Violence, 7–9
Nigeria, 286
Vulnerability, 134, 140, 238, 239, 357
Vulnerable groups, 101, 103, 105
Vulnerable population
business shutdown on, 101

W
Western development paradigms and theories
during COVID-19 pandemic
COVID-19 and development, 404–406
defining development, 401, 402
post COVID-19, alternative development agenda for, 407
structural adjustment programmes and underdevelopment, 404
underdevelopment, 402
Western traits, 400
Women
mobility, and violence, 7–9
Women migrant workers (WMWs), 17, 18
Women's and children's situation, 230, 231
World Bank, 299

X
Xenophobia, 146, 147

Y
YOLRED, 361, 362
Youth bulg, 134
Youth empowerment, 445

Z
Zimbabwe
mobility-based livelihoods, precarity, and the lockdown, 59–61
physical space, personal hygiene, and COVID-19, 61–63
social workers' perspectives, Freirean analysis of, 307, 308
critical social work practice, implications for, 318, 319
critical views, suppression of, 312–314
Freire and, 310–312
horizontal violence, 316, 317
methods, 312
oppressive practice, 317, 318
political neutrality, 314–316
politics and social justice nexus, 309, 310
and social justice mission, 308, 309
socioeconomic status, 57–59
Zimbabwe's reaction, 55–57
Zimbabwean migrants, 146

The manufacturer's authorised representative in the EU is Springer Nature Customer Service Centre GmbH, Europaplatz 3, 69115 Heidelberg, Germany. If you have any concerns regarding our products, please contact ProductSafety@springernature.com

Printed and bound by CPI Group (UK) Ltd, Croydon, CR0 4YY
30/09/2026
02225687-0020